Bedside Pain Management Interventions

Dmitri Souza • Lynn Kohan
Editors

Bedside Pain Management Interventions

Springer

Editors
Dmitri Souza
Center for Pain Medicine
Western Reserve Hospital
Cuyahoga Falls, OH, USA

Lynn Kohan
Dept of Anesthesiology, Pain
Medicine division
University of Virginia
Charlottesville, VA, USA

Associate Editor
Imanuel R. Lerman
Electrical and Computer Engineering, and
Anesthesiology Departments
University of California San Diego School
of Medicine
La Jolla, CA, USA

ISBN 978-3-031-11187-7 ISBN 978-3-031-11188-4 (eBook)
https://doi.org/10.1007/978-3-031-11188-4

This Springer imprint is published by the registered company Springer Nature Switzerland AG
The registered company address is: Gewerbestrasse 11, 6330 Cham, Switzerland

To my best friend, my beautiful wife Natasha, who supports and inspires me. To my brilliant children, Dariya, Nicole, and Tim, who make me feel accomplished. To my mentors, especially Dr. Samer Narouze, from whom I learn continuously. And lastly, to the men and women who devote their lives to help those in need.

Dmitri Souza

This book is dedicated to my family. Thank you to my husband Nick and my daughters Alexandra and Lauren for all your support.

Lynn Kohan

I would like to dedicate this book to my amazing wife Natasha, and my three daughters Ava, Eliana, and Aleah. Thanks for your continuous support and for keeping the ship even keeled!

Imanuel R. Lerman

Preface

It is a challenge to treat hospitalized pain patients. Core to inpatient pain care, pain management interventions can dramatically improve patient satisfaction, decrease the length of stay, decrease opioid requirements, and improve outcomes by providing effective multimodal analgesia. These pain management procedures, including occipital nerve blocks, fascial plain blocks, intercostal nerve blocks, and many others, can be conveniently performed at the bedside. The current literature on bedside interventions is limited to clinical trials, observational studies, and case reports. This project, intended to fill the current knowledge gap, aims to provide clinicians with real-world practical information including patient selection, required equipment, and procedure guidance that will optimize the bedside interventions. In aggregate, the authors united to provide a concise guide on commonly performed bedside interventions. The editors' and contributors' expertise and enthusiasm are sure to benefit our readers and their patients.

Respectfully,

Cuyahoga Falls, OH, USA — Dmitri Souza
Charlottesville, VA, USA — Lynn Kohan
La Jolla, CA, USA — Imanuel R. Lerman

Contents

Part I

Challenges of Pain Management and Types of Bedside Interventions

Challenges of Pain Management and the Role of Bedside Interventions

Arjun Ramesh and Jianguo Cheng

Essential Concepts

- Acute and chronic pain is a growing concern and leads to healthcare costs exceeding $500 billion annually.
- While opioid medication was a mainstay in the treatment of both acute and chronic pain, concerns about opioid overuse has led to the use of multimodal anesthesia to improve efficacy and safety of patient care.
- Bedside pain interventions, as parts of multimodal analgesia regimens, can be performed to effectively treat pain, as well as spare opioid use in these patients.

1 Overview

Pain, defined as "An unpleasant sensory and emotional experience associated with actual or potential tissue damage, or described in terms of such damage" [1], is generally classified into acute pain and chronic pain on the basis of duration, with pain lasting greater than 3 months being considered chronic. While acute pain is generally associated with a specific disease or injury and is usually self-limited and serves a protective function, many forms of chronic pain are associated with

A. Ramesh
Department of Pain Management, Cleveland Clinic, Cleveland, OH, USA

J. Cheng (✉)
Departments of Pain Management and Neurosciences, Cleveland Clinic Anesthesiology Institute and Lerner Research Institute, Cleveland, OH, USA
e-mail: CHENGJ@ccf.org

D. Souza et al. (eds.), *Bedside Pain Management Interventions*,
https://doi.org/10.1007/978-3-031-11188-4_1

pathological changes in the peripheral and/or central nervous systems and can be a category of disease in its own right. Chronic pain is generally mediated by the interplay of the nervous, immune, and endocrine systems, and results from the body's inability to return to homeostasis after an acute insult [2, 3]. As such, acute pain management should be focused on addressing the underlying cause of the pain with a multimodal analgesic approach and preventing progression to a chronic pain state, while chronic pain is best managed through comprehensive, individualized, and multidisciplinary approaches [4]. While medication is a mainstay for the treatment of both acute and chronic pain in the inpatient setting, bedside interventions also play an important role in providing better pain control, preventing the progression from acute to chronic pain, and on limiting reliance of opioid therapy.

2 Historical Aspects

Pain has historically been considered an undertreated condition [5]. In fact, there have been calls for improved treatment of pain since the 1990s. Recommendations to improve the treatment of pain included making pain more "visible," and the therapeutic use of opioids, among others [6]. An article from 1980 was often quoted to support the safe use of "narcotics" as rarely leading to addiction [7]. Ultimately this led to the adoption of pain as "the fifth vital sign" in 2000, with an increase in the prescription of opioid medication [8]. This increase may have contributed to the "opioid epidemic," which has a yearly death toll greater than the total deaths in any armed conflict since World War II [9]. Although opioid-related deaths are most commonly associated with heroin, synthetic opioids such as fentanyl, and polydrugs, prescription opioids may also contribute in some cases. As such there is now a greater emphasis on opioid sparing therapies, such as multimodal analgesia with bedside procedures as a critical component.

3 Recent Developments

The cost of pain is estimated to be over $500 billion annually, which is greater than the cost of heart disease, cancer, or diabetes [10]. The prevalence of chronic pain is anywhere from 11% to 47% depending on the source [11]. This incidence will likely increase over the next several years as the incidence of chronic illness with associated pain increases [11]. There has also been an increased cost associated with increased prescription of opioid pain medications. Between 2006 and 2010 there were over 250,000 emergency department visits associated with opioid poisoning, with over $4 billion in associated hospital costs [12]. This has led to a heightened interest in pain management strategies which will decrease the burden of chronic pain while also reversing the trend of increasing opioid usage.

As many as 35% of patients presenting for surgeries will have concurrent chronic pain [13]. As such it is important to have an appreciation for pain management strategies in these patients. Currently, multimodal therapy is recommended for the inpatient management of chronic pain as well as acute postoperative pain. However, there are no well accepted combinations of medications which have been shown to be superior. Nonsteroidal anti-inflammatory drugs and selective cyclooxygenase-2 inhibitors have shown the most consistent decrease in opioid consumption [14], however some recent trials have shown smaller reductions in pain with the use of NSAIDs than was previously seen [15]. N-methyl-D-aspartate (NMDA) antagonists and alpha-2 adrenergic agonists have shown variable results when used postoperatively. Skeletal muscle relaxants can be used, although research is equivocal on their efficacy [16]. Anticonvulsant medications have shown benefit in treating chronic neuropathic pain and are now commonly used in the treatment of acute perioperative pain [11]. Antidepressant medications have shown benefit in the treatment of chronic pain disorders such as fibromyalgia and complex regional pain syndrome [11]. Opioid pain medications play an important role in the management of acute pain [14], cancer pain, and patients with chronic pain that are refractory to other treatments. Bedside interventions/procedures not only provide quality analgesia but also offer opioid sparing effects.

4 Role of Bedside Interventions

As there are no clearly superior medical therapies, bedside interventions are useful for both preventing pain, as well as controlling breakthrough pain. These therapies are generally targeted at blunting the response to pain, either by blocking the conduction and/or transmission of pain more centrally, or by suppressing the pain signals at the site of injury. The longer the pain is allowed to persist, the more common the transition to chronic pain. This is thought to be due to central and peripheral sensitizations [17]. Central sensitization results from an interplay of pain projecting neurons, inhibitory interneurons, and glial cells that leads to increased excitability of pain pathways and processing matrix within the central nervous system. Peripheral sensitization results from changes in more peripheral structures such as muscle, nerves, and fascia that lead to increased excitability of nociceptors [11]. To prevent central sensitization, some have argued for pre-emptive preoperative analgesia. However, it is now understood that the development of central sensitization may be due not only to surgical incision and other intraoperative insults such as retraction and visceral manipulation, but also to inflammatory changes that can extend into the postoperative period. As such, treatments are now aimed at modulating the response to these factors through the entire perioperative period [17].

Several nonpharmacological, nonsurgical conservative pain management modalities may be considered in select patients to help with the treatment of acute and chronic pain. Acupuncture therapy is being investigated for its utility in the treatment of both acute and subacute low back pain. A randomized controlled trial found acupuncture to be superior to parenteral morphine for patients presenting to the emergency department with acute pain [18]. Physical therapy, massage therapy, and mindfulness therapies including yoga and tai chi have also been shown to be beneficial in the treatment of chronic pain. These therapies are generally performed on a daily basis and are able to provide patients with increased pain relief compared to pharmacologic and interventional techniques alone [11]. Noninterventional techniques, while having limited side effects, often require an experienced practitioner for performance of the service (i.e. an acupuncturist or a massage therapist). These may not be readily available at all institutions, and may be difficult to continue as an outpatient.

Nonsurgical interventional techniques have gained traction for the control of acute and chronic pain (Table 1). Historically, regional nerve blockade was performed by landmark-based techniques utilizing nerve stimulation to ensure injection of anesthetic near the nerve of interest. However, ultrasound guidance has increased the success of regional nerve blockade as well as decreased the rate of complications associated with these blocks [19]. Commonly utilized techniques include saphenous nerve block, femoral nerve block, popliteal sciatic nerve block, and brachial plexus blocks to allow for regional anesthesia of the extremity of interest. In addition, paravertebral blocks may be utilized for the management of rib fractures and thoracic and abdominal surgeries. The use of ultrasound guidance has also allowed for the performance of fascial plane blocks which would have been difficult or impossible without real time image guidance. These include the

Table 1 Benefits and challenges of different bedside techniques

Type of intervention	Benefits	Challenges
Neuraxial blockade	Excellent and predictable analgesia with the ability to prolong blockade with catheter placement	Sympathectomy leading to hypotension Weakness Contralateral analgesia which may be unnecessary May be technically challenging Contraindicated in the setting of anticoagulation
Peripheral nerve blockade	Excellent regional anesthesia Preservation of sensation proximal to the level of blockade Isolated analgesia at the region of injury Ability to prolong duration of blockade with catheter placement	Facility with ultrasound or nerve stimulation guidance is often required Higher incidence of failed blockade when using landmark based techniques May cause motor weakness which can interfere with recovery Relatively contraindicated in the setting of anticoagulation
Fascial plane blockade	Excellent analgesia Fewer injections required to provide larger regions of coverage Ability to prolong duration of blockade with catheter placement More likely to be acceptable risk in the setting of anticoagulation	Facility with ultrasound guidance is often required
Conservative interventions	Minimal side effects	Poor patient acceptance Requires specially trained staff

transversus abdominis plane block, erector spinae plane block, as well as pectoralis and sartorius plane blocks. Innovations in drug delivery including liposomal formulations, as well as increasing awareness and use of adjunctive medications with local anesthetics allow for longer acting analgesia with single injection techniques [20]. The field is currently undergoing an era of growth, with ongoing investigation into novel ultrasound based regional approaches and less reliance on landmark based and nerve stimulation techniques.

While peripheral nerve blockade and fascial plane blocks have been growing in popularity, neuraxial blockade is still a commonly used modality. This allows for excellent analgesia and is generally very predictable in region of blockade, as well as duration. Catheters can be employed to provide continuous nerve block or neuraxial block by continuous infusion of medications.

5 Challenges of Inpatient Pain Management

The challenges of bedside interventions are multifold (Table 1). Initial identification of patients with pain may be difficult. As mentioned previously, pain has been a historically undertreated condition [5]. While increased vigilance and documentation of a patient's pain scores have helped bring this to light, it is important for early involvement of pain management teams because early treatment of acute pain may help minimize the risk of transition to chronic pain [21].

While there are many new bedside interventions that can be offered to patients, these techniques do not always result in lasting relief. Nerve blockade is limited by the duration of action of the local anesthetics with commonly used "long acting" local anesthetics having a maximum duration of about 18 h, although there are now commercially available preparations with longer durations of action [20]. Catheters can also be placed to prolong the duration of analgesia by allowing for continuous infusion of medication. However, catheter dislodgement may occur depending on the location of insertion, which could potentially interrupt therapy and require additional procedures for replacement. In addition, the ideal blockade would provide analgesia without concomitant weakness. However, in many cases this is not possible and the weakness produced by peripheral blockade may result in increased hospitalization time or may increase the risk of falls.

Neuraxial techniques may also cause significant weakness. Efforts should be directed at striking a balance between adequate analgesia and minimizing weakness by adjusting the concentration of anesthetic medication. Neuraxial techniques also cause a sympathectomy with resulting decreases in vascular tone, which may be poorly tolerated and not suitable for certain patients. Due to these side effects, some practitioners may avoid the use of neuraxial techniques after surgery. However, with prudent dosing these side effects can be mitigated with excellent results for the patient.

Both neuraxial techniques and peripheral nerve blockade, and to a lesser extent fascial plane blocks are contraindicated in the setting of anticoagulation. While anticoagulation may be held to allow for the performance of these interventions, it is not always feasible in the inpatient setting. The American Society or Regional Anesthesia and Pain Medicine has released a set of guidelines for when to hold and resume anticoagulation for commonly used anticoagulants and interventions, which is now in its fourth edition [22].

6 Conclusion

Pain is a natural response to injury but can progress to a pathological state. There are several modalities to treat pain, but a multimodal approach to treating acute pain and a multidisciplinary approach to treating chronic pain are most beneficial. Medication is the most commonly used treatment modality, but increasing awareness of the risks of opioid use and misuse have sparked interest in alternate treatment modalities. Alternate treatment modalities including acupuncture, physical therapy, cognitive behavioral therapy, massage therapy, and mindfulness exercises have also shown utility in the treatment of both acute and chronic pain. Ultrasound guidance has increased the utility of bedside nerve blocks which can effectively control pain in the short term. The placement of catheters can prolong the duration of analgesia. As our understanding of the pathophysiology of acute and chronic pain increases, increasingly targeted therapies can start to be utilized and current interventions can be refined to decrease side effects and improve efficacy in pain control. Bedside interventions are becoming an integral part of the practice of pain management.

References

1. Merskey H, Bogduk N, editors. Part III: pain terms: a current list with definitions and notes on usage. In: Classification of chronic pain. 2nd ed. Seattle, WA: IASP Press; 1994. p. 209–14.
2. Chapman CR, Tuckett RP, Song CW. Pain and stress in a systems perspective: reciprocal neural, endocrine, and immune interactions. J Pain. 2008;9(2):122–45.
3. Loeser JD, Melzack R. Pain: an overview. Lancet. 1999;353(9164):1607–9.
4. Grichnik KP, Ferrante FM. The difference between acute and chronic pain. Mt Sinai J Med. 1991;58(3):217–20.
5. Harstall C, Ospina M. How prevalent is chronic pain? Pain Clin Updat. 1991;58(3):217–20.
6. Max MB. Improving outcomes of analgesic treatment: is education enough? Ann Intern Med. 1990;113(11):885–9.
7. Porter J, Jick H. Addiction rare in patients treated with narcotics. N Engl J Med. 1980;302(2):123.
8. Levy N, Sturgess J, Mills P. "Pain as the fifth vital sign" and dependence on the "numerical pain scale" is being abandoned in the US: why? Br J Anaesth. 2018;120(3):435–8.
9. National Academies of Sciences E, Division H and M, Policy B on HS, Abuse C on PM and RS to APO, Phillips JK, Ford MA, et al. Trends in opioid use, harms, and treatment. National Academies Press (US); 2017 [cited 2019 Oct 5]. https://www.ncbi.nlm.nih.gov/books/NBK458661/.
10. Gaskin DJ, Richard P. The economic costs of pain in the United States. J Pain. 2012;13(8):715–24.

11. Tick H, Nielsen A, Pelletier KR, Bonakdar R, Simmons S, Glick R, et al. Evidence-based nonpharmacologic strategies for comprehensive pain care: the consortium pain task force white paper. Explore (NY). 2018;14(3):177–211.
12. Tadros A, Layman SM, Davis SM, Davidov DM, Cimino S. Emergency visits for prescription opioid poisonings. J Emerg Med. 2015;49(6):871–7.
13. Apfelbaum JL, Chen C, Mehta SS, Gan TJ. Postoperative pain experience: results from a national survey suggest postoperative pain continues to be undermanaged. Anesth Analg. 2003;97(2):534–40, table of contents.
14. Buvanendran A, Kroin JS. Multimodal analgesia for controlling acute postoperative pain. Curr Opin Anaesthesiol. 2009;22(5):588–93.
15. Chou R, Deyo R, Friedly J, Skelly A, Weimer M, Fu R, et al. Systemic pharmacologic therapies for low Back pain: a systematic review for an American College of Physicians clinical practice guideline. Ann Intern Med. 2017;166(7):480–92.
16. Chou R, Peterson K, Helfand M. Comparative efficacy and safety of skeletal muscle relaxants for spasticity and musculoskeletal conditions: a systematic review. J Pain Symptom Manag. 2004;28(2):140–75.
17. Vadivelu N, Mitra S, Schermer E, Kodumudi V, Kaye AD, Urman RD. Preventive analgesia for postoperative pain control: a broader concept. Local Reg Anesth. 2014;7:17–22.
18. Grissa MH, Baccouche H, Boubaker H, Beltaief K, Bzeouich N, Fredj N, et al. Acupuncture vs intravenous morphine in the management of acute pain in the ED. Am J Emerg Med. 2016;34(11):2112–6.
19. Gelfand HJ, Ouanes J-PP, Lesley MR, Ko PS, Murphy JD, Sumida SM, et al. Analgesic efficacy of ultrasound-guided regional anesthesia: a meta-analysis. J Clin Anesth. 2011;23(2):90–6.
20. Beiranvand S, Moradkhani MR. Bupivacaine versus liposomal bupivacaine for pain control. Drug Res. 2018;68(7):365–9.
21. Tawfic Q, Kumar K, Pirani Z, Armstrong K. Prevention of chronic post-surgical pain: the importance of early identification of risk factors. J Anesth. 2017;31(3):424–31.
22. Horlocker TT, Vandermeuelen E, Kopp SL, Gogarten W, Leffert LR, Benzon HT. Regional anesthesia in the patient receiving antithrombotic or thrombolytic therapy: American Society of Regional Anesthesia and Pain Medicine evidence-based guidelines (fourth edition). Reg Anesth Pain Med. 2018;43(3):263–309.

Clinical Assessment of Pain and Assessment of Outcomes of Bedside Procedures

Ankit Maheshwari and Bradford Jones

Essential Concepts

- Diagnosis of pain is multifaceted, requiring an understanding of the underlying etiology and the use of exam skills with assessment tools to accurately distinguish various types.
- A systematic approach to evaluating patient pain can be beneficial to the initial assessment, diagnosis and treatment of pain; as well as evaluating efficacy of procedures.
- Pain measurement tools can provide subjective detail and further support diagnoses.
- Procedural outcome is essential to monitor in the setting of clinical effectiveness and direction of further therapy.

1 Overview

Clinical examination skills with a methodical approach are indispensable to the practitioner for a complete evaluation and accurate diagnosis of a patient's pain. With the growing number of resources available to assist in diagnostics and treatment, one of the most important assets to a physician remains the history and

A. Maheshwari (✉)
Texas Pain Intervention Clinic, McKinney, TX, USA

B. Jones
Department of Anesthesiology and Perioperative Medicine, University Hospitals Cleveland Medical Center, Cleveland, OH, USA
e-mail: Bradford.Jones@uhhospitals.org

D. Souza et al. (eds.), *Bedside Pain Management Interventions*,
https://doi.org/10.1007/978-3-031-11188-4_2

physical examination. The assessment chapter serves as the framework on which a clinician can continue to integrate knowledge of pain conditions and special testing to become proficient in diagnosing pain. This chapter will outline an approach to utilize the history and physical examination not only for diagnoses, but for assessment of interventions and guiding further clinical course.

2 Initial Encounter

As should be considered with any patient encounter, the physician-patient relationship should be established to create a comfortable environment in which both can interact to produce the best outcome for the patient. Prior workup and imaging should be obtained and reviewed prior to meeting the patient. Effective listening and affirmation of understanding is key to both sides of the conversation. It is also important to concisely define the chief complaint to direct the remainder of the examination.

3 Detailed History

Onset

This question is often first as it can direct diagnoses and further interview questions. Abrupt pain that began with a certain recallable inciting event or activity may relate to an acutely injured area or the need for more urgent treatment. On the contrary, an insidious onset of pain may still relate to a remote acute injury that has been exacerbated, a degenerative process, or a more diffuse pain pathophysiology.

Location

Anatomic location is important, as it directs the physician to an area for further examination and potential areas of treatment. This is usually fairly clear in case of postoperative pain or injured site. Special attention should be paid at this juncture, as to not be misled by radicular pain or referred pain. Location can further hone in on treatment urgency as described above.

Duration

Pain that has been occurring for a few days or weeks may be approached in a different manner than pain that a patient has had for several months or even years. Duration can also further delineate urgency of treatment. Consistent, ongoing pain for years is approached differently than progressively worsening pain over a much shorter duration, especially if alarm symptoms, such as the neurologic sequelae or signs of active infection were present.

Course/Frequency

How often the pain occurs for the patient may be static or dynamic. There may be regularity of the pain in a temporal manner, such as in the morning or worse in the evening. It can also be dynamic in that the intensity changes throughout the day or it comes and goes in spurts. Worsening pain over time can be of greater concern to both the patient and physician.

Character

The description of pain can vary from patient to patient. However, descriptors such as dull, sharp, stabbing, aching, burning, or throbbing are fairly common terms used. Eliciting subjective descriptors can help delineate what type of pain fibers or neurologic components may be affected by the injury or pain syndrome. Descriptions of the pain can clue the physician in to the type of pain the patient may be experiencing.

Aggravating/Alleviating Factors

What makes the pain better or worse can direct diagnosis, treatment, and add suggestions for activity modification. Movement, as well as positions of comfort, provide further insight. Another example would be distinguishing bilateral leg pain of neurogenic claudication, that is above the knee, triggered by standing and relieved by sitting, from vascular claudication that is primarily in the calf and relieved with standing [1]. Other factors may include psychological stress and diet as pain adjuncts. The patient may also have found items that help as well, such as heat/ice, stretching, physical therapy, and medications.

Related Symptoms

Symptoms related to the pain will aid even further in diagnosis. As there are a multitude of pain conditions, some have a constellation of associated symptoms such as vision changes, balance changes, weakness, joints giving way, bowel or bladder changes, weight changes, fever, chills, night sweats, skin changes, and altered sensorium. This list provides examples of such symptoms, but is not intended in any way to be completely comprehensive. The take home message is that each singular or group of related symptoms should bring to mind an association with a particular diagnosis. If not, this may indicate further evaluation is needed.

Severity

Severity is another subjective measure of pain that can vary between patients for the same pain condition. This item does, however, give information regarding the degree of significance the pain has in the patient's life. Examples of pain assessment tools will follow that can be helpful in this matter.

4 Assessment Tools

There is an ever-increasing number of pain assessment tools at the physician's disposal to aid in completely evaluating the patient. These tools can be a helpful addition in the clinical assessment of pain, as well as provide a means for comparison of pain in the same patient over the course of treatment. When selecting assessment tools, a specific clinical question should be in mind. Some are best for rating severity of pain, while others are more involved and provide greater detail with more data points collected. Simple tools can be used that have ordinal data to classify the severity of a patient's pain along a scale that can tell the physician where the pain is currently at and can re-evaluate for change in pain post procedure. Figure 1 depicts different types of pain scales.

These scales are useful not only when the question of pain severity needs to be answered, but also in the scenario of decreased communication. Other scales exist, though, that combine qualitative and quantitative data to either address a barrier to communicate or provide more detail when needed. Young children may represent the former and latter arena as they may not have developed the linguistic skills or understanding to further describe their pain. For children, the Wong-Baker Faces Pain Rating Scale and Visual Analog Scale have proven to be useful tools in assessing pain

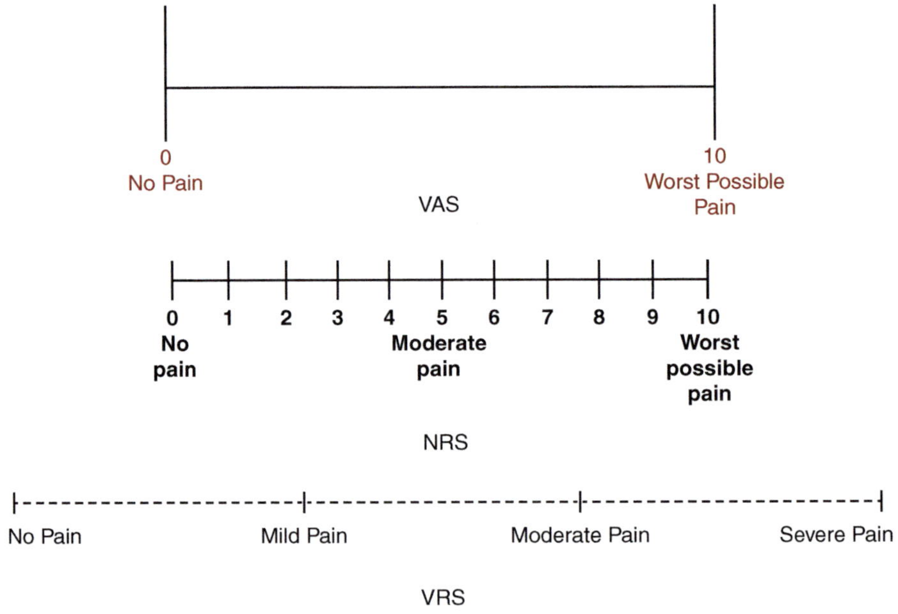

Fig. 1 Commonly used pain scales. *VAS* Visual Analog Scale, *NRS* Numeric Rating Scale, *VRS* Visual Rating Scale

Pain Assessment Tool Guidelines for use: PAINAD

Indicator	Score = 0	Score = 1	Score = 2	Total Score
Breathing:	Normal breathing	Occasional labored breathing Short period of hyperventilation	Noisy labored breathing. Long period of hyperventilation. Cheyne-Stokes respiration	
Negative vocalizations:	None	Occasional moan/groan. Low level, speech with a negative or disapproving quality	Repeated troubled calling out. Loud moaning or groaning. Crying.	
Facial Expression	Smiling or inexpressive	Sad, frightened, frown	Facial grimace	
Body Language	Relaxed	Tense, distressed, pacing fidgeting.	Rigid, fists clenched. Knees pulled up. Striking out. Pulling or pushing away.	
Consolability:	No need to console	Distracted by voice or touch.	Unable to console, distract or reassure.	
			TOTAL:	

Fig. 2 Pain Assessment in Advanced Dementia Scale (PAINAD). (With Permission from Elsevier)

[2]. Another tool for children that has utility in those too young for verbal communication is Crying Requires oxygen Increased vital signs Expression Sleep (CRIES) [3].

Adults with cognitive impairment may provide yet another challenging population for assessment. The Checklist of Non-Verbal Pain Indicators (CNPI) may provide a means of evaluating pain in cognitively impaired adults based on six key elements including: nonverbal vocalizations, facial grimace, bracing, restlessness, rubbing, and verbal complaints [4, 5]. The Pain Assessment in Advanced Dementia Scale (PAINAD) scale is another resource that may be useful in both the cognitively impaired and cognitively intact elderly patient (Fig. 2) [6].

For the standard adult population, additional examples of tools that offer a variety of qualitative and quantitative data include the McGill Pain Questionnaire, SF-12, and WHOQOL-100 with and without Pain Discomfort Module (PDM) addition [7–9]. These examples offer additional data points such as descriptors of pain, physical function, social effects, psychological effects, and many more than can be used if needed to better understand a patient's pain, establish a baseline, and track treatment progress. The assessment of bedside interventions requires time efficiency and the evaluation tool should be selected based on time available for assessment and the patient population as described above. A baseline evaluation is necessary followed by administration of the same measure after the procedure. Timing of assessment should be after the expected onset of pain relief from the intervention and when sedation, if administered has worn off.

5 Physical Examination

After a thorough interview is conducted with the patient, the next step is the physical examination. Each exam component will be briefly discussed and should be modified to the anatomic site on which it is conducted.

Inspection

Observation of the patient should begin as soon as the physician lays eyes on the patient, whether it is entering the room or walking down the hall. Careful attention should be paid to posture, gait, how the patient navigates the door, room, exam table or chair, and any other observable obstacles. Gross visual examination of the entire patient, as well as the specific area of pain and related areas, is also key.

Palpation

Palpation should consist of the soft tissue, bones, joints, and adjacent regions. The physician should be mindful of where the pain is located when palpating as not to worsen pain for the patient. However, the goal is to pinpoint the area of pain and identify sources of radiation, if applicable.

Range of Motion

When applicable, the associated joint and adjacent joints should be assessed for both active and passive range of motion. Limitations in range of motion should be noted as well as pain.

Percussion/Auscultation

Percussing and listening to the area of pain may be appropriate. Specific regions such as the abdomen or thorax would be appropriate to perform this part of the examination. Percussive sounds as well as pertinent positive or negative findings on auscultation can aid diagnosis.

Motor

Both gross and fine motor skills should be thoroughly assessed in the patient. Gross motor should include strength testing and gait. Fine motor skills and ability to manipulate objects in a patient's hands should also be performed.

Sensory

Testing a patient's sensation should be performed to assess for associated neurologic deficits associated with the pain. This portion of the exam should allow the physician to determine if any deficits exist along a dermatome, peripheral nerve, or diffuse anatomic region. Proprioception should also be tested to determine if any deficits exist in the patient's ability to sense and navigate their body in the world. Both motor and sensory testing can be scored using the International Standards for Neurological Classification of Spinal Cord Injury Tool from the American Spinal Injury Association: (Fig. 3) [10].

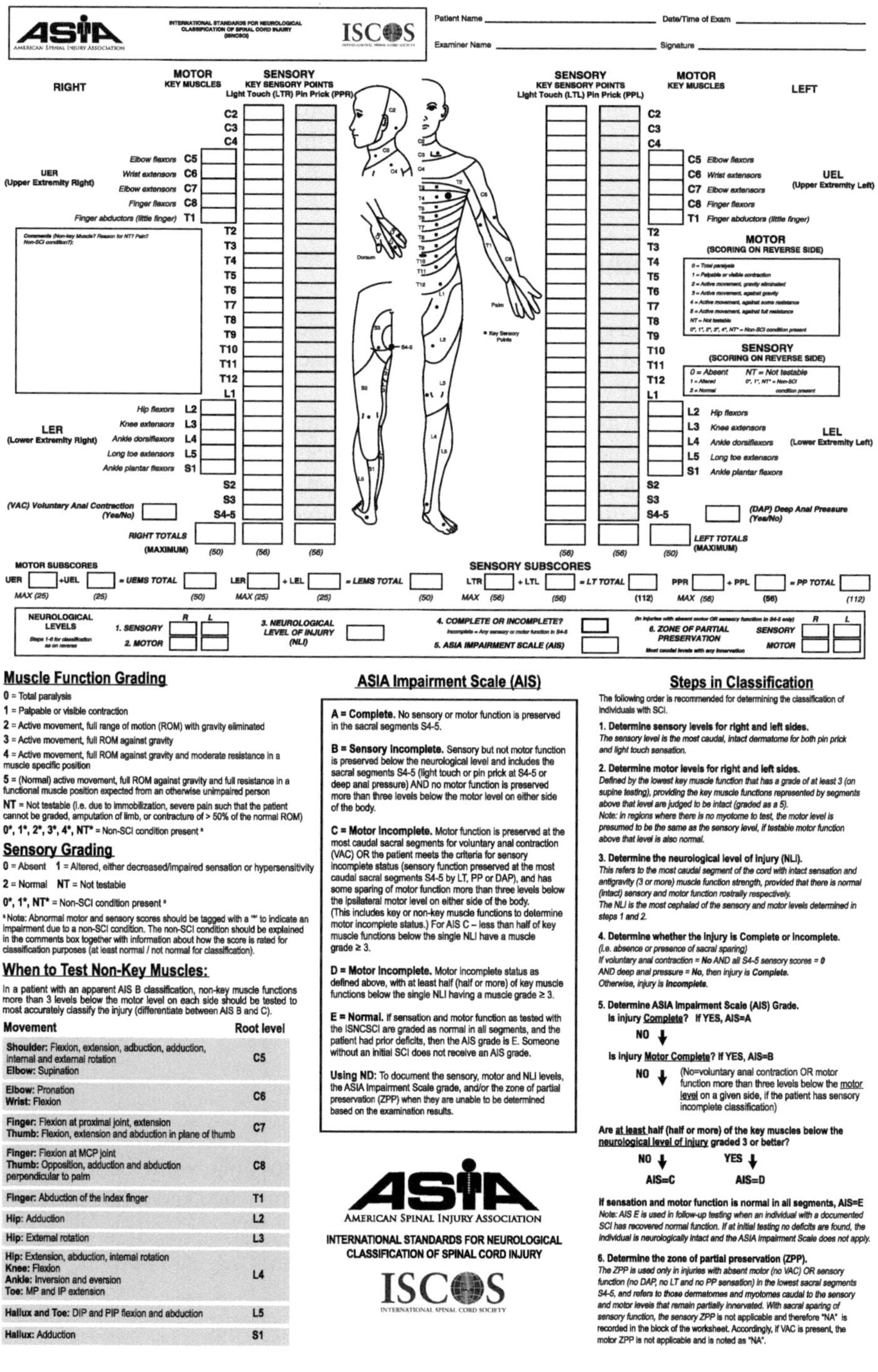

ASIA — American Spinal Injury Association
INTERNATIONAL STANDARDS FOR NEUROLOGICAL CLASSIFICATION OF SPINAL CORD INJURY (ISNCSCI)
ISCOS

Patient Name ______ Date/Time of Exam ______
Examiner Name ______ Signature ______

RIGHT	MOTOR KEY MUSCLES	SENSORY KEY SENSORY POINTS Light Touch (LTR) Pin Prick (PPR)	SENSORY KEY SENSORY POINTS Light Touch (LTL) Pin Prick (PPL)	MOTOR KEY MUSCLES	LEFT
		C2	C2		
		C3	C3		
		C4	C4		
UER (Upper Extremity Right)	Elbow flexors C5			C5 Elbow flexors	UEL (Upper Extremity Left)
	Wrist extensors C6			C6 Wrist extensors	
	Elbow extensors C7			C7 Elbow extensors	
	Finger flexors C8			C8 Finger flexors	
	Finger abductors (little finger) T1			T1 Finger abductors (little finger)	
		T2–T12, L1	T2–T12, L1		
LER (Lower Extremity Right)	Hip flexors L2			L2 Hip flexors	LEL (Lower Extremity Left)
	Knee extensors L3			L3 Knee extensors	
	Ankle dorsiflexors L4			L4 Ankle dorsiflexors	
	Long toe extensors L5			L5 Long toe extensors	
	Ankle plantar flexors S1			S1 Ankle plantar flexors	
		S2	S2		
		S3	S3		
		S4-5	S4-5		

Comments (Non-key Muscle? Reason for NT? Pain? Non-SCI condition?):

(VAC) Voluntary Anal Contraction (Yes/No) | (DAP) Deep Anal Pressure (Yes/No)

RIGHT TOTALS (MAXIMUM) (50) (56) (56) | LEFT TOTALS (MAXIMUM) (56) (56) (50)

MOTOR (SCORING ON REVERSE SIDE): 0 = Total paralysis; 1 = Palpable or visible contraction; 2 = Active movement, gravity eliminated; 3 = Active movement, against gravity; 4 = Active movement, against some resistance; 5 = Active movement, against full resistance; NT = Not testable; 0*, 1*, 2*, 3*, 4*, NT* = Non-SCI condition present

SENSORY (SCORING ON REVERSE SIDE): 0 = Absent; 1 = Altered; 2 = Normal; NT = Not testable; 0*, 1*, NT* = Non-SCI condition present

Key Sensory Points

MOTOR SUBSCORES
UER + UEL = UEMS TOTAL; MAX (25) (25) (50)
LER + LEL = LEMS TOTAL; MAX (25) (25) (50)

SENSORY SUBSCORES
LTR + LTL = LT TOTAL; MAX (56) (56) (112)
PPR + PPL = PP TOTAL; MAX (56) (56) (112)

NEUROLOGICAL LEVELS (Steps 1-6 for classification as on reverse): 1. SENSORY R L; 2. MOTOR R L
3. NEUROLOGICAL LEVEL OF INJURY (NLI)
4. COMPLETE OR INCOMPLETE? (Incomplete = Any sensory or motor function in S4-5)
5. ASIA IMPAIRMENT SCALE (AIS)
6. ZONE OF PARTIAL PRESERVATION (In injuries with absent motor OR sensory function in S4-5 only; Most caudal levels with any innervation): SENSORY R L; MOTOR R L

Muscle Function Grading

0 = Total paralysis

1 = Palpable or visible contraction

2 = Active movement, full range of motion (ROM) with gravity eliminated

3 = Active movement, full ROM against gravity

4 = Active movement, full ROM against gravity and moderate resistance in a muscle specific position

5 = (Normal) active movement, full ROM against gravity and full resistance in a functional muscle position expected from an otherwise unimpaired person

NT = Not testable (i.e. due to immobilization, severe pain such that the patient cannot be graded, amputation of limb, or contracture of > 50% of the normal ROM)

0*, 1*, 2*, 3*, 4*, NT* = Non-SCI condition present *

Sensory Grading

0 = Absent **1** = Altered, either decreased/impaired sensation or hypersensitivity

2 = Normal **NT** = Not testable

0*, 1*, NT* = Non-SCI condition present *

* Note: Abnormal motor and sensory scores should be tagged with a "*" to indicate an impairment due to a non-SCI condition. The non-SCI condition should be explained in the comments box together with information about how the score is rated for classification purposes (at least normal / not normal for classification).

When to Test Non-Key Muscles:

In a patient with an apparent AIS B classification, non-key muscle functions more than 3 levels below the motor level on each side should be tested to most accurately classify the injury (differentiate between AIS B and C).

Movement	Root level
Shoulder: Flexion, extension, adbuction, adduction, internal and external rotation **Elbow:** Supination	C5
Elbow: Pronation **Wrist:** Flexion	C6
Finger: Flexion at proximal joint, extension **Thumb:** Flexion, extension and abduction in plane of thumb	C7
Finger: Flexion at MCP joint **Thumb:** Opposition, adduction and abduction perpendicular to palm	C8
Finger: Abduction of the index finger	T1
Hip: Adduction	L2
Hip: External rotation	L3
Hip: Extension, abduction, internal rotation **Knee:** Flexion **Ankle:** Inversion and eversion **Toe:** MP and IP extension	L4
Hallux and Toe: DIP and PIP flexion and abduction	L5
Hallux: Adduction	S1

ASIA Impairment Scale (AIS)

A = Complete. No sensory or motor function is preserved in the sacral segments S4-5.

B = Sensory Incomplete. Sensory but not motor function is preserved below the neurological level and includes the sacral segments S4-5 (light touch or pin prick at S4-5 or deep anal pressure) AND no motor function is preserved more than three levels below the motor level on either side of the body.

C = Motor Incomplete. Motor function is preserved at the most caudal sacral segments for voluntary anal contraction (VAC) OR the patient meets the criteria for sensory incomplete status (sensory function preserved at the most caudal sacral segments S4-5 by LT, PP or DAP), and has some sparing of motor function more than three levels below the ipsilateral motor level on either side of the body. (This includes key or non-key muscle functions to determine motor incomplete status.) For AIS C – less than half of key muscle functions below the single NLI have a muscle grade ≥ 3.

D = Motor Incomplete. Motor incomplete status as defined above, with at least half (half or more) of key muscle functions below the single NLI having a muscle grade ≥ 3.

E = Normal. If sensation and motor function as tested with the ISNCSCI are graded as normal in all segments, and the patient had prior deficits, then the AIS grade is E. Someone without an initial SCI does not receive an AIS grade.

Using ND: To document the sensory, motor and NLI levels, the ASIA Impairment Scale grade, and/or the zone of partial preservation (ZPP) when they are unable to be determined based on the examination results.

ASIA — American Spinal Injury Association
INTERNATIONAL STANDARDS FOR NEUROLOGICAL CLASSIFICATION OF SPINAL CORD INJURY
ISCOS — International Spinal Cord Society

Steps in Classification

The following order is recommended for determining the classification of individuals with SCI.

1. Determine sensory levels for right and left sides.
The sensory level is the most caudal, intact dermatome for both pin prick and light touch sensation.

2. Determine motor levels for right and left sides.
Defined by the lowest key muscle function that has a grade of at least 3 (on supine testing), providing the key muscle functions represented by segments above that level are judged to be intact (graded as a 5).
Note: in regions where there is no myotome to test, the motor level is presumed to be the same as the sensory level, if testable motor function above that level is also normal.

3. Determine the neurological level of injury (NLI).
This refers to the most caudal segment of the cord with intact sensation and antigravity (3 or more) muscle function strength, provided that there is normal (intact) sensory and motor function rostrally respectively.
The NLI is the most cephalad of the sensory and motor levels determined in steps 1 and 2.

4. Determine whether the injury is Complete or Incomplete.
(i.e. absence or presence of sacral sparing)
*If voluntary anal contraction = **No** AND all S4-5 sensory scores = **0** AND deep anal pressure = **No**, then injury is **Complete**.*
*Otherwise, injury is **Incomplete**.*

5. Determine ASIA Impairment Scale (AIS) Grade.
Is injury Complete? If YES, AIS=A
NO ↓
Is injury Motor Complete? If YES, AIS=B
NO ↓ (No=voluntary anal contraction OR motor function more than three levels below the motor level on a given side, if the patient has sensory incomplete classification)

Are at least half (half or more) of the key muscles below the neurological level of injury graded 3 or better?
NO ↓ AIS=C **YES ↓ AIS=D**

If sensation and motor function is normal in all segments, AIS=E
Note: AIS E is used in follow-up testing when an individual with a documented SCI has recovered normal function. If at initial testing no deficits are found, the individual is neurologically intact and the ASIA Impairment Scale does not apply.

6. Determine the zone of partial preservation (ZPP).
The ZPP is used only in injuries with absent motor (no VAC) OR sensory function (no DAP, no LT and no PP sensation) in the lowest sacral segments S4-5, and refers to those dermatomes and myotomes caudal to the sensory and motor levels that remain partially innervated. With sacral sparing of sensory function, the sensory ZPP is not applicable and therefore "NA" is recorded in the block of the worksheet. Accordingly, if VAC is present, the motor ZPP is not applicable and is noted as "NA".

Fig. 3 American Spinal Injury Association: International Standards for Neurological Classification of Spinal Cord Injury. (With Permission from American Spinal Injury Association ("ASIA"))

Provocative Testing

Special testing specific to the anatomic location can be performed to further delineate causes of pain. Many special tests for each anatomic region exist and are too numerous to list in this chapter. Further reading on this topic is listed at the end of this chapter.

6 Post-procedure Evaluation

Many of the history and examination components described at the beginning of this chapter can be repeated after a procedure to determine if there has been a clinically significant improvement for the patient. Pain assessment tools should also be implemented post-procedure as a means of subjective comparison to the post-procedure state, as information regarding treatment effectiveness can be gleaned from repetition post-procedure. In addition to tools for post-procedure assessment in young children, discussion with the caregiver can also give insight to how the child's behavior and activity has changed. In cognitively impaired adults or elderly, the same holds true in regard to repeating assessments and discussion with caregivers when available. "Additional monitoring should include vital signs of blood pressure and heart rate to determine if sympathetic discharge from pain symptoms is being controlled" [11].

Based on the treatment response and the patient's overall satisfaction, an ongoing treatment plan should be established. If the response is suboptimal, the overall encounter should be reviewed, as the importance of a correct diagnosis to ensure appropriate treatment cannot be stressed enough. If the diagnosis remains after re-evaluation, alternative interventional and/or pharmacologic therapies should be considered if the patient feels treatment was suboptimal. If the procedure is viewed as successful, a plan should be formulated for the event of worsening or return of symptoms. Post-procedure goals should be an adequate reduction in the patient's pain, as well as to provide ongoing treatment for further improvement in pain and overall quality of life. Many of these questions should be asked, and the clinician will likely develop his or her own strategy over time to adequately address the patient's status after a procedure.

Clinical and Technical Pearls

- The initial assessment should be as thorough as possible, while being performed in an efficient manner, which can be accomplished and refined over the course of clinical practice.
- Pain assessment tools should be administered with a targeted purpose and clinical questions in mind.

- Expectations of procedural outcome should be discussed upfront and practitioners should provide appropriate feedback regarding those expectations.
- A pre-procedure patient baseline should be established, then reassessed immediately post-procedure and over time to monitor symptoms; as treatment does not end after the procedure, appropriate follow up and ongoing care are vital to overall patient improvement.

References

1. Nadeau M, Rosas-Arellano MP, Gurr KR, Bailey SI, Taylor DC, Grewal R, et al. The reliability of differentiating neurogenic claudication from vascular claudication based on symptomatic presentation. Can J Surg. 2013;56(6):372–7. https://doi.org/10.1503/cjs.016512.
2. Garra G, Singer AJ, Taira BR, Chohan J, Cardoz H, Chisena E, Thode HC. Validation of the Wong-Baker FACES Pain Rating Scale in pediatric emergency department patients. Acad Emerg Med. 2010;17(1):50–4. https://doi.org/10.1111/j.1553-2712.2009.00620.x.
3. Krechel SW, Bildner J. CRIES: a new neonatal postoperative pain measurement score. Initial testing of validity and reliability. Pediatr Anesth. 1995;5(1):53–61. https://doi.org/10.1111/j.1460-9592.1995.tb00242.x.
4. Feldt KS. The checklist of nonverbal pain indicators (CNPI). Pain Manag Nurs. 2000;1(1):13–21. https://doi.org/10.1053/jpmn.2000.5831.
5. Nygaard HA, Jarland M. The Checklist of Nonverbal Pain Indicators (CNPI): testing of reliability and validity in Norwegian nursing homes. Age Ageing. 2006;35(1):79–81. https://doi.org/10.1093/ageing/afj008.
6. Warden V, Hurley AC, Volicer L. Development and psychometric evaluation of the Pain Assessment in Advanced Dementia (PAINAD) scale. J Am Med Dir Assoc. 2003;4(1):9–15. https://doi.org/10.1097/00130535-200301000-00002.
7. Melzack R. The McGill Pain Questionnaire. In: Melzack R, editor. Pain measurement and assessment. New York: Raven Press; 1983. p. 41–7.
8. Luo X, George ML, Kakouras I, Edwards CL, Pietrobon R, Richardson W, Hey L. Reliability, validity, and responsiveness of the short form 12-item survey (SF-12) in patients with back pain. Spine. 2003;28(15):1739–45. https://doi.org/10.1097/01.brs.0000083169.58671.96.
9. Mason VL, Skevington SM, Osborn M. A measure for quality of life assessment in chronic pain: preliminary properties of the WHOQOL-pain. J Behav Med. 2008;32(2):162–73. https://doi.org/10.1007/s10865-008-9187-y.
10. Burns S, Biering-Sørensen F, Donovan W, Graves D, Jha A, Johansen M, et al. International standards for neurological classification of spinal cord injury, revised 2011. Top Spinal Cord Inj Rehabil. 2012;18(1):85–99. https://doi.org/10.1310/sci1801-85.
11. Tennant F. Evaluating pain intervention effectiveness and compliance. Pract Pain Manag. 2012;8(6). https://www.practicalpainmanagement.com.

Further Reading

Bickley LS. Bate's guide to physical examination and history taking. 11th ed.

Donohoe CD. History and physical examination of the pain patient (Chapter 5). In: Waldman SD, editor. Pain management. 2nd ed. p. 36–49.

Hoppenfeld S. Physical examination of the spine & extremities. 1st ed.

Pharmacotherapy of Pain in the Hospital: Review of Limitations

Alicia Grubich, Michael Pribula, and Dmitri Souza

Essential Concepts

- There are significant limitations for pharmacological therapy of pain in some patients in certain patient populations.
- Familiarity with pharmacological pain management options and their limitations and risks is essential.
- NSAIDs can lead to increased risk of ulcer formation and bleeding and Acetaminophen overuse can lead to liver failure while regular use can mask fever.
- Antidepressants and antiepileptics can have a wide variety of side effects ranging from tachycardia to serotonin syndrome to fatigue and dependence depending on the medication used.
- Skeletal Muscle Relaxants have several central nervous system and respiratory depressant effects.
- Opioids, while effective for acute pain, are not the best choice for certain patients given the risk factors associated with their use and their lack of long-term efficacy.
- Bedside interventional procedures could be a reasonable alternative strategy to help patients who are at risk for polypharmacy or side effects from pharmacological treatment of pain.

A. Grubich · D. Souza (✉)
Center for Pain Medicine, Western Reserve Hospital, Cuyahoga Falls, OH, USA
e-mail: agrubich@westernreservehospital.org; dsouza@westernreservehospital.org

M. Pribula
Department of Family Medicine, Western Reserve Hospital, Cuyahoga Falls, OH, USA
e-mail: mpribula@westernreservehospital.org

D. Souza et al. (eds.), *Bedside Pain Management Interventions*,
https://doi.org/10.1007/978-3-031-11188-4_3

1 Background

Pain is prevalent in the hospital setting and has been shown to occur in 37.7–84% of the patient population. Pain can be difficult to control and, if inadequately treated, it has been shown to produce unwanted clinical outcomes and increase the risk of developing chronic pain [1]. There are various classes of medications that are utilized for pain management. As with any medication, these pharmacologic options come with the risk of adverse effects. It is important to become familiar with the limitations of pharmacotherapy to help guide treatment selection. Understanding these limitations allows one to consider when interventional bedside procedures may be appropriate, with the goal of improving patient outcomes.

2 Pain Medications

Non-steroidal Anti-inflammatory Drugs (NSAIDs)

Non-steroidal anti-inflammatory drugs (NSAIDs), such as Ibuprofen, Naproxen, Ketorolac, and Meloxicam, are commonly used for pain control. They inhibit cyclooxygenase (COX) enzymes and subsequently decrease the formation of prostaglandin precursors. Due to their mechanism of action, NSAIDs carry a risk for various adverse effects. The decrease in prostaglandin production leads to a decrease in mucin and bicarbonate production as well as decreased mucosal proliferation. This puts patients at an increased risk for the development of gastric ulcers. The decrease in prostaglandin production also inhibits platelet aggregation, putting patients at an increased risk for bleeding. NSAIDs exhibit negative effects on the kidneys and cardiovascular system as well. They cause afferent arteriole vasoconstriction in the kidneys leading to an increase in sodium and water reabsorption and a decrease in blood flow. This can lead to acute kidney injury, edema, and hypertension [2].

Acetaminophen

Another commonly used medication to treat pain is Acetaminophen. Although generally thought of as a safe medication, it has its limitations as well. One such limitation is the potential of hepatotoxicity and the risk of overdose at large doses [3]. Acetaminophen is the most common cause of liver transplants in the United States (U.S.) (Fig. 1) . it has been shown to result in 50,000 emergency department visits, 10,000 hospitalizations, and 500 deaths per year [4, 5]. Aside from its analgesic effects, Acetaminophen also has antipyretic effects. The antipyretic effect is a result of COX enzyme inhibition, the rate-limiting step in prostaglandin synthesis, which regulates heat production and fever. This effect can become a limitation in a patient with an undiagnosed infection since fever is a cardinal sign of infection. Masking fever with acetaminophen could lead to delays in diagnosis and treatment [5] (Fig. 1).

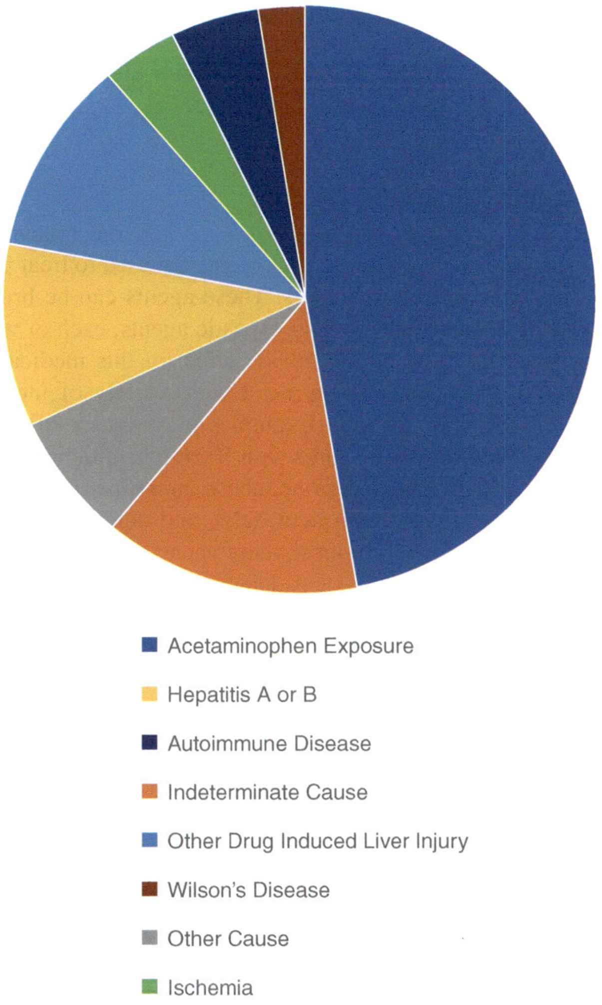

Fig. 1 Causes of acute liver failure [14]

Antidepressants and Antiepileptic Drugs

Select antidepressants and antiepileptic drugs are often used to treat pain. They exhibit their effects by acting on various neurotransmitters and ion channels. A common class of antidepressants used for pain control is tricyclic antidepressants (TCAs), such as Amitriptyline and Nortriptyline. Common side effects associated with TCAs include anticholinergic effects such as dry mouth, urinary retention, blurred vision, and tachycardia. Additional antidepressant agents used for pain control include Bupropion, Venlafaxine, and Duloxetine. Side effects associated with Bupropion include tachycardia, insomnia, agitation, and increased risk of seizures. Venlafaxine and Duloxetine have many drug interactions due to their mechanism of action and cytochrome P450 metabolism. They increase serotonin and should be used with caution in other serotonergic agents to avoid serotonin syndrome. Common antiepileptic drugs that are used for pain control include Gabapentin and Pregabalin. Side effects associated with these agents include sedation, dizziness, weight gain, and physical dependence [6].

Skeletal Muscle Relaxants

Skeletal muscle relaxants are commonly used to treat pain affecting the bone, muscles, tendons, and ligaments. These agents can be broken up into two categories, antispasmodic agents and antispastic agents, each of which comes with its own set of side effects. A common side effect of this medication class is central nervous system depression. There are a wide variety of medication-specific side effects within the class as well. Examples of agent-specific side effects within the class include withdrawal seizures with Baclofen, anticholinergic effects and QTc prolongation with Cyclobenzaprine, abuse, and misuse with Carisoprodol, and increased risk of cognitive impairment, falls, and delirium with Diazepam. Although commonly prescribed long-term, these agents are only recommended for short-term use due to the risk of physical dependence. There is limited data comparing agents within the class and treatment is often selected based on side effect profile and patient-specific factors [7].

Opioids

Opioids are commonly used to treat pain due to their known efficacy in the acute setting [8]. However, evidence of long-term efficacy in non-cancer pain has been insufficient [9]. In 2017, there were more than 191 million opioid prescriptions dispensed in the United States (U.S.). Opioids are associated with serious side effects, including respiratory and central nervous system (CNS) depression, constipation, dependence, and addiction [10].

Opioid-induced ventilatory impairment (OIVI) is a common side effect that occurs when there is a combination of respiratory depression, sedation, and airway obstruction. This combination leads to decreased ventilation and increased carbon dioxide levels. It has been shown that OIVI is associated with an increased risk of mechanical ventilation and death. Patients at an increased risk of respiratory depression and oversedation include the following patient populations: the elderly, the opioid naïve, current or previous smokers, the morbidly obese, those on increased opioid doses, and those with concomitant sedative medications (benzodiazepines, antihistamines, central nervous system depressants, etc.). Additional risk factors include pulmonary disease, cardiac disease, major organ failure, sleep apnea, sleep disorder, snoring, and post-thoracic or upper abdominal surgery [11]. Opioid-induced constipation (OIC) is another common side effect, occurring in 40–95% of non-cancer patients. This side effect is due to the activation of μ receptors in the gastrointestinal tract leading to an inhibition of gastric emptying and peristalsis. If left untreated, it has been shown that OIC can lead to hemorrhoids, fecal impaction, bowel obstruction, bowel rupture, and death [12].

A major concern with opioid medications is the risk of physical dependence and addiction. In 2016, more than 11.5 million patients in the U.S. reported misusing their prescriptions. In 2018, almost 47,000 overdose deaths occurred, 32% of which involved prescription opioids [10]. Due to the opioid epidemic at hand, it is important to limit their use and reserve these agents for patients with a strong indication.

In addition to the previously mentioned side effects, opioids require close monitoring or avoidance in special patient populations. These medications are recommended to be avoided in the elderly population due to the increased risk of respiratory depression and falls. The pediatric population has limited evidence for use and has an increased risk of respiratory depression and future misuse. It is recommended to avoid opioids in pregnant women due to the risk of premature birth, birth defects, and neonatal abstinence syndrome [13]. Patients with renal or hepatic impairment should be monitored closely due to decreased metabolism of these medications leading to increased serum concentrations and increased risk of adverse effects.

3 Pain Consult/Bedside Procedures

Patients with conditions that may benefit from an evaluation for possible bedside pain interventions include: postoperative pain, opioid administration prior to admission or opioid tolerance, frequent admissions for pain control, high opioid requirements (acute injuries, sickle cell disease, abdominal pain, etc.), limited tolerance to pain medications, pain accompanied by anxiety or depression, special populations (elderly, pregnant, history of substance abuse, etc.), change in mental status possibly related to pain medications, and patients with implanted devices (spinal cord stimulators, intrathecal pain pumps, etc.). Patients who may be candidates for alternative treatment such as injections include patients with acute or chronic pain and limited tolerance to medications, patients who may benefit from nerve blockade (acute radicular pain, rib and other fractures, etc.), or patients who are candidates for joint, muscle or tendon sheath injections.

4 Conclusion

Treatment of acute on chronic pain in the hospital setting can be challenging. There are recognized limitations of pharmacological therapy. When selecting a pain medication, it is important to take these limitations into consideration. Bedside pain management interventions may be a reasonable option for patients with actual or potential concerns with pharmacological therapy of pain and should be considered when appropriate.

References

1. Gregory J, McGowan L. An examination of the prevalence of acute pain for hospitalized adult patients: a systematic review. J Clin Nurs. 2016;25(5–6):583–98.
2. Gunaydin C, Bilge SS. Effects of nonsteroidal anti-inflammatory drugs at the molecular level. Eurasian J Med. 2018;50(2):116–21.
3. Kennon-McGill S, McGill MR. Extrahepatic toxicity of acetaminophen: critical evaluation of the evidence and proposed mechanisms. J Clin Transl Res. 2017;3(3):297–310.
4. Gerriets V, Anderson J, Nappe TM. Acetaminophen. StatPearls website. https://www.ncbi.nlm.nih.gov/books/NBK482369/. Updated 11 Aug 2020. Accessed 15 Aug 2020.
5. Lee WM. Acetaminophen (APAP) hepatotoxicity—isn't it time for APAP to go away? J Hepatol. 2017;67(6):1324–31. https://doi.org/10.1016/j.jhep.2017.07.005.
6. Maizels M, McCarberg B. Antidepressants and antiepileptic drugs for chronic non-cancer pain. Am Fam Physician. 2005;71(3):483–90.
7. Witenko C, Moorman-Li R, Motycka C, et al. Considerations for the appropriate use of skeletal muscle relaxants for the management of acute low back pain. P T. 2014;39(6):427–35.
8. Furlan AD, Sandoval JA, Mailis-Gagnon A, et al. Opioids for chronic noncancer pain: a meta-analysis of effectiveness and side effects. Can Med Assoc J. 2006;174(11):1589–94.
9. Chou R, Turner JA, Devine EB, et al. The effectiveness and risks of long-term opioid therapy for chronic pain: a systematic review for a national institutes of health pathways to prevention workshop. Ann Intern Med. 2015;162(4):276.
10. Opioid Overdose. Centers for Disease Control and Prevention website. https://www.cdc.gov/drugoverdose/opioids/prescribed.html. Updated 19 Mar 2020. Accessed 15 Aug 2020.
11. Macintyre PE, Loadsman JA, Scott DA. Opioids, ventilation and acute pain management. Anaesth Intensive Care. 2011;39(4):545–58.
12. Sizar O, Genova R, Gupta M. Opioid induced constipation. StatPearls website. https://www.ncbi.nlm.nih.gov/books/NBK493184/. Updated 10 Aug 2020. Accessed 15 Aug 2020.
13. Pregnancy. Centers for Disease Control and Prevention website. https://www.cdc.gov/pregnancy/opioids/basics.html. Updated 13 Aug 2020. Accessed 15 Aug 2020.
14. Olson KR, Davarpanah A, Schaefer E, Elias N, Misdraji J. Case 2-2017—an 18-year-old woman with acute liver failure. N Engl J Med. 2017;376:268–78. https://doi.org/10.1056/NEJMcpc1613467.

Further Reading

Rosenquist RW, Souzdalnitski D, Urman R. Chronic pain management for hospitalized patient. 1st edition. New York: Oxford University Press; 2016. p. 420.

Sedation and Patient Monitoring for Bedside Pain Management Interventions

Wenyu Pan, Shiragi Patel, and Magdalena Anitescu

Essential Concepts

- Balance patient safety and patient comfort during interventional pain procedures.
- Determine the appropriate choice for sedation (or no sedation) depending on the type of interventional pain procedure and the patient's comorbidities.
- Recognize that sedation may confound the results of diagnostic pain procedures and expose patients to unnecessary and more invasive further procedures.
- Consider which inpatients are not appropriate candidates for invasive pain management techniques (e.g., patients with substance abuse, coagulopathy or systemic pain disorders like sickle cell disease) and utilize other pain management techniques, including ketamine, lidocaine, and dexmedetomidine infusions.
- Identify potential complications of sedation, including airway compromise, hemodynamic collapse, predisposition to nerve injury, and disinhibition/agitation.

W. Pan
Department of Anesthesia and Critical Care, University of Chicago, Chicago, IL, USA
e-mail: wenyu.pan@uchospitals.edu

S. Patel
Department of Anesthesia and Critical Care, University of Chicago Medical Center, University of Chicago, Chicago, IL, USA
e-mail: shiragi.patel@uchospitals.edu

M. Anitescu (✉)
Division of Pain Management, Department of Anesthesia and Critical Care, University of Chicago Medical Center, University of Chicago, Chicago, IL, USA
e-mail: manitescu@dacc.uchicago.edu

D. Souza et al. (eds.), *Bedside Pain Management Interventions*,
https://doi.org/10.1007/978-3-031-11188-4_4

1 Overview

The array of interventional pain procedures is becoming increasingly complex and can occur in many different settings, including pain clinics, procedure rooms, surgery centers, inpatient floors, and intensive care units. Balancing patient comfort during the procedure and risk of sedation is key. Medications for sedation may produce varying degrees of amnesia, anxiolysis, and analgesia for patients undergoing interventions for acute or chronic pain. They may also alter the patient's consciousness and potentially confound the certainty for diagnostic procedures or result in complications such as airway compromise. Therefore, it is essential to balance patient safety and patient comfort during interventional pain procedures and choose the appropriate type and level of sedation.

2 Historical Aspects, Levels of Sedation

The history of interventional pain management began in 1884 with Koller's discovery that cocaine numbs the tongue. Consequently, in the early twentieth century multiple interventional techniques were developed using local anesthetics; these include caudal epidural injections, trigeminal ganglion block, neuraxial anesthesia, epidural diagnostic blockades, and others [1–3]. Over time, procedures became increasingly complex and prolonged, requiring deeper levels of sedation or general anesthesia.

The American Society of Anesthesiologists (ASA) and the Joint Commission consider sedation a continuum that ranges from minimal sedation, through moderate (conscious) sedation, to deep sedation, in addition to general anesthesia (Table 1) [4]. Although sedation may not be needed in simple pain procedures, physicians are utilizing it more often due to the benefit of anxiolysis in ailing patients with high

Table 1 Levels of sedation

	Minimal sedation anxiolysis	Moderate sedation/analgesia ("conscious sedation")	Deep sedation/ analgesia	General anesthesia
Responsiveness	Normal response to verbal stimulation	Purposeful response to verbal or tactile stimulation	Purposeful response following repeated or painful stimulation	Unarousable even with painful stimulus
Airway	Unaffected	No intervention required	Intervention may be required	Intervention often required
Spontaneous ventilation	Unaffected	Adequate	May be inadequate	Frequently inadequate
Cardiovascular function	Unaffected	Usually maintained	Usually maintained	May be impaired

Adapted from [4]. ASA Continuum of Depth of Sedation, ASA Continuum of Depth of Sedation: Definition of General Anesthesia and Levels of Sedation/Analgesia. Committee of Origin: Quality Management and Departmental Administration, 2009 (Approved by the ASA House of Delegates)

levels of pain and discomfort; a "painless" procedure may also distinguish one physician's practice from another's and drive a referral base [5].

3 Anesthesia for Outpatient Procedures

Choosing the appropriate level of sedation and anesthesia depends on the complexity and difficulty of the interventional pain procedure and the patient's comorbidities. Interventions range from simple office procedures to operating room procedures; accordingly, the level of sedation required also varies (Table 2) [6].

Patients tolerate most simple in-office procedures without sedation, such as trigger point injections and major or minor joint or bursa injections and often with minimal local skin infiltration [6]. Infusions with lidocaine or ketamine require standard ASA monitoring due to their potential sedative side effects and potential changes in hemodynamic parameters [6]. In particular, patients undergoing ketamine infusions for various types of neuropathic pain are routinely pre-treated with

Table 2 Common interventional pain procedures and their anesthetic management

Locations	Procedures	Fluoroscopy	Ultrasound	Types of sedation/ anesthesia
Office	Trigger points	–	±	None
	Major/minor joint injection/ bursa injections	–	±	None/local skin infiltration
	Infusions (lidocaine/ketamine)	–	±	None/minimal/ moderate sedation
Pain clinic procedure room/ ambulatory surgery center	Routine procedures: Epidural steroid injections, transforaminal epidural steroid injections, medial branch nerve blocks, etc.	+	±	Local skin infiltration, ± minimal sedation
	Complex procedures: Sympathetic chain blocks, discographies, gasserian ganglion blocks and RF,	+	–	Local skin infiltration, ± minimal sedation
	minimally invasive lumbar decompression, pump trial, spinal cord stimulator trial, bone marrow biopsy	±	±	Local skin infiltration, ± minimal sedation and ± regional anesthesia
Surgery center operating room	Kyphoplasty, spinal cord stimulator, drug delivery system insertion	+	–	Local infiltration, deep sedation, general anesthesia, regional anesthesia

Adapted from [6]. Anitescu M. Chronic pain: anesthesia for procedures. Anesthesiol Clin. 2014;32(2):395–409, with modifications midazolam to blunt the psychotropic effects from ketamine. Adding the hypnotic effects of ketamine, these patients often experience moderate levels of sedation during their outpatient visit to the pain clinic.

Sedation techniques vary depending on the type of pain practice, whether a standalone pain clinic with its own pain procedure rooms or one associated with an ambulatory surgery center with procedures performed in the operating rooms.

Sedation performed in pain clinic procedure rooms and ambulatory surgery centers vary greatly among various practices. In a survey of 61 pain practices giving IV sedation (including 79% anesthesia practices), 46% gave IV sedation for lumbar epidurals, 53% for cervical epidurals [7], 80% for radiofrequency ablation, 65% for intra-articular joint injections, and > 90% for discography and stimulator trials [7]. Other surveys to determine patient satisfaction found no benefit of sedation with epidural, spinal, and zygapophyseal joint injections [8, 9]. There is insufficient evidence regarding whether or not sedation has a role in reducing vasovagal reactions in interventional spine procedures for patients undergoing pain procedures for the first time. Vasovagal reactions are rare and associated with male gender, younger age (<65), lesser pre-procedural pain (<5/10), and larger needle gauge [10]. However, it is suggested that in patients with a confirmed history of vasovagal reactions, mild to moderate sedation may be beneficial [11].

Sedation, especially if it involves opioid medication, may confound the results of diagnostic procedures, such as selective nerve root block, medial branch nerve block, or discography, and may lead to unnecessary and invasive procedures such as radiofrequency ablation of the medial branch nerve, or spine surgery [6]. For patients on home opioid regimens, such as cancer patients who present for celiac plexus block, medications that routinely produce minimal sedation such as midazolam and especially fentanyl can result in deep sedation upon completion of the block as pain relief is instantaneous with local anesthetic. While positioning during the procedure can be especially challenging in these very frail individuals, the lowest dose of sedation medication is recommended to achieve comfort. This difficult situation is further complicated by the recommendation that, when a celiac plexus block is planned, use of home opioids be slightly reduced at least a few hours before the procedure in order to ensure a positive response to the block. Thus, positioning for this procedure may be challenging; completion of the procedure with the least amount of sedative to achieve comfort requires constant evaluation of patient during the procedure with frequent input and assessment of level of consciousness.

Among the longest and most complex pain-relieving interventions are spinal cord stimulator and generator placement, intrathecal pump insertion, and vertebral body augmentation with kyphoplasty and vertebroplasty. These procedures are performed in operating rooms of ambulatory surgical centers where patients undergo deep sedation, general anesthesia, or regional anesthesia. Great care should be taken in patient positioning for vertebral body augmentation procedures as these patients are often frail; a neurological exam should be performed after the procedure [12]. Kyphoplasty is often performed under general anesthesia because active balloon distension can be painful. If the number of vertebrae being treated are greater than three for vertebral augmentation procedures, general anesthesia may also be preferred due to the prolonged time in a potentially uncomfortable position [6]. If the procedure involves fewer than three vertebrae, patients may tolerate the procedure under moderate or deep sedation with infiltration of local anesthetics. A patient's comorbidities should be taken into account [12]. For example, patients with severe chronic obstructive pulmonary disease may benefit from a neuraxial technique with light sedation while maintaining the patient's comfort. Some practices have the capabilities to perform vertebral augmentation procedures and spinal cord stimulator trials in their own offices; in these cases, sedation can be administered and, depending on the patient's comorbidities, it can vary from minimal to deep sedation with propofol and/or dexmedetomidine. Common sedation medications and doses are listed in Table 3.

Placement of a spinal cord stimulator is particularly challenging due to the need for patient input and feedback following lead placement. Short and uneventful trials can be performed in-office with minimal sedation. More challenging cases may require deeper levels of sedation either with dexmedetomidine or propofol that can be easily turned off for intermittent testing of the coverage. Ketamine is not advised as a sedative as it may alter a patient's reaction to common questions.

Intrathecal drug delivery systems can be placed with a patient under general anesthesia or deep sedation; in some instances, regional anesthesia with delivery of local anesthetic through a needle or catheter allows less systemic medication and pain relief that can endure beyond the operating room. When local anesthetic is administered through a catheter, the main reason is primarily to ensure pain relief during tunneling and reservoir placement.

A variety of new and emerging procedures have been described in recent years, including minimally invasive lumbar decompression (mild) and interbody spacers. Both are indirect spine decompression techniques that either remove calcified ligamentum flavum or place a small winged implant between the spinous process to alleviate pain from spinal stenosis. In both cases, minimal to moderate sedation can be used for patient comfort.

In all situations where sedation is administered in outpatient clinics and/or ambulatory surgery centers, ASA monitors need to be applied. In operating rooms, an anesthesia team is necessary for moderate or deep sedation, while in office settings minimal or mild sedation can be administered by nurses under the guidance of a pain provider.

Table 3 Common sedation medications and doses

Drug	Common IV sedation dosage for adults
Midazolam	0.5–2 mg, may repeat every 2–3 min as needed. Total dose 2.5–5 mg
Fentanyl	25–50, may repeat every 5–10 min as needed. Total dose 100 μg
Propofol	0.5 mg/kg loading infusion followed by a maintenance infusion of 25–75 μg/kg/min
Ketamine and propofol (1:10) "Ketofol"	Titrate according to propofol, 25–75 μg/kg/min
Dexmedetomidine	1 μg/kg loading infusion for 10 min followed by a maintenance infusion of 0.2–0.6 μg/kg/h. Usual range 0.2–1 μg/kg/h

4 Anesthesia for Inpatient and ICU Procedures

The use of mild to moderate sedation in inpatient settings for certain pain interventions such as ultrasound guided peripheral nerve blocks remains controversial. Cases of long-term nerve injury have been reported in deeply sedated patients during certain pain procedures [5]. However, it is also important to consider patient comfort, the setting in which the procedure is performed, and the type of pain intervention. For example, in performing regional peripheral nerve blocks, the risk of complications is rare [13]. A study by Perlas et al. further found that only one third of patients noticed needle-to-nerve contact during ultrasound guided nerve localization [14]. Based on these facts, it is reasonable to offer mild sedation to patients undergoing peripheral ultrasound guided nerve blocks (non-diagnostic, neuraxial procedures) as it may increase patient satisfaction without any additional risk. When giving sedation, it is important to monitor patients with standard ASA monitors.

Patients in a hospital setting are also in close proximity to health care professionals who can monitor and intercede if a patient is inadvertently over sedated. Therefore, it is not uncommon for patients to receive mild sedation with small doses of fentanyl and/or midazolam as a means to help with anxiolysis and procedure-related pain during ultrasound guided peripheral nerve blocks.

For inpatients who are not appropriate candidates for invasive pain management techniques (for example, those with substance abuse, coagulopathy or systemic pain disorders such as sickle cell disease), other pain management techniques exist, including ketamine, lidocaine, and dexmedetomidine infusions. These drugs are good substitutes for opioid substances as they do not cause dependence or respiratory depression but do help with analgesia. Table 4 compares the various pharmacological effects of medications used in pain management. Intravenous lidocaine infusions can be effective for analgesia in patients with trigeminal neuralgia, fibromyalgia, cancer pain refractory, opioid therapy, and diabetic neuropathy [16]. However, because of its cardiotoxic and neurological effects, patients on lidocaine infusions must be closely monitored and have blood values drawn within the first 12 h of infusion initiation. Table 5 describes the authors' institutional protocol for lidocaine infusions. When lidocaine infusions are initiated in the operating room, bolus can be administered. However, when lidocaine is started on the floor, it is administered as a simple continuous infusion. Blood levels (therapeutic of 1.5–6 ng/mL) are measured upon arrival in PACU if initiated during a procedure and checked once daily after that; levels at 12 h

Table 4 Pharmacologic spectrum of agents used in interventional pain

Drug	Anxiolysis	Sedation	Analgesia	Amnesia	Dependency
Midazolam	+	+	0	+	+
Propofol	0	+	0	+	+
Ketamine	0	0	+	+	+
Fentanyl	0	+	+	0	+
Remifentanyl	0	+	+	0	+
Dexmedetomidine	0	+	+	+	0/A[a]

Data from [15]. Smith HS, Colson J, Sehgal N. An update of evaluation of intravenous sedation on diagnostic spinal injection procedures. Pain Physician 2013;16(Suppl 2):SE217–28
[a]Attenuates withdrawal symptoms from barbiturates, benzodiazepines, and opioids

Table 5 Lidocaine infusion protocol at The University of Chicago Medical Center

Protocol	Definition	Restrictions	Dosing	Monitoring
Low dose	Continuous infusion for optimal analgesia (max 24 h)	Ordered by acute pain service; available on floors with continuous telemetry	Bolus 1–1.5 mg/kg over 10 min Continuous thereafter at 0.3–0.5 mg/kg/h[a]	Drug level monitoring: First level when patients arrive in PACU, subsequent levels daily with AM labs Therapeutic blood level:1.5–6 mg/mL Monitor side effects every 4 h with continuous telemetry for dysrhythmia
Moderate dose	Continuous infusion >24 h	Ordered by acute pain service Available in PACU, ICU, ED	Bolus 1–1.5 mg/kg over 10 min Continuous thereafter at 0.3–0.5 mg/kg/h[a]	Continuous telemetry Monitor clinical response Monitor blood levels daily Monitor for toxicity every 4 h

PACU post anesthesia care unit, *ICU* intensive care unit, *ED* emergency department
Source: The University of Chicago Protocols. Table adapted from Anitescu M. The patient with substance use disorder. Curr Opin Anaesthesiol. 2019;32(3):427–37
[a]Based on ideal body weight

Table 6 Ketamine infusion protocol at The University of Chicago Medical Center

Restriction	Dosing, dispensing, and administration	Monitoring
APS consultation required to initiate therapy. Low dose ketamine infusion order set managed by APS	Doses 0.06–0.3 mg/kg/h[a] Starting doses: Adult: (assuming normal renal and hepatic function) start at 0.12 mg/kg/h[a] Consider starting at 0.06 mg/kg/h for BMI < 18 Pediatric: 0.06 mg/kg/h[a] Contraindications: Liver failure Changes in infusion rates controlled by APS Consider reducing current opioids, if possible, during ketamine titrations	Continuous pulse oximetry Routine vital signs Pain and sedation score every 2 h ×2 then every 4 h thereafter Monitor closely: Blood pressure changes, mental status changes, RR < 10 breaths/min, difficulty with arousal. If any of the above signs occur, then stop ketamine infusion and notify APS

APS acute pain service, *RR* respiratory rate
Source: The University of Chicago Protocols. Table adapted from Anitescu M. The patient with substance use disorder. Curr Opin Anaesthesiol. 2019;32(3):427–37
[a]Based on ideal body weight

are checked when started on the wards. Ketamine infusions are an alternative option for post-operative pain management. Ketamine is an NMDA antagonist that can be used as an opioid-sparing analgesic; its inpatient protocol is further detailed in Table 6. However, even at subanesthetic doses, ketamine can be associated with side effects such as hallucinations, hemodynamic instability, excessive agitation, and sedation.

5 Potential Complications

The continuum of sedation has the potential to risk patient safety and result in possible complications when attempting to balance patient comfort during interventional pain procedures. Past case reports have demonstrated poor outcomes for patients over sedated during epidural steroid injections or intrathecal catheters [5]. Other drawbacks to sedation include possible airway compromise, hemodynamic collapse, predisposition to nerve injury, and disinhibition/agitation. Also, in situations where mild sedation accidentally progresses to moderate and even further to deep sedation, airway compromise can occur. This can be the case when high doses of hypnotic medications, such as propofol, are administered with sedation [17].

Disinhibition and agitation that can cause uncontrolled movement can also occur during deep sedation [18]. The rise in chronic-pain related claims over the past few decades has expanded the debate over the use of sedation for diagnostic neuraxial procedures as it may increase the risk of needle malposition and thereby neural injury [19].

When describing the risks and complications of sedation during pain management interventions, it is important to note that these risks are related to diagnostic neuraxial pain management techniques associated with deep sedation; they are not related to mild sedation used for ultrasound guided peripheral nerve blocks in outpatient procedures.

All aspects of sedation—including the risks, benefits, challenges, and possible adverse effects—need to be reviewed with patients during discussions related to the procedure being performed. While patients prefer to be comfortable during the procedure, it's important they understand the added risk of excessive sedation.

6 Conclusion and Future Directions

Many factors play a role in determining the use of sedation for pain management interventions. The type of procedure, the setting in which the intervention is performed, and patient comfort and satisfaction are all part of the decision. For outpatient procedures, including epidural steroid injections, joint injections, or other diagnostic neuraxial procedures, the use of sedation is limited, and local infiltration of lidocaine is commonly used. The more complex procedures performed in operating rooms, such as spinal cord stimulators and intrathecal drug delivery systems, moderate or deep sedation or general/regional anesthesia is typically provided by a separate team. For inpatient procedures, including non-diagnostic pain interventions such as peripheral nerve blocks, patients may receive sedation as long as appropriate ASA monitors are used. For pain management in patients unable to tolerate interventional procedures, lidocaine and ketamine infusions are good pain management alternatives. In all instances, it is vital to discuss the risks and benefits of the anticipated sedation with the patient.

References

1. Brown DL, Fink BR. The history of neural blockade and pain management. In: Cousins MJ, Bridenbaugh PO, editors. Neural blockade in clinical anesthesia and management of pain. 3rd ed. Philadelphia: Lippincott Raven; 1998. p. 3–34.
2. Cushing H. On the evidence of shock in major amputations by cocainization of large nerve-trunks preliminary to their division. Ann Surg. 1902;36:36–321.
3. Schloesser H. Heilung periphar Reizzustande sensibler und motorischer Nerven. Klin Monbl Augenheilkd. 1903;41:255.
4. ASA Continuum of depth of sedation: definition of general anesthesia and levels of sedation/analgesia. Committee of Origin: Quality Management and Departmental Administration; 2009 (Approved by the ASA House of Delegates).
5. Prager JP, Aprill C. Complications related to sedation and anesthesia for interventional pain therapies. Pain Physician. 2008;9(S1):S121–7.
6. Anitescu M. Chronic pain: anesthesia for procedures. Anesthesiol Clin. 2014;32(2):395–409.
7. Ahmed SU, Tonidandel W, Trella J, Martin NM, Chang Y. Peri-procedural protocols for interventional pain management techniques: a survey of US pain centers. Pain Physician. 2005;8(2):181–5.
8. Cucuzzella TR, Delport EG, Kim N, Marley J, Pruitt C, Delport AG. A survey: conscious sedation with epidural and zygapophyseal injections: is it necessary? Spine J. 2006;6(4):364–9.
9. Kim N, Delport E, Cucuzzella T, Marley J, Pruitt C. Is sedation indicated before spinal injections? Spine (Phila Pa 1976). 2007;32(25):E748–52.
10. Kennedy DJ, Schneider B, Casey E, Rittenberg J, Conrad B, Smuck M, et al. Vasovagal rates in fluoroscopically guided interventional procedures: a study of over 8,000 injections. Pain Med. 2013;14(12):1854–9.
11. Kennedy DJ, Schneider B, Smuck M, Plastaras CT. The use of moderate sedation for the secondary prevention of adverse vasovagal reactions. Pain Med. 2015;16(4):673–9.
12. Burton AW, Hamid B. Kyphoplasty and vertebroplasty. Curr Pain Headache Rep. 2008;12(1):22–7.
13. Auroy Y, Benhamou D, Bargues L, et al. Major complications of regional anesthesia in France: the SOS regional anesthesia hotline service. Anesthesiology. 2002;97:1274–80.
14. Perlas A, Niazi A, McCartney C, et al. The sensitivity of motor response to nerve stimulation and paresthesia for nerve localization as evaluated by ultrasound. Reg Anesth Pain Med. 2006;31:445–50.
15. Smith HS, Colson J, Sehgal N. An update of evaluation of intravenous sedation on diagnostic spinal injection procedures. Pain Physician. 2013;16(Suppl 2):SE217–28.
16. Marmura M, Rosen N, Abbas M, et al. Intravenous lidocaine in the treatment of refractory headache: a retrospective case series. Headache. 2009;49:286–91.
17. Abram SE, Francis MC. Hazards of sedation for interventional pain procedures. Anesthesia Patient Safety Foundation Newsletter; 2012.
18. Braidy HF, Singh P, Ziccardi VB. Safety of deep sedation in an urban oral and maxillofacial surgery training program. J Oral Maxillofac Surg. 2011;69:2112–9.
19. Metzner J, Posner KL, Lam MS, et al. Closed claims' analysis. Pract Res Clin Anaesthesiol. 2011;25:263–76.

Further Reading

Anitescu M. Chronic pain: anesthesia for procedures. Anesthesiol Clin. 2014;32(2):395–409.

Anitescu M. The patient with substance use disorder. Curr Opin Anaesthesiol. 2019;32(3):427–37.

Bedside Joint, Muscle, and Tendon Injections: Overview

Howard Meng, Priodarshi Roychoudhury, and James S. Khan

Essential Concepts

- Joints, tendons, and muscles are common sources of pain for patients.
- Ultrasound has significantly improved the accuracy and ease of performing a joint, tendon, or muscle injection at the bedside.
- A number of different medications exist for injection into these areas including emerging therapies such as platelet-rich plasma, hyaluronic acid, and mesenchymal stem cells.

1 Overview

Chronic pain is a major public health issue. An investigation of 25,916 consecutive patients attending a primary care clinic at 15 centers in 14 countries indicated that 22% of patients suffer from chronic pain [1]. Similar survey studies in the United States (n = 27,035) and in Canada (n = 2012) report a prevalence of chronic pain of

H. Meng
Department of Anesthesia, Sunnybrook Health Sciences Centre, Toronto, ON, Canada
e-mail: howard.meng@sunnybrook.ca

P. Roychoudhury
Department of Anesthesiology, Pharmacology and Therapeutics, University of British Columbia, Vancouver, BC, Canada

J. S. Khan (✉)
Department of Anesthesia and Pain Medicine, Mount Sinai Hospital, Toronto, ON, Canada

Department of Anesthesiology, University of Toronto, Toronto, ON, Canada
e-mail: James.khan@medportal.ca

D. Souza et al. (eds.), *Bedside Pain Management Interventions*,
https://doi.org/10.1007/978-3-031-11188-4_5

31% and 29%, respectively, suggesting that chronic pain may be more prevalent in North America [2, 3].

Chronic pain is associated with significant psychosocial distress, and there is a high co-occurrence with mood and psychological disorders (e.g., anxiety and depression) [4, 5]. Further, chronic pain places a financial strain on the patient, healthcare system, and society— pain is one of the top causes for work absenteeism and reduced productivity, and approximately one in five patients with chronic pain will lose their job because of their pain [6, 7]. A United Kingdom study identified that chronic pain resulted in 4.6 million visits to a primary care physician, which cost the system approximately £69 million ($100 million USD) a year [8]. The total direct and indirect costs of chronic pain are staggering and is estimated to be in the billions of dollars each year [9, 10].

A significant portion of patients with chronic pain suffer from musculoskeletal (MSK) pain. MSK pain comprises pain from muscles (myofascial pain), joints, or tendons. MSK pain is estimated to affect up to 47% of the general population [11]. Older age, low socioeconomic status, depression, anxiety, sleep disorders, and manual work are potential risk factors for MSK pain. Management options for MSK pain include a number of strategies such as physical therapy, psychological counselling, oral analgesics, and interventional options [12, 13].

There are a number of interventional therapies targeting pain joints, tendons, and muscles. Performing these injections at the bedside can help reduce waiting times for operating room availability, which can be reserved for procedures requiring sedation, increased monitoring, or fluoroscopy. Bedside procedures, whether performed as an inpatient or within an outpatient pain clinic, can facilitate early interval improvement in pain, faster rehabilitation, and mitigate oral pharmacologic use.

2 Historical Aspects

Traditionally, bedside MSK procedures have been performed using landmark-based approaches. This practice relies heavily on normal anatomy and tactile feedback of the injection needle. Challenges that exist with this approach include access to deeper joints or use in patients with a larger body habitus. Success rates with landmark-based approaches have been variable ranging from 16.7% to 100% [14]. However, since it is not possible to visualize the needle tip with a landmark-based approach, it is not possible to guarantee adequate injection at the desired anatomical location and it can pose unnecessary risks with the potential of puncturing nearby tissues (e.g., blood vessels, viscera, lungs).

Ultrasound technology has significantly improved the accuracy of MSK procedures. Numerous studies have demonstrated improved injection accuracy and decreased injection pain with ultrasound guidance [14]. Accuracy of upper and lower extremity injections using ultrasound has consistently resulted in greater than 90% accuracy. Benefits of ultrasound-guided procedures include needle visualization confirming placement in the joint or targeted tissue, real-time visualization of clear spread of the injectate, and improved safety by avoiding neurovascular structures and inflicting less needle trauma [15].

Acquisition of appropriate ultrasound images is highly user-dependent. A learning curve exists for the safe and accurate use of ultrasound-guided injections [16]. Individuals may have difficulties visualizing two dimensional structures while conceptualizing three-dimensional structures. Other challenges with ultrasound use include the presence of acoustic artifacts, optical illusions, and random noise. Patient characteristics including obesity, edema, air, muscle atrophy, and the need to access deeper anatomical targets pose further difficulties for the operator [17].

Types of Injections

A number of procedural options exist for joint, tendon, and muscle-related pain. Muscle pain, otherwise known as myofascial pain, is characterized by regional pain originating from hyperirritable spots known as myofascial trigger points (MTrPs) [18]. Several studies have suggested that myofascial trigger points accounted for the primary source of pain in up to 85% of patients presenting to a primary care clinic for pain evaluation [19]. Several injections exist for MTrPs, which are believed to mechanically disrupt dysfunctional activity in the motor endplates by both direct need placement and by injection of medications [20]. Dry needling is a common technique where a needle is placed into a trigger point with multiple passes, resulting in a local twitch response from rapid depolarization of the involved muscle fibers [21]. Apart from dry needling, injection of medications (wet needling) including local anesthesia, botulinum type A toxin (BoNT-A), and steroids can be used to alleviate myofascial pain [18]. Unfortunately, there are limited evidence to identify whether dry or wet needling is superior and which type of medication is most helpful.

Further, there are a number of joint and tendon injections that can be done at the bedside using ultrasound guidance. A number of tendon dysfunctions such as trigger fingers, rotator cuff tendinopathies, epicondylitis, biceps tendinopathy, and Achilles tendinopathy could be considered for injection therapy [22]. Furthermore, bedside injection of a number of small and large joints (i.e., zygapophyseal, acromio-clavicular, glenohumeral, hip, and knee joints) can also be performed reliably using ultrasound guidance [23].

Types of Injection Medications

Several different types of medications are commonly used in bedside procedures. Selection of these medications are based on both the etiology of pain and the purpose of the injection. Some injectates are combined (i.e. mixture of local anesthetics and steroids) in hopes of providing an additive or synergistic effect, although evidence for this is lacking. Here we discuss commonly used injection medications along with their potential risks and benefits.

Steroids are among the most commonly used medications for joint, tendon, and muscle injections. Most commonly used steroids are methylprednisolone, triamcinolone, betamethasone, and dexamethasone [24]. Steroids have an anti-inflammatory effect acting directly and indirectly to suppress the activity of pro-inflammatory cytokines by inhibition of phospholipase A2 activity [25]. Much of the clinical difference that exists between types of steroids is based on water solubility and aggregation characteristics resulting in the classification of *particulate* (poorly soluble) or *non-particulate* (soluble) steroids. Particulate steroids are ester preparations requiring hydrolysis by cellular esterases to produce the active moiety which results in the benefit of clinically longer duration of effect [26]. Non-particulate steroids may be safer in that regard however, they have shorter duration of anti-inflammatory effects. Systemic effects of steroid use are dose-dependent and commonly manifest as transient hypertension, hyperglycemia, post-injection flare, facial flushing and mood alterations [22]. Higher risk complications include septic arthritis, avascular necrosis, and tendon rupture and repeat steroid injections can result in local tissue atrophy and skin de-pigmentation [27].

Local anesthetics act by blocking sodium channels in the nerve membrane, interfering with the propagation of action potentials along the axon. They are often used for both diagnostic and therapeutic purposes, and often in combination with steroids and with a vasoconstrictor (i.e., epinephrine) which can increase the duration of effect and risk of local anesthetic toxicity [26]. Local anesthetics are synthesized as hydrochloride salts to render them water soluble. Intra-articular local anesthetics can improve postoperative pain scores and reduce narcotic consumption [28]. While local anesthetics appear to be safe when used in tendon, joint, and muscle injections, there are concerns for potential side-effects. Intravascular injections of local anesthetics can cause local anesthesia toxicity, resulting in central nervous system dysfunction and cardiorespiratory collapse—case reports have been published reporting local anesthesia toxicity after a single injection [29]. Further, local anesthesia appears to be toxic to both muscles and chondrocytes [30, 31].

3 Recent Developments

Hyaluronic acid is a glycosaminoglycan that is found within synovial fluid and the cartilage matrix [32]. Normal concentrations of hyaluronic acid as part of synovial fluid provides viscous lubrication during joint movements and provides shock-absorbing effects. Synthetic hyaluronic acid has been developed as a potential therapy for joint injections. It is believed to provide an analgesic effect via several mechanisms including anti-inflammatory, anabolic, analgesic, and chondroprotective mechanisms [33]. Specifically, hyaluronic acid can increase chondrocyte proliferation, decrease chondrocyte apoptosis, and retard the overall osteoarthritic process that results in joint space narrowing. Different products for use exist that vary in molecular weight, hyaluronic acid concentration, elasticity, and viscosity. Intra-articular hyaluronic injections are considered safe with transient local reaction of injection site reaction and injection site pain, with systemic reactions being rare [34].

PRP (platelet-rich plasma) is also another novel injection for MSK pathologies that requires separating the patient's blood to collect a solution that is generally four to six times the baseline concentration of platelets [35]. With injection of platelets, it is believed that they become activated and causes the release of these growth factors leading to an anti-inflammation effect and promotion of healing [36]. Prior studies suggested that 5% was the optimal concentration of platelets required to stimulate chondrocyte proliferation from an intraarticular injection [37]. Preparations of PRP vary considerably and can include leukocyte-rich or leukocyte-poor solutions [38]; leukocyte-rich preparations are preferred for tendon injections while leukocyte-poor preparations are preferred for intraarticular injections. A recent systematic review has evaluated the use of PRP for tendon and ligament pathologies and overall reports positive findings, particularly for lateral epicondylitis and rotator cuff tendinopathy [39]. Several reviews have suggested that PRP may be beneficial for intraarticular injection, particularly in the knee [40, 41].

Mesenchymal stem cells (MSCs) are an emerging therapy used for joint and tendon-related pain. It is believed that since MSCs have pluripotency properties, they can differentiate into different cell lineages, including type II chondrocytes, which can then produce cartilage in deficient joints with osteoarthritis [42]. MSCs can also be derived from bone marrow, adipose tissues, umbilical cord, and from synovium itself, with the greatest yields from adipose tissues [43]. MSCs have been studied in a number of animal models and small human studies and have shown some favorable findings [44]. Apart from stem cell differentiation and release of cartilage, MSCs are believed to possess robust anti-inflammatory properties by antagonizing resident macrophages from secreting pro-inflammatory cytokines [45]. Nonetheless, most studies are small and low-quality and there is a pressing need for more evidence for the use of this therapy.

4 Conclusions and Future Directions

Joint, tendon, and muscle injections are frequently performed procedures to alleviate pain. Bedside procedures can help provide immediate access to these therapies with minimal waiting times to operating room or procedure suites. The wide availability of ultrasound machines has allowed greater availabilities for clinicians to offer bedside procedures; however, there is a learning curve to obtain adequate skills required for ultrasound-guided procedures.

An increasing number of resources are becoming available on different types of joint, tendon, and muscle injections. Further, different injectates are available depending on the type of injection and presumed cause of pain. More evidence is needed on emerging therapies such as hyaluronic acid, platelet-rich plasma, and mesenchymal stem cells to definitively identify the efficacy and safety of these therapies.

References

1. Gureje O, Von Korff M, Simon GE, Gater R. Persistent pain and well-being. JAMA. 2013;280(2):147–52.
2. Johannes CB, Le TK, Zhou X, Johnston JA, Dworkin RH. The prevalence of chronic pain in United States adults: results of an internet-based survey. J Pain. 2010;11(11):1230–9.

3. Moulin D, Clark A, Speechley M, Morley-Forster P. Chronic pain in Canada, prevalence, treatment, impact and the role of opioid analgesia. Pain Res Manag. 2002;7:179–84.
4. Birket-Smith M. Somatization and chronic pain. Acta Anaesthesiol Scand. 2001;11:1114–20.
5. McWilliams LA, Cox BJ, Enns MW. Mood and anxiety disorders associated with chronic pain: an examination in a nationally representative sample. Pain. 2003;106(1):127–33.
6. Allen H, Hubbard D, Sullivan S. The burden of pain on employee health and productivity at a major provider of business services. J Occup Environ Med. 2005;47(7):658–70.
7. Breivik H, Collett B, Ventafridda V, Cohen R, Gallacher D. Survey of chronic pain in Europe: prevalence, impact on daily life, and treatment. Eur J Pain. 2006;10(4):287–333.
8. Belsey J. Primary care workload in the management of chronic pain. A retrospective cohort study using a GP database to identify resource implications for UK primary care. J Med Econ. 2002;5:39–50.
9. Gaskin DJ, Richard P. The economic costs of pain in the United States. J Pain. 2012;13(8):715–24.
10. Coyte PC, Asche CV, Croxford R, Chan B. The economic cost of musculoskeletal disorders in Canada. Arthritis Care Res. 1994;11(5):315–25.
11. Cimmino MA, Ferrone C, Cutolo M. Epidemiology of chronic musculoskeletal pain. Best Pract Res Clin Rheumatol. 2011;25(2):173–83.
12. Bergman S. Management of musculoskeletal pain. Best Pract Res Clin Rheumatol. 2007;21(1):153–66.
13. Babatunde OO, Jordan JL, Van Der Windt DA, Hill JC, Foster NE, Protheroe J. Effective treatment options for musculoskeletal pain in primary care: a systematic overview of current evidence. PLoS One. 2017;12(6):1–30.
14. Daniels EW, Cole D, Jacobs B, Phillips SF. Existing evidence on ultrasound-guided injections in sports medicine. Orthop J Sports Med. 2018;6(2):1–7.
15. Chen CPC, Lew HL, Tsai WC, Hung YT, Hsu CC. Ultrasound-guided injection techniques for the low back and hip joint. Am J Phys Med Rehabil. 2011;90(10):860–7.
16. Deimel GW, Jelsing EJ, Hall MM. Musculoskeletal ultrasound in physical medicine and rehabilitation. Curr Phys Med Rehabil Rep. 2013;1(1):38–47.
17. Henderson M, Dolan J. Challenges, solutions, and advances in ultrasound-guided regional anaesthesia. BJA Educ. 2016;16(11):374–80.
18. Desai MJ, Saini V, Saini S. Myofascial pain syndrome: a treatment review. Pain Ther. 2013;2(1):21–36.
19. Skootsky SA, Jaeger B, Oye RK. Prevalence of myofascial pain in general internal medicine practice. West J Med. 1989;151(2):157–60.
20. Borg-Stein J. Treatment of fibromyalgia, myofascial pain, and related disorders. Phys Med Rehabil Clin. 2006;17(2):491–510.
21. Kalichman L, Vulfsons S. Dry needling in the management of musculoskeletal pain. J Am Board Fam Med. 2010;23(5):640–6.
22. Speed C. Corticosteroid injections in tendon lesions. BMJ. 2002;323:382–6.
23. Narouze S. Atlas of ultrasound-guided procedures in interventional pain management. Springer; 2018.
24. Hwang H, Park J, Lee WK, Lee WH, Leigh JH, Lee JJ, et al. Crystallization of local anesthetics when mixed with corticosteroid solutions. Ann Rehabil Med. 2016;40(1):21–7.
25. McEwen BS, Kalia M. The role of corticosteroids and stress in chronic pain conditions. Metab Clin Exp. 2010;59(Suppl. 1):S9–15.
26. MacMahon PJ, Eustace SJ, Kavanagh EC. Injectable corticosteroid and review for radiologists. Radiology. 2009;252(3):647–61.
27. Sardana V, Burzynski J, Hasan K, Zalzal P. Are non-steroidal anti-inflammatory drug injections an alternative to steroid injections for musculoskeletal pain?: a systematic review. J Orthop. 2018;15(3):812–6.
28. Busch CA, Shore BJ, Bhandari R, Ganapathy S, MacDonald SJ, Bourne RB, et al. Efficacy of periarticular multimodal drug injection in total knee arthroplasty: a randomized trial. J Bone Joint Surg A. 2006;88(5):959–63.

29. Dhir S, Ganapathy S, Lindsay P, Athwal GS. Case report: ropivacaine neurotoxicity at clinical doses in interscalene brachial plexus block. Can J Anesth. 2007;54(11):912–6.
30. Reurink G, Goudswaard GJ, Moen MH, Weir A, Verhaar JAN, Tol JL. Myotoxicity of injections for acute muscle injuries: a systematic review. Sports Med. 2014;44(7):943–56.
31. Dragoo JL, Korotkova T, Kanwar R, Wood B. The effect of local anesthetics administered via pain pump on chondrocyte viability. Am J Sports Med. 2008;36(8):1484–8.
32. Elmorsy S, Funakoshi T, Sasazawa F, Todoh M, Tadano S, Iwasaki N. Chondroprotective effects of high-molecular-weight cross-linked hyaluronic acid in a rabbit knee osteoarthritis model. Osteoarthr Cartil. 2014;22(1):121–7.
33. Altman RD, Manjoo A, Fierlinger A, Niazi F, Nicholls M. The mechanism of action for hyaluronic acid treatment in the osteoarthritic knee: a systematic review. BMC Musculoskelet Disord. 2015;16(1):1–10.
34. Aggarwal A, Sempowski IP. Hyaluronic acid injections for knee osteoarthritis. Systematic review of the literature. Can Fam Physician. 2004;50:249–56.
35. Filardo G, Kon E, Roffi A, Di Matteo B, Merli ML, Marcacci M. Platelet-rich plasma: why intra-articular? A systematic review of preclinical studies and clinical evidence on PRP for joint degeneration. Knee Surg Sports Traumatol Arthrosc. 2015;23(9):2459–74.
36. Anitua E, Andia I, Ardanza B, Nurden P, Nurden AT. Autologous platelets as a source of proteins for healing and tissue regeneration. Thromb Haemost. 2004;91(1):4–15.
37. Spreafico A, Chellini F, Frediani B, Bernardini G, Niccolini S, Serchi T, et al. Biochemical investigation of the effects of human platelet releasates on human articular chondrocytes. J Cell Biochem. 2009;108(5):1153–65.
38. Braun HJ, Kim HJ, Chu CR, Dragoo JL. The effect of platelet-rich plasma formulations and blood products on human synoviocytes: implications for intra-articular injury and therapy. Am J Sports Med. 2014;42(5):1204–10.
39. Kia C, Baldino J, Bell R, Ramji A, Uyeki C, Mazzocca A. Platelet-rich plasma: review of current literature on its use for tendon and ligament pathology. Curr Rev Musculoskelet Med. 2018;11(4):566–72.
40. Laudy ABM, Bakker EWP, Rekers M, Moen MH. Efficacy of platelet-rich plasma injections in osteoarthritis of the knee: a systematic review and meta-analysis. Br J Sports Med. 2015;49(10):657–72.
41. Meheux CJ, McCulloch PC, Lintner DM, Varner KE, Harris JD. Efficacy of intra-articular platelet-rich plasma injections in knee osteoarthritis: a systematic review. Arthroscopy. 2016;32(3):495–505.
42. Marini JC, Forlino A. Replenishing cartilage from endogenous stem cells. N Engl J Med. 2013;366(26):2522–4.
43. Freitag J, Bates D, Boyd R, Shah K, Barnard A, Huguenin L, et al. Mesenchymal stem cell therapy in the treatment of osteoarthritis: reparative pathways, safety and efficacy—a review. BMC Musculoskelet Disord. 2016;17(1):1–13.
44. Jevotovsky DS, Alfonso AR, Einhorn TA, Chiu ES. Osteoarthritis and stem cell therapy in humans: a systematic review. Osteoarthr Cartil. 2018;26(6):711–29.
45. Harrell CR, Markovic BS, Fellabaum C, Arsenijevic A, Volarevic V. Mesenchymal stem cell-based therapy of osteoarthritis: current knowledge and future perspectives. Biomed Pharmacother. 2019;109:2318–26.

Further Reading

Haskins SC, Boretsky K, Boublik J, Bronshteyn Y, Byrne M, Chan V, El-Boghdadly K, Hernandez N, Hogg R, Kalagara H, Kruisselbrink R, Manson W, Nader A, Nejim J, Perlas A, Ramsingh D, Shankar H, Silva M, Souza D, Wilkinson JN, Zimmerman J, Narouze S. American Society of Regional Anesthesia and Pain Medicine expert panel recommendations on point-of-care ultrasound education and training for regional anesthesiologists and pain physicians, part 1. Reg Anesth Pain Med. 2021;46(12):1031–47. https://doi.org/10.1136/rapm-2021-102560. PMID: 33632778

Rosenquist RW, Souzdalnitski D, Urman R, editors. Chronic pain management for hospitalized patient. 1st ed. New York: Oxford University Press; 2016. 420 p. https://global.oup.com/academic/product/chronic-pain-management-for-the-hospitalized-patient-9780199349302?cc=eu&lang=en&. Assessed 31 Jan 2021.

Bedside Peripheral Nerve Blockade: Overview

Andrew T. Burzynski and Jinlei Li

Essential Concepts

- Peripheral nerve blocks and catheters are an effective means of analgesia in the hospitalized patient and clinic patients alike.
- Peripheral nerve blocks and catheters decrease opiate consumption and subsequent side effects including nausea, vomiting, delayed return of bowel function while also decreasing hospital length of stay and development of chronic pain [1, 2].
- Through use of ultrasound guidance, regional anesthesia is a safe, effective, and anatomically specific means of providing analgesia for the surgical and non-surgical patients.

1 Introduction

Regional Anesthesiology is a continuously evolving field of Anesthesiology which is able to provide pain relief for diagnosis and treatment purpose, as well as surgical anesthesia to assist a surgical procedure. Regional Anesthesia allows for a more

A. T. Burzynski
Department of Anesthesiology, Yale University School of Medicine, New Haven, CT, USA

Department of Anesthesiology, Lutheran Medical Center, Physician Anesthesia Services, P.C., Golden, CO, USA
e-mail: Andrew.burzynski@yale.edu

J. Li (✉)
Regional Anesthesia and Acute Pain Medicine, Yale New Haven Health, New Haven, CT, USA
e-mail: Jinlei.li@yale.edu

D. Souza et al. (eds.), *Bedside Pain Management Interventions*,
https://doi.org/10.1007/978-3-031-11188-4_6

localized and specific pain relief modality as compared to systemic opioids, and its use has grown from its original inception more than 100 years ago for a variety of orthopedic procedures, which were very well adapted to benefit from the specificity which regional anesthesia allows [3]. As the field has grown and its clinical benefits became more evident, the application of regional anesthesia techniques broadened to include many other types of surgeries as well as for acute pain management interventions. With the advent of peripheral nerve catheter use, the utilization of regional anesthesia for pain relief was broadened even further as continuous infusions could lengthen the period of pain relief even further than a single shot injection may provide [3]. Ultrasound guidance further improved the safety of performing peripheral nerve blocks as well as allowing for the execution of more technically challenging peripheral nerve blocks as our understanding of the beneficence improved. Today, there are a variety of applications of this ever-evolving field which may help patients in many different clinical scenarios. This brief overview will provide a basic understanding of required materials, patient selection, different examples of specific peripheral nerve blocks, and application of those blocks for the hospitalized patient.

2 Bedside Peripheral Nerve Blockade: Overview

Background

Materials, Location, and Supplies

Settings in which a bedside nerve block could be performed include the clinics, emergency room, perioperative locations, hospital beds, and intensive care units can all be optimized to satisfy the necessities for performing a peripheral nerve block in each of those locations without compromise to patient safety and outcomes (Fig. 1). Of utmost importance is to maintain certain specifications to ensure the safety of the patient at all times [4]. Each location should have the capability to monitor the patient with standard American Society of Anesthesiologists (ASA) monitoring devices including blood pressure, electrocardiogram, and pulse oximetry. [4] Additionally, access to resuscitation supplies including but not limited to emergency medication, intralipid, airway intervention devices and oxygen should be readily available, particularly if IV anxiolytics or opiates are administered to the patient (Table 1). A quiet location with privacy for the patient and team to work will help to alleviate undo stressors to the patient and to allow the team to work expeditiously. As with any bedside procedure, patient consent must be obtained explaining the risks, benefits, and alternatives to the procedure. A timeout should be performed with patient identifiers, procedures and laterality verified.

Ultrasound

The majority of nerve blocks can be done utilizing an 8–16 MHz linear array probe. The linear array ultrasound probe optimizes needle visualization and detailing of superficial structures (less than 4–5 cm). 2–5 MHz Curvilinear probes utilizing a lower frequency have their place for deeper blocks or when necessitated by patient body habitus for deeper tissue penetrance (>5 cm).

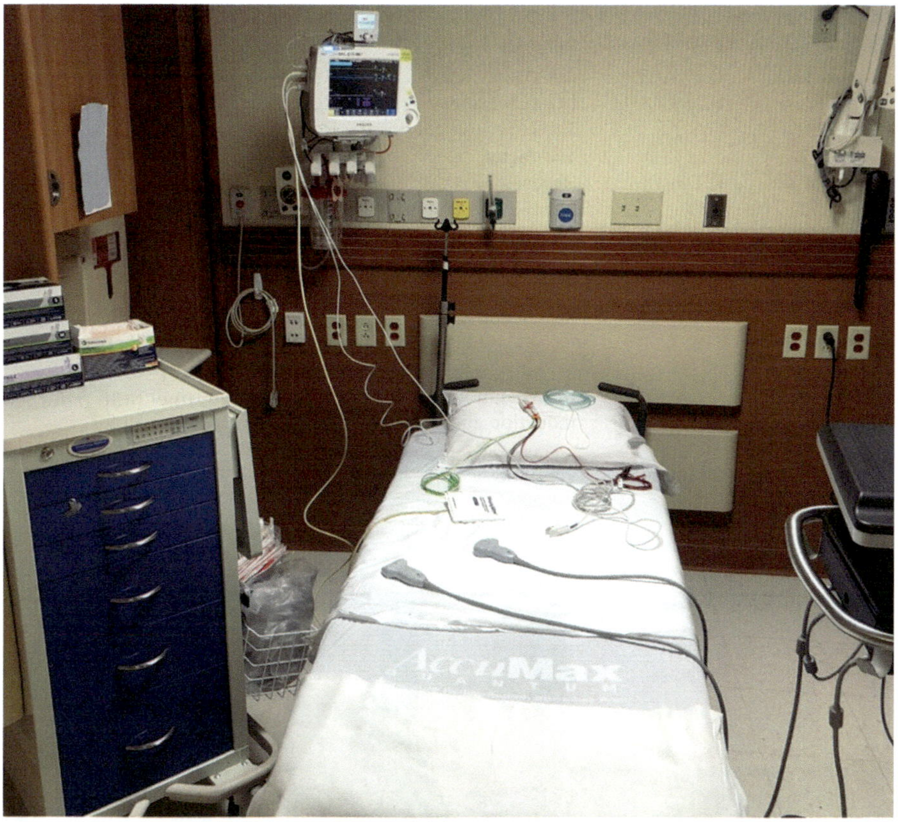

Fig. 1 Block bay set up in a pre-operative hospital bay. Standard ASA monitors including EKG, pulse oximetry, and non-invasive blood pressure monitoring, nasal cannula, ultrasound machine with both linear (6–15 MHz) and curvilinear (2–5 MHz) ultrasound probes, nerve block cart with necessary medications and supplies

Needles and Catheters

The ideal needle for peripheral nerve blocks will be small gauge to avoid tissue trauma, short bevel/non-cutting to avoid injury in the rare event of contact with neural fascicles, insulated when in combination with nerve stimulator devices, and one could consider using echogenic ones to optimize visualization under ultrasound. The majority of upper extremity nerve blocks can be accomplished with 22-gauge × 2-in. needles as the brachial plexus is superficial when compared to other nerves of interest. Lower extremity and truncal nerve blocks can be completed with 20 gauge or 21-gauge × 4-in. needles in the majority of cases, with patient body habitus occasionally requiring a 6-in. needle. If a catheter is to be placed, an 18-gauge × 4-in. short bevel needle with depth markings can be utilized to both administer the original bolus medication and thread the 20-gauge polyamide catheter (ideally poly-orifices) through when in the correct anatomic location (Fig. 2). Catheters can then be utilized with infusion pumps to administer a continuous infusion with optional self-administered bolus titrated to patient need for prolonged analgesic effect.

Table 1 Peripheral nerve block medications

Drug name	Concentration	Purpose	Mechanism of action
Ropivacaine	0.2%/0.5%	Local anesthetic	Reversible Na^+ channel binding
Bupivacaine	0.25%/0.5%	Local anesthetic	Reversible Na^+ channel binding
Lidocaine	1%/2%	Topical anesthetic/local anesthetic	Reversible Na^+ channel binding
Epinephrine	0.1 mg/mL	Resuscitation	Alpha and Beta agonist
Intralipid	20%	Local anesthetic systemic toxicity treatment	"Lipid sink" local anesthetic absorbent
Phenylephrine	100 μg/mL	Resuscitation	Alpha 1-adrenergic agonist
Ephedrine	5 mg/mL	Resuscitation	Increased norepinephrine activity at postsynaptic alpha and beta receptors
Glycopyrrolate	0.2 mg/mL	Resuscitation	Muscarinic anticholinergic
Propofol	10 mg/mL	Induction agent	Decreased GABA-receptor disassociation
Succinylcholine	20 mg/mL	Paralytic	Depolarizing neuromuscular blockade

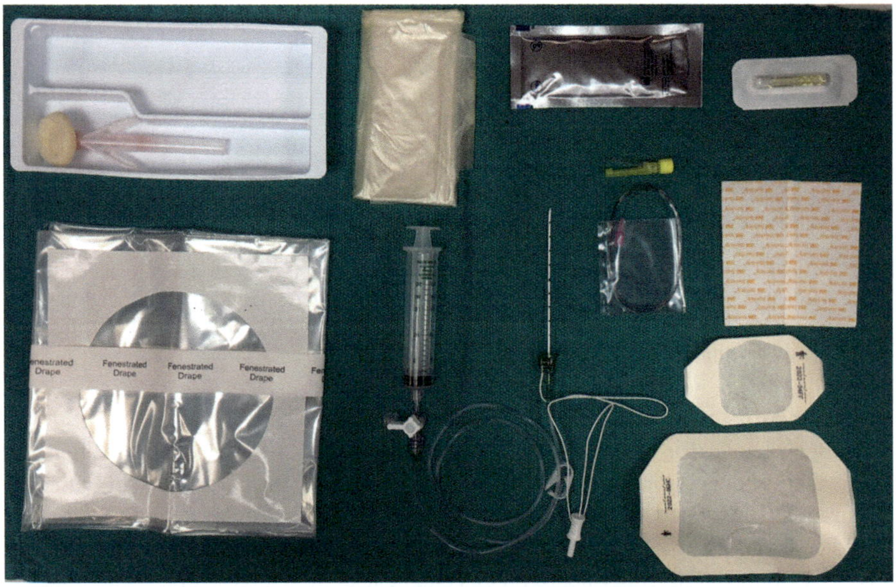

Fig. 2 Sample perineural catheter set up. Items from upper left hand corner, clockwise: (1) Chlorhexidine stick (2) Ultrasound sleeve (3) Ultrasound gel (4) Liquid Adhesive (5) Adhesive bandages (6) Perineural catheter and clasp connector (7) Small transparent medical dressing (8) Large transparent medical dressing (9) 18-gauge Tuohy needle with extension, stopcock, and syringe (10) Fenestrated drape

Local Anesthetics

Local anesthetics disrupt the action potentials coursing along nerve fibers by targeting voltage-gated sodium channels [5]. The degree of nerve blockade is secondary to local anesthetic concentration, potency, and volume, clinically expressing itself differentially, first with temperature distinction, proprioception, then sharp pain, light touch, and motor blockade [5]. A variety of local anesthetics such as 1–2% lidocaine, 0.2–0.75% Ropivacaine, 0.25–0.5% bupivacaine can be used for diagnostic, treatment or surgical anesthesia purposes. Bupivacaine and Ropivacaine are two commonly used local anesthetics for their prolonged and consistent duration of action and efficacy. Common adjuvants such as glucocorticoids have been used with success to augment block effects and prolong analgesic duration.

Local Anesthetic Systemic Toxicity

Local Anesthetic Systemic Toxicity is a most feared complication for which any clinician performing regional anesthesiology should be educated on its clinical presentation and treatment modalities. LAST may cause neurologic and cardiovascular compromise, and can even prove to be fatal [6]. Patients risk factors include extreme age, disease burden, hypoalbuminemia, and impaired cardiac, renal, or hepatic function [6]. Risk factors which are independent of the patient include local anesthetic type, potency, volume, dosage, and location of injection and the systemic absorption from that site [6]. Seizures are the most common symptoms in cases of LAST, with prodromal symptoms such as lightheadedness, dizziness, and auditory or visual disturbances, tinnitus, and perioral numbness have been described [6]. Treatment entails management of the airway including hyperventilation with 100% FiO_2. Convulsions should be abolished with benzodiazepam medications such as diazepam or midazolam. Mainstay of therapy is 20% Intralipids emulsion, dosing is 1.5 mL/kg over 2–3 min (100 mL in patients >70 kg) and then a continuous infusion of 0.25 mL/kg/min (200–250 mL over 20 min in patients >70 kg) [6]. In setting of CPR or ACLS initiation, consideration should be made for cardiopulmonary bypass for the patient who is refractory to ACLS [6].

Upper Extremity Nerve Blocks

Upper extremity nerve blocks can be best organized based on operative site and the nomenclature of each nerve block is based on the anatomic location of the nerve block to be performed. Based on the location of the nerve block, the brachial plexus (C4/5-T1/2) can be blocked at its roots, trunks, divisions, cords, or terminal branches to provide coverage for the specific anatomic area of interest for each specific procedure [7].

Interscalene Block

The Interscalene peripheral nerve block is performed at the level of the roots/trunks of the brachial plexus and provides primarily C5 to C7 blockade with occasional involvement of C3 or C4 [8]. Thus, the Interscalene block provides excellent coverage of the proximal upper extremity, particularly the shoulder [8]. If the distal extremity needs to be covered, the Interscalene block is not suitable for coverage due to its sparing of the Ulnar nerve [7]. Additionally, caution should be used in patients with significant pulmonary compromise due to temporary phrenic nerve involvement which can cause ipsilateral diaphragmatic paresis and decrease lung function by as much as 25% [8, 9]. An appropriate dose for an effective surgical or analgesic block will be around 15–30 mL of choice local anesthetics [8].

Supraclavicular Nerve Block

As we work our way distally along the brachial plexus, the next commonly used upper extremity peripheral nerve block is the supraclavicular block. This is performed at the level of the trunks/divisions of the brachial plexus and can provide reliable coverage of the upper extremity distal to the mid upper arm [8]. In fact, evidence suggests that high supraclavicular nerve blocks/superior trunk brachial plexus block [10] are associated with less incidence of dyspnea, Horner's syndrome, or hoarseness and no greater need for rescue analgesia when compared to the classic interscalene block for shoulder surgery [10, 11]. 20–30 mL of choice local anesthetics of different concentrations can be used to achieve anesthesia or analgesia respectively [8].

Infraclavicular Nerve Block

The infraclavicular peripheral nerve block is where the lateral, medial, and posterior cords can be found along the axillary artery [7]. Similarly as supraclavicular block, infraclavicular nerve block will produce analgesia of the distal upper extremity [7]. There is much less likelihood of phrenic nerve involvement in comparison with the interscalene or supraclavicular nerve block and so this may be a suitable alternative for a patient with compromised lung function [7, 8]. 20–40 mL of choice local anesthetics will provide appropriate surgical anesthesia or analgesia [8]. If necessary for post-operative analgesia, interscalene, supraclavicular or infraclavicular catheters can also be placed for prolonged analgesic coverage [12].

Axillary Nerve Block

Continuing to traverse down the upper extremity at the location of the terminal branches of the brachial plexus, an axillary peripheral nerve block can be performed for analgesia of the hand, wrist, and forearm [7, 8]. Care must be taken to additionally block the musculocutaneous nerve, which may lie in a separate fascial plane from the terminal branch median, ulnar, and radial nerves found clockwise around the axillary artery in order to ensure coverage of the lateral forearm [8]. Due to the distal location, it is highly unlikely to develop phrenic nerve involvement or pneumothorax during the axillary nerve block, however, risk of arterial puncture, hematoma, and inadvertent local anesthetic systemic toxicity must be considered when performing this peripheral nerve block [7].

Lower Extremity Nerve Blocks

Lower extremity nerve blocks, similarly to the upper extremity nerve blocks, can be organized proximally to distally along the extremity depending on the area of need for local anesthetic effect and expectant results of the nerve block being performed at particular sites. Similarly, the lower extremity can also be simplified by dividing it into its origins of the lumbar plexus, which gives rise to the femoral nerve, and sacral plexus, which gives rise to the sciatic nerve, respectively. Some of the more common lower extremity blocks will be further detailed below.

Femoral Nerve Block

The femoral nerve is the largest branch of the lumbar plexus composed of L2, L3, and L4 nerve roots [13]. The femoral nerve supplies sensation to the anterior medial thigh as well as the medial lower leg which is supplied by the saphenous nerve branch of the femoral nerve. Femoral nerve block will have motor blockade of the anterior thigh, including the vastus medialis, vastus lateralis, vastus intermedius, as well as the sartorius muscle and the rectus femoris leading to quadriceps weakness [8]. The femoral nerve block can be used acutely for analgesia for patients suffering from femoral neck or shaft fractures, for surgery of the knee, distal thigh or medial leg and foot [8, 13]. A catheter can be placed at the femoral nerve block for prolonged duration of analgesic coverage. Depending on the clinical situation, the femoral nerve block can be combined with a sciatic nerve block, an obturator nerve block, or a lateral femoral cutaneous nerve block for complete analgesia in the clinical setting which may arise [13]. When performing the femoral nerve block, care must be made to avoid femoral artery puncture due to the proximity of the nerve, at the inguinal crease underneath the fascia lata and fascia iliaca, 1–2 cm lateral to the femoral artery. Likewise, consideration for the expectant quadriceps motor weakness and its implications must be addressed when considering the femoral nerve block [8].

Adductor Canal Block

Continuing distally along the anterior thigh, the adductor canal is an anatomic compartment whose borders are composed of the vastus medialis muscle laterally, the adductor magnus muscle posteriorly, and the sartorius muscle medially [8]. An adductor canal block is an effective means of providing similar sensory nerve block via the largest sensory branch of the femoral nerve, the saphenous nerve, while maintaining greater motor function and quadriceps strength [14]. While the adductor canal block does have motor effect on the vastus medialis muscle, its overall effect on post procedure mobility is diminished in comparison to the femoral nerve block [14]. In fact, moving to the mid distal thigh will further isolate the saphenous nerve and decrease motor effect even further while maintaining similar sensory efficacy along the distal medial thigh, knee, and leg [8]. Like, the femoral nerve block, a continuous catheter can be placed in the adductor canal for prolonged analgesic effect.

Popliteal Sciatic Nerve Block

The sciatic nerve is the largest branch of the sacral plexus composed of L4-S3 nerve roots. While the saphenous branch of the femoral nerve provides cutaneous innervation to the medial ankle and foot, the sciatic nerve and its branches provide sensory and motor components to the rest of the foot and leg distal to the knee [5]. As the sciatic nerve approaches the popliteal fossa of the posterior knee, the sciatic nerve separates into the tibial nerve medially and the common peroneal nerve laterally [5]. While the sciatic nerve can be blocked by the gluteal, subgluteal, or popliteal fossa approaches, due to its more superficial location and easily identifiable popliteal artery as identified under ultrasound, the popliteal approach to the sciatic nerve block is utilized for any surgical procedure from the knee distally, enhanced by the addition of the corresponding saphenous nerve block for complete analgesic coverage [8]. A catheter can be placed in the sciatic nerve block via popliteal approach for distal lower extremity analgesia, combined with an adductor canal or femoral nerve block anteriorly.

Truncal Nerve Blocks

Truncal nerve blocks can be utilized for a variety of perioperative, acute traumatic indications and non-surgical pain management. There is wide variety of techniques and clinical application continues to be studied and modified, but the more popular clinical techniques will be briefly described.

Paravertebral Nerve Block

Thoracic paravertebral nerve blocks provide analgesia along a consistent dermatomal distribution [8]. This can be utilized for a variety of surgical procedures involving the chest and abdomen in addition to as a bedside intervention for painful conditions such as rib fractures, chest tube placement [15]. Rib fracture pain, in particular, has shown recovery to be dependent on amount of internal injuries, but also, how well pain is controlled due to the fact that inadequate pain management can lead to respiratory compromise including splinting, poor respiratory toilet, and shallow breathing leading to pneumonia which can lead to increased ventilatory requirements and even death [16]. This is in addition to the respiratory depressant effects of opioids used for acute rib fracture pain. Paravertebral nerve blocks and catheters have been shown to decrease opiate requirements and improve ventilatory status and mobility in the patients most at risk for respiratory compromise, namely, the elderly patient with more than three rib fractures [16].

The paravertebral space is a triangle immediately lateral to the spine who's borders include the superior costotransverse ligament posteriorly, the parietal pleura anterolaterally, and the vertebra, vertebral disks, and the intervertebral foramina medially [8, 16]. Paravertebral nerve blocks can be single bolus doses in the perioperative setting but clinically more commonly catheters are placed for prolonged analgesia. According to the American Society for Regional Anesthesia coagulation guidelines, Paravertebral catheters should be treated similarly to neuraxial guidelines for respective anticoagulation medications and must be considered in their implementation clinically.

Erector Spinae Block

The erector spinae block is an interfascial plane block which deposits local anesthetic below the erector spinae fascia [8]. This block was first described in 2016 and since that time has clinically been applied to assist with pain following ventral hernia repair, thoracic surgery, breast surgery, rib fractures, chronic shoulder pain, back surgery and post thoracotomy pain syndrome [17]. Despite its broad clinical efficacy, there is controversy when comparing cadaveric studies in regards to spread of the local anesthetic along the dorsal and ventral rami in the paravertebral space or if an alternative mechanism of local anesthetic spread involved the dorsal rami and lateral cutaneous branches of the intercostal nerves given the pronounced lateral distribution of local anesthetic spread [17, 18]. A benefit to performing the erector spinae block at bedside in comparison to the paravertebral block, whose injectate spread is three-fifths caudad and two-fifths cephalad, is due to the significant cranial spread of local anesthetic, catheters can be placed remotely from surgical fields or dressing and still provide clinical coverage to the distal cephalad affected areas [8, 19].

Transverse Abdominal Plane Block

The Transverse Abdominal Plane Block successfully covers the ventral rami of spinal nerves T6-L1 along the lateral abdominal wall providing analgesia to the anterolateral abdominal wall [15]. Local anesthetic can be successfully deposited under direct visualization in the fascial plane below the external and internal oblique muscles of the abdominal wall and above the transversus abdominus muscle plane [15]. This is a useful block for patients with incisional site pain along the abdominal wall as well as following cesarean delivery for prolonged pain relief of the abdominal incision. 15–20 mL of local anesthetic per side will appropriately expand the potential space between the muscle layers and appropriately cover the intended area [8]. Care must be made to avoid peritoneal injury which can be a potential complication of this procedure [8].

Rectus Sheath Blocks

As the nerve roots of T6-L1 advance medially, the nerve roots lie between the rectus abdominus muscle and the posterior rectus sheath, continuing to enter the rectus muscle close to midline [15]. For midline incisions, the rectus sheath block can be performed by depositing local anesthetic in this potential space for effective analgesia in doses of 10–20 mL per side.

3 Conclusion

Peripheral nerve blocks and catheters are a safe and effective means of providing patients with localized anesthesia and/or analgesia for surgical procedures and pain management. Regional anesthesia has the benefit of anatomic specificity and diminished systemic opiate dosing. This has proven to provide the patient with fewer side effects of opiates including nausea, vomiting, delayed return of bowel function, improved acute pain control and decreased hospital length of stay as well decreased development of chronic pain [1, 2]. Ultrasound adoption has increased the block success rate, sped up performance, and improved safety profile. Peripheral nerve blocks performed under ultrasound guidance are safe and effective in bedside pain management interventions to aid with the pain control of the hospitalized patient and patients in the clinic. Bedside nerve block should be performed with proper monitors and resuscitation supplies readily available and with proper documentation including image storage.

References

1. Fredrickson MJ, Krishnan S, Chen CY. Postoperative analgesia for shoulder surgery: a critical appraisal and review of current techniques. Anaesthesia. 2010;65(6):608–24.
2. Lenart MJ, Wong K, Gupta RK, Mercaldo ND, Schildcrout JS, Michaels D, et al. The impact of peripheral nerve techniques on hospital stay following major orthopedic surgery. Pain Med. 2012;13(6):828–34.
3. Hadzic A. Hadzic's textbook of regional anesthesia and acute pain management. 2nd ed. New York: McGraw-Hill Education LLC; 2017. https://accessanesthesiology.mhmedical.com/book.aspx?bookid=2070.
4. Equipment for regional anesthesia. https://www.nysora.com/foundations-of-regional-anesthesia/equipment/equipment-regional-anesthesia/.
5. Barash PG. Clinical anesthesia. 6th ed. Philadelphia: Wolters Kluwer/Lippincott Williams & Wilkins; 2009. xviii, 1640 p.
6. Gitman M, Fettiplace MR, Weinberg G, Neal JM, Barrington MJ. Local anesthetic systemic toxicity: a narrative literature review and clinical update on prevention, diagnosis and management. Plast Reconstr Surg. 2019;144(3):783–95.
7. Mian A, Chaudhry I, Huang R, Rizk E, Tubbs RS, Loukas M. Brachial plexus anesthesia: a review of the relevant anatomy, complications, and anatomical variations. Clin Anat. 2014;27(2):210–21.
8. Ardon AE, Prasad A, McClain RL, Melton MS, Nielsen KC, Greengrass R. Regional anesthesia for ambulatory anesthesiologists. Anesthesiol Clin. 2019;37(2):265–87.
9. Urmey WF, McDonald M. Hemidiaphragmatic paresis during interscalene brachial plexus block: effects on pulmonary function and chest wall mechanics. Anesth Analg. 1992;74(3):352–7.
10. Kang R, Jeong JS, Chin KJ, Yoo JC, Lee JH, Choi SJ, et al. Superior trunk block provides non-inferior analgesia compared with interscalene brachial plexus block in arthroscopic shoulder surgery. Anesthesiology. 2019;131(6):1316–26.
11. Guo CW, Ma JX, Ma XL, Lu B, Wang Y, Tian AX, et al. Supraclavicular block versus interscalene brachial plexus block for shoulder surgery: a meta-analysis of clinical control trials. Int J Surg. 2017;45:85–91.
12. Ahsan ZS, Carvalho B, Yao J. Incidence of failure of continuous peripheral nerve catheters for postoperative analgesia in upper extremity surgery. J Hand Surg Am. 2014;39(2):324–9.

13. Kasibhatla RD, Russon K. Femoral nerve blocks. J Perioper Pract. 2009;19(2):65–9.
14. Gao F, Ma J, Sun W, Guo W, Li Z, Wang W. Adductor canal block versus femoral nerve block for analgesia after total knee arthroplasty: a systematic review and meta-analysis. Clin J Pain. 2017;33(4):356–68.
15. Abrahams MS, Horn JL, Noles LM, Aziz MF. Evidence-based medicine: ultrasound guidance for truncal blocks. Reg Anesth Pain Med. 2010;35(2 Suppl):S36–42.
16. Ho AM, Ho AK, Mizubuti GB, Klar G, Karmakar MK. Regional analgesia for patients with traumatic rib fractures—a narrative review. J Trauma Acute Care Surg. 2020;88(1):e22–30.
17. Ivanusic J, Konishi Y, Barrington MJ. A cadaveric study investigating the mechanism of action of erector spinae blockade. Reg Anesth Pain Med. 2018;43(6):567–71.
18. Adhikary SD, Bernard S, Lopez H, Chin KJ. Erector spinae plane block versus retrolaminar block: a magnetic resonance imaging and anatomical study. Reg Anesth Pain Med. 2018;43(7):756–62.
19. Melvin JP, Schrot RJ, Chu GM, Chin KJ. Low thoracic erector spinae plane block for perioperative analgesia in lumbosacral spine surgery: a case series. Can J Anaesth. 2018;65(9):1057–65.

Further Reading

Capek A, Dolan J. Ultrasound-guided peripheral nerve blocks of the upper limb. BJA Educ. 2015;15(3):160–5.

Salinas FV. Evidence basis for ultrasound guidance for lower-extremity peripheral nerve block: update 2016. Reg Anesth Pain Med. 2016;41:261–74.

Manual Medicine Interventions for Bedside Pain Management

Emily Hillaker, Jacob Boomgaardt, Joseph Amalfitano, and Michael Lockwood

Essential Concepts

- There are two overarching methods for osteopathic treatment of dysfunctional regions or body parts. Those techniques that engage biomechanical restrictive barriers are termed Direct Methods and those where the dysfunctional tissues are moved from a point of increased tissue tensions to a point of equalized tensions on all planes and directions are grouped as Indirect Methods. In the acute phase of illness or injury, the indirect approach is generally preferred and reduces the inflammatory process, edema, and favorably alters nociception as a source of pain. The direct techniques, including articulatory, muscle energy, and direct thrust techniques, may be needed for restoration of range of motion and joint function. Modalities such as myofascial release, muscle energy, counter-strain, inhibitory pressure, and articulatory technique are common, relatively easy and quick to perform at bedside, and can be beneficial treatments or adjuvants to pain management for patients.
- Myofascial release (MFR) is a technique that employs continual palpatory feedback to achieve release of myofascial tissues. The technique uses either direct or indirect gentle, sustained pressure into the connective tissue matrix to relieve tension, ease pain, and restore motion and function while improving blood and lymphatic circulation (Fig. 4).

E. Hillaker · J. Boomgaardt · J. Amalfitano (✉)
Department of Physical Medicine and Rehabilitation, University of Virginia, Charlottesville, VA, USA
e-mail: eh9hx@hscmail.mcc.virginia.edu; jab5cq@hscmail.mcc.virginia.edu; ja4ay@virginia.edu

M. Lockwood
Department of Osteopathic Manipulative Medicine, Liberty University College of Osteopathic Medicine, Lynchburg, VA, USA

D. Souza et al. (eds.), *Bedside Pain Management Interventions*,
https://doi.org/10.1007/978-3-031-11188-4_7

- Counter-strain is an indirect, passive technique that inhibits aberrant neuromuscular reflexes by putting the targeted tissue in a position of maximal ease. In other words, a painful muscle in spasm is placed in its shortest position by approximating the origin and insertion in order to inhibit firing of the neuromuscular reflex. The method is described in Fig. 2.
- Paraspinal inhibition decreases sympathetic output from the sympathetic chain ganglia that causes muscle hypertonicity induced by viscerosomatic reflex pathways. The technique utilizes the application a gentle consistent pressure to paraspinal muscles (Fig. 3).
- Articulatory technique uses a low velocity, high amplitude force to carry a restricted joint through its full ROM in order to restore normal joint function (Fig. 5).

1 Overview

The diagnostic approach to neuromusculoskeletal dysfunction can be complex, however for simple techniques, the diagnosis of dysfunction can be made by examining a patient to identify any of the four criteria for somatic dysfunction [1]: Tissue texture abnormalities, Asymmetry of position, Restricted motion, and Tenderness (TART). By understanding normal physiologic motion of that structure and recognizing dysfunction utilizing the TART criteria, you can use several modalities to attempt to gently restore normal ROM or decrease painful abnormal neuromuscular reflexes. Taking the painful structure or its fascia through passive ROM can help determine the pathologic barrier in three planes of motion. The techniques selected for this chapter can be safely and effectively utilized in many aspects of patient care. For more complex or refractory cases, however, the patient may need referral to an osteopathic physician having the appropriate skill set or Board Certified in Osteopathic Neuromuscular Medicine. For proper documentation, osteopathic treatments are considered as procedures and CPT codes for medical record keeping are discussed.

2 Historical Aspects and Introduction to Osteopathic Manipulative Treatment

Manual medicine has been a modality of treatment for millennia, dating back to ancient Egypt [2]. There is documentation that supports Hippocrates used manual techniques for the spine as well [3]. Since then, there have been many practitioners of manual medicine. In the nineteenth century, Dr. Andrew Taylor Still and Daniel David Palmer were primary contributors to the growth of manual medicine in the United States. Palmer founded the chiropractic approach and Dr. Still founded osteopathic medicine.

Andrew Taylor Still formed the first School of Osteopathy in 1892 and since that time, the profession has grown exponentially [4]. His philosophical approach to the art and science of medicine was founded on four basic tenants. The first is that the human body is a functional unit. Second, the human body has self-regulatory mechanisms and an innate ability to heal itself. Third, structure and function are interrelated. And finally, the use of osteopathic manipulative treatment (OMT) is based upon the application of the previous tenants [5–7]. Therefore, OMT is a facet of medicine that emphasizes the interrelated function and structure of each body system and uses that knowledge to facilitate healing.

OMT uses hands-on techniques to address structural components of pain including, bones and their articulations, muscles fascia, ligaments, dura, fluids, viscera, and neural circuitry. It is used to diagnose, treat, and remove barriers to healing from illness or injury with emphasis on the lymphatic and neuromusculoskeletal systems. OMT has been shown to improve healing and decrease morbidity in conditions such as pneumonia, otitis media, post-op ileus, headache, cervical/thoracic/lumbar pain, pelvic pain, carpal tunnel syndrome, dysmenorrhea, and fibromyalgia, and in other clinical scenarios [8]. For the purpose of this chapter, we will discuss techniques that focus on the neuromusculoskeletal system and how they can be utilized to reduce pain and enhance function.

Somatic dysfunction, defined as impaired function of the neuromusculoskeletal system, is a pathological or restricted range of motion due to mechanical causes, tissue damage, or disease. OMT can be used alone or in conjunction with other modalities to relieve or resolve somatic dysfunction, and in some cases, reduce the need for medications or surgery.

Clinical studies have shown OMT to be an effective complement with, or alternative to, medication or other therapies in a variety of clinical scenarios including postoperative pain, neck and low back pain, headaches, and musculoskeletal injuries [9–11]. Patients reported decreased pain, need for pain medications, anxiety, an increased overall comfort level after receiving OMT treatment and decreased length of hospital stays [12, 13]. Not only are these treatments beneficial for patients, but many of these techniques take very little time to perform and results are often apparent immediately or shortly after treatment, resulting in enhanced physician career satisfaction.

Treatment of acute and chronic pain has grown in complexity. Treatment options for patients may range from OMT, to medication management, to interventional procedures under fluoroscopy and surgery. Admittedly, there is not a single treatment option that fits best for all patients; therefore, a comprehensive approach is often required in acute or chronic pain management. This chapter serves as an introduction to pain management using OMT, which at times is *the* treatment of choice. We present simple techniques in an ever-evolving complex world of pain management that can help relieve pain and optimize overall function and well-being. Traditionally these techniques have been taught in licensed osteopathic medical schools across the country. In the recent decades, more allopathic physicians, manual physical therapists, and other providers have also adapted these techniques in their practice of medicine. There are several accredited continuing medical education courses offered that lead to certification, although this certification does not apply to licensure or board certification. We encourage the reader, however, to further investigate educational opportunities to enhance their physical assessment and manual medicine techniques.

3 Osteopathic Manipulative Treatment for the Head and Neck, Low Back, Hip and Sacrum

Headaches are one of the most common causes of pain complaints in general practice clinics. Socioeconomic costs of treatment and work time lost are estimated at $14 billion per year in the US [14]. This frames the importance of cost-effective prevention and treatment. Somatic dysfunction in the cervical spine and supporting musculature can lead to various cervicogenic, migraine, and tension type headaches [15]. Studies have shown that OMT is an effective treatment for headache and can be utilized for both abortive and preventative therapy [16, 17].

In the acute phase of a headache, active or passive manipulation of the head may aggravate the symptoms, which is why inhibitory pressure or indirect techniques are generally preferred [18]. For example, sub-occipital release is a soft tissue technique used for reducing tissue tension in the suboccipital musculature. It can also help to regulate autonomic nervous system activity via effects on the vagus nerve (Fig. 1).

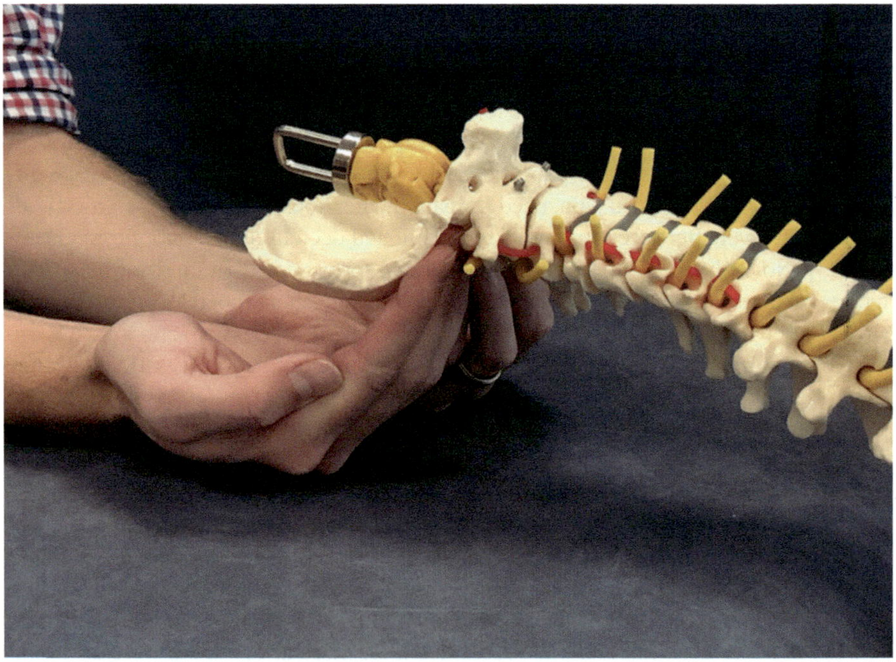

Fig. 1 Suboccipital Release. (1) With patient supine, place your fingertips just caudally to occiput. (2) Cradle the head by gently placing pressure through only the fingertips, lifting the head and neck. (3) Hold pressure until tissue starts to release and soften, at least 30 s to 1 min. As the tissue relaxes, the head will release back and rest on the practitioner's palms

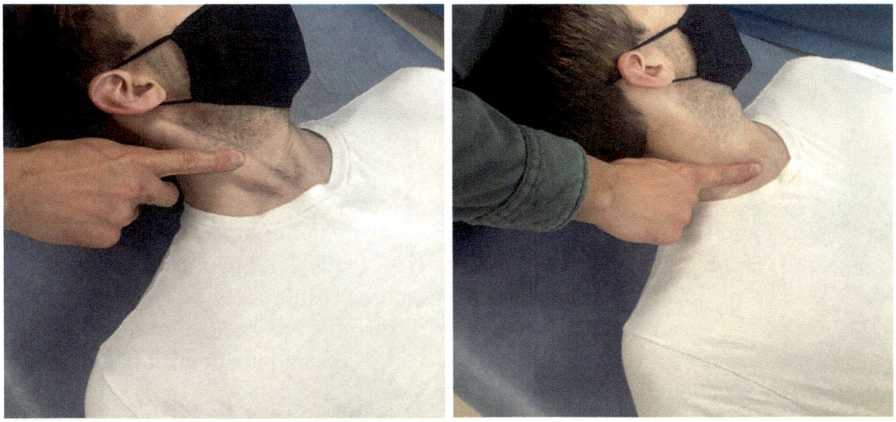

Fig. 2 Counter strain, demonstrated on the sternocleidomastoid muscle. (1) Palpate the muscle to find the point of most pain and determine the level of pain (scale 1–10). (2) Attempt to approximate the origin and insertion of the muscle to shorten it while your finger remains over the tender point. With the SCM, this involves head flexion, ipsilateral side-bending and contralateral rotation. (3) Determine level of pain with the muscle shortened and adjust movements until there is a significant reduction in pain. (4) Hold this position for at least 90 s before returning to neutral, and then reassess for pain

Neck pain, similar to headache, is a common condition and is often very disabling and functionally limiting to the patient. OMT can be an effective treatment in the management of acute or chronic neck pain [19, 20]. Although aggressive neck manipulation could be harmful in a small subset of patients, as detailed further below in the complications section, the techniques described here are safe and can be easily used to treat patients in clinic or at the bedside presenting with neck pain or headaches.

Counter-strain, as described earlier, can be utilized for the deep and superficial musculature of the head and neck. Figure 2 demonstrates counter strain technique for the sternocleidomastoid muscle. This technique can also be used for common neck pain generators such as splenius capitus, scalenes, upper trapezius, levator scapulae, and deeper muscles. Figure 3 demonstrates paraspinal inhibitory pressure to relieve hyperactive sympathetic facilitation. The technique can be applied to the cervical, thoracic, and lumbar paraspinal muscles.

Myofascial release is another gentle technique depicted in Fig. 4 and described earlier in this chapter, which can be used for restrictions of the paraspinal musculature or on tissues that are more lateral to the spine, unlike inhibitory pressure, which can be painful over the ribs if applied too laterally. Figure 5 demonstrates the use of an articulatory technique for the sacroiliac joints.

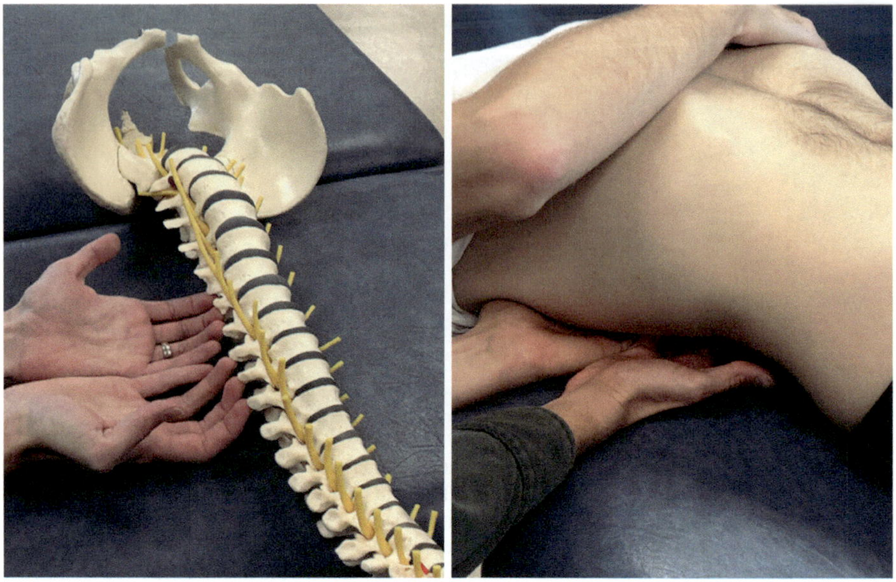

Fig. 3 Paraspinal Inhibitory Pressure. (1) With the patient supine, place your fingertips just medial to the paraspinal musculature. (2) Apply anterolateral traction. This can be either a series of tractions or a single long traction. (3) Perform this technique for about 3–5 min, or until relaxation of the muscle is felt. For provider comfort, it is recommended that you use your forearms as a fum fulcrum to apply the sustained pressure and traction. This technique can be used along the entire spine

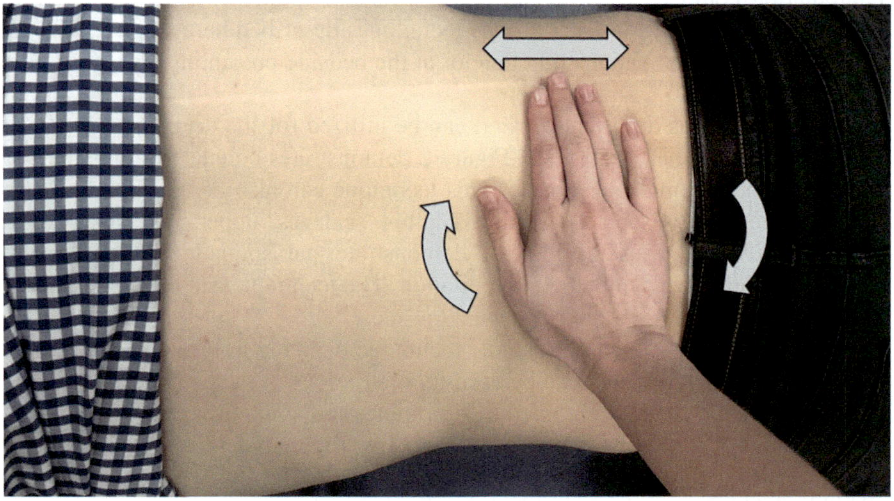

Fig. 4 Direct myofascial release. (1) With very gentle pressure, place your hands over the area of pain. (2) Determine the tissue restrictions with flexion and extension (up and down), side-bending (side to side) and rotation (twisting). (3) Once the restriction is noted in the three planes of motion, carry the tissue directly into each barrier simultaneously. (4) Hold this position until you feel a relaxation of the tissues, then slowly return to neutral

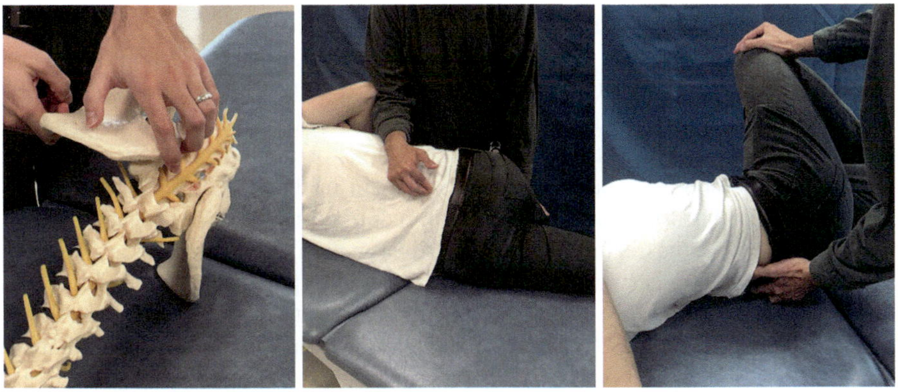

Fig. 5 Sacral Articulatory. (1) Place the patient on their side with the painful SI joint facing up. (2) Place one hand on the sacrum and grasp the top leg just below the knee, flex the knee and hip while palpating for motion at the SI joint. (3) Abduct the thigh until you reach the restrictive barrier. (4) Have the patient to take in a deep breath in and hold it. The practitioner then carries the hip through extension while maintaining hip abduction. This may produce an audible or palpable articulation

4 Potential Complications

OMT is considered a safe, non-invasive treatment modality, with severe side effects being exceedingly rare. Because of its safety profile, OMT can be particularly useful in those who are more prone to medication side effects such as the elderly or those with polypharmacy [21]. A recent study of 884 patients receiving OMT documented a rate of adverse events at 2.5%, the majority of which were increased pain or discomfort at the site of treatment with no serious adverse events recorded and, in most cases, these symptoms resolved within 7 days of treatment. Temporary adverse effects were low but more common with direct techniques such as high-velocity-low-amplitude (HVLA) which uses a thrusting motion to articulate a joint. Adverse events with gentle techniques such as myofascial release were less common [22, 23]. The most feared complications with OMT is vertebral artery dissection leading to stroke. In particular, high velocity thrusts of the cervical spine especially with rotation movement, seemed to be associated with severe adverse events. While serious adverse effects are rare, HVLA to the cervical spine should only be performed by experienced practitioners in carefully selected patients.

There are very few absolute contraindications to OMT. Absolute contraindications include spinal cord compression, unstable fracture, joint or ligamentous instability, or open wounds. Lymphatic techniques are contraindicated in necrotizing fasciitis and certain kinds of infection or cancer due to the risk of seeding infection or neoplastic cells by mobilizing lymph fluid. Also consider condition-specific risk factors such as atlantoaxial instability in rheumatoid arthritis or Down Syndrome, or in vertebral artery insufficiency or dissection, where forceful cervical manipulation should be avoided.

5 Documentation of Osteopathic Treatment

Proper documentation for OMT is straightforward and simple. There needs to be objective evidence of somatic dysfunction. Use the TART acronym as a guide. Record asymmetry of position, motion restrictions or motion preferences, altered tissue textures, and associated tenderness or pain in the Objective portion of the medical record. For the Assessment section, record typical E & M diagnoses. Then include the body areas exhibiting somatic dysfunction and are coded as M99.00-head region, M99.01-cervical spine, M99.02-thoracic spine, M99.03-lumbar spine, M99.04 sacrum, M99.05 pelvis, M99.06-lower extremity, M99.07-upper extremity, M99.08-rib cage, and M99.09 abdomen and other regions. For the Plan, list that the patient consented to osteopathic treatment, common possible side effects and likely outcomes were discussed, and include post treatment instructions such as increasing fluids, avoiding strenuous activities for 24 h and follow-up. Since a separate service was provided by the same physician on the same day add a −25 modifier. If a Resident performed all or part of the supervised procedure, also add a -PC modifier. Then bill according to number of body regions treated (not complexity of techniques or patient problems) using codes 98925 for treatment of 1–2 areas, 98926 for 3–4, 98927 for 5–6, 98928 for 8, and 98929 for 9–10 body areas. Record objective results such as increased range of motion, reduction in tissue hypertonicity, and subjective reduction in pain and improvement in mood and affect. Favorable patient responses, which are common and often spontaneous, reflect heightened patient satisfaction and afford the physician with enhanced job satisfaction.

6 Conclusion and Future Directions

Osteopathic manipulative treatment remains a safe, efficient, and cost-effective treatment for patients with acute and chronic pain, with its clinical utility and practicality spanning across specialties and in a wide variety of clinical settings [24, 25]. This chapter provides a simple introduction to OMT and demonstrates a small number of techniques that could be readily employed by a pain management physician with proper training.

References

1. Somatic and segmental dysfunction is the necessary and sufficient diagnosis [ICD 10 code M99.xx] which allows for the provision of Osteopathic Manipulative Treatment [CPT codes 98921-29]. Somatic dysfunction is defined as the impaired or altered function of related components of the somatic (bodywork) system, including: the skeletal, arthrodial, and myofascial structures, and their related vascular, lymphatic, and neural elements.
2. DeStefano LA. Principles of manual medicine. 5th ed. Philadelphia: Lippincott Williams & Wilkins; 2017. p. 2–11.

3. Fraix MP, Wieting M, Lipton JA. Osteopathic considerations in physical medicine and rehabilitation. In: Seffinger MA, editor. Foundations of osteopathic medicine. 4th ed. Philadelphia: Lippincott Williams & Wilkins; 2018.
4. Jones JM III, Peterson BP. History of osteopathic profession. In: Seffinger MA, editor. Foundations of osteopathic medicine. 4th ed. Philadelphia: Lippincott Williams & Wilkins; 2018. p. 19–43.
5. Seffinger MA, Hollins HK, Ward RC, Jones JM III, Rogers FJ, Patterson MM. Osteopathic philosophy. In: Ward RC, editor. Foundations of osteopathic medicine. 2nd ed. Philadelphia: Lippincott Williams & Wilkins; 2003. p. 3–18.
6. Seffinger MA, Hruby RJ, Hollins HK, Willard FH, LIcciardone J, Jones JM III, King HH. Philosophy of osteopathic medicine. In: Seffinger MA, editor. Foundations of osteopathic medicine. 4th ed. Philadelphia: Lippincott Williams & Wilkins; 2018. p. 2–18.
7. Jones BE. The difference a D.O makes. Millenium. 2nd ed. Oklahoma City: Oklahoma educational foundation; 2001. p. 1–16.
8. Papa L, Mandara A, Bottali M, Gulisano V, Orfei S. A randomized control trial on the effectiveness of osteopathic manipulative treatment in reducing pain and improving the quality of life in elderly patients affected by osteoporosis. Clin Cases Miner Bone Metab. 2012;9(3):179–83.
9. Tick H, Nielsen A, Pelletier KR, et al. Evidence-based nonpharmacologic strategies for comprehensive pain care: the Consortium Pain Task Force white paper. Explore (NY). 2018;14(3):177–211. https://doi.org/10.1016/j.explore.2018.02.001.
10. Assendelft WJ, Bouter LM, Knipschild PG. Complications of spinal manipulation: a comprehensive review of the literature. J Fam Pract. 1996;42(5):475–80.
11. Gross A, Langevin P, Burnie SJ, et al. Manipulation and mobilisation for neck pain contrasted against an inactive control or another active treatment. Cochrane Database Syst Rev. 2015;(9):CD004249. https://doi.org/10.1002/14651858.CD004249.pub4.
12. Pomykala M, McElhinney B, Beck BL, Carreiro JE. Patient perception of osteopathic manipulative treatment in a hospitalized setting: a survey-based study. J Am Osteopath Assoc. 2008;108(11):665–8.
13. Nicholas AS, Oleski SL. Osteopathic manipulative treatment for postoperative pain. J Am Osteopath Assoc. 2002;102(9 Suppl 3):S5–8.
14. Rizzoli P, Mullally WJ. Headache. Am J Med. 2018;131(1):17–24. https://doi.org/10.1016/j.amjmed.2017.09.005.
15. Kidd RF, Nelson R. Musculoskeletal dysfunction of the neck in migraine and tension headache. Headache. 1993;33(10):566–9. https://doi.org/10.1111/j.1526-4610.1993.hed3310566.x.
16. Smith MS, Olivas J, Smith K. Manipulative therapies: what works. Am Fam Physician. 2019;99(4):248–52.
17. Cerritelli F, Lacorte E, Ruffini N, Vanacore N. Osteopathy for primary headache patients: a systematic review. J Pain Res. 2017;10:601–11. https://doi.org/10.2147/JPR.S130501.
18. Gallagher RM. Headache pain. J Am Osteopath Assoc. 2005;105(9 Suppl 4):S7–11.
19. Giles PD, Hensel KL, Pacchia CF, Smith ML. Suboccipital decompression enhances heart rate variability indices of cardiac control in healthy subjects. J Altern Complement Med. 2013;19(2):92–6. https://doi.org/10.1089/acm.2011.0031.
20. Franke H, Franke J-D, Fryer G. Osteopathic manipulative treatment for nonspecific low back pain: a systematic review and meta-analysis. BMC Musculoskelet Disord. 2014;15:286. https://doi.org/10.1186/1471-2474-15-286.
21. Degenhardt BF, Johnson JC, Brooks WJ, Norman L. Characterizing adverse events reported immediately after osteopathic manipulative treatment. J Am Osteopath Assoc. 2018;118(3):141–9. https://doi.org/10.7556/jaoa.2018.033.
22. Ernst E. Manipulation of the cervical spine: a systematic review of case reports of serious adverse events, 1995–2001. Med J Aust. 2002;176(8):376–80.

23. Assendelft WJJ, Morton SC, Yu EI, Suttorp MJ, Shekelle PG. Spinal manipulative therapy for low back pain. Cochrane Database Syst Rev. 2004;(1):CD000447. https://doi.org/10.1002/14651858.CD000447.pub2.
24. McReynolds TM, Sheridan BJ. Intramuscular ketorolac versus osteopathic manipulative treatment in the management of acute neck pain in the emergency department: a randomized clinical trial. J Am Osteopath Assoc. 2005;105(2):57–68.
25. Verhaeghe N, Schepers J, van Dun P, Annemans L. Osteopathic care for low back pain and neck pain: a cost-utility analysis. Complement Ther Med. 2018;40:207–13. https://doi.org/10.1016/j.ctim.2018.06.001.

Further Reading

Nicholas, Oleski. Osteopathic manipulative treatment for postoperative pain.
Smith et al. Manipulative therapies: what works.

Bedside Electro-Acupuncture

Joseph Walker III

Essential Concepts
- Electro-acupuncture can modulate pain (1) locally, (2) regionally, (3) segmentally, and (4) non-segmentally.
- Low frequency, high-intensity electrical stimulation modulates pain at the level of the spinal cord, midbrain, and pituitary hypothalamus while high-frequency, low-intensity electrical stimulation modulates pain at the level of the spinal cord and midbrain.
- For clinically effective acupuncture analgesia, type 2 afferent muscles fibers need to be stimulated to produce a sensation of numbness.
- Clinical variables to consider while delivering electro-acupuncture are (1) intensity, (2) frequency, (3) waveform, (4) length of treatment, and (5) location of needle input.

1 Overview

Electro-acupuncture was developed in concurrently in China, Russia, Japan, and Korea during the mid-twentieth century and it involves applying an electric current to acupuncture needles for the purpose of strengthening or altering the nature of the

J. Walker III (✉)
Department of Orthopedic Surgery, University of Connecticut School of Medicine, Farmington, CT, USA

UCONN Comprehensive Spine Center, UCONN Health, Farmington, CT, USA

UCONN Musculoskeletal Institute & John Dempsey Hospital, UCONN Health, Farmington, CT, USA
e-mail: jwalker@uchc.edu

D. Souza et al. (eds.), *Bedside Pain Management Interventions*,
https://doi.org/10.1007/978-3-031-11188-4_8

needle stimulation [1]. Electroacupuncture is clinically utilized for numerous reasons including (1) to provide stronger and more continuous stimulation to an area than manual acupuncture can provide, (2) to modulate pain messages to the brain, (3) to initiate and regulate release of endogenous opiates from the central nervous system, and/or (4) to affect local neuro-metabolic and biomechanical processes [2, 3]. Specifically, electro acupuncture is indicated for acute pain, neuralgia, limb and joint pain, soft tissue injuries, and post-surgical pain [4, 5].

2 Background and Mechanism of Action

Much of the contemporary research on electro acupuncture is done in laboratory settings on animals and has focused on the basic science and the mechanisms of action. Although further research needs to be done in human clinical settings and with larger sample sizes, basic science and mechanistic studies have clarified a lot of clinically useful information on the basic science behind electro acupuncture. This information includes (1) the type of nerves that are stimulated, (2) the neurotransmitters secreted as a result, and (3) the effector structures/organs of the nerve stimulation or secreted neurotransmitter.

Table 1 Traditional Chinese Medicine (TCM) acupuncture point correlation with peripheral/cranial nerve location [6, 41–43]

Upper extremity		Lower extremity	
TCM acupuncture point	Nerve	TCM acupuncture point	Nerve
Yu Yao	Supraorbital Nerve	Yao Yan	Cuneal Nerves
Stomach 2	Infraorbital Nerve	Bladder 40	Medial Popliteal Nerve
Triple Warmer 17	Greater Auricular Nerve	Stomach 36	Recurrent Genicular Nerve
Small Intestine 19	Trigeminal-Facial Nerve	Gallbladder 34	Common Fibular Nerve
Governor Vessel 26	Philtrum Point	Spleen 9	Saphenous Nerve
Bladder 10	Greater Occipital Nerve	Bladder 57	Sural Nerve
Gallbladder 20	Lesser Occipital Nerve	Spleen 6	Tibial Nerve
Gallbladder 21	Spinal Accessary Nerve	Bladder 60	Tibial Nerve
Large Intestine 11	Lateral Antebrachial Nerve		
Large Intestine 10	Deep Radial Nerve	Kidney 3	Sural Nerve
Lung 7	Superficial Radial Nerve	Gallbladder 41	Sural Nerve
Triple Warmer 5	Radial Nerve	Liver 3	Deep Fibular Nerve
Pericardium 6	Median Nerve		
Heart 7	Ulnar Nerve	Stomach 9	Vagus Nerve
Small Intestine 3	Ulnar Nerve	Concha of the Ear	Vagus Nerve
Large Intestine 4	Radial/Median/Ulnar Nerve		

Anatomically about 309 acupuncture points are situated on or very close to nerves [6] (Table 1). The types of stimulated nerves are (1) small myelinated fibers (A-delta—sensory), (2) small unmyelinated fibers (C-fibers—pain and temperature), and/or (3) large myelinated fibers (A-beta—motor) [7]. Muscle fibers are also affected by needle and electrical stimulation [8]. For clinically effective acupuncture analgesia, type 2 afferent muscles fibers need to be stimulated to produce a sensation of numbness. Stimulation of type 3 muscle fibers creates a sensation of distension, heaviness, and aching. Simulation of type 4 afferent muscle fibers creates a sensation of soreness. Acupuncture analgesia is blocked by intramuscular injection of procaine but not subcutaneous injection of procaine [9].

In 1965, Ronald Melzack, Ph.D and Patrick D. Wall, Ph.D developed their first iteration Gate Control theory of pain [10]. This theory helps to explain the effect nerve stimulation has on pain sensation propagation within the central nervous system. Electro acupuncture modulates pain control because electrical stimulation of the large myelinated nerve fibers inhibits the pain information transmission from the small myelinated/unmyelinated nerve fibers at the spinal cord level particularly at the substantia gelatinosa (Fig. 1).

Over the next 30 years later, the Gate Control theory of pain was refined and clarified by Melzack and Wall [11–13]. In the later iterations, the same process of pain modulation occurred: stimulation of the large myelinated fibers inhibis pain information transmission from the smaller myelinated/unmyelinated nerve fibers. In this iteration, however, the inhibitory effect does not happen directly at the substantia gelatinosa but rather through (1) inhibitory transmitting cells and (2) at the cortical level (thalamus, cerebrum) via a descending inhibitory control (Fig. 2).

As described by Dr. Bruce Pomeranz, Ph.D, electro acupuncture stimulation works at various levels of the central nervous system including (1) at the spinal cord level, (2) at the midbrain level, and (3) at the pituitary hypothalamus level [14] (Fig. 3).

At the level of the spinal cord, low-frequency, high intensity electrical stimulation causes enkephalins and dynorphins to be secreted [15]. This creates an inhibitory loop in which released enkephalins decrease calcium in flow which in turn

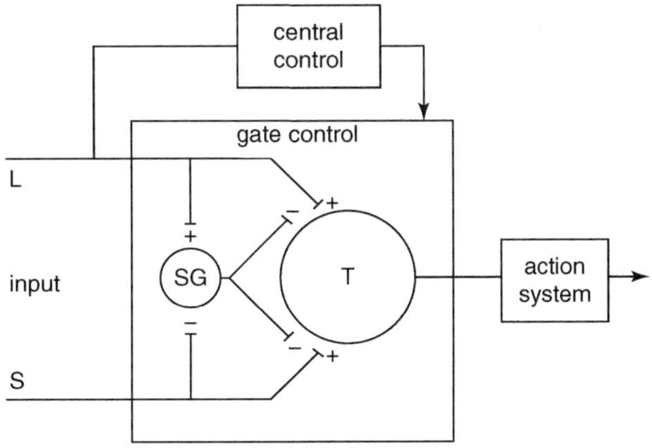

Fig. 1 *SG* substantia gelatinosa, *T* central transmission cell, *L* large diameter, *S* small diameter (Melzack and Wall, 1963)

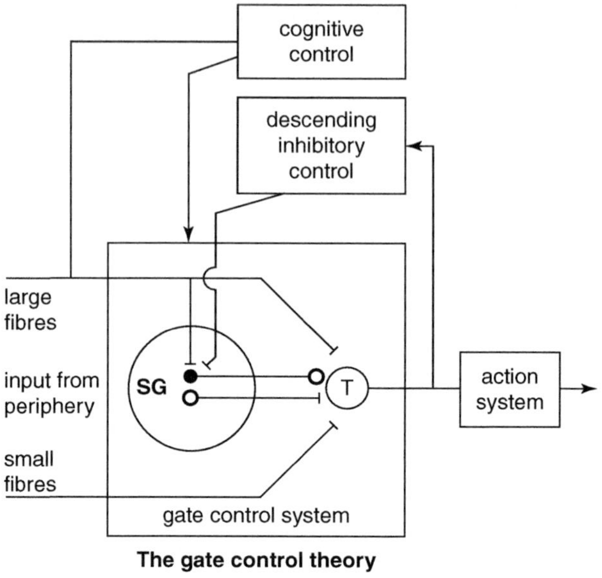

Fig. 2 *SG* substantia gelatinosa, *T* central transmission cell, ● excitatory link, ○ inhibitory link (Melzack and Wall, 1993)

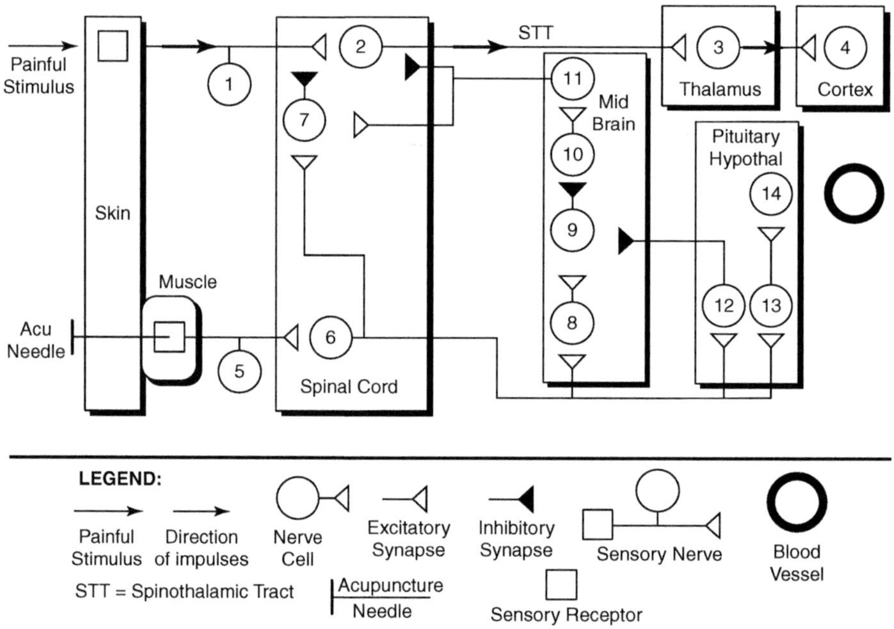

Fig. 3 Overall pain pathway schematic

decreases substance P release. At the level of the spinal cord, high-frequency electrical stimulation promotes the release of GABA which inhibit pain information transmission (Fig. 4).

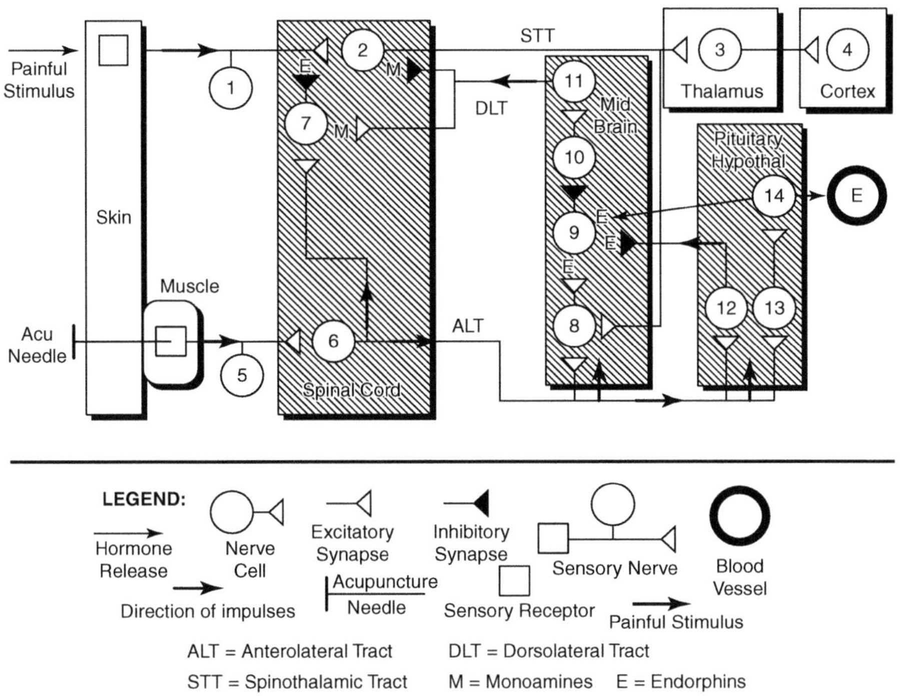

Fig. 4 Low frequency electroacupuncture stimulation pain pathway schematic

At the level of the midbrain, low-frequency, high intensity electrical stimulation activates the dorsolateral tract (raphe descending system) and stimulates monoamines like serotonin and norepinephrine to create an inhibitory effect back at the spinal cord level. This type of stimulation also promotes the release of enkephalins. At the level of the midbrain, high-frequency, low intensity electrical stimulation works synergistically with monoamines such as serotonin and via the raphe descending system (dorsolateral tract) produces spinal cord inhibition. It also has a norepinephrine effect. This effect is enhanced by tryptophan. This type of stimulation bypasses the enkephalin system (Fig. 5).

At the level of the pituitary-hypothalamus axis, low-frequency, high intensity electrical stimulation promotes the release of beta-endorphins and ACTH [16]. These hormones produce an inhibitory effect back at the midbrain level and when secreted into the body produce systemic physiological effects. When secreted into the cerebral spinal fluid via the periaqueductal gray, these hormones/neurotransmitters travel through the midbrain and the raphe descending system to have an inhibitory influence at these respective levels. When secreted into the circulation, these hormones/neurotransmitters cause distant analgesia. High frequency, low intensity electrical stimulation does not have an effect at the pituitary-hypothalamus axis. Locally acupuncture needles have the following mechanical effects: release of

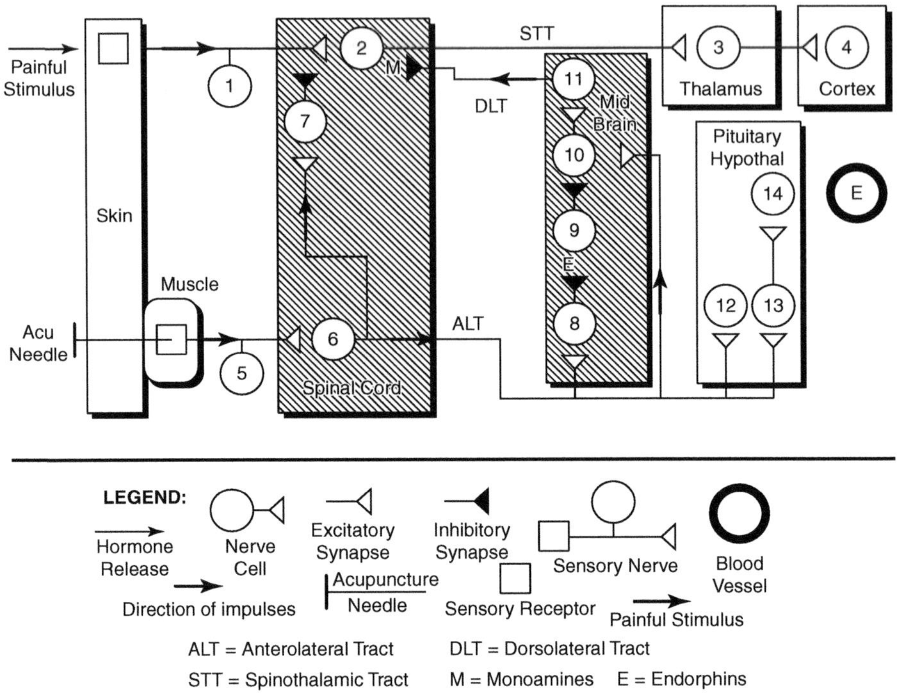

Fig. 5 High frequency electroacupuncture stimulation pain pathway schematic

spasm, disruption of fibrosis, stimulation of blood flow, and diffuse noxious inhibitory control.

3 Clinical Application and Presentation of Techniques

The clinical variables to consider while delivering electro acupuncture are (1) intensity, (2) frequency, (3) waveform, (4) length of treatment, and (5) location of needle input. Currently, there are no standard clinical guidelines for electro-acupuncture yet there is some consistency regarding the setup of the clinical variables. These are presented below:

Intensity

The level of intensity of stimulation should be determined by the patient's tolerance and the condition being treated. Stimulation level should neither be painful or uncomfortable to the patient. When stimulating a motor point, the stimulation intensity should just enough to illicit a non-noxious muscle contraction. When stimulating a sensory nerve, the stimulation intensity should just enough to illicit a non-noxious paresthesia along the dermatomal distribution of the nerve. One way to assess if the intensity of e-stim is appropriate for the patient is to gauge the patient's verbal and non-verbal response and adjust to tolerance. Another way to assess the intensity of e-stim is to monitor the patient's pulse/heart rate before and during the treatment. If the pulse/heart rate becomes rapid after applying e-stim, it is a sign to reduce the intensity.

Frequency

Frequency is the number of pulses delivered per second. It is measured in Hertz (Hz).

(a) High frequency is 80–100 pulses per second. High-frequency stimulation mainly affects the sensory nerve fibers which are associated with pain, temperature, pressure and touch [17]. High-frequency stimulation can be effective for acute pain, paresthesia, dysesthesias, and neuropathies with sensory deficit, such as those that occur with median nerve entrapment seen with carpal tunnel syndrome.
(b) Low frequency is 1–10 pulses per second. Low-frequency stimulation mainly affects motor nerve fibers [17]. Low-frequencies can effective for motor inhibition (weakness), joint proprioceptive dysfunction, and myofascial trigger points. Low-frequency stimulation is also effective for chronic nociceptive pain (Table 2).

Generally high frequency is considered sedating, low frequency more tonifying. Overall acupuncture is a sedating technique. Clinically, one recommendation is to match the frequency of electro acupuncture to the frequency that the practitioner would use during manual needle manipulation.

Table 2 Differences between high frequency stimulation (TENS) and low frequency stimulation (electro acupuncture)

TENS like stimulation (High frequency, low intensity)	Electro acupuncture like stimulation (Low frequency, high intensity)
Gate Theory	De Qi Empiricism
Large Muscle (I) and Skin Nerves (Aβ) activation	Small Muscle Nerves (III/Aδ) release endocrine
Segmental Effect	Segmental & Extra segmental Effect
Burning on skin, no DeQi in muscle	Activate small muscle nerves (III) with DeQi
Spasm at high frequency	No spasm at low frequency
Analgesia is rapid but short lasting	Analgesia slow onset (30min), longer lasting
Tolerance from continuous use	No tolerance from short 30 min use
Vasoconstriction (sympathetic)	Vasodilation (parasympathetic)
Treats nerve and neuropathic pain	Treats myofascial pain
Produces dynorphin	Produces endorphin and enkephalin

Waveform

A waveform is basically the pattern of the electrical current flow. There are three main categories of waveforms: continuous, intermittent, and dense/disperse.

Continuous

A continuous pattern is a constant and equally spaced sequence of pulses that can be increased or decreased by adjusting the wave frequency. The body quickly acclimates to the continuous waveform, so it is advisable to change the intensity every 5 min in order to achieve the best therapeutic effect. This waveform can be uncomfortable for some patients (Fig. 6).

Intermittent

An intermittent pattern of stimulation is a sequence of equally spaced pulsations with equal periods of no activity. This wave form simulates manual manipulation of the acupuncture needle where stimulation is alternated with periods of rest. Like the continuous waveform, the body quickly acclimates to intermittent stimulation so the practitioner will need to change the intensity of the stimulation approximately every 5 min (Fig. 7).

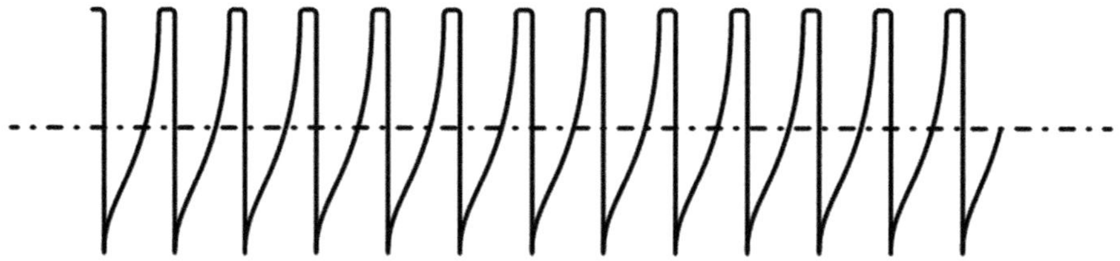

Fig. 6 Continuous waveform

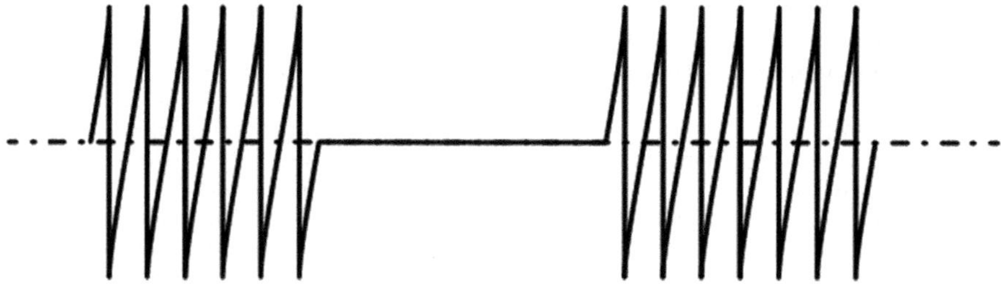

Fig. 7 Intermittent waveform

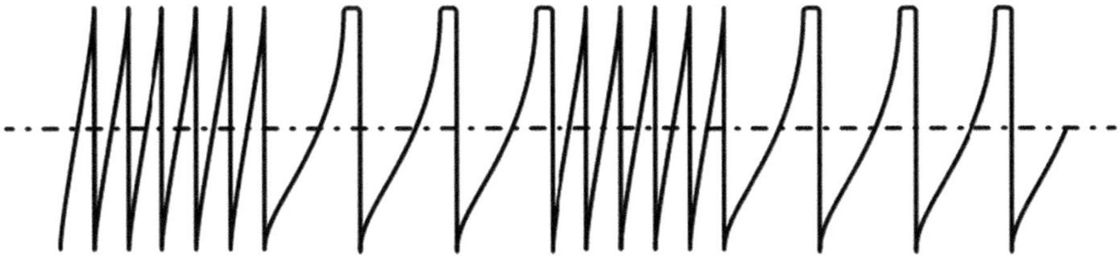

Fig. 8 Dense-disperse waveform

Dense/Disperse

This pattern refers to equally proportion periods of high-frequency and low-frequency pulsations. Dense waveforms, which is high frequency (80–100 Hz) with low intensity, alternate with disperse waveforms, which are low frequency (1–10 Hz) and high intensity. Because of the alternating current, the body does not act limit to the electric pattern like the two previous waveforms. It has been suggested that dense disperse waveform provides the longest lasting pain relief for musculoskeletal injury and sensory deficits (Fig. 8).

Duration of Treatment

A stimulation time of less than 20 min generally increases sympathetic tone. A stimulation time of more than 20 min increases parasympathetic tone after the treatment is complete. This change can last around 8–12 h after the first treatment. Generally, in treatments for reducing pain, increasing parasympathetic tone is the clinical goal. Cheing et al. tested the effect of EA for the treatment of osteoarthritic pain, and found that EA for 40 min achieved the strongest and longest lasting therapeutic effect [18]. Continuous acupuncture stimulation for more than 1–2 h may lead to a diminution of analgesic effect, known as 'acupuncture tolerance [1, 19]. Therefore, excessive duration of acupuncture stimulation is not recommended.

Location of Needle Input

There are many different strategies for needle placement in electro acupuncture. Needles can be placed subcutaneously, myotomally, or sclerotomally. A few pertinent needle input protocols for pain management are presented in this section.

Craig Percutaneous Electrical Nerve Stimulation (PENS)

This technique, developed by William Craig, MD, affects the central nervous system via dermatomes, myotomes, sclerotomes, peripheral nerve, and autonomic nervous system [20]. With this technique, the needles are strategically placed at selected

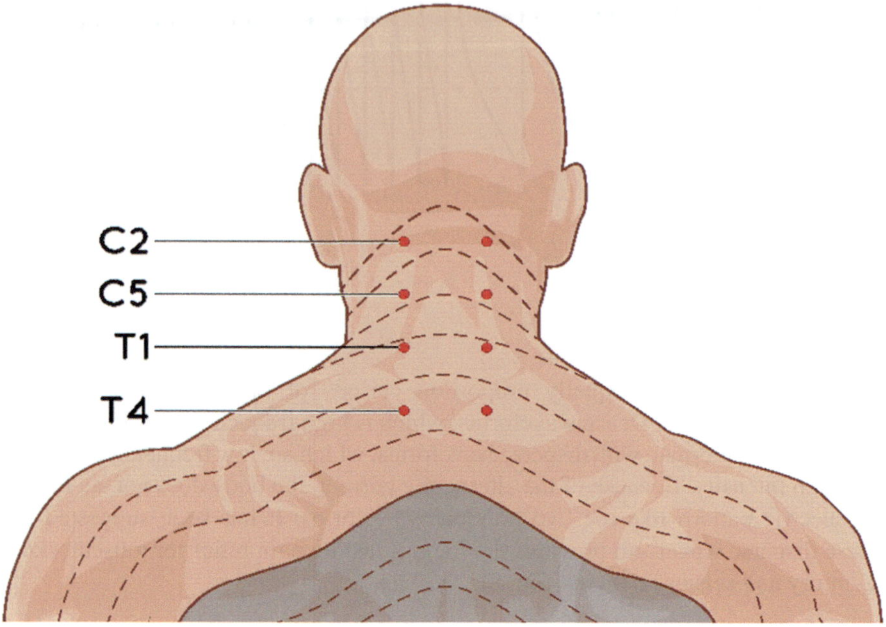

Fig. 9 CraigPENs—cervical array pattern

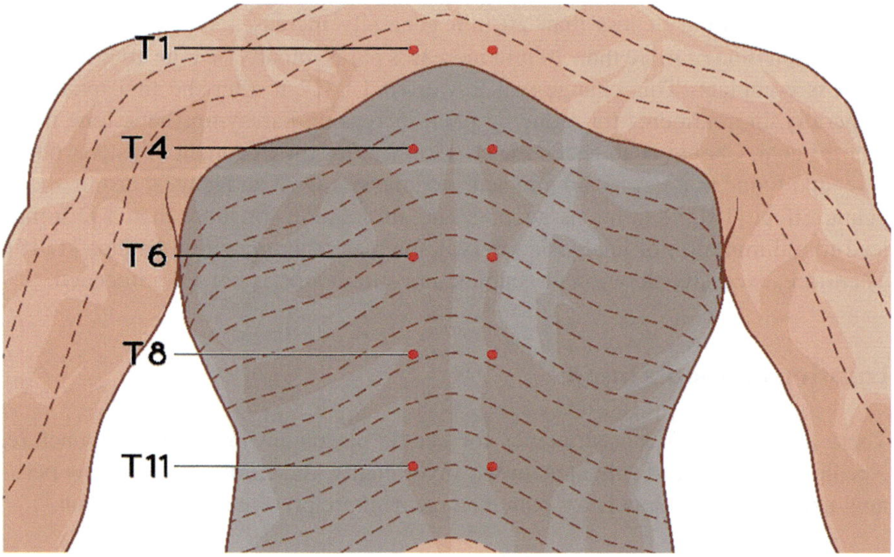

Fig. 10 CraigPENs—thoracic array pattern

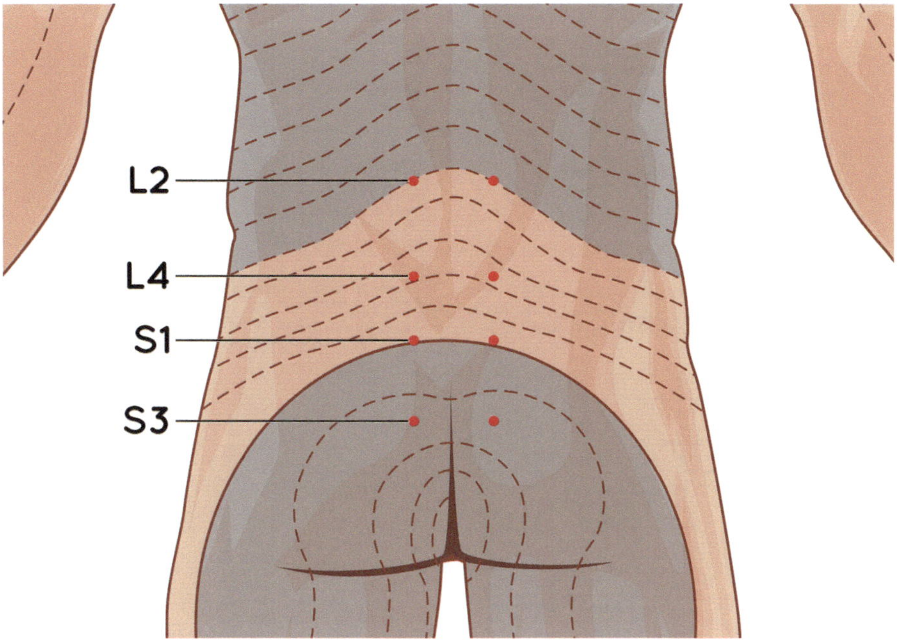

Fig. 11 CraigPENs—lumbar array pattern

inputs along the axial spine [21]. There is a cervical, thoracic, and lumbar array pattern (Figs. 9, 10 and 11).

The needles are inserted 0.5–1 cm lateral to the spinous process. The direction of needle placement depends on the spinal region the treatment is taking place and is either (1) perpendicular or (2) 45° to the perpendicular towards the spinous process. To influence the dermatomal level the needles are inserted subcutaneously. To influence the myotome level, the needles are inserted to the multifidus muscles. To influence the sclerotome level, the needles are inserted to the lamina of the respective vertebral level. The clinical influence on pain is by electrical stimulation at various selected frequency montages. These montages are selected sequentially and depend on the patient's clinical response. Initially, the following frequency montage is selected for treatment: 2 Hz and 4 Hz. If the patient has good pain relief, than this frequency is repeated for the other remaining sessions. If, on subsequent treatment sessions, the patient does not have good relief, the frequency montage is increased sequentially to the following: 4 Hz and 15 Hz [22], 4 Hz and 40 Hz, 4 Hz and 80 Hz, and lastly 4 Hz and 150 Hz. The treatments typically are 20–40 min once a week for 4–8 treatments. There are a variety of versions of Craig PENS treatment protocols. These variable protocols adjust both the frequencies and needle inputs to increase treatment specificity. For example, for neck pain, the motor points of the trapezius and levator scapulae muscles can be added to the cervical array pattern. The motor points of the gluteus medius and gluteus maximus can be added to the lumbar array

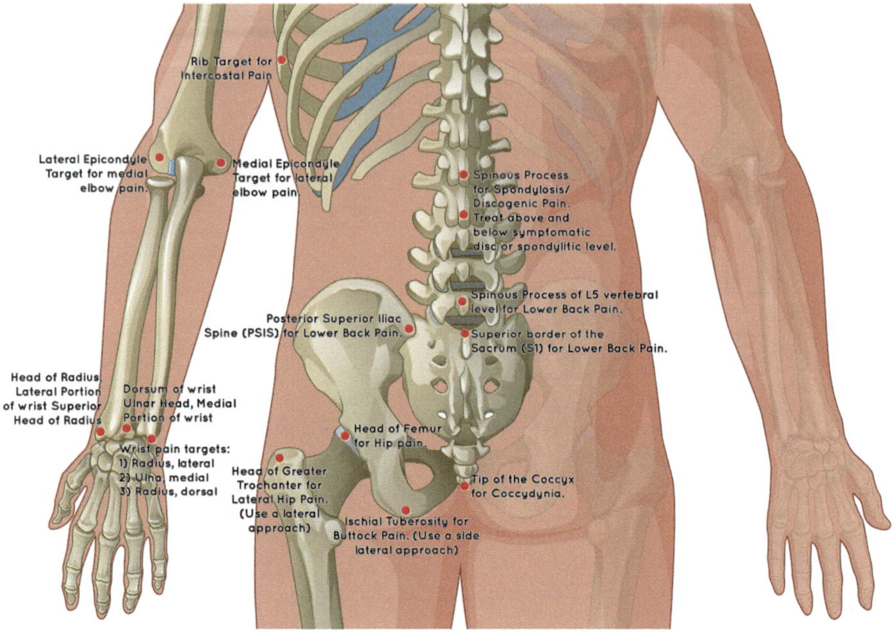

Fig. 12 Osteopuncture common point locations

pattern for lower back pain. A low frequency, continuous waveform pattern is used for these motor points, either 1 Hz or 10 Hz.

Osteopuncture

This technique, developed by Ronald Lawrence MD and Felix Mann MD, affects pain via the sclerotomes and the autonomic nervous system [23, 24]. The periosteum is rich in sympathetic nerve fibers. The treatment goal is to increase local tissue blood flow, to modulate the autonomic nervous system at the sclerotome level, and to modulate pain at the spinal cord level [25, 26]. The C fibers are a slow link to the thalamic nuclei. With this technique the needles are inserted on to the periosteum. The selected inputs maybe either anatomical points or acupuncture points (Fig. 12). The needle is than stimulated at a high frequency, greater than 100 Hz. Typically, 500 Hz or higher is used. The treatments typically are 20–40 min once a week for 4–8 treatments. To avoid the body acclimating to the high frequency stimulation, frequency variation can be done via the dense-disperse settings on the electrical stimulation unit. This treatment can be used alone as a local treatment or in combination with other acupuncture techniques such as CraigPENS, Gokavi technique, or systemic regulatory points. Complementary modalities such as infrared heat can be used during the osteopuncture treatment as appropriate.

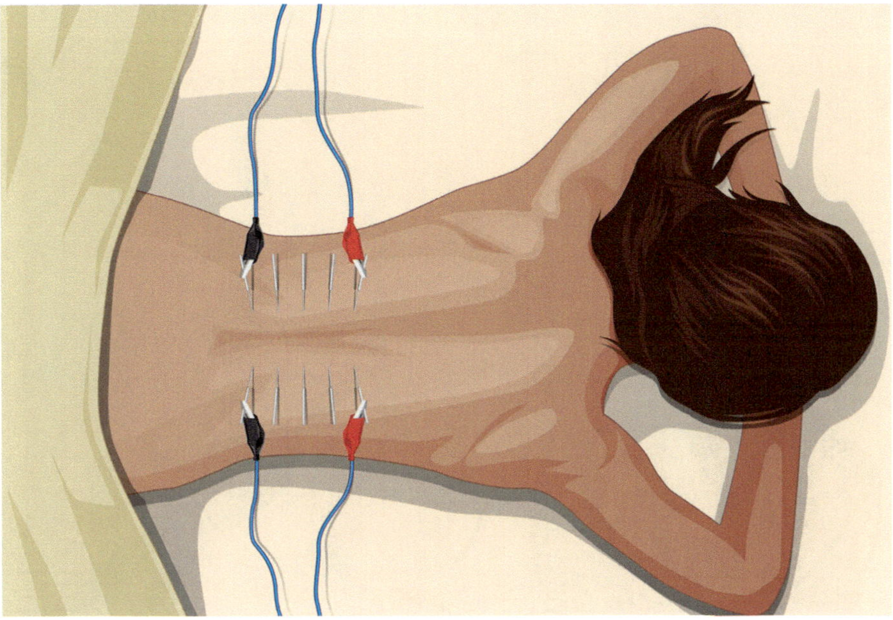

Fig. 13 Gokavi technqiue—high freqency technique on the spine

Gokavi Transverse Technique (GTT)

This technique, developed by Cynthia Gokavi, MD, is used to affect pain at the myotome level utilizing both (1) high frequency stimulation and (2) dry needling [27]. Clinically this technique is used in the treatment and management of chronic myofascial pain. Within the region of the patient's pain complaint, needles are inserted to the myotome level in a transverse direction to envelop this area. This part of the treatment is a regional and segmental treatment (Fig. 13). The needles are then stimulated at two different high-frequencies (dense-disperse)—typically 100–500 Hz is used. The level of intensity is such that the patient feels paresthesia and tingling but there is no motor contraction or fasciculation. The clinical goal of the high frequency stimulation is analgesia and relaxation of the target muscles. The analgesia produced is enkephalin mediated. Treatment time is 20–40 min. The high-frequency electro acupuncture is followed by local dry (trigger point) needling to the same region (Fig. 14). The muscle is dry needled transversely to release spasms and trigger points. The initial high-frequency analgesia helps with patient tolerance during the dry needling session. The clinical goal of the dry needling is to improve any functional deficits such as reduced mobility, pain, and motor inhibition (weakness) as a result of trigger points. Typical regions of treatment include the cervical spine, shoulder girdle (trapezius/levator scapula), and the thoracic spine.

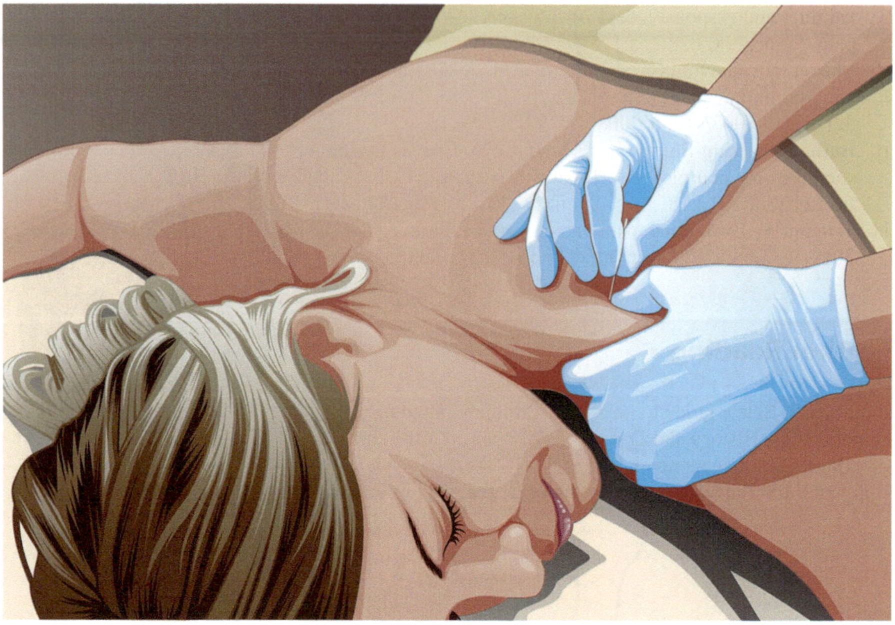

Fig. 14 Gokavi technqiue—dry needling technique on trapezius

Systemic Regulatory Points

Non or extra segmental acupuncture points can be used to treat pain as well. These inputs are located at distal areas of the lower extremity and ankle, typically close to joints. Extrasegmental analgesia is a systemic effect therefore point selection is not critical. LI 4, LI 11, ST 36 and LV 3 are commonly used [28–30] (Table 3). For rapid pain relief, strong input producing DeQi sensation is critical. Most of these distal extra segmental treatment protocols signals influence the autonomic nervous system [31]. By augmenting the autonomic nervous system, mainly the sympathetic side, these protocols help to treat pain [32]. These protocols are generally treated with low frequency stimulation, 1–2 Hz, for 20–40 min duration. Below highlights a few of these protocols:

(a) Four Gates

This is a traditional Chinese medicine point combination. The four gates are the combination of Large Intestine 4 and Liver 3. Various research studies have shown that these inputs help to regulate the autonomic nervous system. The

Table 3 Systemic regulatory acupuncture points and indications [44]

Point	Location	Indications	Visual representation
Large Intestine 4	Dorsum of hand, between first and second metacarpal bones, in middle of second metacarpal bone on radial side	Diseases of the head and face, ex: headache, toothache, swelling of face, dizziness, congestion. Cold, flu, febrile disease, dysmenorrhea [18]	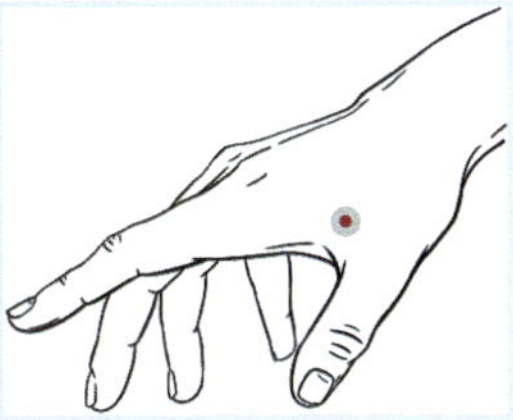
Large Intestine 11	With the elbow flexed, lateral end of transverse cubital crease	Febrile diseases, pain of eye, teeth, shoulder, or abdomen, dysmenorrhea	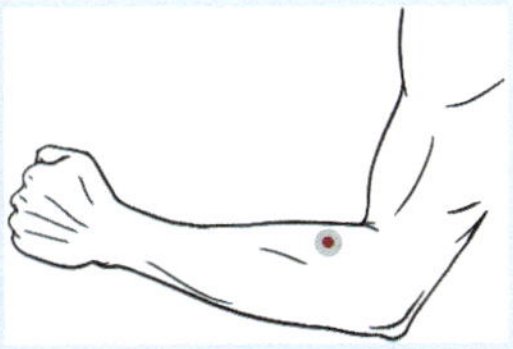
Small Intestine 3	Ulnar aspect of the hand, proximal to the fifth metacarpophalangeal joint, at the junction of light and dark skin	Pain and rigidity of head and neck. Pain of the lumbar and sacrum spine. Spasm of hand and arm	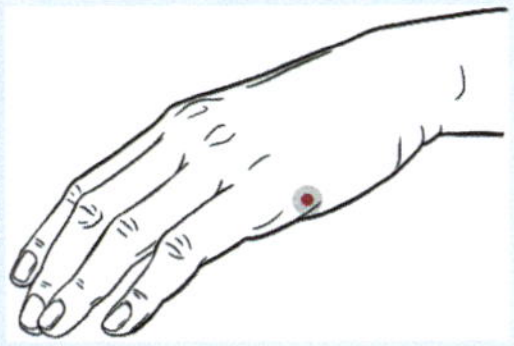
Liver 3	Distal to the junction of the bases of the first and second metatarsal	Low back pain, high blood pressure, genital pain, menstrual cramps, limb pain, anxiety	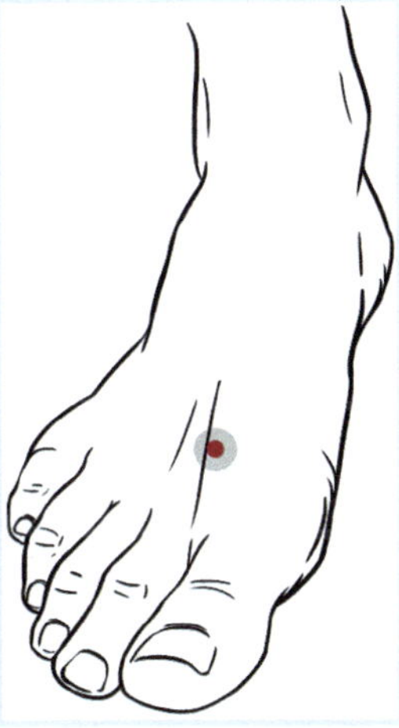

(continued)

Table 3 (continued)

Point	Location	Indications	Visual representation
Stomach 36	One finger width lateral to the anterior crest of the tibia	Cough, asthma, Pain in the knee point, gastric pain, vomiting, dysphagia, diarrhea	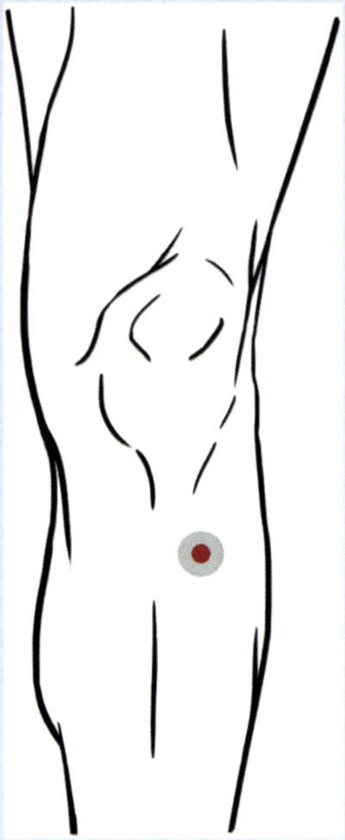
Triple Warmer 5	2 fingerbreadths proximal to the dorsal wrist crease in the interosseous space	Migraine, facial pain/ paralysis, tinnitus, headache, hand tremor, abdominal pain	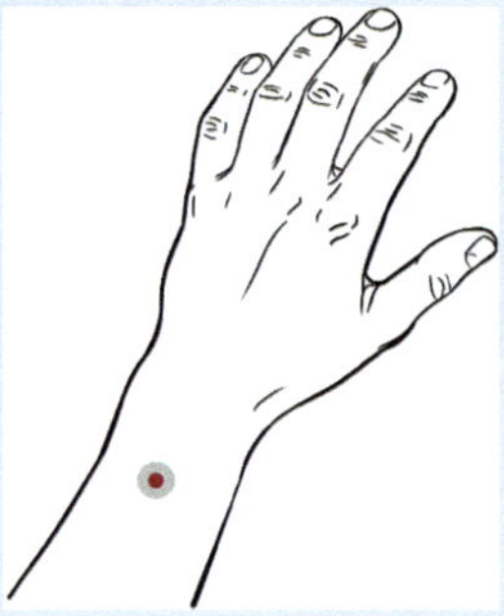
Gall Bladder 41	On the lateral side of the dorsum of the foot. Proximal to the fourth metatarsophalangeal joint	Pain of the eye, foot & toe. Mastitis & irregular menstruation	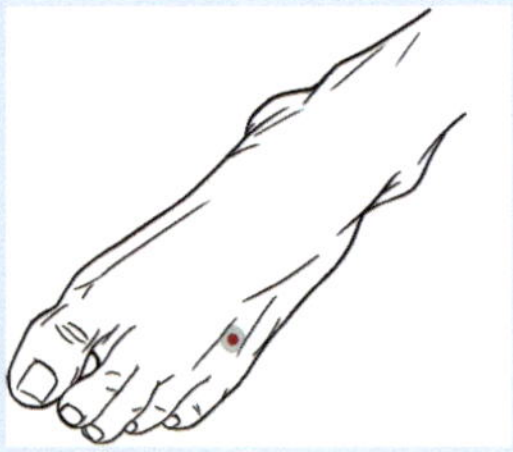

Table 3 (continued)

Point	Location	Indications	Visual representation
Bladder 60	On the foot, posterior to the external malleolus	Acute lumbar pain, pain of the heel, neck stiffness, headache, difficult labor	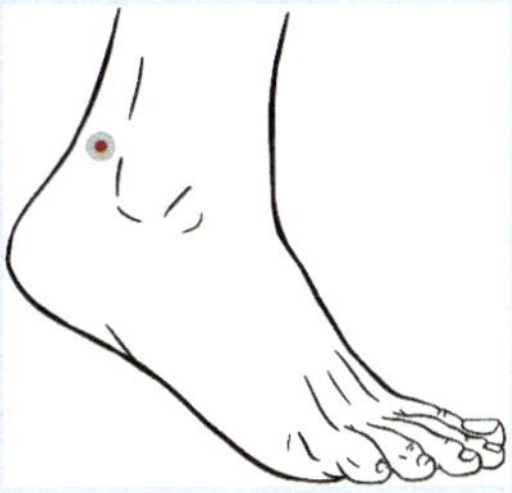
Bladder 62	In the depression, directly below the external malleolus	Insomnia, epilepsy, headache, neck rigidity, lumbar or leg pain	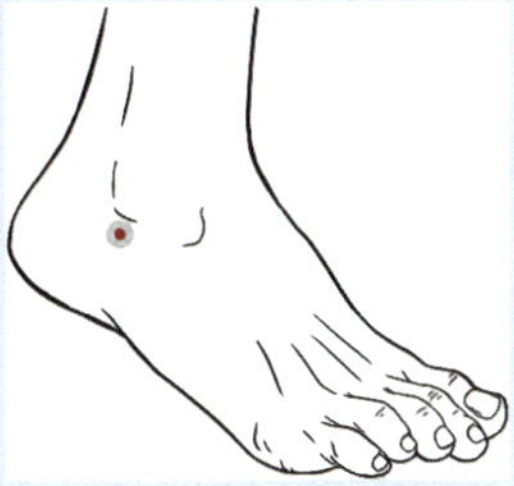
Lung 7	Proximal to the radial styloid, in the depression between tendons of brachioradialis and abductor pollicis longus	Headache, stiffness of neck, cough, asthma, sore throat, weakness of wrist	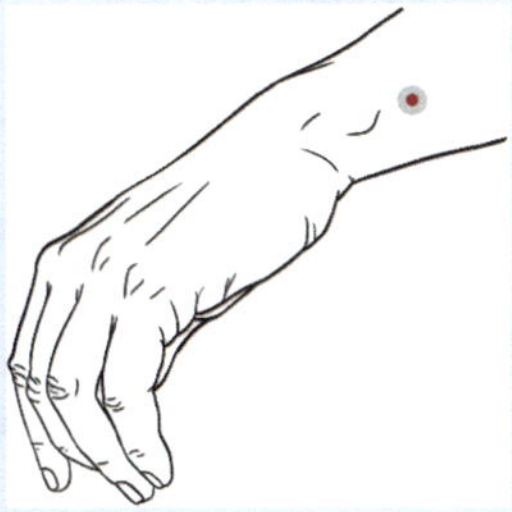
Spleen 4	Medial aspect of the foot, inferior to the base of the first metatarsal bone	Gastric pain, abdominal pain, poor appetite	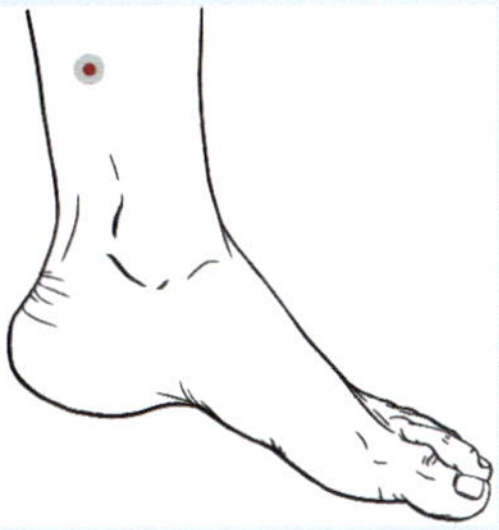

indication for this point combination is headaches and general pain conditions, acute and chronic. These points are used bilaterally.

Point Prescription: Bilateral Large Intestine 4 and Liver 3

(b) Inner and Outer Gates

This is a traditional Chinese medicine point combination. The inner and outer gate expands upon the four gates treatment noted above. In addition to bilateral Liver 3 and Large intestine 4, bilateral Large Intestine 11 and Stomach 36 are added to the treatment protocol. Once again, these points are systemic

Table 4 Influential points [45]

Qi	Governor Vessel (Ren) 17
Blood	Bladder 17
Tendons	Gall Bladder 34
Bone	Bladder 11
Marrow	Gall Bladder 39
Blood Vessels/Pulse	Lung 9

regulatory points which work via the mechanism described in the earlier section. The indications are the same as the four gates treatment.

Point Prescription: Bilateral Large Intestine 4, Large Intestine 11, Stomach 36, and Liver 3

(c) Koffman Cocktail

This point combination, developed by US Navy Captain Robert Koffman, MD, utilizes a combination of systemic regulatory points to help with chronic pain conditions [33]. This treatment also expands upon the four gates treatment. In addition to Liver 3 and Large Intestine 4 bilaterally, Governor Vessel (GV) 20 and Governor Vessel (GV) 24.5 without electrical stimulation are added. Indications for this combination of points include headaches, insomnia, anxiety and other symptoms commonly seen in patients with PTSD [34, 35].

Point Prescription: Bilateral Large Intestine 4, Liver 3, Governor Vessel (GV) 20, and Governor Vessel (GV) 24.5

(d) Miriam Lee 10 Point Protocol

Miriam Lee 10-point protocol also known as 'Miriam Lee's Great 10 Needles' is a combination of systemic regulatory points which are used for generalized systemic complaints, acute pain, and chronic pain [36, 37]. The protocol is a combination of five points in the upper and lower extremity used bilaterally: Liver 4, Lung 7, Large Intestine 11, Stomach 36, and Spleen 6. Additional inputs, such influential points, can be added or subtracted depending on the patient's specific presenting complaint.

Point Prescription: Bilateral Liver 4, Lung 7, Large intestine 11, Stomach 36, and Spleen 6

(e) Influential Points

The influential points are eight important acupuncture points that have close relationships with physiological functions of a specific tissue. And treating pain conditions, the influential points that are especially effective are those that pertain to muscle, blood, tendons, marrow, and Bone. These points are added to the above point prescriptions according to patient underlying diagnosis or pathological injury. For example, for a patient presenting with low back pain with a diagnosis if facet joint mediated pain, UB 11, the influential point for bone can be used (Table 4).

4 Cautions and Contraindications

The practitioner should exercise caution when applying e-stim in the needles over the thoracic, pleural, and abdominal cavities. Muscle contractions can cause the needle to penetrate deeper than initially inserted. In the thoracic cavity this can mean entrance into the lungs or heart. While in the abdominal cavity this can mean entrance into the vital organs/viscera such as the intestine or liver. Electro acupuncture can create a strong sensation. Distal input locations such as the hands and feet are more sensitive than other body locations and the e-stim intensity should be adjusted for patient comfort. Electro acupuncture also creates vasoconstriction and muscle tension which can aggravate muscle spasms in some cases. Contraindications to electro-acupuncture include: patients with blood dyscrasias, cardiac arrhythmias, cardiac pacemakers, autonomic dysregulation, pregnant women, through malignant tumors, and transcranial in patients with seizure disorders.

5 Conclusion and Future Directions

As there is a shift away from opioid management for chronic pain conditions, the research into the clinical utility for electroacupuncture has room for growth. Future directions with this modality would include research into physical examination techniques for determining needle inputs, such as through functional assessment, research into treatment outcome measurement, such as using heart rate variability for measurement of autonomic nervous system status [38, 39], and lastly, research into how best to incorporate this modality into established treatment pathways for pain conditions [40].

References

1. Mayor D. Electroacupuncture: a practical manual and resource. Churchill Livingstone; 2006.
2. Lin JG, Chen WL. Acupuncture analgesia: a review of its mechanisms of actions. Am J Chin Med. 2008;36(4):635–45.
3. Yang JW, Li QQ, Li F, Fu QN, Zeng XH, Liu CZ. The holistic effects of acupuncture treatment. Evid Based Complement Alternat Med. 2014;739708.
4. Patil S, Sen S, Bral M, et al. The role of acupuncture in pain management. Curr Pain Headache Rep. 2016;20(4):22.
5. Zhang R, Lao L, Ren K, Berman B. Mechanisms of acupuncture–electroacupuncture on persistent pain. Anesthesiology. 2014;120(2):482–503.
6. Robinson NG. Interactive medical acupuncture anatomy. Teton NewMedia; 2016.
7. Chan S. What is being stimulated in acupuncture? Evaluation of the existence of a specific substrate. Neurosci Biobehav Rev. 1984;8:25–33.
8. Liu YK, Varela M, Oswald R. The correspondence between some motor points and acupuncture loci. Am J Chin Med. 1975;3:347–58.
9. Wang SM, et al. Acupuncture analgesia: I. The scientific basis. Anesth Analg. 2008;106:602–10.
10. Melzack R, Wall PD. Pain mechanisms: a new theory. Science. 1965;150(3699):971–9.
11. Nathan PW. The gate control theory of pain: a critical review. Brain. 1976;99(1):123–58.
12. Melzack R. Pain: past, present and future. Can J Exp Psychol. 1993;47(4):615–29.

13. Wall PD. The gate control theory of pain mechanisms. A re-examination and re-statement. Brain. 1978;101(1):1–18.
14. Stux G, Pomeranz B. Basics of acupuncture. Berlin: Springer; 1995. p. 281.
15. Wang Y, Zhang Y, Wang W, Cao Y, Han JS. New evidence for synergistic analgesia produced by endomorphin and dynorphin. Chin J Pain Med. 2002;8:118–9.
16. Cheng RS, Pomeranz B. Electroacupuncture analgesia could be mediated by at least two pain-relieving mechanisms; endorphin and non-endorphin systems. Life Sci. 1979;25(23):1957–62.
17. Silvério-lopes, Sandra. "Electroacupuncture and stimulatory frequencies in analgesia." (2011).
18. Cheing GLY, Tsui AYY, Lo SK, Hui-Chan CWY. Optimal stimulation duration of tens in the management of osteoarthritic knee pain. J Rehabil Med. 2003;35:62–8.
19. Han JS, Ding XZ, Fan SG. Cholecystokinin octapeptide (CCK-8)—antagonism to electroacupuncture analgesia and a possible role in electroacupuncture tolerance. Pain. 1986;27:101–15.
20. Niemtzow R. Interview with Dr William Craig, inventor of Craig-PENS. Med Acupunct. 2007;19(4):165–8.
21. Ghoname EA, Craig WF, White PF, et al. Percutaneous electrical nerve stimulation for low back pain. JAMA. 1999;281:818–23.
22. Chen XH, Han JS. All three types of opioid receptors in the spinal cord are important for 2/15 Hz electroacupuncture analgesia. Eur J Pharmacol. 1992;211(2):203–10.
23. Mann F. Reinventing acupuncture: a new concept of ancient medicine. 2nd ed. Oxford: Butterworth Heinemann; 2000.
24. Hansson Y, Carlsson C, Olsson E. Intramuscular and periosteal acupuncture in patients suffering from chronic musculoskeletal pain—a controlled trial. Acupunct Med. 2008;26:214–23.
25. Weiner DK, Rudy TE, Morone N, Glick R, Kwoh CK. Efficacy of periosteal stimulation therapy for the treatment of osteoarthritis-associated chronic knee pain: an initial controlled clinical trial. J Am Geriatr Soc. 2007;55(10):1541–7.
26. Dunning, et al. Periosteal electrical dry needling as an adjunct to exercise and manual therapy for knee osteoarthritis. A multicenter randomized clinical trial. Clin J Pain. 2018;34(12).
27. Gokavi C. The treatment and management of chronic myofascial pain release: Gokavi transverse technique. Gokavi Publications; 2000.
28. Ernst M, Lee M. Sympathetic effects of manual and electrical acupuncture of the Tsusanli knee point: comparison with the Hoku hand point sympathetic effects. Exp Neurol. 1986;94:1310.
29. Filshie J, White A, Cummings M. Medical acupuncture: a western scientific approach. Elsevier; 2016.
30. Wong YM. An understanding of anatomy under the LI4 acupuncture point. Acupunct Med. 2013;31(3):333.
31. Hui, et al. Acupuncture, the limbic system, and the anticorrelated networks of the brain. Auton Neurosci. 2010;157:81–90.
32. da Silva MA, Dorsher PT. Neuroanatomic and clinical correspondences: acupuncture and vagus nerve stimulation. J Altern Complement Med. 2014;20(4):233–40.
33. Koffman RL. Downrange acupuncture. Med Acupunct. 2011;23:4.
34. Abanes J, et al. Feasibility and acceptability of a brief acupuncture intervention for service members with perceived stress. Mil Med. 2020;185(1–2):e17–22.
35. Ritchie EC. Posttraumatic stress disorder and related diseases in combat veterans. 1st ed. Cham: Springer; 2015.
36. Lee M. Insights of a senior acupuncturist. Blue Poppy Printing; 1992.
37. Fan AY, Fan Z. Dr. Miriam Lee: a heroine for the start of acupuncture as a profession in the State of California. J Integr Med. 2014;12(3):182–6.
38. Alraek T, Ozan Tan C. Acupuncture and heart rate variability. Acupunct Med. 2011;29:7–8.
39. Lee S, et al. Acupuncture and heart rate variability: a systematic review. Auton Neurosci. 2010;155:5–13.
40. Wang SM, et al. Acupuncture analgesia: II. Clinical considerations. Anesth Analg. 2008;106:611–21.

41. Dorsher PT, Chiang P. Neuroembryology of the acupuncture principal meridians: part 3. The head and neck. Med Acupunct. 2018;30(2):80–8.
42. Lee M, Longenecker R, Lo S, Chiang P. Distinct neuroanatomical structures of acupoints kidney 1 to kidney 8: a cadaveric study. Med Acupunct. 2019;31(1):19–28.
43. Ortiz D, Chiang P. Neuroanatomical significance of acupuncture points TE1–TE10 based on the systematic classic. Med Acupunct. 2017;29(2):66–76.
44. Jin S, Jin W, Jin P. A practical handbook of acupuncture points. People's Medical Publishing House; 2008.
45. Helms JM. Acupuncture energetics: a clinical approach for physicians. Medical Acupuncture Publishers; 1995.

Further Reading

Filshie J, White A, Cummings M, editors. Medical acupuncture: a western scientific approach. 2nd ed. Elsevier; 2016.
Mayor D. Electroacupuncture: a practical manual and resource. Churchill Livingstone; unknown edition; 2006.
Robinson NG. Interactive medical acupuncture anatomy. 1st ed. Teton NewMedia; 2016.
Wancura-Kampik I. Segmental anatomy: the key to mastering acupuncture, neural therapy and manual therapy. 1st ed. Urban & Fischer; 2019.
Wong J. A manual of neuro-anatomical acupuncture, vol. III: east meets west. Redwing Book Co; 2003.

Bedside Pain Psychology, Spiritual and Complementary Medicine Interventions

Daniel Adams, Shayan Azizi, Matthew Steiner, and Dmitri Souza

Essential Concepts

- Many behavioral, spiritual, and complementary interventions have been shown to be effective within multimodal pain management models and can be easily adapted to the bedside.
- These therapies are not a substitute for a psychological consultation performed by behavioral health practitioners who specialize in the treatment of pain.
- Education, cognitive therapy, relaxation therapy, guided imagery, breathing exercises, art, music, massage, aromatherapy, Reiki, mindfulness, and spiritual interventions have been shown to improve clinical outcomes safely and at little cost.
- Interventions should be selected based on an evaluation of the patient's motivation and preferences as well as practical considerations.
- Patient education is especially important in modifying expectations, improving compliance with treatment plans, and increasing an understanding of the mind-body connection.

D. Adams
Western Reserve Hospital –Center for Pain Medicine, Cuyahoga Falls, OH, USA
e-mail: dadams@westernreservehospital.org

S. Azizi
Northeast Ohio Medical University, Rootstown, OH, USA
e-mail: sazizi@neomed.edu

M. Steiner
Northeast Ohio Medical University, Rootstown, OH, USA

Department of Family Medicine, St. Vincent Hospital, Erie, OH, USA
e-mail: msteiner@neomed.edu

D. Souza (✉)
Center for Pain Medicine, Western Reserve Hospital, Cuyahoga Falls, OH, USA
e-mail: dsouza@westernreservehospital.org

D. Souza et al. (eds.), *Bedside Pain Management Interventions*,
https://doi.org/10.1007/978-3-031-11188-4_9

1 Introduction

It is now widely recognized that pain is a psychological phenomenon as well as a physical one given the wide variation in both objective and subjective responses to painful stimuli and tissue damage [1]. This is because mood, expectations, and beliefs all play a role in descending pain pathways as well as the neurotransmitters dopamine, serotonin, and other endogenous ligands [2]. As a result, psychotherapeutic treatment of pain has a firm basis in the biopsychosocial model of pain alongside procedural, pharmacologic, and rehabilitative approaches [3, 4]. The purpose of this chapter is to discuss interventions that can be delivered in the same settings as the interventional procedures covered elsewhere in this book. The term "behavioral" is more appropriate than "psychological" or "psychotherapeutic" for these approaches, as the latter imply treatments initiated by a psychological specialist [5].

2 Benefits, Risks, and Limitations of Behavioral Interventions

The behavioral interventions described below all have few side effects or contraindications, and they carry none of the risks of invasive procedures such as radiation exposure, blood loss, or infection. They do not require a high degree of specialized training or equipment and can be administered in almost any setting such as a small, curtained space within an emergency department, nursing home, or hospital bed. Providers may be physicians, psychologists, social workers, nurse practitioners, physician assistants, nurses, medical assistants, family members, or even the patients themselves. They are usually applicable regardless of the type of pain (i.e., neuropathic, somatic) and are opioid-sparing, cost-effective, and easily incorporated with other modalities. Nevertheless, there are risks of any therapy and it is recommended that the provider know the legal aspects and standards of care. The risks of individual therapies are discussed below.

There are significant limitations of the interventions described below. First, they cannot replace or approximate a psychological consultation. There is simply no way for a non-specialist to assess the many factors which determine treatment, employ standardized assessment tools or deliver interventions such as traditional cognitive behavioral therapy (CBT), biofeedback, or hypnosis. Neither is there usually sufficient time at the bedside to build the rapport and trust of a strong therapeutic relationship. Another limitation is the lack of evidence for some interventions at the bedside. Though the benefits of psychotherapeutic approaches are well demonstrated, studies of them in short-term acute pain are often few and inconsistent in protocol design, interventional methods, and reported outcomes [6, 7].

3 Patient Evaluation

If no psychological consultation is required and the provider feels these therapies are indicated instead, their implementation is relatively simple. Not only is the evaluation time much shorter, but there is less risk of triggering defensiveness or suspicion from patients when they are asked to speak with a psychological specialist [5]. Nonetheless, there are some common-sense tools of the conventional psychological interview which can be applied here.

As with any proposed intervention, first, it is necessary to inform the patient as to the purpose of the visit and ask them if they are interested in hearing about their options. In these first moments, the provider/educator should attempt to establish rapport and trust by showing empathy and acknowledging the patient's pain, especially in chronic pain patients [8]. This caring attitude can be shown by asking simple questions, actively listening, and allowing patients to express what is important to them. Even negative interactions or complaints may serve as opportunities to introduce behavioral therapies and solve immediate problems. Throughout this conversation, one can often determine these predictors of success: Do they have realistic expectations of pain control? Are they willing to try new approaches? Are they simply in too much pain to participate in a certain therapy? Do they have difficulties with communication, cognition, or emotional lability? Are there cultural, ethnic, or religious factors to consider?

4 Interventions

The purpose of this section is to summarize interventions that are non-invasive, easily delivered at the bedside, and can improve outcomes within one or two sessions. They are not likely to be contraindicated by injury, interfere with concurrent therapies, or require specialized training (i.e., massage, acupuncture, yoga). Not included are pharmacologic, manipulative or exercise/movement modalities, which may also be beneficial.

Many of the following therapies share potential positive outcomes: reducing pain level and duration, shortening hospital stays, reducing as-needed opioid use, increasing functionality, and improving patient satisfaction. They also overlap in methods of action including increased parasympathetic stimulation, reduction of sympathetic tone, release of pain-reducing neurotransmitters, distraction/refocusing, better mind-body awareness, and social support.

There is no clear consensus about when to consider these interventions. Some authors, respecting the current paradigms of pain control, recommend them when requested by patients or when adequate pain control is not achieved through more conventional methods [9]. Another perspective is that given the relative benefit versus risk ratio of these therapies, it is reasonable to introduce them earlier. This more forward-leaning view better reflects the current climate in which more non-pharmacologic (i.e., non-opioid) options are needed [10].

Patient Education

Education is the most recommended behavioral intervention for both acute and chronic pain according to several guidelines and meta-analyses [11]. This may take the form of verbal instruction, written materials, videos, audio programs, or web-based content. The information provided may consist of how to score pain, the use of opioids on an as-needed basis, expectations of pain control, the effects of pre-operative opioid use, understanding of the mind-body connection, and possible side effects and interactions of pain medications. Many high-quality materials are available online at no cost (see Further Reading). Education is most effective when tailored to individual patient characteristics: age, health literacy, pregnancy status, addiction history, cultural background, and linguistic requirements.

Even single sessions have been effective and in one randomized controlled study, whiplash injury patients were shown a 12-min educational video once during their emergency department (ED) stay. They subsequently reported 70% less pain, 85% less narcotic use, and 85% fewer subsequent ED visits at 1 month. These dramatic results indicate not only improvement in these clinical outcomes, but strongly suggest cost-saving and quality of life benefits as well [12].

Music and Art

Music can modulate oxytocin and endogenous opioid pathways to improve pain and more subjective/affective qualities like well-being and satisfaction. Easily incorporated with other therapies, it can be delivered in almost any care environment, though some modifications to the environment may be necessary to optimize the effect (dimming lights, limiting interruptions, etc.). Patients should be encouraged to choose the pieces themselves [13]. Application at the bedside has been well studied and strong evidence exists not only for its ability to reduce opioid use, anxiety, and pain scores but also to improve blood pressure and respiratory rate [7, 14]. Specific protocols and recommendations have even been made in terms of duration, tempo, and how to incorporate music into multimodal pain control [15].

The making of visual art is also easy to introduce and it is not necessary for the patient to have any instruction or experience. Coloring books for children and adults are now available in a variety of themes if they are not able to create their own images. One review of visual art-making in cancer care found that individual art-making works through several mechanisms: "learning about self, diversion and pleasure, self-management of pain, a sense of control, and enhanced social relationships" [16].

Guided Imagery

The goal of guided imagery is for the patient to refocus by imagining relaxing environments. This is usually accomplished with audio programs but can also involve reading a script to them. Though the visual sense is often the primary target, all of the other senses can be utilized. As with music therapy, manipulation of the environment can reduce distractions and aid concentration. The program may invoke a natural environment such as a beach or other pleasing locations such as an amusement park. Another approach is to visualize the body ridding itself of pain or disease. Though guided imagery is generally well-tolerated, caution should be used with psychotic or demented patients who may have difficulty distinguishing real from imagined environments [17]. There is strong evidence for the effectiveness of guided imagery at the bedside [18].

Breathing Exercises

Relaxation breathing is familiar to many patients and has, of course, been used for decades in childbirth. Patients can perform breathing therapy by taking deep, even and slow breaths from the abdomen. Slow counting can be incorporated to ensure that the duration of expiration exceeds that of inspiration, thus enhancing parasympathetic tone [19]. This type of breathing increases the patient's sense of emotional well-being, moderates vital signs, and can decrease pain immediately. Benefits to the bedbound patient also include increased perfusion of oxygen and improved gastric motility through mechanical stimulation by the diaphragm. It is usually safe but may be contraindicated in painful conditions of the thorax or seizure disorders.

Recreation and Journaling

Distraction with various media can be a powerful tool to refocus and patients may benefit from access to their usual books, laptops or other materials. They may also benefit from doing their school or professional work (provided these are not stressful). Alternatively, keeping a journal of events during their stay such as conversations with the medical team, their medication regimen, and how they're feeling may also lessen anxiety and keep them distracted. The simple act of putting their thoughts and concerns in writing can be cathartic, provided the journal is not a tool to obsess over negative thoughts.

Solution-Focused

Helping patients gain a sense of agency over their surroundings and treatment is crucial: "Of all the psychological factors affecting a pain patient, perhaps the greatest and most distressing is the perception of a loss of control" [8]. The provider should look for opportunities to respond to patients' loss of independence or dignity. Some causes may be immediately apparent such as a distressing roommate, late or distasteful food, fear of upcoming procedures, or anxiety about test results. Others may relate to life outside of the visit: financial stress, medical bills, pet care, family stressors, missing work, uncertainty about discharge times, etc. Simply listening and validating their concerns can convey a willingness to help. They may also be lonely, so facilitating their normal contacts, even if only by phone, may be beneficial. Social support increases endogenous endorphins such as dopamine and the social bonding hormone, oxytocin.

Spiritual Interventions

Chaplains may act as spiritual denizens to help patients cope and confront their illnesses and circumstances. Unlike most beside interventions discussed, spiritual care has historically been a more pervasive and utilized facet of clinical care.

Mindfulness

Mindfulness relies upon an individual's abilities to utilize a degree of personal control to attempt to center their thoughts and perceptions. More broadly, it can incorporate purposeful thought, meditation, and many other techniques to reframe an individual's illness and its manifestations. Though mindfulness may not be utilized as a cure, it has been widely documented that providing a patient the means to focus their thoughts may act as a powerful force to cope or confront a disease or illness.

Such techniques may be easily incorporated at the bedside and require only a patient's willingness and informed healthcare professional. Mindfulness may be utilized as an initial treatment or co-therapy in the treatment of depression, anxiety, post-traumatic stress disorder, and many others [20]. Patients may also see the benefit in the reduction of stress and increase in coping abilities. When combined with cognitive behavior therapy and/or pharmaceuticals, mindfulness has shown great benefit in reducing the perception of pain [21, 22].

Service Animals

Service animals have gained a great deal of popularity as a therapeutic adjunct. Specifically, dogs have been utilized to assist individuals suffering blindness, deafness, and numerous other disabilities. More recently, the idea of pet therapy; that is, utilizing the companionship animals provide to help feelings of depression, anxiety, and isolation, has gained increasing acceptance and practice. In fact, animals have even utilized in the academic sphere to positively impact the mental health of students to reduce anxiety and burnout [23].

Recent research has demonstrated the positive impact of dogs on the mental health of patients in the clinical setting [24]. Often, but not in all cases, dogs must be certified to ensure they are well behaved and can appropriately interact with patients and hospital staff. Although other benefits exist, the most significant benefit appears to be the impact of service dogs on the mental health of patients. Moreover, benefits are seen over a wide array of patients and disease states from terminal to innocuous [25] (Fig. 1).

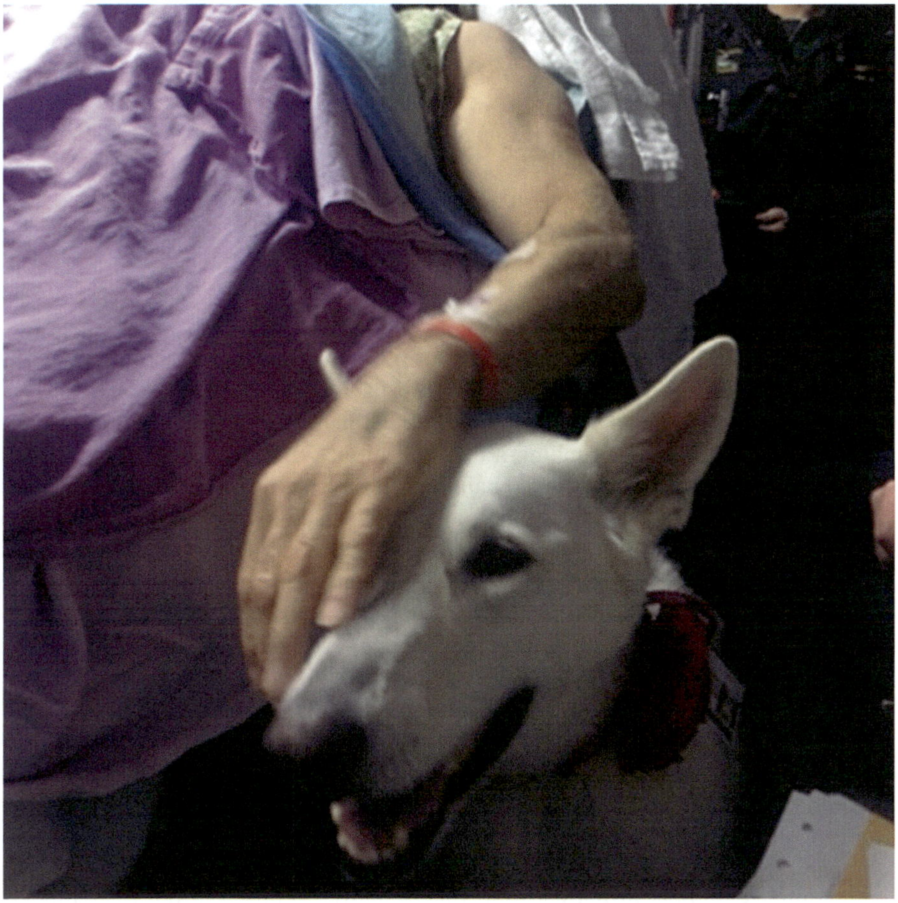

Fig. 1 Service dog

Reiki

Reiki, despite its inception almost a century ago, has remained a seldom discussed and poorly understood aid to standard therapies. Briefly, it is the belief that qi, the universal life force, may be utilized to heal through the hands of a practitioner. The debate regarding the efficacy of Reiki as a treatment notwithstanding, its addition as co-therapy has certainly not been demonstrated to be of harm to patients [26].

Massage

Although Reiki does not incorporate physical touch as the conveyance for energy transfer, there are numerous other methods that do rely on touch. As mentioned previously, chiropractic manipulation is one such example of a touch-based care technique. Worth elucidating here, massage therapy has likewise been utilized to provide pain relief, redistribute blood and fluid in the body, and provide a sense of comfort [27, 28]. Massage is typically not utilized at the patient's bedside, though protocols do exist for its utility in a clinical setting [29]. Based on the minimal adverse events from trials on massage therapy to treat pain, it is reasonable for patients who choose to pursue it, given their understanding that its researched efficacy is only in short-term follow-up [30].

Aromatherapy

Aromatherapy is an ancient practice that utilizes aromatic materials for improved psychological and/or physical well-being. It is usually from an essential oil derived from a plant source. It can be done by the patient themselves by simply inhaling the scent of an essential oil or rubbing it onto the surface of their skin. The efficacy of aromatherapy in reducing perceived pain in a research setting has been mixed based on limited sample size, context of use, conjunctive use of massage, type of oil, and type of pain studied. It has shown to have a transient reduction in pain rating, but more studies need to be done on the long-term benefit [31]. A meta-analysis of 12 studies determined that aromatherapy has been shown to reduce pain. Namely, aromatherapy showed the most potential in reducing post-operative and obstetrical and gynecological pain [32].

Care should be taken in using aromatherapy as an adjunctive therapy considering the potential for adverse reactions to the essential oils used, including phototoxicity and dermatitis [33]. Patients should be aware of the source of essential oils, both the plant source and the manufacturer, given the variation of physiologic of effects of the compounds present and the lack of rigorous regulation compared to pharmaceutical medications. Considering the risks discussed, aromatherapy is a cost-effective tool that usually requires little oversight in application.

5 Summary

Behavioral and complementary interventions for chronic and acute pain are well-established as stand-alone or adjunct therapies. Many of these have been demonstrated to be effective, safe, and cost-effective at the bedside and can play an important role in multimodal pain control. Others have less evidence to support their use in this setting, but their success in other areas suggests them as valid. The development and prevalence of behavioral and complementary therapies are likely to increase as more non-opioid solutions to pain control are sought. This will occur along several tracks including awareness, training, research, and reimbursement. Technology will play a role as virtual-reality relaxation programs and internet-delivered pain-coping skills training (PCST) develop [11].

References

1. Songer D. Psychotherapeutic approaches in the treatment of pain. Psychiatry. 2005;2(5):19–24. PubMed PMID: 21152145; PubMed Central PMCID: PMC3000182.
2. Argoff C. Mechanisms of pain transmission and pharmacologic management. Curr Med Res Opin. 2011;27(10):2019–31. https://doi.org/10.1185/03007995.2011.614934. Epub 2011 Sep 14. Review. PubMed PMID: 21916528.
3. Turk D, Meichenbaum D, Genest M. Pain and behavioral medicine: a cognitive-behavioral perspective. New York: Guilford Press; 1983.
4. Tajerian M, Clark JD. Nonpharmacological interventions in targeting pain-related brain plasticity. Neural Plast. 2017;2017:2038573. https://doi.org/10.1155/2017/2038573. Epub 2017 Feb 16. PubMed PMID: 28299206; PubMed Central PMCID: PMC5337367.
5. Myerscough R. Chapter 17. Role of clinical psychologist.
6. Chou R, Gordon DB, de Leon-Casasola OA, Rosenberg JM, Bickler S, Brennan T, Carter T, Cassidy CL, Chittenden EH, Degenhardt E, Griffith S, Manworren R, McCarberg B, Montgomery R, Murphy J, Perkal MF, Suresh S, Sluka K, Strassels S, Thirlby R, Viscusi E, Walco GA, Warner L, Weisman SJ, Wu CL. Management of postoperative pain: a clinical practice guideline from the American Pain Society, the American Society of Regional Anesthesia and Pain Medicine, and the American Society of Anesthesiologists' Committee on Regional Anesthesia, Executive Committee, and Administrative Council. J Pain. 2016;17(2):131–57. https://doi.org/10.1016/j.jpain.2015.12.008. PubMed PMID: 26827847.
7. Sakamoto JT, Ward HB, Vissoci JRN, Eucker SA. Are nonpharmacologic pain interventions effective at reducing pain in adult patients visiting the emergency department? A systematic review and meta-analysis. Acad Emerg Med. 2018; https://doi.org/10.1111/acem.13411. PubMed PMID: 29543359.
8. Mushkat J. Chapter 3. Psychological and social markers of chronic pain.
9. Hamlin AS, Robertson TM. Pain and complementary therapies. Crit Care Nurs Clin North Am. 2017;29(4):449–60. https://doi.org/10.1016/j.cnc.2017.08.005. Epub 2017 Sep 20. Review. PubMed PMID: 29107307.
10. Schoomaker E, Buckenmaier C III. Call to action: "if not now, when? If not you, who?". Pain Med. 2014;15(Suppl 1):S4–6. https://doi.org/10.1111/pme.12385. PubMed PMID: 24734858.
11. Tick H, Nielsen A, Pelletier KR, Bonakdar R, Simmons S, Glick R, Ratner E, Lemmon RL, Wayne P, Zador V. Evidence-based nonpharmacologic strategies for comprehensive pain care: the Consortium Pain Task Force white paper. Explore (NY). 2018;14(3):177–211. https://doi.org/10.1016/j.explore.2018.02.001. Epub 2018 Mar 1. PubMed PMID: 29735382.
12. Oliveira A, Gevirtz R, Hubbard D. A psycho-educational video used in the emergency department provides effective treatment for whiplash injuries. Spine (Phila Pa 1976). 2006;31(15):1652–7. https://doi.org/10.1097/01.brs.0000224172.45828.e3. PubMed PMID: 16816758.
13. Cole LC, LoBiondo-Wood G. Music as an adjuvant therapy in control of pain and symptoms in hospitalized adults: a systematic review. Pain Manag Nurs. 2014;15(1):406–25.
14. Bernatzky G, Presch M, Anderson M, Panksepp J. Emotional foundations of music as a non-pharmacological pain management tool in modern medicine. Neurosci Biobehav Rev. 2011;35(9):1989–99. https://doi.org/10.1016/j.neubiorev.2011.06.005. Epub 2011 Jun 16. Review. PubMed PMID: 21704068.
15. Poulsen MJ, Coto J. Nursing music protocol and postoperative pain. Pain Manag Nurs. 2018;19(2):172–6. https://doi.org/10.1016/j.pmn.2017.09.003. Epub 2017 Nov 16. Review. PubMed PMID: 29153918.
16. Ennis G, Kirshbaum M, Waheed N. The beneficial attributes of visual art-making in cancer care: an integrative review. Eur J Cancer Care (Engl). 2018;27(1) https://doi.org/10.1111/ecc.12663. Epub 2017 Feb 21. Review. PubMed PMID: 28220543.
17. Felix MMDS, Ferreira MBG, da Cruz LF, Barbosa MH. Relaxation therapy with guided imagery for postoperative pain management: an integrative review. Pain Manag Nurs.

2019;20(1):3–9. https://doi.org/10.1016/j.pmn.2017.10.014. Epub 2017 Dec 15. Review. PubMed PMID: 29249618.
18. Carpenter JJ, Hines SH, Lan VM. Guided imagery for pain management in postoperative orthopedic patients: an integrative literature review. J Holist Nurs. 2017;35(4):342–51. https://doi.org/10.1177/0898010116675462. Epub 2016 Oct 23. Review. PubMed PMID: 30208778.
19. Busch V, Magerl W, Kern U, et al. The effect of deep and slow breathing on pain perception, autonomic activity, and mood processing—an experimental study. Pain Med. 2012;13(2):215–28.
20. Goyal M, Singh S, Sibinga EM, Gould NF, Rowland-Seymour A, Sharma R, Berger Z, Sleicher D, Maron DD, Shihab HM, Ranasinghe PD, Linn S, Saha S, Bass EB, Haythornthwaite JA. Meditation programs for psychological stress and well-being: a systematic review and meta-analysis. JAMA Intern Med. 2014;174(3):357–68. https://doi.org/10.1001/jamainternmed.2013.13018. Pubmed PMID: 24395196.
21. Cherkin DC, Sherman KJ, Balderson BH, Cook AJ, Anderson ML, Hawkes RJ, Hansen KE, Turner JA. Effect of mindfulness-based stress reduction vs cognitive behavioral therapy or usual care on back pain and functional limitations in adults with chronic low back pain: a randomized clinical trial. JAMA. 2016;315(12):1240–9. https://doi.org/10.1001/jama.2016.2323. PMID: 27002445.
22. Morone NE, Greco CM, Moore CG, Rollman BL, Lane B, Morrow LA, Glynn NW, Weiner DK. A mind-body program for older adults with chronic low back pain: a randomized clinical trial. JAMA Intern Med. 2016;176(3):329–37. https://doi.org/10.1001/jamainternmed.2015.8033. PubMed PMID: 26903081.
23. Pendry P, Carr AM, Vandagriff JL, Gee NR. Incorporating human–animal interaction into academic stress management programs: effects on typical and at-risk college students' executive function. AERA Open. 2021; https://doi.org/10.1177/23328584211011612.
24. Olsen C, Pedersen I, Bergland A, Enders-Slegers MJ, Patil G, Ihlebaek C. Effect of animal-assisted interventions on depression, agitation and quality of life in nursing home residents suffering from cognitive impairment or dementia: a cluster randomized controlled trial. Int J Geriatr Psychiatry. 2016;31(12):1312–21. https://doi.org/10.1002/gps.4436. Epub 2016 Jan 25. PubMed PMID: 26807956.
25. Lundqvist M, Carlsson P, Sjödahl R, Theodorsson E, Levin LÅ. Patient benefit of dog-assisted interventions in health care: a systematic review. BMC Complement Altern Med. 2017;17(1):358. https://doi.org/10.1186/s12906-017-1844-7. PubMed PMID: 28693538.
26. Billot M, Daycard M, Wood C, Tchalla A. Reiki therapy for pain, anxiety and quality of life. BMJ Support Palliat Care. 2019;9(4):434–8. https://doi.org/10.1136/bmjspcare-2019-001775. Epub 2019 Apr 4. PubMed PMID: 30948444.
27. Frey Law LA, Evans S, Knudtson J, Nus S, Scholl K, Sluka KA. Massage reduces pain perception and hyperalgesia in experimental muscle pain: a randomized, controlled trial. J Pain. 2008;9(8):714–21. https://doi.org/10.1016/j.jpain.2008.03.009. Epub 2008 May 2. PubMed PMID: 18455480.
28. Chatchawan U, Jarasrungsichol K, Yamauchi J. Immediate effects of self-Thai foot massage on skin blood flow, skin temperature, and range of motion of the foot and ankle in type 2 diabetic patients. J Altern Complement Med. 2020;26(6):491–500. https://doi.org/10.1089/acm.2019.0328. Epub 2020 Apr 28. PubMed PMID: 32349513.
29. Dreyer NE, Cutshall SM, Huebner M, Foss DM, Lovely JK, Bauer BA, Cima RR. Effect of massage therapy on pain, anxiety, relaxation, and tension after colorectal surgery: a randomized study. Complement Ther Clin Pract. 2015;21(3):154–9. https://doi.org/10.1016/j.ctcp.2015.06.004. Epub 2015 Jun 12. PubMed PMID: 26256133.
30. Furlan AD, Giraldo M, Baskwill A, Irvin E, Imamura M. Massage for low-back pain. Cochrane Database Syst Rev. 2015;2015(9):CD001929. https://doi.org/10.1002/14651858.CD001929.pub3. PubMed PMID: 26329399.

31. Cassileth BR, Vickers AJ. Massage therapy for symptom control: outcome study at a major cancer center. J Pain Symptom Manage. 2004;28(3):244–9. https://doi.org/10.1016/j.jpainsymman.2003.12.016. PubMed PMID: 15336336.
32. Lakhan SE, Sheafer H, Tepper D. The effectiveness of aromatherapy in reducing pain: a systematic review and meta-analysis. Pain Res Treat. 2016;2016:8158693. https://doi.org/10.1155/2016/8158693. Epub 2016 Dec 14. PubMed PMID: 28070420.
33. Farrar AJ, Farrar FC. Clinical aromatherapy. Nurs Clin North Am. 2020;55(4):489–504. https://doi.org/10.1016/j.cnur.2020.06.015. Epub 2020 Sep 28. PubMed PMID: 33131627.

Further Reading

International Association for the Study of Pain. https://www.iasp-pain.org/PatientResources?navItemNumber=678. Assessed 14 Jan 2022.

The American Holistic Nurses Association. Pain relief tools for patients & self-care. https://www.ahna.org/Home/Resources/Holistic-Pain-Tools. Assessed 14 Jan 2022.

The American Psychological Association. https://www.apa.org/helpcenter/pain-management. Assessed 14 Jan 2022.

Patient Safety Considerations for Bedside Interventions

Nicholas Alvey and Narayana Varhabhatla

Essential Concepts

- The primary concern of bedside procedures is to avoid doing any harm to the patient while providing relief from pain.
- Understanding the anatomy of the procedure being done is paramount. Understanding the adjacent structures can help to diagnose complications if they arise.
- Knowing the potential complications unique to each procedure can help the injecting physician respond quickly should a complication arise.
- In a busy pain practice, it is easy to skip simple steps such as universal protocol, time out, and meticulous antisepsis. But these are critical in keeping the physician and the patient safe.

1 Overview

Keeping patients safe and avoiding complications are critical goals when performing bedside interventional procedures [1]. Knowing the patient, pertinent anatomy, indications for the procedure, and doing procedures with the most up-to-date techniques are critical for patient safety. This chapter reviews aspects of patient safety that are most pertinent to bedside interventions.

N. Alvey · N. Varhabhatla (✉)
Department of Anesthesiology, University of Colorado Medical Center, Aurora, CO, USA
e-mail: Nicholas.alvey@usap.com; Narayana.varhabhatla@cuanschutz.edu

D. Souza et al. (eds.), *Bedside Pain Management Interventions*,
https://doi.org/10.1007/978-3-031-11188-4_10

2 Procedure Preparation

Preparation is key to safety, and each clinic's process should be standardized as much as possible to minimize the possibility of missing critical steps.

Informed Consent

The patient should have a clear understanding of the procedure they are having done, what it entails, and the potential risks, benefits and alternatives [2]. Barriers to getting an appropriate consent may include language issues, health literacy, and the use of medical terminology [3, 4]. An appropriate consent may require having a medical interpreter, eliminating medical jargon, allowing ample time for patient questions, and ensuring patient understanding before obtaining the patient's signature [5].

The Universal Protocol

Pain clinics tend to move at a fast pace and it is critical to follow the Universal Protocol adopted by JHACO to avoid errors of wrong site, wrong procedure, and wrong patient [6]. Just before starting the procedure, the patient's name, procedure being done, side of the procedure, and matching information on the consent should be confirmed. This process was initially developed to avoid surgical errors, but the same concerns apply to bedside procedures. It is not known the rate at which these errors occur during bedside procedures, but the risk can be minimized by following the Universal Protocol every time [7].

Hand Hygiene

Hand hygiene can include handwashing with an antiseptic wash, alcohol-based hand rubs, or surgical hand wash [8, 9]. For alcohol-based rubs to be effective the solution must contact all surfaces of the hand. For handwashing with soap and water, hands should be rubbed vigorously together for 15 s after the application of soap under lukewarm water, then dried completely [8]. Before a bedside procedure, an alcohol-based hand rub should be used before wearing gloves. An alcohol-based hand rub should then be used again after removing gloves at the end of the procedure and again before contact with the next patient [9].

Procedure Site Antisepsis

Procedure site and skin antisepsis are critical for preventing surgical and procedure site infections. The most common agents employed for skin antisepsis are chlorhexidine gluconate and iodophors solutions in either alcohol-based or aqueous-based solvents [10]. Alcohol-based compounds are superior to aqueous-based ones [11]. The only exception would be if the procedure were to occur on a mucosal surface in which case the only safe solution to use is an aqueous-based iodophor [11].

3 Adverse Events During Bedside Procedures

All procedures carry a risk of adverse events, thus all clinicians performing procedures must have deep knowledge and understanding of the specific adverse events for each procedure.

Provider Needlestick

The National Institute for Occupational Safety and Health (NIOSH) estimates that between 600,000 and 800,000 needle stick injuries occur every year [12]. The estimated seroconversion rate after a needlestick injury from an infected patient is approximately 30% with HBV, 1.8% with HCV, and 0.3% with HIV [13]. Recapping a used needle, transferring body fluid between containers, and not disposing of used needles in proper storage containers are the most common times when a needle stick injury occurs.

Both the source patient and the employee should be tested for HBC, HCV, and HIV, with their consent. Post-exposure prophylaxis for HBV and HIV may be needed [13].

Infection

There are no specific studies on the risk of infection in bedside pain procedures. A survey by Surgical Outcomes Information Exchange in 2010 of pain management clinics at ASC's reported no infections from around the country. This may be due to the minimally invasive nature of most bedside procedures. However, universal precautions and proper antisepsis should always be followed.

Peripheral Nerve Injury

Peripheral nerve injury after nerve blocks can be divided into mechanical or traumatic injury from the procedure (such as intraneural injection), toxic injury from the injected medication (as with highly concentrated solutions), and ischemic injury from vascular supply disruption to the nerve [14, 15]. The most significant factors for the risk of nerve injury are pre-existing nerve damage, location of the needle tip at the time of injection as well as the opening injection pressure [16].

Multiple steps can be taken to help prevent peripheral nerve injury. Ultrasound can show the presence of intra-neural injection but has not been shown consistently to reduce the incidence of peripheral nerve injury [15]. Longer bevel and wider diameter needles are more likely to cause a nerve injury [15]. Finally, preexisting peripheral neuropathy or spinal canal stenosis and procedure positioning can also increase the risk of a peripheral nerve injury [17]. If the patient reports paresthesia or intense pain with injection, the injection needs to be stopped and the needle should be adjusted even if the ultrasound picture looks appropriate. The patient is the first and best indicator of an intra-neural injection.

Pneumothorax

Procedures done in the thoracic region carry a risk of pneumothorax. These include intercostal nerve blocks, trigger point injections, PECS blocks, serratus plane blocks, and brachial plexus blocks via the supraclavicular approach. Before the use of ultrasound technology, the incidence of pneumothorax from these blocks was estimated as high as 6%. However, the use of ultrasound has reduced the incidence to 0.06%, a 100-fold reduction [18]. Skillful ultrasound guidance is key, and the needle should be seen clearly and accurately during the entire procedure to avoid causing a pneumothorax.

Patients reporting dyspnea and nothing evidence of hypoxia after a thoracic procedure should be evaluated. 100% oxygen should be administered and a chest radiograph obtained. Most can be treated conservatively, but more severe cases may require a chest tube placement, hospitalization, and potential ICU stay.

Vascular Injection and LAST

Local Anesthetic Systemic Toxicity, or LAST, can occur from a vascular injection of local anesthetic. The American Society of Regional Anesthesia provides updated practice advisories and checklists for suspected LAST [19]. LAST should be suspected in any patient with acute neurologic changes and/or hemodynamic instability following the injection of a local anesthetic. There are no measures to prevent LAST. Ultrasound can reduce the risk, but doesn't eliminate it. To minimize the risk, use the lowest effective dose of local and inject incrementally. Aspiration carries an approximately 2% false-negative rate, so direct visualization on ultrasound may be the most effective way.

Maintain the patient's airway with 100% oxygen and assisted ventilation if needed. Seizures should be treated with benzodiazepines. Hypotension and bradycardia should be treated. Advanced Cardiac Life Support (ACLS) may be necessary. Finally, a 20% lipid emulsion therapy should be initiated as soon as possible with a weight-based bolus followed by an infusion. In the case of ACLS measures, epinephrine doses should be reduced to less than 1 μg/kg. Propofol is not useful in LAST since it's more dilute than the lipid emulsion and it won't be as effective, and it may lead to further cardiovascular instability.

4 Conclusion

Interventional procedures carry an inherent risk that cannot be eliminated, but the risk can be minimized by cleaning one's hands and injection sites, being up-to-date on the latest and safest ways to perform procedures, and recognizing complications unique to each procedure.

References

1. Committee on Quality Health Care in America IoM. Crossing the quality chasm: a new health system for the 21st century. Washington, DC: National Press Academy; 2001.
2. Kinnersley P, Phillips, K, Savage, K, Kelly, MJ, Farrell, E, Morgan, B, Whistance, R, Lewis, V, Mann, MK, Stephens, BL, Blazeby, J, Elwyn, G, Edwards, AGK. Interventions to promote informed consent for patients undergoing surgical and other invasive healthcare procedures (Review). The Cochrane Library. 2013(7).
3. Schyve P. Language differences as a barrier to quality and safety in health care: the Joint Commission perspective. J Gen Intern Med. 2007;22(2):1.
4. Schenker Y, Fernandez A, Sudore R, Schillinger D. Interventions to improve patient comprehension in informed consent for medical and surgical procedures: a systematic review. Med Decis Making. 2011;31(1):23.
5. Schenker Y, Meisel A. Informed consent in clinical care: practical considerations in the effort to achieve ethical goals. JAMA. 2011;305(11):1.
6. The Joint Commission. Universal protocol. https://www.jointcommission.org/standards_information/up.aspx. Published 2019. Accessed 29 Nov 2019.
7. Kwaan M, Studdert DM, Zinner MJ, Gawande AA. Incidence, patterns, and prevention of wrong-site surgery. Arch Surg. 2006;141(4):5.
8. Healthcare Infection Control Practices Advisory Committee. Guideline for hand hygiene in health-care settings. MMWR. 2002;51(RR-16):48.
9. World Health Organization. Global guidelines on the prevention of surgical site infection. https://www.who.int/gpsc/ssi-prevention-guidelines/en/. Published 2016. Accessed 29 Nov 2019.
10. Berrios-Torres S, Umscheid CA, Bratzler DW, Leas B, Stone EC, Kelz RR, et al. Centers for Disease Control and Prevention guideline for the prevention of surgical site infection, 2017. JAMA Surg. 2017;152(8):8.
11. Hemani M, Lepor H. Skin preparation for the prevention of surgical site infection: which agent is best? Rev Urol. 2009;11(4):6.
12. US Public Health Service. Updated U.S. Public Health Service guidelines for the management of occupational exposures to HBV, HCV, and HIV and recommendations for postexposure prophylaxis. MMWR. 2001;50(RR11):42.
13. Center for Disease Control. Updated guidelines for antiretroviral postexposure prophylaxis after sexual, injection drug use, or other nonoccupational exposure to HIV—United States, 2016. https://www.cdc.gov/hiv/pdf/programresources/cdc-hiv-npep-guidelines.pdf. Published 2016. Accessed 29 Nov 2019.
14. Hogan Q. Pathophysiology of peripheral nerve injury during regional anesthesia. Reg Anesth Pain Med. 2008;33(5):7.
15. Brull R, Hadzic A, Reina MA, Barrington MJ. Pathophysiology and etiology of nerve injury following peripheral nerve blockade. Reg Anesth Pain Med. 2015;40(5):12.
16. Steinfeldt T, Nimphius W, Werner T, Vassiliou T, Kill C, Karakas E, Wulf H, Graf J. Nerve injury by needle nerve perforation in regional anaesthesia: does size matter? Br J Anaesth. 2010;104(2):9.

17. Hebl J, Kopp SL, Schroeder DR, Horlocker TT. Neurologic complications after neuraxial anesthesia or analgesia in patients with preexisting peripheral sensorimotor neuropathy or diabetic polyneuropathy. Anesth Analg. 2006;103(5):6.
18. Gauss A, Tugtekin I, Georgieff M, Dinse-Lambracht A, Keipke D, Gorsewski G. Incidence of clinically symptomatic pneumothorax in ultrasound-guided infraclavicular and supraclavicular brachial plexus block. Anaesthesia. 2014;69(4):10.
19. Neal J, Barrington MJ, Fettiplace MR, Gitman M, Memtsoudis SG, Mörwald EE, Rubin DS, Weinberg G. The Third American Society of Regional Anesthesia and Pain Medicine practice advisory on local anesthetic systemic toxicity: executive summary 2017. Reg Anesth Pain Med. 2018;43(2):11.

Further Reading

Morello RT, Lowthian JA, Barker AL, McGinnes R, Dunt D, Brand C. Strategies for improving patient safety culture in hospitals: a systematic review. BMJ Qual Saf. 2013;22(1):11–8. https://doi.org/10.1136/bmjqs-2011-000582. Epub 2012 Jul 31. PMID: 22849965.

Part II

Technology and Tools for Bedside Interventions

Imaging Vs Landmark Techniques for Bedside Interventions: Which Modality to Choose

Robert P. Owens, Maged Guirguis, Gassan Chaiban, and Yashar Eshraghi

Essential Concepts

- Most bedside pain procedures can be done with or without image guidance.
- Imaging modalities for pain management interventions include ultrasound, fluoroscopy, or computed tomography, however only ultrasound-guided procedures can be performed at the bedside. Therefore it is the imaging modality of choice for bedside procedures.
- Research identifying guidance techniques and which modality to choose is largely procedure-specific.
- Practitioner experience, cost, time, and efficacy are all factors that should be considered when planning bedside pain procedures.

R. P. Owens
Southeast Louisiana VA Healthcare System, New Orleans, LA, USA

Department of Medicine, Section of Physical Medicine and Rehabilitation, LSU Health Sciences Center, New Orleans, LA, USA
e-mail: Rowen3@lsuhsc.edu

M. Guirguis
Ochsner Clinic, New Orleans, LA, USA
e-mail: maged.guirguis@ochsner.org

G. Chaiban
Allied Health, Lake Charles, LA, USA
e-mail: gassan.chaiban@ochsner.org; gassanchaiban@gmail.com

Y. Eshraghi (✉)
Ochsner Clinic, New Orleans, LA, USA

Department of Anesthesiology and Critical Care Medicine, Ochsner Health System University of Queensland Ochsner Medical School, Louisiana State University School of Medicine, New Orleans, LA, USA
e-mail: yashar.eshraghi@ochsner.org

D. Souza et al. (eds.), *Bedside Pain Management Interventions*,
https://doi.org/10.1007/978-3-031-11188-4_11

1 Overview

Interventional procedures at the bedside to treat chronic pain have evolved significantly in the past century, and like many other aspects of medicine, these interventions are evolving every year. The improvement in imaging guidance technologies is responsible for much of the evolution in interventional pain medicine. The advent of fluoroscopy ushered in an era of more accurate and safe interventional procedures. Later, computed tomography (CT) and then ultrasound were adopted by pain specialists. Ultrasound is now increasingly used for many bedside pain interventions. In the modern era, pain medicine practitioners must weigh the benefits and drawbacks of utilizing imaging guidance for bedside procedures as an alternative to using time-honored anatomic landmark guidance. The available research on efficacy and outcomes is particularly important in guiding strategy.

2 Available Imaging Modalities

Fluoroscopy is currently the most widely used technology practitioners employ for interventional pain procedures [1]. Fluoroscopy allows clear images in real-time of bony anatomy to allow accurate needle or device placement. The main disadvantage is the exposure of the patient and physician to ionizing radiation. In addition, soft tissues are not well visualized with fluoroscopy. Computed tomography (CT) is also utilized by some pain medicine practitioners. CT allows cross-sectional imaging of bone and soft tissue but requires even more ionizing radiation to produce images and is not as widely available. Ultrasound is the most recently developed imaging modality that is increasingly used for pain procedures. Interest in using ultrasound in place of fluoroscopy for many interventional pain management procedures has grown significantly in recent years [2]. The portability of ultrasound imaging makes it attractive for bedside use. Ultrasound allows imaging of soft tissue including muscle, tendon, ligament, nerves, and blood vessels. It can produce real-time images of needles and injectate, and there is no radiation exposure or other patient risk. Ultrasound is limited when imaging bone and structures deep to the bone since sound waves are not able to penetrate dense structures. It is also limited when trying to image deep structures or tissue, as there is image degradation from sonographic attenuation.

Prior to the development of these imaging technologies, all pain procedures were performed entirely by anatomic landmark-based guidance. These techniques utilize palpable anatomic landmarks to allow guidance of needles and medication. Currently, fluoroscopy remains the gold standard for all neuraxial procedures given its superior ability to define deep anatomy and reliability to detect possible intravascular injection [3]. In contrast to neuraxial procedures, using anatomic landmarks remains the first learned and primary technique for most performing peripheral procedures such as joint injections, tendon sheath injections, and some nerve blocks. The use of imaging for many bedside procedures then becomes an optional adjunct, and current research continues to emerge regarding pros and cons of using imaging for each specific procedure. Increased cost, increased time requirement, user dependent learning curve, and unnecessary complexity are often cited downsides of utilizing imaging modalities in place of anatomic landmark guidance for those bedside procedures.

3 Which Modality to Choose for Bedside Interventions

For non-spinal pain procedures, fluoroscopy is indicated at times, but most of these procedures can be performed at the bedside using either ultrasound guidance or anatomic landmark guidance. The evidence supporting use of imaging versus anatomic landmarks varies for each specific procedure. Available research evaluating increased cost, increased time, and the impact use of imaging has on efficacy varies widely amongst different types of procedures. The remaining portion of this chapter will focus on a discussion of the most commonly performed bedside pain procedures, with a specific discussion regarding imaging modalities for each type of procedure.

Shoulder Girdle Injections

When evaluating patients with chronic neck pain, shoulder pathology is frequently coincident. Thus, procedures to treat shoulder pain can be quite useful in a pain physician's practice. A review of current literature shows general favorability towards using ultrasound guidance for these injections. A 2015 review showed that acromioclavicular, biceps tendon sheath, and glenohumeral joint injections performed under ultrasound were significantly more accurate than anatomic landmark-based techniques [4]. Subacromial bursa injections using ultrasound were not found to be more accurate but did provide significantly improved pain relief and improvement in function compared to blind techniques [4]. Another study found that ultrasound-guided injections are the most cost-effective choice for steroid injection in patients with adhesive capsulitis [5] (Figs. 1 and 2).

Hip Injections

Similarly to coinciding shoulder pathology in neck pain, hip pathology can be a confounding factor in the workup and treatment of chronic low back pain. Hip joint injections were originally performed using anatomic landmark guidance, but in modern times they are performed almost exclusively with ultrasound or fluoroscopic guidance. Ultrasound-guided hip injections have been shown to be more accurate than blind techniques in a systematic review [6]. Byrd et al.'s study found that ultrasound-guided hip injections were associated with higher patient satisfaction scores and lower pain scores than fluoroscopic injections [7].

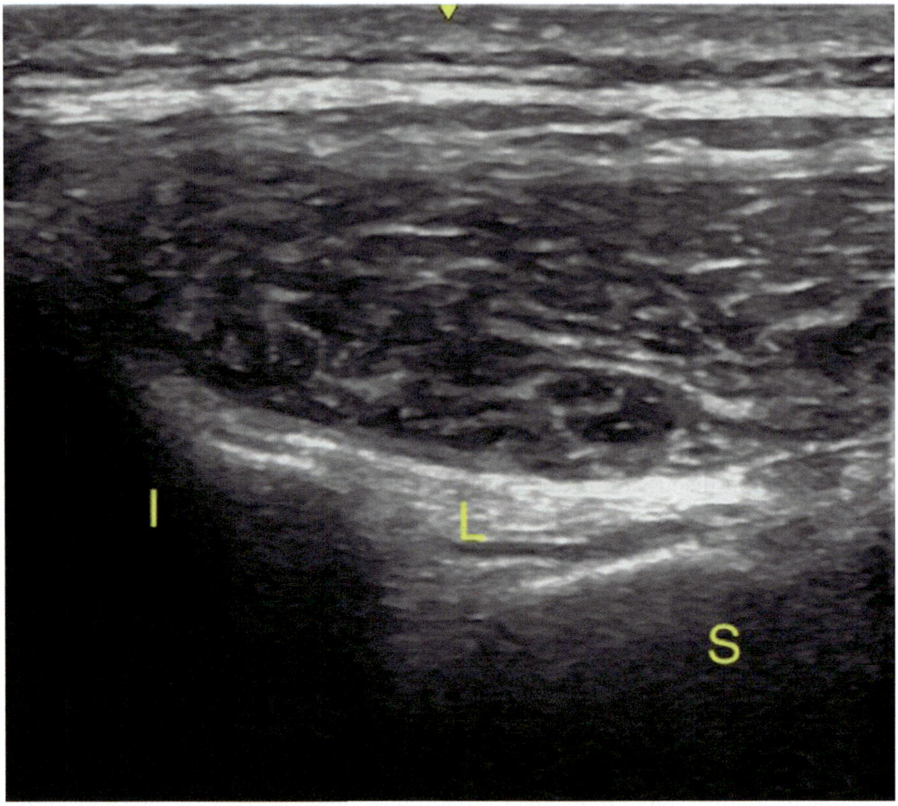

Fig. 1 Ultrasound image of a glenohumeral injection. The tip of the needle has entered the joint capsule just superficial to the labrum. *G* glenoid, *HH* humeral head, *L* labrum

Sacroiliac Joint Injections

Sacroiliac joint pain is believed to be responsible for 10–25% of low back pain [8]. Sacroiliac joint injections are performed for both diagnostic and therapeutic purposes. Fluoroscopic guidance has been the standard technique, since anatomic landmark based injections have reported accuracy rates for placing the needle into the sacroiliac joint of around 20% [9]. Ultrasound guided sacroiliac joint injections have been reported to have accuracy ranging from 40 to 90%, and are not considered superior to fluoroscopically guided injections by some studies [9]. Of note, however, is the study by Hartung et al. which established that there are no differences in efficacy whether the needle tip is peri-articular or intra-articular [10]. If true, this would seem to negate the need for absolute accuracy in placing the needle tip. Another study comparing outcomes between ultrasound guided SIJ injections and fluoroscopic SIJ injections did not identify any significant differences in pain relief and overall satisfaction [11]. Furthermore, Cohen et al. showed through a

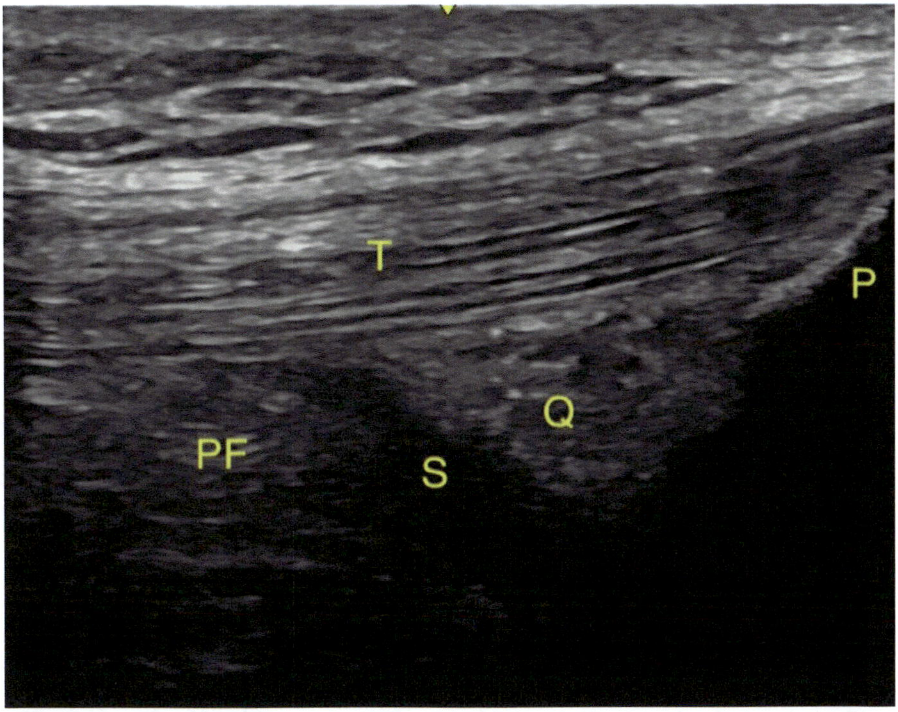

Fig. 2 The notoriously difficult to palpate acromioclavicular joint is easily visualized on ultrasound. *A* acromion, *C* clavicle

randomized control trial that when compared to fluoroscopic guided injections, landmark based injections were able to provide more immediate pain relief, with no difference in outcome at 1 month, and slight improvements in some outcome measures at 3 months for the fluoroscopic guided sacroiliac joint injections [12]. Detailed discussion in this study also discussed the much higher cost for fluoroscopic procedures, and relative cost benefit ratio [12] (Fig. 3).

Knee Injections

Peripheral joint osteoarthritis is a commonly encountered condition in the outpatient pain clinic setting. Knee joint injections have traditionally been performed with good efficacy using landmark-based techniques. Some providers began using fluoroscopic guidance for knee injections, and ultrasound has become popular more recently. In a 2010 review [13], ultrasound guidance for injections into the knee was found to increase accuracy from 77.8% to 95.8% when compared to landmark based techniques. In the same study, patients reported decreased procedural pain, better reduction in pain scores, and improved function when injections were performed

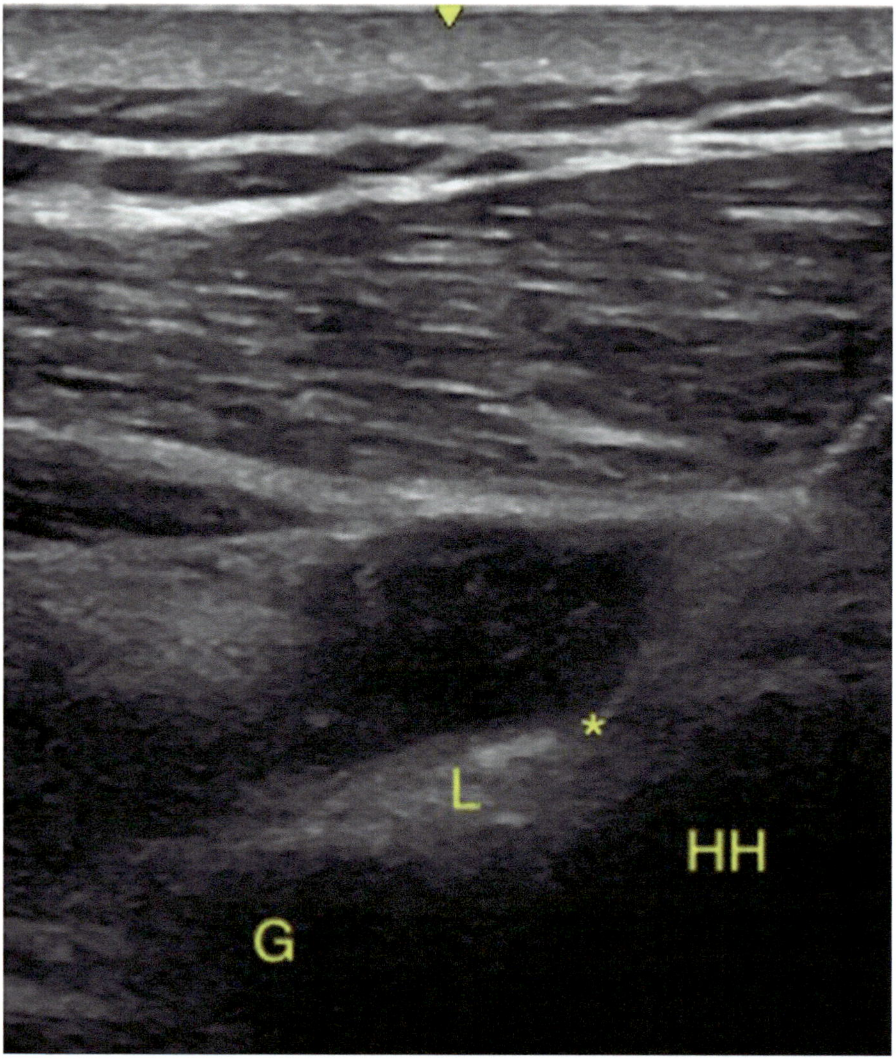

Fig. 3 Ultrasound visualization of the sacroiliac joint just distal to the posterior superior iliac spine. The sacroiliac ligament complex is clearly visible. *I* ilium, *S* sacrum, *L* sacroiliac ligament complex. [fileSIjoint02]

with ultrasound guidance [13]. A randomized controlled trial performed in 2018 reported significant improvements in pain and function of the subscales of the WOMAC scale at 6 and 12 weeks in patients who underwent ultrasound-guided viscosupplementation compared to anatomic landmark guided injection [14]. The authors postulated that use of ultrasound guidance may improve clinical outcomes for knee viscosupplementation (Fig. 4).

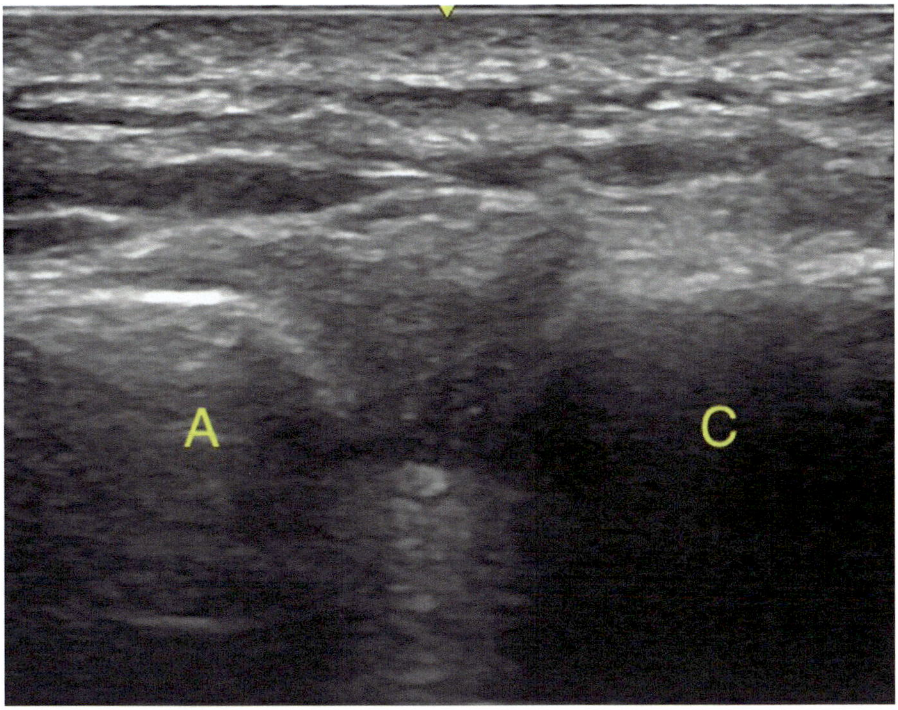

Fig. 4 Ultrasound visualization of the suprapatellar recess, an excellent target for knee injection since it is an extension of the knee joint. Image is in plane to the patellar ligament, with the patella on the right and the suprapatellar recess seen between the prefemoral and quadriceps fat pads. *PF* prefemoral fat pad, *Q* quadriceps fat pad, *P* patella, *T* quadriceps tendon, *S* suprapatellar recess

Greater Trochanteric Pain/Bursa Injections

Greater trochanteric pain syndrome often accompanies lumbosacral radiculopathies as well as chronic axial low back pain. In many cases, an injection at the greater trochanter is performed with anatomic landmark guidance, but some providers utilize fluoroscopic guidance to confirm needle placement. An important study found that fluoroscopic guided injections did not provide any improvement in outcome but dramatically increased cost when compared to landmark guided injections for greater trochanteric pain syndrome [15]. This study recommended fluoroscopic greater trochanteric injection only when patients have failed landmark guided injections and conservative treatment [15]. There is scant evidence evaluating ultrasound versus landmark guidance for greater trochanteric injections.

Piriformis Muscle Injections

Piriformis syndrome is a less common cause of buttock and leg pain, but it should remain in the differential as piriformis muscle injections can be highly successful. This procedure has frequently been performed under fluoroscopic guidance, but a notable cadaveric study performed by Finnoff et al. reported significantly more accurate needle placement with ultrasound guidance (95%) versus fluoroscopic guided (30%) [16]. Due to the deep nature of the muscle and the proximity to the sciatic nerve, anatomic landmark guided piriformis injections are generally not advised.

Lateral Femoral Cutaneous Nerve Block

Used for blockade of the lateral femoral cutaneous nerve in meralgia paresthetica, the traditional technique has utilized anatomic landmarks such as the anterior superior iliac spine to target the nerve. A study comparing ultrasound guidance versus anatomic landmark guidance for lateral femoral cutaneous nerve block in cadavers and volunteers found much higher accuracy of needle placement with ultrasound guidance (16 of 19 cadavers and 16 of 20 volunteers) versus landmark guidance (1 of 19 cadavers and 0 of 20 volunteers) [17].

Greater Occipital Nerve Block

Blockade of the Greater and/or Lesser Occipital Nerves are frequently performed by the pain practitioner for diagnostic and therapeutic treatment of headache. These can be performed with anatomic landmark guidance, with fluoroscopy, and with ultrasound. A 2013 randomized controlled trial by Finlayson et al. determined that both fluoroscopic and ultrasound guidance provided similar success rates, but that ultrasound guidance was associated with improved efficiency (decreased performance time and fewer needle passes) [18]. There are sparse studies comparing image guidance to anatomic guided injections, but some have suggested higher success rates with ultrasound guidance compared to none [19].

Ilioinguinal/Iliohypogastric Block

Ilioinguinal and Iliohypogastric nerve blocks can be helpful in evaluation and management of chronic groin and pelvic pain. Historically, landmark based approaches have been used. In regional anesthesia literature, failure rates of landmark based blocks is suggested to be as high as 30%. Ultrasound has been suggested to allow lower volumes of medication and improved efficacy and pain control in a paper by Willschke and colleagues [20].

Table 1 Advantages and disadvantages of using image guidance in comparison to anatomic landmark guidance

	Advantages	Disadvantages
Anatomic landmark guidance	• Low cost • Fast • No additional equipment required • No additional training needed	• Decreased accuracy • Decreased functional response in some studies
Ultrasound guidance	• Improved accuracy • Improved functional response in some studies	• Increased cost • Increased time requirement • User dependent learning curve • More complexity

Pudendal Nerve Block

Pudendal nerve blocks have been used for diagnosis and treatment of pelvic and perineal pain. Traditionally, landmark based techniques were utilized. Fluoroscopic and ultrasound guided approaches are now frequently used. A 2012 randomized controlled trial showed no difference in degree of neural blockade between ultrasound and fluoroscopically guidance, although ultrasound required significantly longer procedural time [21] (Table 1).

4 Conclusion

For non-spinal pain procedures including most bedside procedures, there is varying evidence specific to each procedure supporting use of image guidance with ultrasound as opposed to anatomic landmark guidance. While fluoroscopy allows advantage in some cases, most of the procedures discussed in this chapter can be safely performed at the bedside. Pain practitioners must make their own evaluation of many factors when choosing whether to use ultrasound guidance. Consideration should be given to efficacy of image guidance on outcome, cost, increased time requirement for image guidance, as well as user dependent experience and comfort level. Another important consideration is patient habitus, as image guidance for obese patients seems to be an obvious advantage. Future research should focus on outcomes rather than just accuracy when evaluating the use of image guidance for bedside pain procedures.

Clinical Pearls

- Ultrasound guidance can increase efficacy for some bedside procedures such as shoulder girdle, hip, knee, and piriformis injections. It has also been found to improve efficacy for lateral femoral cutaneous nerve, ilioinguinal, and iliohypogastric nerve blocks.
- For other procedures such as occipital nerve block, sacroiliac joint injection, and greater trochanteric injections, landmark guidance seems to be equally effective.
- The decision to utilize ultrasound guidance should be dependent on practitioner experience, as there is a steep learning curve.
- Ultrasound guidance may be especially helpful in patients with challenging body habitus.

References

1. Wang D. Image guidance technologies for interventional pain procedures. Curr Pain Headache Rep. 2018;22(1):6. https://doi.org/10.1007/s11916-018-0660-1.
2. Perrinea D, Votta-Velisa G, Borgeat A. Ultrasound indications for chronic pain: an update on the most recent evidence. Pain Med. 2016;29(5).
3. Perrinea D, Votta-Velisa G, Borgeat A. Ultrasound indications for chronic pain management: an update on the most recent evidence. Curr Opin Anesthesiol. 2016;29:600–5.
4. Aly A, Rajasekaran S, Ashworth N. Ultrasound-guided shoulder girdle injections are more accurate and more effective than landmark-guided injections: a systematic review and meta-analysis. Br J Sports Med. 2015;49:1042–9.
5. Gyftopoulos S, Abballe V, Virk M, Koo J, Gold H, Subhas N. Comparison between image-guided and landmark-based glenohumeral joint injections for the treatment of adhesive capsulitis: a cost-effectiveness study. Am J Radiol. 2018;210:1279–87.
6. Hoeber S, Aly A, Ashworth N, Rajasekaran S. Ultrasound-guided hip joint injections are mor accurate than lanmark-guided injections: a systematic review and meta-analysis. Br J Sports Med. 2016;50:392–6.
7. Byrd J, Potts E, Allison R, Jones K. Ultrasound-guided hip injections: a comparative study with fluoroscopy-guided injections. Arthroscopy. 2014;30(1):42–6.
8. Schwarzer A, Aprill C, Bogduk N. The sacroiliac joint in chronic low back pain. Spine. 1995;10(1):31–7.
9. Korbe S, Udoji E, Ness T, Udoji M. Ultrasound-guided interventional procedures for chronic pain management. Pain Manag. 2015;56:465–82.
10. Hartung W, Ross C, Straub R, Feuerbach S, Schölmerich J, Fleck M, Herold T. Ultrasound-guided sacroiliac joint injection in patients with established sacroiliitis: precise IA injection verified by MRI scanning does not predict clinical outcome. Rheumatology. 2010;49(8):1479–82.
11. Jee H, Lee J, Park K, Ahn J, Park Y. Ultrasound-guided versus fluoroscopy-guided sacroiliac joint intra-articular injections in the noninflammatory sacroiliac joint dysfunction: a prospective, randomized, single-blinded study. Arch Phys Med Rehabil. 2014;95(2):330–7.
12. Cohen S, Bicket M, Kurihara C, Griffith S, Fowler I, Jacobs M, Liu R, White M, Verdun A, Hari S, Fisher R, Pasquina P, Vorobeychik Y. Fluoroscopically guided vs landmark-guided sacroiliac joint injections: a randomized controlled study. Mayo Clin Proc. 2019;94(4):628–42.
13. Berkoff D, Miller L, Block J. Clinical utility of ultrasound guidance for intra-articular knee injections: a review. Clin Interv Aging. 2012;7:89–95.

14. Kianmehr N, Hasanzadeh A, Naderi F, Khajoie S, Haghighi A. A randomized blinded comparative study of clinical response to surface anatomy guided injection versus sonography guided injection of hyaloronic acid in patients with primary knee osteoarthritis. Int J Rheum Dis. 2018;21:134–9.
15. Cohen S, Strassels S, Foster L, Marvel J, Williams K, Crooks M, Gross A, Kurihara C, Nguyen C, Williams N. Comparison of fluoroscopically guided and blind corticosteroid injections for greater trochanteric pain syndrome: multicentre randomised controlled trial. Br Med J. 2009;338:b1088.
16. Finnoff JT, Hurdle MF, Smith J. Accuracy of ultrasound-guided versus fluoroscopically guided contrast-controlled piriformis injections: a cadaveric study. J Ultrasound Med. 2008;27:1157–63.
17. Tagliafico A, Serafini G, Lacelli F, Perrone N, Valsania V, Martinoli C. Ultrasound-guided treatment of meralgia paresthetica (lateral femoral cutaneous neuropathy): technical description and results of treatment in 20 consecutive patients. J Ultrasound Med. 2011;30:1341–6.
18. Finlayson R, Etheridge J, Vieira L, Gupta G, Tran D. A randomized comparison between ultrasound- and fluoroscopy-guided third occipital nerve block. Reg Anesth Pain Med. 2013;38(3):212–7.
19. Palamar D, Uluduz D, Saip S, Erden G, Unalan H, Akarirmak U. Ultrasound guided greater occipital nerve block: an efficient technique in chronic refractory migraine without aura? Pain Physician. 2015;18:153–62.
20. Willschke H, Marhofer P, Bosenber A, et al. Ultrasonograpy for ilioinguinal/iliohypogastric nerve blocks in children. Br J Anaesthesiol. 2005;95(2):226–30.
21. Bellingham F, Bhatia A, Chan C, Peng P. Randomized controlled trial comparing pudendal nerve block under utrasound and fluroscopic guidance. Reg Anesth Pain Med. 2012;37(3):262–6.

Further Reading

Jacobson J. Fundamentals of musculoskeletal ultrasound. Philadelphia: Elsevier; 2013.
Malanga G, Mautner K. Atlas of ultrasound guided musculoskeletal injections. New York: Springer; 2014.

Point-of-Care Ultrasound

Isaac A. Zoch, Mostafa Maita, William D. Kang, Emily A. Vail,
and Ameet Nagpal

Essential Concepts

- Medical ultrasound is crucial to bedside diagnostics, monitoring, resuscitation, screening, and procedural guidance.
- Compared to other imaging modalities, ultrasonography does not utilize ionizing radiation, is relatively cost-effective, and allows for quick visualization of anatomical structures.

I. A. Zoch
Department of Anesthesiology, UT Health San Antonio, San Antonio, TX, USA
e-mail: zoch@uthscsa.edu

M. Maita
Department of Anesthesiology, UT Health San Antonio, San Antonio, TX, USA

Department of Pain Management, Mayo Clinic Hospital, Phoenix, AZ, USA
e-mail: maita@uthscsa.edu; maita.mostafa@mayo.edu

W. D. Kang
Department of Anesthesiology, UT Health San Antonio, San Antonio, TX, USA

Department of Anesthesiology, University of Texas Health Science Center Houston, Houston, TX, USA
e-mail: william.d.kang@uth.tmc.edu

E. A. Vail
Department of Anesthesiology, UT Health San Antonio, San Antonio, TX, USA

Department of Anesthesiology & Critical Care, University of Pennsylvania Perelman School of Medicine, Philadelphia, PA, USA
e-mail: emily.vail@pennmedicine.upenn.edu

A. Nagpal (✉)
Department of Anesthesiology, UT Health San Antonio, San Antonio, TX, USA

Department of Orthopaedics & Physical Medicine, Medical University of South Carolina, Charleston, SC, USA
e-mail: nagpala@uthscsa.edu; nagpal@musc.edu

D. Souza et al. (eds.), *Bedside Pain Management Interventions*,
https://doi.org/10.1007/978-3-031-11188-4_12

- 3-D mechanical scanning offers the advantage of shorter imaging and reconstruction times and more accurate 3-D images. However, its bulkiness and weight sometimes make it inconvenient to use.
- During interventional procedures, needles may be advanced in one of two planes, (1) an in-plane (longitudinal) approach, where a needle is inserted parallel to the long axis of the transducer, and (2) an out-of-plane approach, in which the needle is directed perpendicular to the ultrasound beam.
- Ultrasound technology comes with several drawbacks, including but not limited to insufficient tissue windows, artifacts, and high cost of equipment.

1 Overview

Ultrasound is a widely used imaging modality in clinical medicine that allows for real-time anatomical visualization. The applications of ultrasound are extensive and valuable due to its portability, affordability, and flexibility. Advancements in ultrasound technology have produced high-end ultrasound machines that are easily transportable to the patient bedside. In addition, unlike other commonly used imaging modalities such as computed tomography, magnetic resonance imaging, and nuclear imaging, ultrasound does not utilize ionizing radiation, is relatively cost-effective, and allows for quick visualization of anatomical structures. Although ultrasound technology does have inherent limitations, the images acquired can provide immediate real-time guidance for clinical diagnosis and many interventional procedures.

The following chapter will focus on its portability and needle visualization in the context of bedside diagnostics and intervention.

2 Historical Aspects and Traditional Approaches

The history of ultrasound technology is based on the fundamental principles of the Doppler effect. These concepts were applied to build the first hydrophone during World War II-era when French physicist Paul Langevin refined the phenomenon of echolocation for underwater detection of submarines and navigation [1, 2]. During the 1950s, Donald and colleagues at the University of Glasgow introduced ultrasonography to the medical field as a diagnostic tool [3]. Early designs for more compact and affordable ultrasound machines were developed in the 1990s; however, they were hampered by poor image quality.

Further advances in ultrasound technology have propelled its regular use in bedside diagnostics and interventional pain practice [4]. Bedside POCUS is increasingly being used to facilitate accurate diagnoses, assist procedures, and triage patients in emergency settings. In addition, it offers a portable, inexpensive, and radiation-free method of diagnosis [5], and real-time visual guidance for minimally invasive interventional procedures [4].

3 Recent Developments

Portable ultrasound devices are not just used for diagnostic imaging but also aid with monitoring, resuscitation, screening, and procedural guidance. As these devices have become more portable in recent years, practitioners have increasingly incorporated their use in bedside interventions. Studies have documented numerous benefits when ultrasound is used for interventional procedures, including a reduction in systemic local anesthetic toxicity [6], recognition of abnormal anatomy, fewer block-related complications such as pneumothorax or a failed block [7], and shortened procedure times [8].

As ultrasound devices rapidly evolve to become smaller, more affordable, and more user-friendly, they expand opportunities for usage and teaching for multiple practitioners and trainees. A novel category of smaller handheld devices has recently emerged, providing increased portability and affordability [5]. These ultra-portable devices are lightweight, battery-powered, and growing increasingly affordable. Recent improvements in ultrasound technology include 2-D phased array transducers, 3-D real-time ultrasound, harmonic tissue imaging, and spatial compound imaging, all potentially offering improvements in diagnosis and treatment [4].

3-D ultrasound images are reconstructed using multiple acquired 1-D or 2-D images. The scanning technique must be rapid or gated to avoid motion artifact. Additionally, geometric distortions can occur in the 3-D image if the location and orientation of the 1-D or 2-D images are not accurately obtained. 3-D mechanical scanning offers the advantage of shorter imaging and reconstruction times, and more accurate 3-D images. However, the bulkiness and weight of 3-D ultrasound consoles reduce their portability and convenience [5].

Tissue harmonic imaging and spatial compound imaging are two recent innovations that have improved image resolution and have been available in most ultrasound units for the past decade. When an ultrasound pulse travels through tissues, the original wave shape becomes distorted. Harmonic frequencies are generated by the reflected echoes of different frequencies of many higher order harmonics. Harmonic imaging captures both the fundamental frequency and its secondary harmonic component to reduce artifact and clutter at the surface tissue. Harmonic imaging technology is especially beneficial for visualization of deep and complex anatomic structures, for which harmonic imaging can improve image resolution [4].

Spatial compound, or multibeam, imaging utilizes parallel beams oriented at different directions to image tissue multiple times. The average of these echoes is compounded to produce a single composite image with reduced levels of "clutter" and "noise" but improved contrast and margin definition, which can aid in needle visualization. This also helps to increase the lateral resolution and decrease the "graininess" of the image [4].

Table 1 Ultrasound-guided interventional pain injections

Neuraxial
• Intra-articular facet blocks/medial branch nerve blocks
• Epidural injections
Joints
• Elbow
• Hip
• Knees
• Sacroiliac
• Shoulder
• Wrist
Peripheral/other
• Stellate ganglion block
• Greater occipital nerve
• Branches of brachial plexus
• Branches of lumbosacral plexus
• Intercostal nerve
• Lateral femoral cutaneous nerve
• Suprascapular nerve
• Ilioinguinal nerve
• Iliohypogastric nerve
• Genitofemoral nerve

Traditionally, interventional pain specialists performed procedures using surface landmarks or imaging guidance from computational tomography, magnetic resonance imaging, or fluoroscopy. The use of ultrasound in interventional pain management has become increasingly popular, as practitioners favor its ease of use, lack of radiation exposure, and real-time visualization of anatomic structures, needle advancement, and spread of injectate. Interventional pain specialists have reported use of ultrasound-guidance for multiple procedures: these are summarized in Table 1.

Studies have demonstrated that ultrasound guidance is safer by bolstering a practitioner's ability to avoid intravascular injections as opposed to with fluoroscopy [4, 9]. Comparative effectiveness data with interventional pain procedures under ultrasound versus fluoroscopy are lacking [4, 9].

Ultrasound-guided interventional procedures may employ one of two approaches for needle insertion: guided and freehand [10]. With a guided needle insertion, a mechanical guide attached to the probe restricts the path of the needle, while the ultrasound screen displays its predicted path. Although the guided needle technique may provide greater precision of needle insertion, needle visualization may be limited in tissues with high echogenicity and artifact. Conversely, freehand needle insertion is more challenging but offers greater flexibility for needle insertion and manipulation.

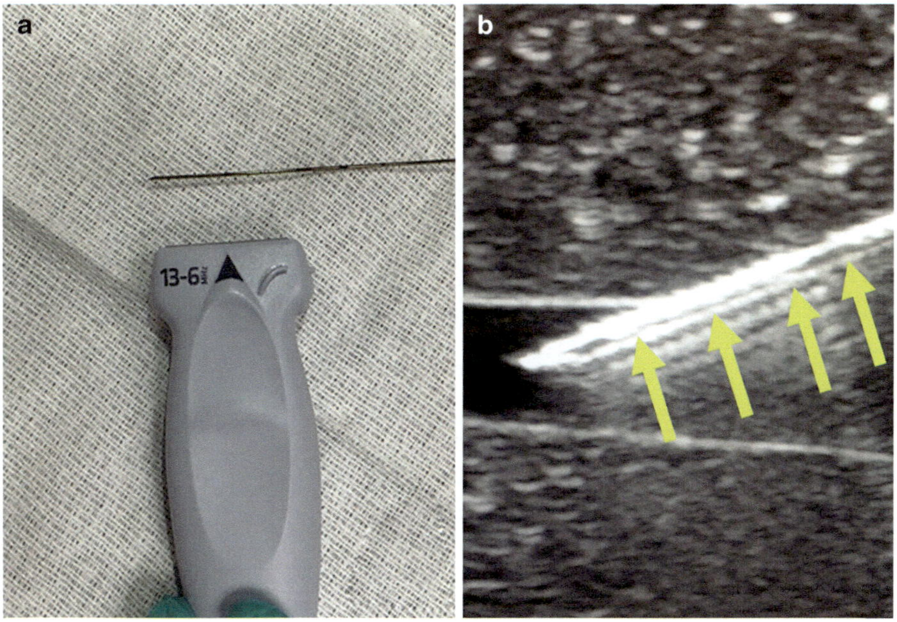

Fig. 1 In-plane approach for ultrasound-guided interventions. The needle is parallel to the probe, which is the in-plane (longitudinal) approach. (**a**) In the in-plane method, the needle is inserted lateral and parallel to the long axis of the transducer, allowing the clinician to visualize the movement of the needle without repositioning the ultrasound probe. (**b**) Ultrasonogram demonstrating the in-plane approach. Yellow arrows—needle shaft

Ultrasound-guided needle advancement may be performed in one of two orthogonal planes, (1) parallel to the ultrasound probe, which is the in-plane (longitudinal) approach and, (2) perpendicular to the probe (the out-of-plane approach). In the in-plane method, the needle is inserted lateral and parallel to the long axis of the transducer, allowing the clinician to visualize the movement of the needle without repositioning the ultrasound probe (Fig. 1). In an out-of-plane approach, the needle is directed perpendicular to the ultrasound probe at its midline, revealing a hyperechoic dot as the needle passes through the ultrasound beam (Fig. 2). In some instances, a procedure may be reasonably performed using both approaches; clinicians may favor one over the other because of personal experience, the location of the needle target in the ultrasound image, or the location of anatomic structures, such as blood vessels, in the path of the needle. Regardless of the approach used, the needle tip should be visualized at all times to minimize the risk of damage to adjacent tissues [11].

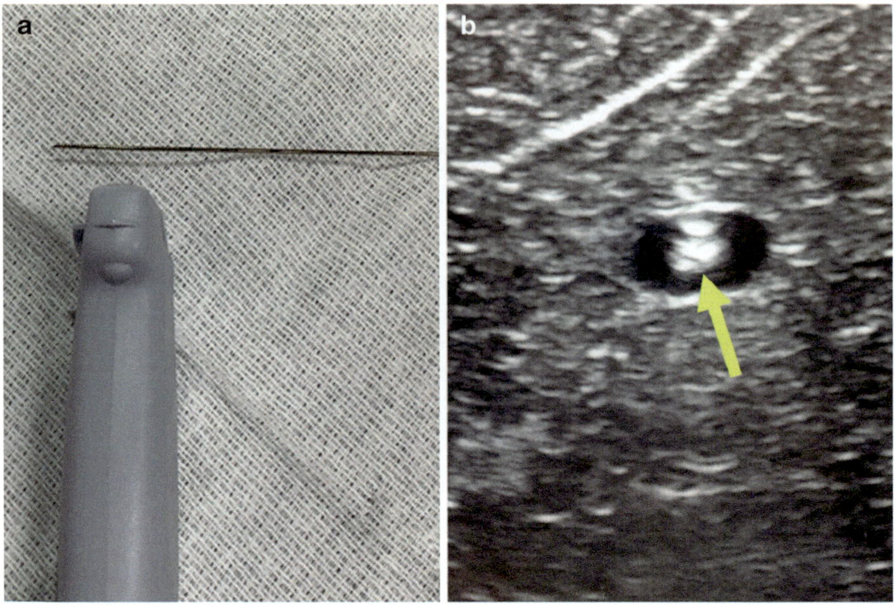

Fig. 2 Out-of-plane approach for ultrasound-guided interventions. In an out-of-plane approach, the needle is directed perpendicular to the ultrasound probe at its midline, revealing a hyperechoic dot as the needle passes through the ultrasound beam. Note that the fluid around the needle tip enhances the visualization. (**a**) In the out-of-plane method, the needle is inserted lateral and parallel to the long axis of the transducer, allowing the clinician to visualize the movement of the needle without repositioning the ultrasound probe. (**b**) Ultrasonogram demonstrating the out-of-plane approach. Yellow arrow—needle shaft. Note that the fluid around the needle tip enhances the visualization

4 Concerns and Drawbacks

Although ultrasound has several practical applications with advantages over other imaging modalities, clinicians should be aware of its limitations. These include but are not limited to the generation of 2-D images, variation in practitioner skill level, and presence of artifact. Measurements obtained using multiple 2-D images can lead to variable, and at times, inaccurate measurements [12]. The physical properties of ultrasound prevent accurate imaging of some body tissues and can generate significant visual artifacts including specular reflection, acoustic shadowing, and image refraction. As a result, the object's location in the displayed image can be misinterpreted and misrepresented, especially to an inexperienced sonographer. High-frequency ultrasound probes emit waves that generate images with superior axial resolution but have low penetrance, limiting their ability to image deeper structures. The opposite is true with low-frequency probes. Additionally, as an ultrasound pulse travels through tissues, the intensity can be attenuated by scattering, friction-like losses, and absorption through the conversion of the original mechanical energy into heat [4].

5 Conclusion and Future Directions

Modern ultrasound equipment is based on many of the same fundamental principles applied in the original devices used over 50 years ago [4]. In comparison to other imaging modalities, ultrasound is relatively inexpensive, portable, safe, and may be used for real-time procedural guidance. Continued improvements in image quality and resolution have expanded the use of ultrasound to many areas of medicine beyond traditional diagnostic imaging, particularly in regional anesthesia and pain medicine. Ultrasound technology has evolved into a safe imaging modality with both diagnostic and procedural utility. When comparing ultrasound to traditional imaging techniques, increased numbers of randomized controlled trials are still needed. Nonetheless, proceduralists recognize the safety and utility of ultrasound and have incorporated its use for many interventional procedures [4].

References

1. Campbell S. A short history of sonography in obstetrics and gynaecology. Facts Views Vis Obgyn. 2013;5(3):213–29.
2. Schellpfeffer MA. Ultrasound imaging in research and clinical medicine. Birth Defects Res C Embryo Today Rev. 2013;99(2):83–92.
3. Johnson G, Kirkpatrick AW, Gillman LM. Ultrasound in the surgical ICU: uses, abuses, and pitfalls. Curr Opin Crit Care. 2019;25(6):675–87.
4. Narouze SN. In: Narouze SN, editor. Atlas of ultrasound-guided procedures in interventional pain management. Springer; 2018. 325 p.
5. Moore C, Copel J. Point-of-care ultrasonography. N Engl J Med 364(8):749–57 (Feb 24). N Engl J Med. 2011;364:749–57.
6. Marhofer P, Schrogendorfer K, Wallner T, Koinig H, Mayer N, Kapral S. Ultrasonographic guidance reduces the amount of local anesthetic for 3-in-1 blocks. Reg Anesth Pain Med. 1998;23(6):584–8.
7. Marhofer P, Greher M, Kapral S. Ultrasound guidance in regional anaesthesia. Br J Anaesth. 2005;94(1):7–17.
8. Gray AT. Ultrasound-guided regional anesthesia: current state of the art. Anesthesiology. 2006;104(2):368–73, discussion 5A.
9. Narouze S, Peng PW. Ultrasound-guided interventional procedures in pain medicine: a review of anatomy, sonoanatomy, and procedures. Part II: axial structures. Reg Anesth Pain Med. 2010;35(4):386–96.
10. Arif M, Moelker A, van Walsum T. Needle tip visibility in 3D ultrasound images. Cardiovasc Intervent Radiol. 2018;41(1):145–52.
11. Jones CD, McGahan JP, Clark KJ. Color Doppler ultrasonographic detection of a vibrating needle system. J Ultrasound Med. 1997;16(4):269–74.
12. Suri JS. Advances in diagnostic and therapeutic ultrasound imaging. Artech House; 2008.

Further Reading

Campbell S. A short history of sonography in obstetrics and gynaecology. Facts Views Vis Obgyn. 2013;5(3):213–29.

Narouze SN. In: Narouze SN, editor. Atlas of ultrasound-guided procedures in interventional pain management. Springer; 2018. 325 p.

Moore C, Copel J. Point-of-care ultrasonography. N Engl J Med 364(8):749–57 (Feb 24). N Engl J Med. 2011;364:749–57.

Neuromodulation at the Bedside

Tuan Tang and Alaa Abd-Elsayed

Essential Concepts

- Non-invasive portable, inexpensive, and overall safe neuromodulation could be a reasonable pain management option at the bedside.
- Most of the techniques, including transcutaneous neurostimulation (TENS) are widely available and there are few barriers to its application.
- Exclusion criteria for candidacy for most of the neuromodulation techniques for bedside applications include (but are not limited to) pregnancy, recent head trauma, prior seizure history, or history of adverse side effects with transcutaneous neuromodulation.

1 Bedside Transcutaneous Electrical Nerve Stimulation

Overview

Transcutaneous Electrical Nerve Stimulation (TENS) is a non-invasive neuromodulatory technique that utilizes electrical currents delivered transcutaneously through electrodes to dermatomal sites or according to auricular therapy mobs for potential localized or systemic analgesia [1]. The main modalities of TENS include conventional TENS, which uses high-frequency, low-intensity electrical current to inhibit

T. Tang
University of Texas HSC at Houston, Houston, TX, USA

A. Abd-Elsayed (✉)
Chronic Pain Medicine, Anesthesiology Department, University of Wisconsin, Madison, WI, USA

D. Souza et al. (eds.), *Bedside Pain Management Interventions*,
https://doi.org/10.1007/978-3-031-11188-4_13

Table 1 Characteristics and mehanism of action of conventional and acupuncture-like TENS

	Characteristics[a]	Mechanism of action
Conventional TENS	• High-frequency (50–100 Hz) • Low-intensity • Small pulse width (50–200 μs)	Stimulate large diameter, low threshold non-noxious afferent (A-beta) in dermatomes, which inhibits the segmental pathway (via inactivation of nociceptors and sensitization in the central nervous system (CNS)
Acupuncture-like TENS	• Low-frequency (2–4 Hz) • High-intensity • Long pulse width (100–400 μs)	Stimulate small diameter, high threshold peripheral afferent (A-delta) fibers, which activates the inhibitory extrasegmental pathway (via activation of midbrain peri-aqueductal grey and rostral ventromedial medulla)

[a]Defined by The International Association for the Study of Pain (IASP)

the segmental pathway, and acupuncture-like TENS (ALTENS) which uses low-frequency, high-intensity electrical current to activate the inhibitory extrasegmental pathway [2]. In terms of clinical effectiveness, some randomized controlled trial publications have shown that TENS has greater pain relief for post-operative pain than placebos, particularly with high-frequency high-intensity stimulation; however early systematic reviews have not confirmed benefits [2–4]. Other considered indications explored have yielded weak evidence for labor pain, insufficient evidence for dysmenorrhea, and inconclusive evidence for chronic pain, therefore further investigation is warranted to verify any benefits of TENS [4–6] (Table 1).

Indications and Contraindications

Similar to other forms of neuromodulation, the indication for TENS therapy would be central pain symptoms however it is better fit to address localized central pain [7–9] (Fig. 1). Because of its cutaneous approach, TENS should not be used on open wounds, skin pathology including malignancies, nor non-sensate dermatomal areas affected by tactile allodynia and hyperesthesia. Important dangerous considerations for electrode placement location include HEENT (carotid sinus stimulation, laryngeal spasms, increase ocular pressure) and in the anterior and posterior chest (cardiac conduction abnormalities, pulmonary compromise via intercostal muscles overstimulation) [1, 3, 10]. Contraindications for electrotherapies such as TENS include cardiac pacemakers and implantable cardioverter-defibrillators, pregnancy and epilepsy, however TENS use can be considered in certain situations under professional supervision [9].

Equipment and Supplies

While many TENS kits exists with different variations and capacities, generally they contain: TENS unit (dual channel), two wires with a total of 4

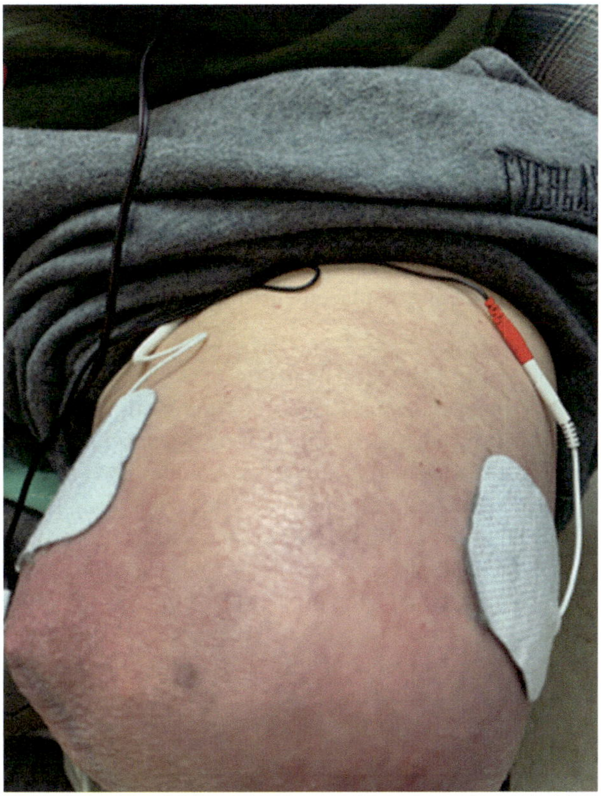

Fig. 1 Bedside transcutaneous neuromodulation procedure for the patient with intractable stump pain. The patient developed intractable lower extremity pain after the amputation. Reported more than 50% relief of his pain with transcutaneous electrical nerve stimulation (TENS)

connectors, four electrode patches, power source/batteries and a belt clip. The user can adjust pulse amplitude (mA), frequency (Hz), pulse width (μs), and pattern of current. Placement of the TENS device is dependent on the location of pain.

Technique

Electrodes should be placed on healthy skin without neuropathies on the dermatomes of interest. However, alternative placements can include larger proximal nerves.

After making sure the contact site is clean and dry, place the two sets of electrodes onto the specific pain site (e.g. neck pain, back pain) and attach the lead wires into the connectors and the TENS unit [9]. With a reliable power source such as batteries or outlet connection, initiate the TENS unit and input the desired settings. Since each device has different settings options, seek the manual or professional assistance in correctly managing the input. Patients can modify settings in accordance with their physician (Fig. 1).

Potential Complications and Adverse Effects

Potential use-dependent analgesic tolerance may occur. This may be offset by N-methyl-D-aspartate blockade, which may prevent tolerance of spinal opioid receptors [1, 4, 10]. Use of mixed frequencies (modulating between high-frequency and low-frequency bursts in the same session) or alternating frequencies (in different sessions) have been shown as a possible tolerance deterrent due to the simultaneous activation of mu-opioids and sigma-opioid receptors [6]. Severe adverse effects are rare with most common side effects reported as skin irritation and dermatitis at the electrode placement side.

Clinical and Technical Pearls

- Transcutaneous Electrical Nerve Stimulation (TENS) is a non-invasive, inexpensive technique that uses a portable, battery-powered pulse generator that is available over-the-counter and can be self-administered and self-titrated with minimal side effects and drug interactions.
- Its effect is often rapid in onset but short-term, requiring multiple and frequent sessions for chronic pain control.
- While there are no predictors of success for TENS, effective trials of TENS can be used to predict the success of dorsal column stimulation devices such as spinal cord stimulation (SSC) implants.

References

1. Verma N, Mudge JD, Kasole M, Chen RC, Blanz SL, Trevathan JK, et al. Auricular vagus neuromodulation—a systematic review on quality of evidence and clinical effects. Front Neurosci. 2021;15:664740. [cited 2022 Feb 5]. http://www.ncbi.nlm.nih.gov/pubmed/33994937.
2. Thuvarakan K, Zimmermann H, Mikkelsen MK, Gazerani P. Transcutaneous electrical nerve stimulation as a pain-relieving approach in labor pain: a systematic review and meta-analysis of randomized controlled trials. Neuromodulation. 2020;23(6):732–46.
3. Tirlapur SA, Vlismas A, Ball E, Khan KS. Nerve stimulation for chronic pelvic pain and bladder pain syndrome: a systematic review. Acta Obstet Gynecol Scand. 2013;92(8):881–7.
4. Hofmeister M, Memedovich A, Brown S, Saini M, Dowsett LE, Lorenzetti DL, et al. Effectiveness of neurostimulation technologies for the management of chronic pain: a systematic review. Neuromodulation. 2020;23(2):150–7.
5. Patel ABU, Weber V, Gourine AV, Ackland GL. The potential for autonomic neuromodulation to reduce perioperative complications and pain: a systematic review and meta-analysis. Br J Anaesth. 2022;128(1):135–49.
6. Zeng H, Pacheco-Barrios K, Cao Y, Li Y, Zhang J, Yang C, et al. Non-invasive neuromodulation effects on painful diabetic peripheral neuropathy: a systematic review and meta-analysis. Sci Rep. 2020;10(1):19184.
7. Cardinali A, Celini D, Chaplik M, Grasso E, Nemec EC. Efficacy of transcutaneous electrical nerve stimulation for postoperative pain, pulmonary function, and opioid consumption following cardiothoracic procedures: a systematic review. Neuromodulation. 2021;24(8):1439–50.

8. Mahran A, Baaklini G, Hassani D, Abolella HA, Safwat AS, Neudecker M, et al. Sacral neuromodulation treating chronic pelvic pain: a meta-analysis and systematic review of the literature. Int Urogynecol J. 2019;30(7):1023–35.
9. Wu LC, Weng PW, Chen CH, Huang YY, Tsuang YH, Chiang CJ. Literature review and meta-analysis of transcutaneous electrical nerve stimulation in treating chronic Back pain. Reg Anesth Pain Med. 2018;43(4):425–33.
10. Reuter U, McClure C, Liebler E, Pozo-Rosich P. Non-invasive neuromodulation for migraine and cluster headache: a systematic review of clinical trials. J Neurol Neurosurg Psychiatry. 2019;90(7):796–804.

Further Reading

DeSantana J, et al. Effectiveness of transcutaneous electrical nerve stimulation for treatment of hyperalgesia and pain. Curr Rheumatol Rep. 2008;10(6):492–9.

Johnson M. Transcutaneous electrical nerve stimulation: mechanisms, clinical application and evidence. Br J Pain. 2007;1(1):7–11.

Mendonca ME, et al. Transcranial DC stimulation in fibromyalgia: optimized cortical target supported by high-resolution computational models. J Pain. 2011;12(5):610–7.

Viscosupplementation for Osteoarthritic Pain

Russell R. Lambert and Steven B. Jackson

Essential Concepts

- Viscosupplementation can be used for pain secondary to the osteoarthritis of the knee.
- There are reports indicating the other large joints, joints including hip, shoulder, and ankle, as well as temporomandibular joints can be treated as well.
- Cross-linked formulations of HA with higher molecular weights are recommended
- Viscosupplementation is a cost-effective treatment of pain secondary to osteoarthritis.
- Clinical significance of symptomatic relief provided by viscosupplementation remains debated and must be evaluated on a case to case basis.

1 Overview

Viscosupplementation (VS) refers to the use of hyaluronic acid (HA) formulations as an injectable solution used to provide intra-articular pain relief. HA is a naturally occurring polysaccharide found within synovial fluid that has multiple functions including lubrication, "shock absorption", anti-inflammation, and even analgesia. Over the past 20 years, VS has gained significant notoriety as a nonsurgical treatment for knee osteoarthritis. Clinical benefits of VS have been described elsewhere including the hip and glenohumeral joints, and even in the treatment of temporomandibular dysfunctions [1–3].

R. R. Lambert (✉) · S. B. Jackson
Department of Orthopedic Surgery, Western Reserve Hospital, Cuyahoga Falls, OH, USA
e-mail: rlambert@altru.org; rlambert@westernreservehospital.org; sjackson@westernreservehospital.org

D. Souza et al. (eds.), *Bedside Pain Management Interventions*,
https://doi.org/10.1007/978-3-031-11188-4_14

From a clinician's perspective, VS can be offered and safely administered to patients with relative ease, utilizing basic technical skills with or without the use of additional imaging modalities. Fluoroscopy, ultrasound, and traditional injection techniques can be used to administer VS. While the clinical benefits continue to be investigated, current consensus statements suggest VS can be a safe non-operative form of treatment for patients complaining of joint pain.

2 Historical Aspects

The commercial development of VS has largely been marketed towards the treatment of knee osteoarthritis. In 1997, HA was approved in the United States as an intra-articular biologic device [4]. Since that time, numerous formulations have been developed, each with varying molecular weights and concentrations of HA., and the number injections in each series often varies between 1 and 5 depending on the manufacturers recommendations [4–6]. VS can be safely administered in the out-patient setting when injected into the knee via a variety of techniques including a lateral mid-patellar site [7]. Intra-articular shoulder injections may be offered based on the providers experience [2, 8]. Other joints including, but not limited to the ankle, hip, and thumb-metacarpal joint should be localized with fluoroscopy [9]. Though widely considered safe, the magnitude of clinical improvement provided by this treatment modality has come into question and has been carefully scrutinized across several different medical disciplines.

3 Recent Developments

As the population continues to age, providers are treating more and more patients complaining of debilitating major joint pain from numerous conditions including osteoarthritis. For example, a patient with knee osteoarthritis will often present complaining of knee pain that is exacerbated by activities of daily living and unrelieved with activity modifications, Non-Steroidal Anti-Inflammatory (Drugs NSAIDs), physical therapy, and even corticosteroid injections. At this point, many patients fear that surgical intervention remains the only available modality left. However, VS may be offered as another treatment option in patients whom wish to avoid surgery or may not yet be ideal surgical candidates.

The clinical benefits of VS are attributed to the multiple mechanisms of actions of HA. VS provides mechanical support by providing added viscosity to the native synovial fluid and stimulates the proliferation and reduces the apoptosis of chondrocytes. HA also promotes the synthesis of naturally occurring proteoglycans to further nourish the articular cartilage while decreasing the inflammatory processes which are inherently chondrotoxic [10] (see Table 1). Furthermore, it has been widely demonstrated that VS can be a safe, and cost-effective treatment option for select patients with major joint pain.

Table 1 Hyaluronic acid mechanisms of action

Area of influence	HA Mechanism of action
Chondroprotection	Stimulates chondrocyte proliferation
Proteoglycan synthesis	Promotes synthesis of aggrecan, the main proteoglycan within articular cartilage
Anti-inflammation	Inhibits IL-1β, IL-8, IL-6, PGE_2, TNF-α, and downregulates MMPs
Mechanical support	Adds viscosity to synovial fluid and buffers physical stresses such as vibrations
Subchondral bone	Preserves bony trabecular structure to maintain subchondral bone density
Analgesia	Binds mechanosensitive ion channels and inhibits joint nociceptors

When VS is chosen as a treatment option for periarticular pain, the technique and means of application are patient and provider specific. Injection techniques for VS supplementation mirror those used with other intra-articular injectables, such as corticosteroids. Traditionally, intra-articular injections of the knee, shoulder, and ankle have been provided by utilizing spatial awareness of specific anatomical landmarks. As mobile imaging modalities, including ultrasound, have become more readily available, providers are finding they are able to provide accurate delivery of injectables including VS, with relative ease. However, the lack of fluoroscopy and or ultrasound should not deter the provider from offering VS. While detailed instructions for each potential injection site are beyond the scope of this chapter, basic injection techniques of the shoulder, knee, and ankle are provided below, each demonstrated without the use of ultrasound.

Figure 1 demonstrates the lateral mid patellar approach for injection of VS in the knee. The patient is often laid supine with the knee extended. The superior, inferior, and lateral aspects of the patella are palpated.

The midpoint of the patella is identified. The patella can be slightly everted and translated laterally to allow better access into the patellofemoral joint. The needle should then be inserted into the patellofemoral joint space, perpendicular to the long axis of the extremity [11]. Figure 2 demonstrates the posterior approach for entry into the glenohumeral joint. This site utilizes a natural soft spot between the humeral head and glenoid which exists approximately 2–3 cm inferior and 1–2 cm medial to the posterolateral corner of the acromion [12].

With the patient facing away from the provider, the needle is introduced through the skin and soft tissues, aiming towards the coracoid process which can sometimes be palpated simultaneously with the providers opposite hand to aid in triangulation. Figure 3 demonstrates an easily accessible site for injection of VS into the ankle. This technique utilizes another naturally occurring soft spot which exists between the tibialis anterior tendon and the medial malleolus at the level of the tibiotalar joint line [13]. The patient may be seated with the extremity hanging off the exam table, or comfortably laying supine. The provider then palpates the soft spot as mentioned above, and introduces the needle into the ankle, parallel to the tibiotalar joint line.

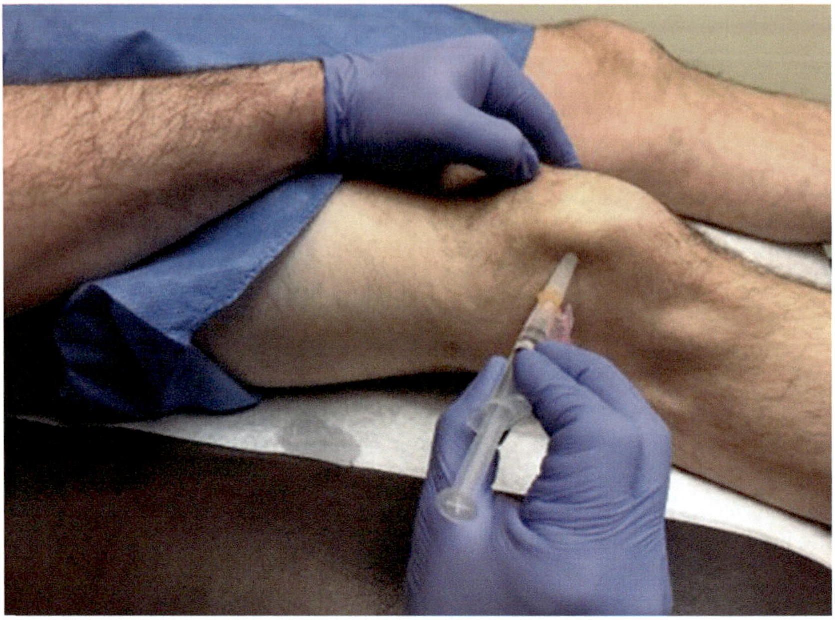

Fig. 1 Lateral mid patellar approach for intra-articular injection of the knee

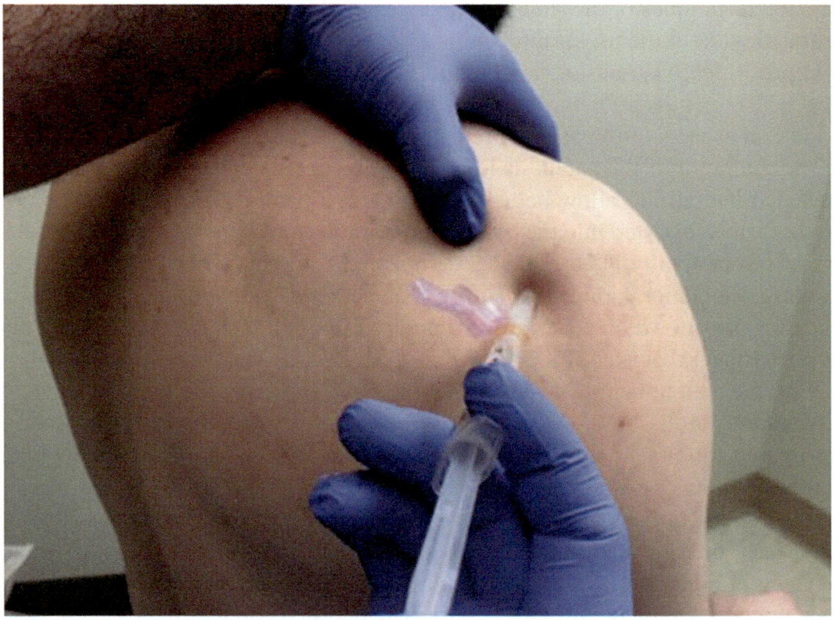

Fig. 2 Posterior entry into the glenohumeral joint is accomplished by palpating the natural "soft spot" between the humeral head and glenoid which is located approximately 2–3 cm inferior, and 1–2 cm medial to the posterolateral aspect of the glenoid. The needle is then introduced through the skin and soft tissues towards the coracoid process which can be palpated simultaneously by the free hand

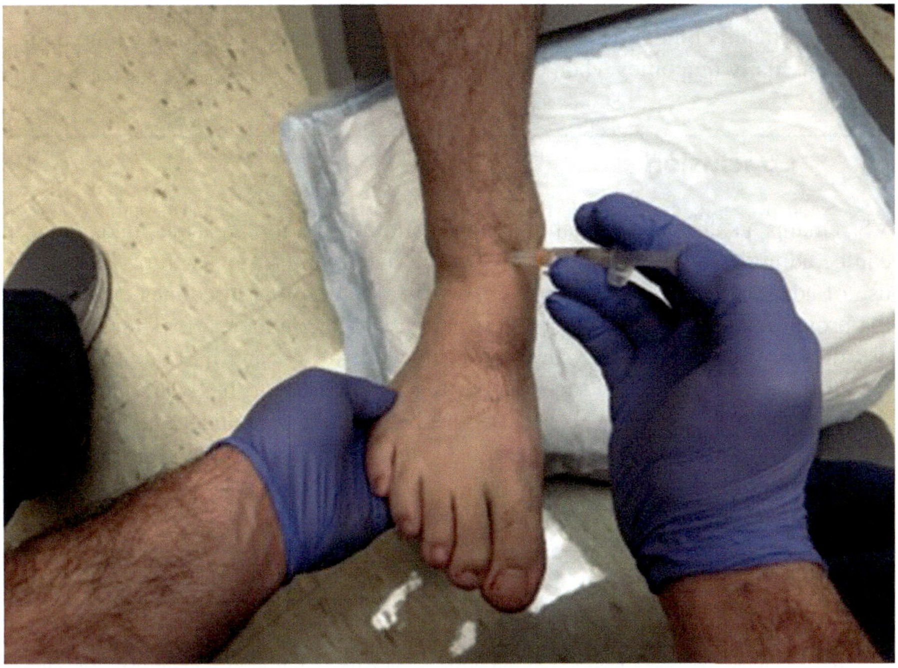

Fig. 3 Needle entry into the ankle joint can be accomplished by placing the needle into a naturally occurring soft spot that exits and the ankle joint line lateral to the medial malleolus and medial the tibialis anterior tendon. The needle can then be introduced into through the skin and soft tissues perpendicular to the tibiotalar joint line

Furthermore, the product used is often dictated by the patient's health insurance provider. Numerous formulations have been developed and refined over the years, each claiming advantages over the competitors. However, consensus statements were summarized by Henrotin et al. and include evidence-based dosing recommendations, single injection regimens must be performed with products specifically developed for such, and highly cross-linked products increase the time of intra-articular residence [9]. The clinical indications for VS continue to evolve and remain the subject of continued debates.

4 Potential Concerns

While widely considered a safe, non-surgical option for the treatment of joint pain, much debate exists regarding the degree of clinical benefit provided by VS. The minimal clinically important difference, MCID, is a metric used to detect the minimum change in patient reported outcomes that is perceived as clinically important. Herman et al. [4] reviewed numerous reports of VS with respect to MCID and reported that despite reported pain relief, evidence of significant clinical benefit is lacking. Furthermore, the American Academy of Orthopedic Surgeons (AAOS) reversed its recommendation regarding the use of VS in the treatment of knee OA in 2013, now stating the academy is unable to recommend the use of HA for patients with symptomatic knee osteoarthritis citing a general lack of evidence demonstrating a significant clinical benefit [14]. Thus, patients need to be educated and understand the likely outcomes when considering VS.

5 Conclusion

VS remains a safe non-surgical treatment option for joint pain as detailed above. It can be administered with relative ease in the outpatient setting with or without the use of advanced imaging modalities. However, conflicting guidelines exist among the professional colleges and societies that publish recommendations regarding the use of VS. Current research surrounding the use of VS and its potential clinical benefit is ever changing and providers offering VS need to be aware and counsel their patients appropriately based on the best available evidence. Thus, patient selection is critical and may be the most critical factor when considering VS as a treatment option for joint pain.

References

1. Leite VF, Daud Amadera JE, Buehler AM. Viscosupplementation for hip osteoarthritis: a systematic review and meta-analysis of the efficacy on pain and disability, and the occurrence of adverse events. Arch Phys Med Rehabil. 2018;99(3):574–83.
2. Kwon YW, Eisenberg G, Zuckerman JD. Sodium hyaluronate for the treatment of chronic shoulder pain associated with glenohumeral osteoarthritis: a multicenter, randomized, double-blind, placebo-controlled trial. J Shoulder Elb Surg. 2013;22(5):584–94.
3. Ferreira N, Masterson D, Lopes de Lima R, de Souza Moura B, Oliveira AT, Kelly da Silva Fidalgo T, et al. Efficacy of viscosupplementation with hyaluronic acid in temporomandibular disorders: a systematic review. J Craniomaxillofac Surg. 2018;46(11):1943–52.
4. Johal H, Devji T, Schemitsch EH, Bhandari M. Viscosupplementation in knee osteoarthritis: evidence revisited. JBJS Rev. 2016;4(4):1–11.
5. Jevsevar D, Donnelly P, Brown GA, Cummins DS. Viscosupplementation for osteoarthritis of the knee. J Bone Jt Surg Am. 2015;97:2047–60.
6. Bedard NA, DeMik DE, Glass NA, Burnett RA, Bozic KJ, Callaghan JJ. Impact of clinical practice guidelines on use of intra-articular hyaluronic acid and corticosteroid injections for knee osteoarthritis. J Bone Jt Surg Am. 2018;100(10):827–34.
7. Douglas RJ. Aspiration and injection of the knee joint: approach portal. Knee Surg Relat Res. 2014;26(1):1–6.
8. Blaine T, Moskowitz R, Udell J, Skyhar M, Levin R, Friedlander J, et al. Treatment of persistent shoulder pain with sodium hyaluronate: a randomized, controlled trial. J Bone Jt Surg Am. 2008;90(5):970–9.
9. Henrotin Y, Raman R, Richette P, Bard H, Jerosch J, Conrozier T, et al. Consensus statement on viscosupplementation with hyaluronic acid for the management of osteoarthritis. Semin Arthritis Rheum. 2015;45(2):140–9.
10. Altman R, Manjoo A, Fierlinger A, Niazi F, Nicholls M. The mechanism of action for hyaluronic acid treatment in the osteoarthritic knee: a systematic review. BMC Musculoskelet Disord. 2015;16(1):321.
11. Jackson DW, Evans NA, Thomas BM. Accuracy of needle placement into the intra-articular space of the knee. J Bone Jt Surg Am. 2002;84(9):1522–7.

12. Paxton ES, Backus J, Keener J, Brophy RH. Shoulder arthroscopy: basic principles of positioning, anesthesia, and portal anatomy. J Am Acad Orthop Surg. 2013;21(6):332–42.
13. Chiodo CP, Logan C, Blauwet CA. Aspiration and injection techniques of the lower extremity. J Am Acad Orthop Surg. 2018;26(15):e313–20.
14. Brown GA. AAOS clinical practice guideline: treatment of osteoarthritis of the knee: evidence-based guideline, 2nd edition. J Am Acad Orthop Surg. 2013;21(9):577–9.

Further Reading

Hunt C, Provenzano DA, Eshraghi Y, Mittal N, Souza D, Buchheit T. Should intra-articular hyaluronic acid be used routinely for knee osteoarthritis pain? PM R. 2021; https://doi.org/10.1002/pmrj.12740. PMID: 34837674.

Bedside Physiotherapy: Therapeutic Ultrasound and Other Physical Factors

Danielle L. Sarno and Erika T. Yih

Essential Concepts

- Therapeutic ultrasound is a low-risk intervention in the treatment of acute and chronic pain from a variety of musculoskeletal conditions.
- Repetitive transcranial magnetic stimulation generates induced electric current in the targeted brain parenchyma. rTMS performed at high frequency over the primary motor cortex seems to have the best efficacy in pain relief.
- Low level laser therapy modulates inflammatory mediators to produce analgesic effects in the treatment of various musculoskeletal conditions.
- Millimeter waves therapy is thought to modify the function of peripheral nerve receptors and induce changes in the endogenous opioid system.
- More robust studies investigating the efficacy and specific treatment protocols for therapeutic ultrasound, repetitive transcranial magnetic stimulation, low level laser therapy, and millimeter waves therapy are needed.

D. L. Sarno (✉)
Department of Physical Medicine and Rehabilitation, Department of Neurosurgery, Spaulding Rehabilitation Hospital, Brigham and Women's Hospital, Harvard Medical School, Boston, MA, USA
e-mail: dsarno@bwh.harvard.edu

E. T. Yih
Department of Physical Medicine and Rehabilitation, Department of Anesthesiology, Spaulding Rehabilitation Hospital, Brigham and Women's Hospital, Harvard Medical School, Boston, MA, USA
e-mail: eyih@partners.org

D. Souza et al. (eds.), *Bedside Pain Management Interventions*,
https://doi.org/10.1007/978-3-031-11188-4_15

1 Therapeutic Ultrasound

Ultrasound has been applied for medical purposes since the 1950s, when it was first used as a diagnostic tool in obstetrics and gynecology [1]. Over the years, its application has expanded to include not only widespread use for diagnosis of soft tissue pathology, imaging guidance during injections and line placements, and fetal monitoring, but also for myriad therapeutic purposes. Ultrasound has most classically been used to treat musculoskeletal conditions such as osteoarthritis, soft tissue shoulder injuries, and myofascial pain [2, 3], but its use has also extended to treatments for atrial fibrillation, nephrolithiasis, fractures, and benign and malignant soft tissue tumors [4, 5].

Low-Intensity Therapeutic Ultrasound/Ultrasound Diathermy

Therapeutic ultrasound involves use of an ultrasound machine that conducts an electric signal through crystals in the head of a handheld transducer. In a phenomenon called the piezoelectric effect, the crystals in the ultrasound probe vibrate, creating mechanical waves at frequencies outside the range of human hearing. The pressure, amplitude, frequency, and propagation length can be adjusted. A coupling medium, usually a hypoallergenic gel, is placed on the skin to help with wave transduction to the target tissue [5]. The energy of the waves produced causes vibration and heating of the tissues under the probe, which can induce vasodilation and increased blood flow and oxygen delivery, thereby accelerating healing [4]. When ultrasound is used for diagnostic purposes, temperature elevations are kept relatively low or negligible [6]. In contrast, therapeutic applications of ultrasound use longer durations of heating with unfocused beams or focused beams at higher intensities.

Physical therapists harness the thermal energy produced by therapeutic ultrasound at low powers to treat stretch pain and shoulder pathologies [7]. The transducer is applied in a circular motion over the injured or painful area in order to warm tendons, muscles, and other tissue and improve the blood flow and healing rate of these regions. There is level III evidence for the use of low-intensity ultrasound to treat pain in degenerative disorders of the musculoskeletal system [4]. Studies investigating the level of clinical benefit from physical therapy ultrasound treatment have conflicting results [3, 8–11], and more robust studies with clearer indications and techniques are needed. However, the risk of harm, such as burns, is low when the technique is applied properly, and overall, therapeutic ultrasound at low intensity provides a modest level of efficacy at a low level of risk.

High-Intensity Focused Ultrasound

High-intensity focused ultrasound (HIFU) is used for uterine fibroid ablation [12, 13], cardiac ablation [14], visceral soft tissue ablation [15], management of prostate cancer [16–18], treatment of glaucoma [19], and aesthetic treatment to lift the eyebrows [20]. HIFU uses a curved transducer probe to create a focal point of the ultrasonic waves several millimeters to centimeters away from the transducer plane. High local intensities of greater than 1 kW/cm^2 of 0.5- to 7-MHz are used to produce lesions in the tissue usually a few millimeters in diameter and length [5]. Before the focal point of the ultrasound beam can be moved to additional locations to complete the planned volume of treatment, tissue changes in the treatment zone must be monitored to ensure adequate treatment effects have been achieved. Imaging modalities such as ultrasound and magnetic resonance imaging (MRI) are used for image guidance and treatment monitoring, and when used in conjunction with therapeutic ultrasound, can increase the safety, accuracy, and efficacy of treatment [21]. Ultrasound imaging confers the benefits of live views, wider compatibility with implanted devices, and lower cost, but MRI is still the preferred imaging modality due to its higher image resolution and wider field of view [21].

2 Other Physical Modalities

Transcranial Magnetic Stimulation (TMS)

TMS is a non-invasive technique that has been used to treat pain since the 1990s [22]. It initially emerged as a non-invasive, less expensive treatment alternative to invasive brain stimulation through epidural motor cortex stimulation and deep brain stimulation, which have both shown efficacy in treating chronic pain of multiple etiologies [23–29]. In TMS, a coil is placed on the patient's scalp, and capacitors in a pulse generator are rapidly charged and discharged to send brief electrical currents through a wiring system within the coil to generate an electromagnetic field. This electromagnetic field produces an induced electric current in the brain parenchyma a few centimeters away, thereby allowing stimulation of specific cortical areas (approximately 5 mm^3 of cortex affected at a time) based on positioning of the coil [22]. The current depolarizes neurons, creates evoked responses, and changes neuronal plasticity in the affected area.

Studies of repetitive transcranial magnetic stimulation (rTMS) have shown that repetitive pulses of TMS produce local changes outlasting the stimulation period [30, 31]. Previous work has suggested that stimulation of the primary motor cortex and prefrontal cortex activates distant brain regions implicated in the integration and modulation of pain stimuli [32], and in healthy subjects, high-frequency unilateral rTMS of the primary motor cortex induces bilateral increase in pain thresholds [33]. In a systematic review of 33 randomized trials on the analgesic effect of rTMS, most studies reported significant pain relief (frequently >30% compared to control) after rTMS [22]. In particular, rTMS performed at high frequency (10 Hz) over the primary motor cortex with the induced electric current delivered in the posterior/anterior direction seemed to have the best efficacy [22]. However, few studies have investigated the efficacy of maintenance sessions of rTMS [22].

Low Level Laser Therapy (LLLT)

LLLT, also known as cold laser therapy, is a low-cost, non-invasive modality that uses low-frequency continuous laser of typically 600–1000 nm wavelength to treat pain and inflammation [34]. This form of light therapy acts on mitochondrial photoreceptors to increase oxidation velocity and accelerate cellular metabolism. Its mechanism of action is thought to be related to its role in modulating inflammatory mediators [35, 36], reducing bradykinin levels [37, 38], and increasing synthesis of endorphins [39–42]. Both experimental and clinical trials have shown analgesic and anti-inflammatory effects of photobiomodulation with few contraindications and rare side effects [43–45]. Specifically, clinical studies have shown promising results for LLLT in the management of Achilles tendonitis [46], neck pain [43, 47], OA [48], and other chronic musculoskeletal pain disorders [49]. However, existing studies have a high variation in LLLT application parameters (laser type, wavelength, power, energy density, etc.), and further research is needed to determine the ideal dose targets for treatment applications [34, 50].

Millimeter Waves Therapy (MWT)

MWT is a non-invasive modality developed in the former USSR in the mid-1980s and reported to be effective in the treatment of numerous diseases, particularly those associated with pain and inflammation [51–54]. MWT consists of repetitively exposing regions of the body to electromagnetic radiation with frequencies of 30–300 GHz and corresponding wavelengths from 10 to 1 mm [55]. Low-intensity MWT penetrates less than 1 mm into soft tissue and is thought to modify the function of peripheral nerve receptors, as well as induce changes in the endogenous opioid system [56–58]. Side effects of MWT include temporary paresthesias, headache, changes in blood pressure, rash, and general fatigue and sleepiness during treatment sessions [51–53, 59–61]. A systematic review of existing literature found that the most commonly used parameters of MWT were frequencies between 30 and 70 GHz and power density up to 10 mW cm^{-2} [62]. Small randomized controlled trials and pilot studies have shown promising results, but higher-quality, larger studies are lacking [62].

References

1. Newman PG, Rozycki GS. The history of ultrasound. Surg Clin North Am. 1998;78(2):179–95.
2. Analan PD, Leblebici B, Adam M. Effects of therapeutic ultrasound and exercise on pain, function, and isokinetic shoulder rotator strength of patients with rotator cuff disease. J Phys Ther Sci. 2015;27(10):3113–7.
3. Robertson VJ, Baker KG. A review of therapeutic ultrasound: effectiveness studies. Phys Ther. 2001;81(7):1339–50.
4. Matthews MJ, Stretanski MF. Ultrasound therapy. Treasure Island, FL: StatPearls; 2019.
5. Miller DL, Smith NB, Bailey MR, et al. Overview of therapeutic ultrasound applications and safety considerations. J Ultrasound Med. 2012;31(4):623–34.

6. Fowlkes JB, Bioeffects Committee of the American Institute of Ultrasound in M. American Institute of Ultrasound in Medicine consensus report on potential bioeffects of diagnostic ultrasound: executive summary. J Ultrasound Med. 2008;27(4):503–15.
7. Morishita K, Karasuno H, Yokoi Y, et al. Effects of therapeutic ultrasound on range of motion and stretch pain. J Phys Ther Sci. 2014;26(5):711–5.
8. Alexander LD, Gilman DR, Brown DR, Brown JL, Houghton PE. Exposure to low amounts of ultrasound energy does not improve soft tissue shoulder pathology: a systematic review. Phys Ther. 2010;90(1):14–25.
9. Muftic M, Miladinovic K. Therapeutic ultrasound and pain in degenerative diseases of musculoskeletal system. Acta Inform Med. 2013;21(3):170–2.
10. Shanks P, Curran M, Fletcher P, Thompson R. The effectiveness of therapeutic ultrasound for musculoskeletal conditions of the lower limb: a literature review. Foot. 2010;20(4):133–9.
11. van der Windt DA, van der Heijden GJ, van den Berg SG, ter Riet G, de Winter AF, Bouter LM. Ultrasound therapy for musculoskeletal disorders: a systematic review. Pain. 1999;81(3):257–71.
12. Fennessy FM, Tempany CM. MRI-guided focused ultrasound surgery of uterine leiomyomas. Acad Radiol. 2005;12(9):1158–66.
13. Taran FA, Tempany CM, Regan L, et al. Magnetic resonance-guided focused ultrasound (MRgFUS) compared with abdominal hysterectomy for treatment of uterine leiomyomas. Ultrasound Obstet Gynecol. 2009;34(5):572–8.
14. Ninet J, Roques X, Seitelberger R, et al. Surgical ablation of atrial fibrillation with off-pump, epicardial, high-intensity focused ultrasound: results of a multicenter trial. J Thorac Cardiovasc Surg. 2005;130(3):803–9.
15. Klingler HC, Susani M, Seip R, Mauermann J, Sanghvi N, Marberger MJ. A novel approach to energy ablative therapy of small renal tumours: laparoscopic high-intensity focused ultrasound. Eur Urol. 2008;53(4):810–6; discussion 817–18.
16. Gelet A, Chapelon JY, Bouvier R, et al. Transrectal high-intensity focused ultrasound: minimally invasive therapy of localized prostate cancer. J Endourol. 2000;14(6):519–28.
17. Thuroff S, Chaussy C, Vallancien G, et al. High-intensity focused ultrasound and localized prostate cancer: efficacy results from the European multicentric study. J Endourol. 2003;17(8):673–7.
18. Zini C, Hipp E, Thomas S, Napoli A, Catalano C, Oto A. Ultrasound- and MR-guided focused ultrasound surgery for prostate cancer. World J Radiol. 2012;4(6):247–52.
19. Burgess SE, Silverman RH, Coleman DJ, et al. Treatment of glaucoma with high-intensity focused ultrasound. Ophthalmology. 1986;93(6):831–8.
20. Alam M, White LE, Martin N, Witherspoon J, Yoo S, West DP. Ultrasound tightening of facial and neck skin: a rater-blinded prospective cohort study. J Am Acad Dermatol. 2010;62(2):262–9.
21. Li S, Wu PH. Magnetic resonance image-guided versus ultrasound-guided high-intensity focused ultrasound in the treatment of breast cancer. Chin J Cancer. 2013;32(8):441–52.
22. Galhardoni R, Correia GS, Araujo H, et al. Repetitive transcranial magnetic stimulation in chronic pain: a review of the literature. Arch Phys Med Rehabil. 2015;96(4 Suppl):S156–72.
23. Bittar RG, Kar-Purkayastha I, Owen SL, et al. Deep brain stimulation for pain relief: a meta-analysis. J Clin Neurosci. 2005;12(5):515–9.
24. Cruccu G, Aziz TZ, Garcia-Larrea L, et al. EFNS guidelines on neurostimulation therapy for neuropathic pain. Eur J Neurol. 2007;14(9):952–70.
25. Fontaine D, Hamani C, Lozano A. Efficacy and safety of motor cortex stimulation for chronic neuropathic pain: critical review of the literature. J Neurosurg. 2009;110(2):251–6.
26. Hamani C, Schwalb JM, Rezai AR, Dostrovsky JO, Davis KD, Lozano AM. Deep brain stimulation for chronic neuropathic pain: long-term outcome and the incidence of insertional effect. Pain. 2006;125(1–2):188–96.
27. Nguyen JP, Nizard J, Keravel Y, Lefaucheur JP. Invasive brain stimulation for the treatment of neuropathic pain. Nat Rev Neurol. 2011;7(12):699–709.
28. Owen SL, Green AL, Nandi D, Bittar RG, Wang S, Aziz TZ. Deep brain stimulation for neuropathic pain. Neuromodulation. 2006;9(2):100–6.

29. Rasche D, Rinaldi PC, Young RF, Tronnier VM. Deep brain stimulation for the treatment of various chronic pain syndromes. Neurosurg Focus. 2006;21(6):E8.
30. Pascual-Leone A, Tormos JM, Keenan J, Tarazona F, Canete C, Catala MD. Study and modulation of human cortical excitability with transcranial magnetic stimulation. J Clin Neurophysiol. 1998;15(4):333–43.
31. Pascual-Leone A, Valls-Sole J, Wassermann EM, Hallett M. Responses to rapid-rate transcranial magnetic stimulation of the human motor cortex. Brain. 1994;117(Pt 4):847–58.
32. Hasan M, Whiteley J, Bresnahan R, et al. Somatosensory change and pain relief induced by repetitive transcranial magnetic stimulation in patients with central poststroke pain. Neuromodulation. 2014;17(8):731–6; discussion 736.
33. Maarrawi J, Peyron R, Mertens P, et al. Motor cortex stimulation for pain control induces changes in the endogenous opioid system. Neurology. 2007;69(9):827–34.
34. Dima R, Tieppo Francio V, Towery C, Davani S. Review of literature on low-level laser therapy benefits for nonpharmacological pain control in chronic pain and osteoarthritis. Altern Ther Health Med. 2018;24(5):8–10.
35. Aimbire F, Albertini R, Pacheco MT, et al. Low-level laser therapy induces dose-dependent reduction of TNFalpha levels in acute inflammation. Photomed Laser Surg. 2006;24(1):33–7.
36. Alcantara CC, Gigo-Benato D, Salvini TF, Oliveira AL, Anders JJ, Russo TL. Effect of low-level laser therapy (LLLT) on acute neural recovery and inflammation-related gene expression after crush injury in rat sciatic nerve. Lasers Surg Med. 2013;45(4):246–52.
37. Chow R, Armati P, Laakso EL, Bjordal JM, Baxter GD. Inhibitory effects of laser irradiation on peripheral mammalian nerves and relevance to analgesic effects: a systematic review. Photomed Laser Surg. 2011;29(6):365–81.
38. Jimbo K, Noda K, Suzuki K, Yoda K. Suppressive effects of low-power laser irradiation on bradykinin evoked action potentials in cultured murine dorsal root ganglion cells. Neurosci Lett. 1998;240(2):93–6.
39. Hagiwara S, Iwasaka H, Hasegawa A, Noguchi T. Pre-irradiation of blood by gallium aluminum arsenide (830 nm) low-level laser enhances peripheral endogenous opioid analgesia in rats. Anesth Analg. 2008;107(3):1058–63.
40. Hagiwara S, Iwasaka H, Okuda K, Noguchi T. GaAlAs (830 nm) low-level laser enhances peripheral endogenous opioid analgesia in rats. Lasers Surg Med. 2007;39(10):797–802.
41. Hawkins D, Houreld N, Abrahamse H. Low level laser therapy (LLLT) as an effective therapeutic modality for delayed wound healing. Ann N Y Acad Sci. 2005;1056:486–93.
42. Laakso EL, Cabot PJ. Nociceptive scores and endorphin-containing cells reduced by low-level laser therapy (LLLT) in inflamed paws of Wistar rat. Photomed Laser Surg. 2005;23(1):32–5.
43. Chow RT, Johnson MI, Lopes-Martins RA, Bjordal JM. Efficacy of low-level laser therapy in the management of neck pain: a systematic review and meta-analysis of randomised placebo or active-treatment controlled trials. Lancet. 2009;374(9705):1897–908.
44. de Morais NC, Barbosa AM, Vale ML, et al. Anti-inflammatory effect of low-level laser and light-emitting diode in zymosan-induced arthritis. Photomed Laser Surg. 2010;28(2):227–32.
45. Ferreira DM, Zangaro RA, Villaverde AB, et al. Analgesic effect of He-Ne (632.8 nm) low-level laser therapy on acute inflammatory pain. Photomed Laser Surg. 2005;23(2):177–81.
46. Bjordal JM, Lopes-Martins RA, Iversen VV. A randomised, placebo controlled trial of low level laser therapy for activated Achilles tendinitis with microdialysis measurement of peritendinous prostaglandin E2 concentrations. Br J Sports Med. 2006;40(1):76–80; discussion 76–80.
47. Gur A, Sarac AJ, Cevik R, Altindag O, Sarac S. Efficacy of 904 nm gallium arsenide low level laser therapy in the management of chronic myofascial pain in the neck: a double-blind and randomize-controlled trial. Lasers Surg Med. 2004;35(3):229–35.
48. Baltzer AW, Ostapczuk MS, Stosch D. Positive effects of low level laser therapy (LLLT) on Bouchard's and Heberden's osteoarthritis. Lasers Surg Med. 2016;48(5):498–504.
49. Bjordal JM, Couppe C, Chow RT, Tuner J, Ljunggren EA. A systematic review of low level laser therapy with location-specific doses for pain from chronic joint disorders. Aust J Physiother. 2003;49(2):107–16.

50. de Andrade AL, Bossini PS, Parizotto NA. Use of low level laser therapy to control neuropathic pain: a systematic review. J Photochem Photobiol B. 2016;164:36–42.
51. Pakhomov AG, Akyel Y, Pakhomova ON, Stuck BE, Murphy MR. Current state and implications of research on biological effects of millimeter waves: a review of the literature. Bioelectromagnetics. 1998;19(7):393–413.
52. Rojavin MA, Ziskin MC. Medical application of millimetre waves. QJM. 1998;91(1): 57–66.
53. Ryan KL, D'Andrea JA, Jauchem JR, Mason PA. Radio frequency radiation of millimeter wave length: potential occupational safety issues relating to surface heating. Health Phys. 2000;78(2):170–81.
54. Skurikhina LA. [The therapeutic use of electromagnetic millimeter waves of nonthermal intensity—millimeter-wave therapy]. Vopr Kurortol Fizioter Lech Fiz Kult. 1988;(5):65–72.
55. Gandhi OP. Some basic properties of biological tissues for potential biomedical applications of millimeter waves. J Microw Power. 1983;18(3):295–304.
56. Enin LD, Akoev GN, Potekhina IL, Oleiner VD. [Effect of extremely high-frequency electromagnetic radiation on the function of skin sensory endings]. Patol Fiziol Eksp Ter. 1992;(5–6):23–5.
57. Radzievsky AA, Rojavin MA, Cowan A, Alekseev SI, Radzievsky AA Jr, Ziskin MC. Peripheral neural system involvement in hypoalgesic effect of electromagnetic millimeter waves. Life Sci. 2001;68(10):1143–51.
58. Rojavin MA, Radzievsky AA, Cowan A, Ziskin MC. Pain relief caused by millimeter waves in mice: results of cold water tail flick tests. Int J Radiat Biol. 2000;76(4):575–9.
59. Radzievsky AA, Rojavin MA, Cowan A, Ziskin MC. Suppression of pain sensation caused by millimeter waves: a double-blinded, cross-over, prospective human volunteer study. Anesth Analg. 1999;88(4):836–40.
60. Usichenko TI, Herget HF. Treatment of chronic pain with millimetre wave therapy (MWT) in patients with diffuse connective tissue diseases: a pilot case series study. Eur J Pain. 2003;7(3):289–94.
61. Usichenko TI, Ivashkivsky OI, Gizhko VV. Treatment of rheumatoid arthritis with electromagnetic millimeter waves applied to acupuncture points—a randomized double blind clinical study. Acupunct Electrother Res. 2003;28(1–2):11–8.
62. Usichenko TI, Edinger H, Gizhko VV, Lehmann C, Wendt M, Feyerherd F. Low-intensity electromagnetic millimeter waves for pain therapy. Evid Based Complement Alternat Med. 2006;3(2):201–7.

Bedside Transcutaneous Drug Delivery

Nicholas Capaldo, Glenn Rech, and Dmitri Souza

Essential Concepts

- Transcutaneous drug delivery for bedside analgesia presents many unique features including the application of analgesic medications directly to the greatest site of pain.
- Transcutaneous drug delivery minimizes undesirable effects from administration via oral and systemic routes.
- Transcutaneous during delivery could be especially helpful in elderly, or debilitated patients who are typically sensitive to medication-related adverse effects.
- Transcutaneous drug delivery options include creams, patches, phonophoresis, iontophoresis, transcutaneous patient-controlled analgesia, and others.

1 Overview

Transcutaneous drug delivery for analgesia presents many unique features that make clinicians think about it as a preferable choice to treat pain at the bedside. It allows patients to apply analgesic medications directly to the greatest site of pain. It

N. Capaldo
Internal Medicine Program, Western Reserve Hospital, Cuyahoga Falls, OH, USA
e-mail: nicholas.capaldo@rockets.utoledo.edu; ncapaldo@westernreservehospital.org

G. Rech
Western Reserve Hospital, Cuyahoga Falls, OH, USA

D. Souza (✉)
Center for Pain Medicine, Western Reserve Hospital, Cuyahoga Falls, OH, USA
e-mail: dsouza@westernreservehospital.org

D. Souza et al. (eds.), *Bedside Pain Management Interventions*,
https://doi.org/10.1007/978-3-031-11188-4_16

minimizes undesirable effects from administration via oral and systemic routes. It can deliver more of the medication to the target site by eliminating the first-pass metabolism associated with several oral medications. It may be preferable in some cases, especially in elderly patients who are commonly sensitive to medications-related adverse effects. It may be helpful for patients with a low tolerance for pills. Important to differentiate between topical therapies in which patients apply medication to the most painful area locally for pain relief at the application site and transdermal therapies in which patients apply transcutaneous medication for absorption and systemic treatment of pain symptoms.

Because skin presents a formidable barrier, topical pain creams often contain enhancers, or chemicals, such as DMSO (dimethyl sulfoxide), contained in a topical product, Pennsaid. DMSO is designed to help move a drug from the surface through the skin (epidermis and dermis) to regional areas below with the goal of reaching a muscle group or joint for treating pain. Drug absorption into and through the skin into painful areas depends on the physical and chemical characteristics of the drug. The most important is the size of the drug. Some novel technologies allow for maximized transcutaneous absorption, such as heat and/or covering with a barrier such as saran wrap.

2 Topical Creams

The use of both prescription and over-the-counter topical creams has been a longstanding popular analgesic option. Classes of available drugs for topical creams are NSAIDs, lidocaine, capsaicin, clonidine, and opioids. Diclofenac is the only topical NSAID commercially available in the US. While the FDA requires box warnings for topical NSAIDs of adverse cardiovascular and GI effects, this is controversial due to its limited systemic availability [1]. Phase III studies of topical clonidine gel for diabetic neuropathy were discontinued in the US in 2016 due to inefficacy [2]. In case reports topical opioids are effective in the palliative treatment of painful skin ulcers. However, they are compounded medications, which are not covered by many third-party payers [1].

In recent reviews there was moderate- and high-quality evidence to support a number of topical creams based on efficacy compared to placebo for specific pain indications. Selected preparations of diclofenac and ketoprofen received favorable reviews in both acute musculoskeletal pain such as sprains or strains, and chronic musculoskeletal pain such as osteoarthritis of the hands and knees. In postherpetic neuralgia capsaicin had moderate-quality evidence to support some limited effectiveness. Different formulations of the same topical analgesic at similar concentrations produce a wide range of efficacies. In topical diclofenac, NNTs range from 1.8 to 8 depending on the formulation used. In general, gels are superior to creams for treating acute pain. Moreover, the efficacy of analgesics consists of more factors than rubbing into the skin. Although the perceived efficacy does tend to support that rubbing is beneficial, there is low objective evidence to support this. In double blind studies the study method de-confounds rubbing from the objective assessment of drug efficacy, including a rubbed placebo that contains no active ingredient.

However this may not entirely remove rubbing from the analgesic experience and it may potentially explain the relatively high placebo response rates of 20–57% [3].

3 Patches

Patches are designed with permeation enhancers to facilitate drug delivery. Concentration-dependent reservoirs and multi-layer patches contain a membrane to control drug release from a single reservoir or from multiple layers within the patch [4]. A typical single-layer drug-in-adhesive patch is shown in Fig. 1.

NSAID patches provide pain relief at 3 h after application, with plasma levels detectable 4.5 h after application removal. This creates a skin depot with a reservoir effect that extends the half-life of elimination after patch removal compared to oral NSAIDs. Limited systemic absorption makes adverse systemic effects such as GI bleeding and ulcers very rare with topical administration. The most common adverse effects are application site redness, itching, rash, and rarely allergic dermatitis [4].

Lidocaine 5% patch (Lidoderm) is approved by the FDA for post-herpetic neuralgia. When used properly systemic absorption is 3 ± 2% of the applied dose, while at least 95% of the drug stays in the patch. The average maximum plasma concentration is roughly 10% of the concentration needed to treat cardiac arrhythmias [4]. Limit application to three or less patches to avoid this adverse effect.

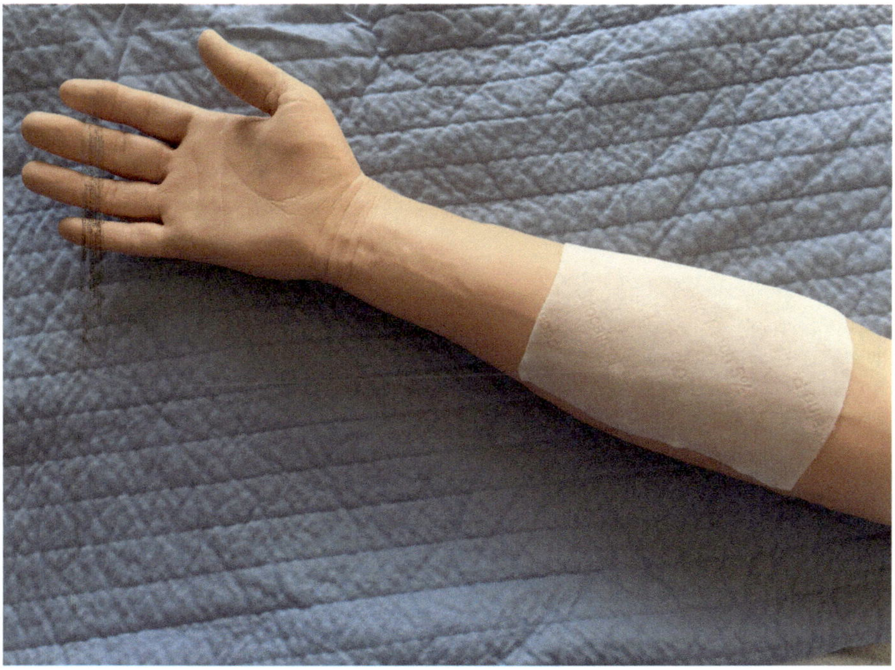

Fig. 1 Model of placement of topical lidocaine patch

Transdermal fentanyl is indicated for palliative treatment of malignant and noncancer pain. Patches designed for a safe rate of absorption reach maximum plasma concentration at 12–24 h and maintain it over a 72-h application. Heat and increased body temperature can increase rate of delivery. The initial slow increase in plasma concentrations, due to forming a depot before entering the systemic circulation, delays the onset of analgesia until 24 h after application and requires supplementation for initial relief. However, the depot creates a reservoir effect on elimination half-life after patch removal. Fentanyl is reserved for opioid-tolerant patients due to the risk of respiratory depression in opioid-naïve patients. There are multiple case reports of unintentional overdose due to accidental exposure, errors in dosing, and heat sources that highlight the narrow therapeutic and toxic window [4].

4 Phonophoresis

Phonophoresis utilizes low-frequency pulsations of ultrasound to increase skin barrier permeability in order to facilitate faster drug absorption. A typical phonophoresis machine and an illustration of its use are shown in Fig. 2a, b.

The topical drug and its carrying agent should both transmit ultrasound to maximize clinical efficacy. In general, drugs suspended in aqueous gels are more suitable conduits for the transmission of ultrasound energy while cream-based preparations (including many often-used topical analgesic creams) are less effective vehicles for this technology, particularly at 1 MHz frequency. Agents that reduce ultrasound transmission during phonophoresis may produce poor therapeutic results [5, 6]. Additional measures to increase efficacy include skin pretreatment, patient positioning to maximize blood flow for systemic uptake, post-treatment occlusive dressings to seal the area and prevent moisture from escaping, and an intensity of 1.5 W/cm^2 that utilizes both thermal and non-thermal properties. Low-intensity ultrasound (0.5 W/cm^2) is used for open wounds and acute injuries [5].

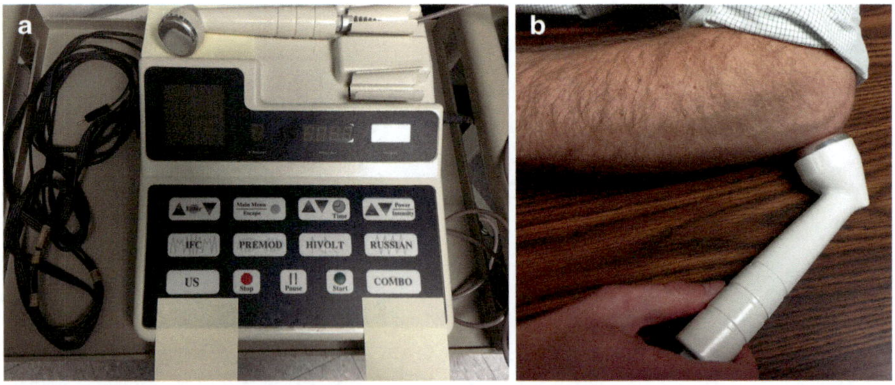

Fig. 2 (**a**) Example of a typical phonophoresis machine and ultrasound transducer. (**b**) Example of phonophoresis technology in use

Phonophoresis significantly accelerates the rate of drug delivery when applied using an occlusive dressing. Saliba et al. [7] found that phonophoresis led to a significantly elevated transdermal absorption rate and total plasma concentration of dexamethasone applied using an occlusive dressing when compared with sham ultrasound which produced only trace plasma concentrations. The researchers noted a phonophoretic effect when the delivered drug saturates the skin.

The procedure is generally well tolerated. There is a minor risk of burns from ultrasound that can be prevented by proper setup and use of the equipment. There are no known contraindications apart from allergic drug reactions.

5 Iontophoresis

Iontophoresis utilizes electrical pulsations to create aqueous pores in the skin and increase drug molecule energy, leading to faster absorption. The iontophoresis patch is prepared with cationic drugs in the positive anode port of the patch and anionic drugs in the negative cathode port of the patch, both together with a saline solution. This aqueous environment facilitates the movement of drug ions from one port to the other within the skin. Active drug transport expedites the onset of action, accelerates the creation of skin depots, and helps promote reaching blood vessels for earlier systemic absorption [8].

Iontophoresis significantly increases the effectiveness of delivery of lidocaine and epinephrine for local analgesia. Additionally, NSAIDs can be used in the TMJ for RA, joint injuries and dislocations, masticatory dysfunction, bruxism, inflammatory conditions, neuralgias, lockjaw, tooth hyperalgesia, and postoperative pain. Topical NSAIDs are well tolerated in patients with GI disease and dysfunction [9].

The main adverse effects are skin tingling during therapy and transient local erythema of the skin. There is also a risk of burn due to improper use of the equipment and improper choice of the electrodes or formulation composition. Bare metal and carbon-based electrodes use hydrolysis of water to generate H^+ and OH^- at the positively charged anode and negatively charged cathode, respectively, and any alteration in pH outside the skin's normal buffering capacity is likely to cause burns. OH^- production is more likely to cause serious burns than H^+ production as the alkaline phase erodes the skin and reduces skin resistance, making burns and skin erosion worse. The risk of burns can be prevented by correctly preparing and setting up the equipment to avoid pressure on the electrodes and prevent either skin-to-metal contact or uneven charge concentration over the skin, avoiding skin defects that have inherently lower skin resistance, and using a current intensity less than 0.5 mA/cm^2. Additionally, Ag-AgCl is a more electrochemically compatible electrode buffer with a lower risk of skin irritation as it works at a lower potential and without using hydrolysis of water [8].

Select contraindications to iontophoresis apart from allergic drug reactions are superficial and deep sensory disorders, pregnancy, and lactation [9].

6 Patient-Controlled Transcutaneous Fentanyl

The fentanyl iontophoretic transdermal system (ITS) is the only transdermal opioid given for acute pain. It is approved in US and Europe for inpatient treatment of acute and moderate-to-severe postoperative pain in the hospital setting. The system consists of a small patch placed on the upper outer arm or chest. Pressing the on-demand button twice within 3 s activates the patch to deliver a pre-programmed dose of 40 μg of transdermal fentanyl over a period of 10 min. The system can deliver a maximum of six doses every hour without exception, and it can also be interrogated for the number of doses that have been given. A system lasts for 24 h or 80 doses, whichever comes first, and is discarded [4]. Patients can receive a maximum of 72 h of treatment on fentanyl ITS [10]. Trade name Ionsys, is available through a restricted program called the Ionsys REMS Program. Healthcare facilities that dispense Ionsys must be certified in this program and comply with the REMS requirements.

Active fentanyl delivery greatly reduces average time to peak plasma concentration compared to fentanyl patch (see discussion on fentanyl patches above), as low as 39 min in one study of the system. After fentanyl PCA is discontinued, the plasma elimination half-life is similar to that following IV administration, which suggests that there is no creation of a skin depot with this route of administration [4].

In randomized controlled trials fentanyl ITS was superior to placebo for moderate-to-severe postoperative pain [4, 10, 11]. In active-comparator trials it provides equivalent analgesia to the standard IV PCA morphine [4, 10, 11]. It helps facilitate postoperative recovery and de-escalation to standard enteral pain regimens when used within a multimodal analgesia plan that includes titration to comfort level before ITS initiation and closely monitored breakthrough medication as needed. In case studies the system provides sufficient analgesia for most patients without requiring breakthrough supplementation, and it is easy and safe to use in appropriate patients within trained medical staff environments [10]. The most frequent adverse effects are opioid-related nausea, vomiting, and pruritus. There are no reported incidences of respiratory depression to date. Application site reactions occurred in 13% of patients [4].

7 Conclusion

Topical analgesics are an appealing option for providing targeted, effective analgesia with reduced adverse effects and drug–drug interactions compared to systemic therapies and lower overall pill requirements. Potential disadvantages can be the requirement for repeated applications during the day, absorption variability depending on skin integrity, and the unavailability of commercial formulations in some cases [1]. Research continues to focus on expanding the applications of emerging technologies for active transcutaneous drug delivery in both topical and transdermal therapy.

References

1. Wang K, LaBeff L, Thomas AM, Raouf M. Topical analgesics for chronic pain conditions. Pract Pain Manag. 2018;18(5):2019. https://www.practicalpainmanagement.com/treatments/pharmacological/opioids/topical-analgesics-chronic-pain-conditions. Accessed 8 Oct 2019.
2. Clonidine topical gel—BioDelivery Sciences International. 2017. https://adisinsight.springer.com/drugs/800027667. Accessed 11 Oct 2019.
3. Derry S, Wiffen PJ, Kalso EA, Bell RF, Aldington D, Phillips T, Gaskell H, Moore RA. Topical analgesics for acute and chronic pain in adults—an overview of Cochrane reviews. Cochrane Database Syst Rev. 2017;5(5):CD008609.
4. Bajaj S, Whiteman A, Brandner B. Transdermal drug delivery in pain management. Contin Educ Anaesth Crit Care Pain. 2011;11(2):39–43. https://doi.org/10.1093/bjaceaccp/mkq054.
5. Byl NN. The use of ultrasound as an enhancer for transcutaneous drug delivery: phonophoresis. Phys Ther. 1995;75(6):539–53. https://doi.org/10.1093/ptj/75.6.539.
6. Cage SA, Rupp KA, Castel JC, Saliba EN, Hertel J, Saliba SA. Relative acoustic transmission of topical preparations used with therapeutic ultrasound. Arch Phys Med Rehabil. 2013;94:2126–30. https://doi.org/10.1016/j.apmr.2013.03.020.
7. Saliba S, Mistry D, Perrin D, Gieck J, Weltman A. Phonophoresis and the absorption of dexamethasone in the presence of an occlusive dressing. J Athl Train. 2006;42:349–54. https://www.researchgate.net/publication/5788203_Phonophoresis_and_the_Absorption_of_Dexamethasone_in_the_Presence_of_an_Occlusive_Dressing. Accessed 8 Oct 2019.
8. Roustit M, Blaise S, Cracowski JL. Trials and tribulations of skin iontophoresis in therapeutics. Br J Clin Pharmacol. 2014;77(1):63–71. https://doi.org/10.1111/bcp.12128.
9. Karpinski TM. Selected medicines used in iontophoresis. Pharmaceutics. 2018;10(4):E204. https://doi.org/10.3390/pharmaceutics10040204.
10. Poplawski S, Johnson M, Philips P, Eberhart LH, Koch T, Itri LM. Use of fentanyl iontophoretic transdermal system (ITS) (IONSYS®) in the management of patients with acute postoperative pain: a case series. Pain Ther. 2016;5(2):237–48. https://doi.org/10.1007/s40122-016-0061-2.
11. Viscusi ER, Siccardi M, Damaraju CV, Hewitt DJ, Kershaw P. The safety and efficacy of fentanyl iontophoretic transdermal system compared with morphine intravenous patient-controlled analgesia for postoperative pain management: an analysis of pooled data from three randomized, active-controlled clinical studies. Anesth Analg. 2007;105(5):1428–36. https://doi.org/10.1213/01.ane.0000281913.28623.fd.

Kinesio Taping for Bedside Pain Management

Matthew B. Noble, Stephanie K. Noble, Stephen R. Shively, and Steven B. Jackson

Essential Concepts

- Billions of dollars are spent each year on pharmacologic pain management and disability compensation. Kinesio Tape is a safe, effective, and affordable alternative.
- Kinesio Tape affects five major physiologic systems: skin, fascia, circulatory/lymphatic systems, muscle, and joint.
- Kinesio Tape is appropriate for any stage of healing, is used to prevent re-injury, and returns the body to homeostasis.
- Evidence suggests that Kinesio Taping provides benefits for a maximum of 3 days.
- Kinesio Tape is a treatment modality that is to be used in conjunction with other treatment methods, such as physical therapy, and is not meant to be a stand-alone treatment. When used as an adjunct therapy, it has been shown to improve functional scores, disability scores, and pain.

M. B. Noble (✉) · S. R. Shively · S. B. Jackson
Western Reserve Hospital, Cuyahoga Falls, OH, USA
e-mail: mnoble@westernreservehospital.org; sshively@westernreservehospital.org; SJackson@Westernreservehospital.org

S. K. Noble
Akron Children's Hospital, Akron, OH, USA
e-mail: snoble@akronchildrens.org

D. Souza et al. (eds.), *Bedside Pain Management Interventions*,
https://doi.org/10.1007/978-3-031-11188-4_17

1 Overview

The pharmaceutical industry makes approximately $16.4 billion annually on pain medications while the reported disability compensation secondary to conditions related to pain is estimated to be $18.9 billion [1]. This is a prime example of the importance of finding non-operative and non-opioid pain relief treatment plans for our society. With a growing opioid crisis in this country, it is important now, more than ever, to find effective treatments for pain control. Kinesio Taping, as a theory, was first introduced in the late 1970s by Dr. Kenzo Kase [2, 3]. It first gained international attention during the 1988 Olympics. In recent years, its growing popularity can be seen at any given nationally televised professional sporting event. Kinesio Tape works by cueing the cutaneous mechanoreceptors on the skin to give the underlying muscle or joint proprioceptive feedback as to how it should be correctly aligned. Kinesio Tape provides a positional hold and inhibits pathological movement. The authors believe that taping provides biomechanical feedback when the physiologic barrier of a joint is reached in order to inhibit overstretching or overuse of a joint or muscle. It is the authors' opinion, which is heavily supported by research, that Kinesio Taping should be used in conjunction with other pain management techniques. The purpose of this chapter is to introduce Kinesio Taping as an effective, affordable, and safe pain relief option [4, 5].

2 Historical Aspects

In the late 1970s, the Kinesio Taping Method was founded by Dr. Kenzo Kase, Doctor of Chiropractic, who was looking for ways to prolong the effects of his hands-on treatments between clinic visits. He then developed Kinesio Tex Tape, which was a combination of cotton and acrylic, similar thickness and weight to skin, latex free, and a 100% medical grade adhesive, which is heat activated. Kinesio Tex Tape itself and Dr. Kase's techniques differ from traditional athletic tape as it addresses more than joint stabilization. Traditional athletic tape is rigid, requires pre-wrap to avoid skin irritation, is meant for acute injuries or as a preventative measure, and is recommended for short-term use only. As described in this chapter, the Kinesio Taping Method, in conjunction with the properties found in the Kinesio Tex Tape, affects five major physiologic systems and has lasting effects of up to 5 days [2, 5, 6].

3 Theories

- Kinesio Tape cues the cutaneous mechanoreceptors on the skin to give a joint proprioceptive feedback as to how it should be correctly aligned [3]. Kinesio Tape provides a positional hold and inhibits pathological movement [5].
- Applying Kinesio Tape from the muscle insertion (anchor) to the muscle origin causes a concentric pull eliciting muscle activation. Applying Kinesio Tape from the muscle origin (anchor) to the muscle insertion causes an eccentric pull eliciting muscle relaxation [3].
  - Kinesio Tape will recoil towards the anchor point [5].
- Creating skin convolutions under the Kinesio Tape lifts the skin allowing interstitial fluid to move more freely, reducing inflammation and swelling, reducing interstitial pressure, creating channels in which lymph can flow, and drawing blood flow to the area [3].

4 Application of Tape

In this section, three Kinesio Taping techniques are outlined.

Definitions

Anchor: Starting point of the tape.

Tail: End point of the tape.

I strip: Single strip of tape with rounded edges.

Paper-off tension: 10% stretch (Figs. 1, 2 and 3).

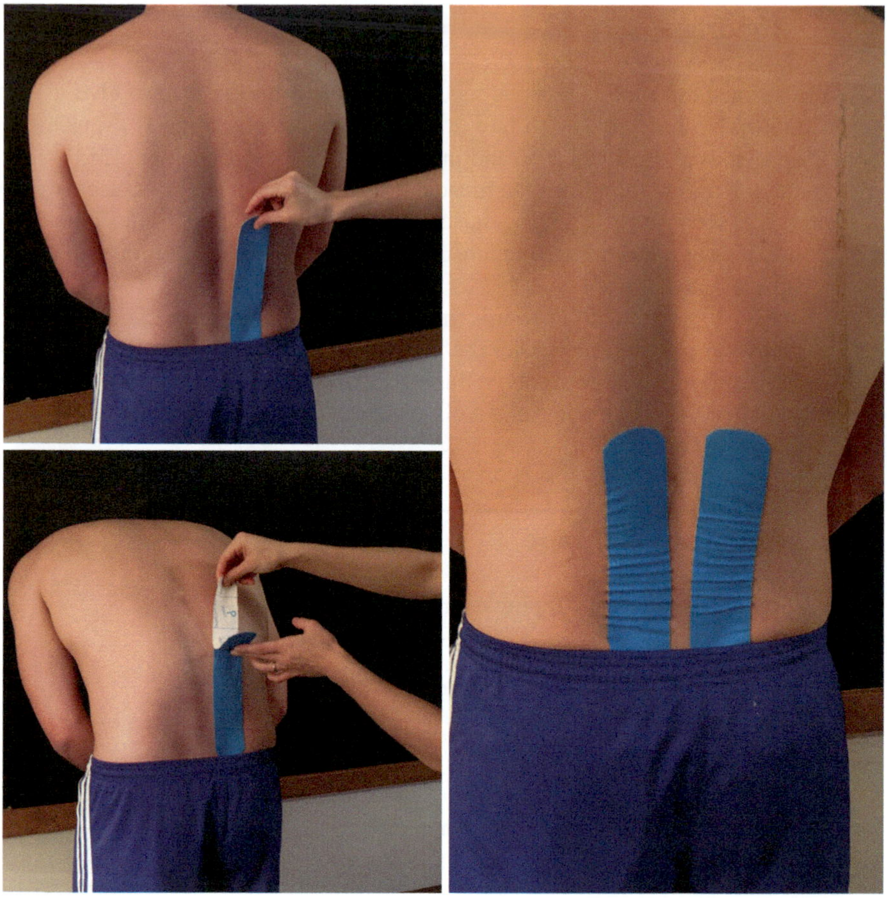

Fig. 1 This figure demonstrates the creation of Kinesio Tape convolutions on lumbar paraspinals to lift the skin to promote free movement of interstitial fluid, reduce interstitial inflammation and/or pressure, allow lymph flow, and draw blood to the area. One or two I strips can be used, pending where the patient is experiencing pain or restriction. In order to apply, the I strip is anchored in the sacroiliac joint region. The patient flexes forward and paper off tension is applied along the I strip. No tension should be applied to the anchor or the tail of the I strip

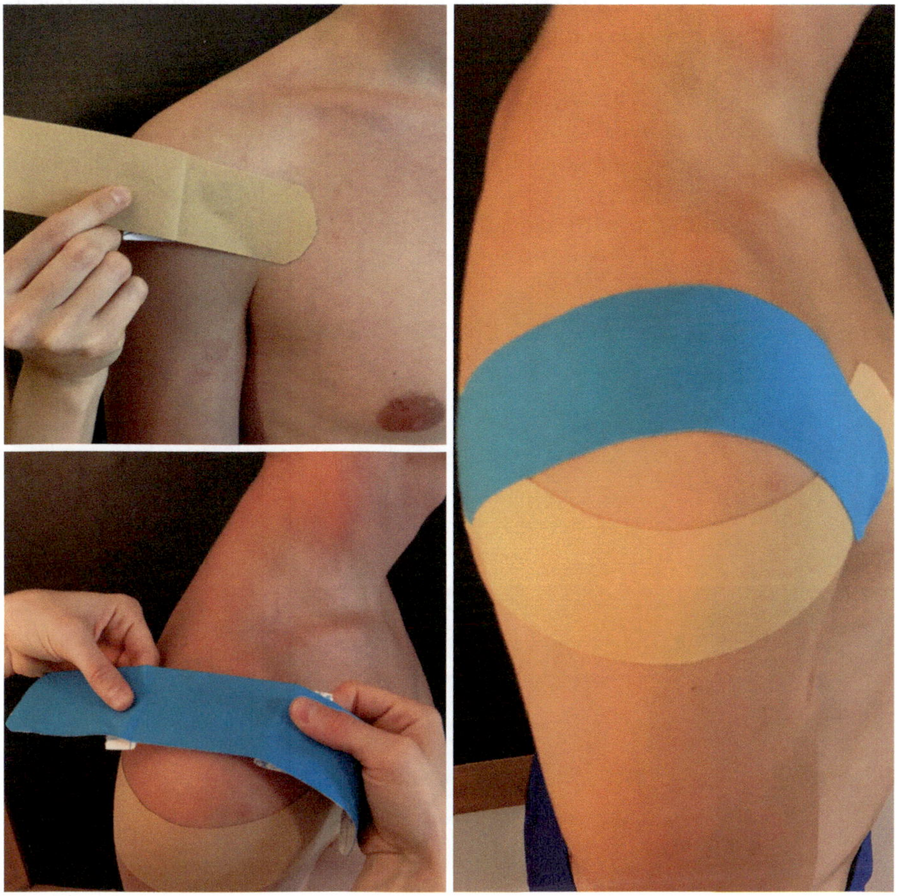

Fig. 2 This figure demonstrates a mechanical correction technique for shoulder instability. In order to apply, two I strips are used. In this figure, the tan tape is anchored to the lateral aspect of the right pectoralis muscle. An inward/downward pressure is applied by the provider's hand as the tape is applied at a 50–75% stretch. The blue tape is anchored in the middle, over the acromion or the humeral head, with a 50–75% stretch. An inward/downward pressure is applied as the tape is applied. No tension should be applied to the anchors or the tails of the I strips

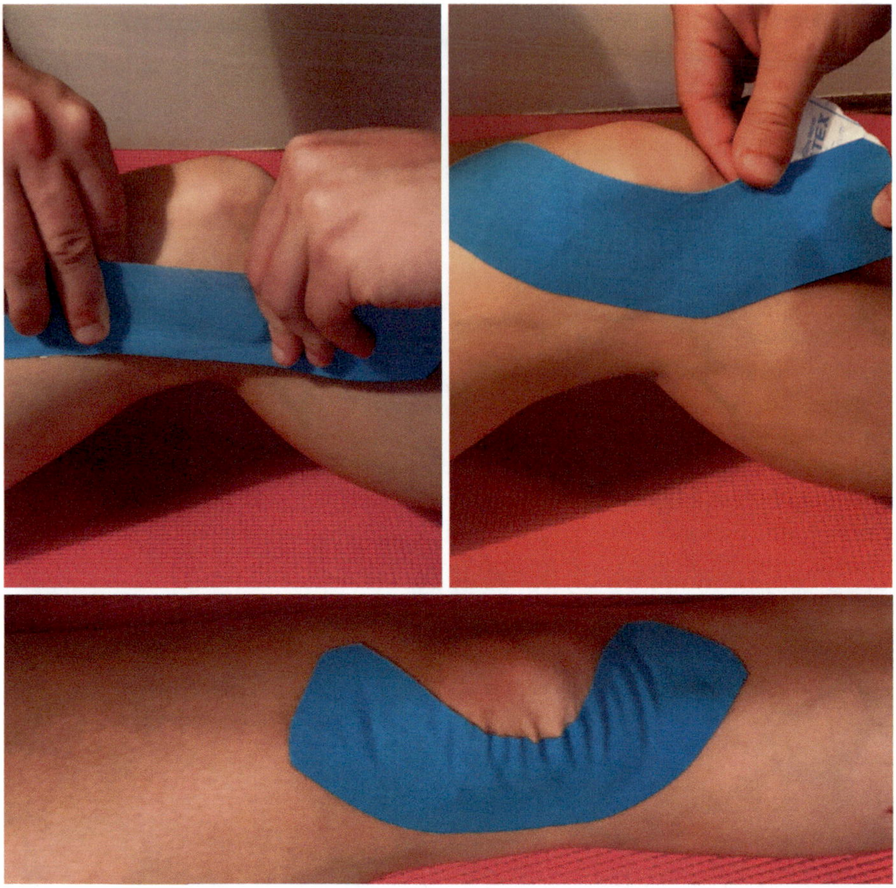

Fig. 3 Demonstrates a mechanical correction technique of the knee to address patellofemoral pain. In order to apply, an I strip is anchored in the middle, lateral to the patella, at a 50–75% stretch. A downward/inward pressure is applied as the patient actively flexes the knee. No tension should be applied to the anchor or the tail of the I strip

5 Research

Kinesio Taping, in combination with structured physical therapy, has been shown in multiple studies to improve disability scores, satisfaction scores, and to provide pain relief in various regions of the body [7, 8]. For example, chronic low back pain affects an overwhelming portion of the population without significant and reliable treatment options [9]. In a 2016 systematic review, Nelson evaluated the effectiveness of Kinesio Taping in patients with chronic low back pain [10]. As an isolated treatment modality, taping had no significant effects on patient symptoms. When used as an adjunctive therapy to traditional physical therapy and exercise, authors reported improved pain and disability scores. As an adjunct to traditional methods,

Kinesio Taping for chronic low back pain may have improved results and reduction of symptoms. In 2018, Li et al. reviewed a series of studies evaluating the use of Kinesio Tape for chronic low back pain. In their evaluation, they noted that there was no statistically significant difference in pain or disability with taping alone or in conjunction with physical therapy, although both trended towards improvement. There was a statistically significant difference between Kinesio Taping alone and sham taping alone. This finding suggests there is certainly some symptomatic benefit to Kinesio Taping in the setting of low back pain. Given its low cost, ease of application, and low risk profile, it should be considered as an adjunctive measure in patients with chronic low back pain [7].

In comparison to chronic low back pain, there are few studies evaluating Kinesio Taping in the acute low back pain setting. Kelle et al., in 2015, evaluated 109 patients with acute, nonspecific low back pain with either Kinesio Taping or education [4]. Both groups were also given as needed use of paracetamol. Patients were evaluated after 12 days and then again after 4 weeks for pain, disability and paracetamol use. Patients in the Kinesio Taping group reached adequate pain control at day 6 compared to day 12 on average, and consumed less medication. At 4 weeks patients in the Kinesio Taping group showed statistically significant improvements in pain scores. Disability scores were no different at 12 weeks. This study strongly suggests that Kinesio Taping may be beneficial in the patient with acute, nonspecific low back pain [4].

Kinesio Taping methods have also been used effectively in relation to shoulder pain. In 2008, Thelen et al. evaluated the effectiveness of Kinesio Taping on patients with shoulder impingement or rotator cuff tendonitis [11]. In their evaluation, they identified pain scores both while the Kinesio Tape was applied as well as each day following its removal. They found a reduction in pain scores after Kinesio Tape removal until day 3 after removal at which time pain scores returned to baseline. As an adjunct, this evaluation supports Kinesio Tape wear as a short-term therapy, and may provide relief up to day 3 after tape removal in patients with chronic pain from shoulder impingement [10]. Kinesio Taping has also been shown to have beneficial effects in treating shoulder impingement syndrome that are similar to the effects of conventional physical therapy. Kul et al., in 2019, compared conventional physical therapy techniques for shoulder impingement syndrome to Kinesio Taping alone. At 1 month follow up, both Kinesio Taping and physical therapy showed statistically significant improvement with the exception of night pain. Kinesio Taping was inferior to physical therapy when it comes to controlling nocturnal symptoms. This study did not evaluate the two treatment modalities in combination however. This study does not specifically support Kinesio Taping in isolation for subacromial impingement syndrome, however the data support its use as an adjunctive measure to conventional physical therapy techniques [6].

Kinesio Taping has been evaluated as a treatment modality for patellofemoral pain syndrome. In 2017, Logan et al. reviewed 5 randomized control trials using Kinesio Tape for patellofemoral pain. All studies evaluated in this review found statistically significant improvement in pain scores compared to both sham taping and taping alone without formal physical therapy. Once again, this review supports the use of Kinesio Tape as an adjunctive measure to formal therapy techniques for the treatment of patella femoral pain syndrome [8]. In the authors' experiences, as seen intra-operatively, a laterally tracking patella can be caused by adhesions between subcutaneous tissues and deeper fascial planes. One method is to surgically release these adhesions to correct the line of pull of the patella. It is the author's belief that the Kinesio Tape correction technique used for a laterally tracking patella may provide a stretch on the adhesions, altering the adhesion tissue properties, in order to redirect the pull on the patella.

6 Concerns/Drawbacks

Contraindications

- Fragile skin
- Tape allergies
- Sunburn
- Infection
- Irritated skin
- Open wound
- Poor circulation
- Arterial insufficiency
- Venous insufficiency

Precautions

- Malignancies
- Congestive heart failure
- Lymphedema

Side effects

- Rash
- Pruritus
- Ecchymosis

7 Conclusion

Kinesio Taping, in conjunction with structured physical therapy, is an effective non-operative method for pain relief. It is the authors' belief that taping provides biomechanical feedback when the physiologic barrier of a joint is reached in order to inhibit overstretching or overuse of a joint or muscle. It is suggested that taping in the presence of instability, secondary to a patulous joint capsule, allows for the closure of anatomic dead space leading to increased stability. Kinesio Taping, in instances like anterior knee pain, can change the mechanical pull and the vector of force on the tendinous attachment. It is the authors' opinion, which is heavily supported by research, that Kinesio Taping should be used in conjunction with other pain management techniques. In a world of growing medical costs and societal burden, Kinesio Taping is an effective, affordable, and safe pain relief option for the correct patient.

References

1. Turk DC, Theodore BR. Epidemiology and economics of chronic and recurrent pain. In: Clinical pain management: a practical guide. New York: Wiley; 2010. p. 6–13. https://doi.org/10.1002/9781444329711.ch2.
2. Bandyopadhyay A, Mahapatra D. Taping in sports: a brief update. J Hum Sport Exerc. 2012;7(2):544–52. https://doi.org/10.4100/jhse.2012.72.17.
3. Bassett KT, Lingman SA, Ellis RF. The use and treatment efficacy of kinaesthetic taping for musculoskeletal conditions: a systematic review. NZ J Physiother. 2010;38(2):56–63.
4. Kelle B, Güzel R, Sakallı H. The effect of Kinesio taping application for acute non-specific low back pain: a randomized controlled clinical trial. Clin Rehabil. 2016;30(10):997–1003. https://doi.org/10.1177/0269215515603218.
5. Kinesio Taping Association International. KT1: fundamental concepts of the Kinesio Taping® Method and KT2: advanced concepts and corrective techniques of the Kinesio Taping® Method. Albuquerque: Kinesio Taping Association International; 2013.
6. Kul A, Ugur M. Comparison of the efficacy of conventional physical therapy modalities and kinesio taping treatments in shoulder impingement syndrome. Eurasian J Med. 2019;51(2):138–43. https://doi.org/10.5152/eurasianjmed.2018.17421.
7. Li Y, Yin Y, Jia G, Chen H, Yu L, Wu D. Effects of kinesiotape on pain and disability in individuals with chronic low back pain: a systematic review and meta-analysis of randomized controlled trials. Clin Rehabil. 2018;33(4):596–606. https://doi.org/10.1177/0269215518817804.
8. Logan CA, Bhashyam AR, Tisosky AJ, Haber DB, Provencher MT. Systematic review of the effect of taping techniques on patellofemoral pain syndrome. Sports Health. 2017;9(5):456–61. https://doi.org/10.1177/1941738117710938.
9. Morris D, Jones D, Ryan H, Ryan CG. The clinical effects of Kinesio® Tex taping: a systematic review. Physiother Theory Pract. 2012;29(4):259–70. https://doi.org/10.3109/09593985.2012.731675.
10. Nelson NL. Kinesio taping for chronic low back pain: a systematic review. J Bodyw Mov Ther. 2016;20(3):672–81. https://doi.org/10.1016/j.jbmt.2016.04.018.
11. Thelen M, Dauber J, Stoneman P. Clinical efficacy of kinesio tape for shoulder pain: a randomized, double-blinded, clinical trial. J Orthop Sports Phys Ther. 2008;38:389–95.

Further Reading

Araya-Quintanilla F, Gutiérrez-Espinoza H, Sepúlveda-Loyola W, Probst V, Ramírez-Vélez R, Álvarez-Bueno C. Effectiveness of kinesiotaping in patients with subacromial impingement syndrome: a systematic review with meta-analysis. Scand J Med Sci Sports. 2022;32(2):273–89. https://doi.org/10.1111/sms.14084.

Part III

Bedside Interventions for Special Patient Populations

Special Considerations for Bedside Pain Management Interventions for Elderly

Jung Hoon Kim, Christopher Alexander,
and Katherine Dawn Travnicek

Essential Concepts
- Multi-modal and interdisciplinary pain management is recommended
- For patients with deficiencies in communication, cognitive decline or dementia, normal methods of elucidating pain are often not adequate
- Sedation and adverse effects are more common in elderly patients

1 Overview

With the advances in society and medicine, the population of Americans aged 65 and older continues to increase. However, while patients are now living longer than ever before, the prevalence of chronic pain in the elderly has been suggested to be as high as 80% [1]. Chronic pain not only interferes with normal functioning for the elderly, but can lead to depression, social isolation, immobility, and sleep disturbances [2]. Compounding this issue are studies that suggest elderly patients under report pain due to misconceptions that it is a normal part of aging or out of fear of addiction [3]. Understandably, they are concerned about the significant side effects

J. H. Kim · C. Alexander
Dartmouth-Hitchcock Medical Center, Lebanon, NH, USA
e-mail: Jung.h.kim@hitchcock.org; Christopher.E.Alexander@hitchcock.org

K. D. Travnicek (✉)
Pain Institute of Nevada, Las Vegas, NV, USA
e-mail: kdt@paininstitute.com

D. Souza et al. (eds.), *Bedside Pain Management Interventions*,
https://doi.org/10.1007/978-3-031-11188-4_18

given the change in their physiology and sensitivity to medications [4]. These aspects pose challenges to effective pain management in the elderly which further deteriorates their quality of life.

2 Historical Aspects and Recent Developments

Effective pain management in the elderly requires a holistic, multimodal, multidisciplinary approach. Treatment prescriptions must correctly identify the source of pain and the severity of its impact, understand the physiological changes of the elderly, and reduce side effects of medications. Moreover, given the age-related changes to pain perception and medication metabolism, incorporation of both pharmacologic and non-pharmacologic approaches should be utilized to optimize pain management for this population.

With normal aging, various changes occur in our organ systems which alter the pharmacokinetics and pharmacodynamics of medications [5]. These changes include reductions in renal and hepatic metabolism and clearance which results in increased sensitivity to several drug classes. Of particular importance is the decreased ventilatory responses to hypoxia and hypercapnia which places the elderly at risk for respiratory failure when exposed to opioid medications.

Accurate assessment of pain in the elderly must correctly identify the source of the pain, the type of pain the patient is experiencing, and also take into consideration the functional limitations brought on by pain. To that end, each patient's unique symptoms and its impact must be elucidated through thorough questioning. Examples may include: Describe to me the type of pain you're experiencing and the impact it has on your life? Do you have pain you experience at baseline? What have you found to be the most helpful solution to your pain? Do you have any reservations about taking medications? What kind of worries do you have about this pain and why? Further functional assessment should include assessment of activities of daily living.

For patients with deficiencies in communication (difficulty hearing, speech impediment, etc.) or those with cognitive decline or dementia, normal methods of elucidating pain are often not adequate. Their inability to effectively communicate pain frequently leads to under treatment [4]. Moreover, cognitive decline may also alter pain perception and pharmacodynamics, which results in increased pain with decreased effectiveness of pain medications [6]. To combat these challenges, providers must use three ways to systematically measure the presence of pain: direct questioning, behavioral observation, and caregiver reports [1]. The American Geriatrics Society has published guidelines on observing common behaviors that correlate with pain: facial expressions, verbalizations, body movements, changes in interpersonal interactions, changes in activity patterns or routines, and mental status changes [7]. Behavioral observations should occur during times of activity as pain may be absent at rest.

Upon accurate assessment, correct diagnosis, and correct classification of the pain (i.e. neuropathic pain versus nociceptive pain versus mixed pain syndrome), interdisciplinary and multimodal pain regimen should be devised. Speaking with the patient to highlight the importance of restoring function over sole reduction in pain score should be emphasized.

3 Non Pharmacologic Interventions

Decreased physiologic reserve, polypharmacy, and altered drug metabolism can make the utilization of pharmacologic agents for pain management in the elderly quite challenging. It is therefore imperative that a multimodal approach including non-pharmacologic modalities be incorporated into the treatment plan. This is especially true in the hospital setting, where elderly patients are particularly susceptible to developing delirium which can precipitate injury/falls.

Pain management should focus on restoration of function and improvement of quality of life, rather than on the complete abolition of pain. Acute inactivity due to illness and hospitalization can lead to significant loss of strength, mobility, and ability to perform activities of daily living. Immobilized elderly patients demonstrate an accelerated loss of muscle mass and functional capacity in comparison to younger populations [8]. In order to combat this, patients should participate in physical and occupational therapies to preserve functionality unless medically contraindicated. This can include gait training, compensatory techniques for functional deficits, and activity modifications for pain-invoking tasks.

While physical therapy and exercise aid in facilitating functional restoration, the concurrent use of therapeutic physical modalities can also attenuate pain. Modalities involve application of some form of cold, heat, light, electromagnetic, acoustic energy, electrical stimulation, and desensitization techniques. Additionally, patients may also be candidates for bedside interventional procedures. Commonly performed bedside procedures include landmark or ultrasound-guided dry needling, trigger point injections, peripheral nerve blocks. There is a role for various joint injections and axial procedures.

Depending on the interventional procedure, there may be important risks to consider. Many elderly patients have multiple comorbid conditions which frequently necessitate the use of anticoagulants or other sedating medications. As such, it is imperative to consider the risks of discontinuing these medications prior to recommending a procedure as well as proper informed consent concerns. Likewise, with the aforementioned physiological changes, patients may have an exaggerated response to sedation which may be required for the procedures. Careful titration of medications is necessary in these situations.

Pain is a subjective experience, and perception of pain can vary significantly across different cultures and belief systems. Moreover, research suggests significant association between psychological distress and the manifestation of physical pain [9]. Because of this, psychological, spiritual, and religious support services may be warranted as part of the treatment plan. Discussing this with patients is paramount to understanding what other services to involve, such as a chaplain.

4 Pharmacologic Interventions

Pharmacologic treatments can be divided into opioids versus non-opioids. As aforementioned, the physiologic changes of the elderly make them more susceptible to the adverse effects of opioids and other sedating medications. Adverse effects include the following: respiratory depression, addiction/dependence, nausea, constipation, sedation, urinary retention, and dizziness. In particular, opioid naive elderly patients have a heightened risk of respiratory depression, so careful patient selection and vigilant monitoring for side effects are imperative [10]. Prior to initiation of opioids, a trial of non-opioid medications and alternative therapies should be completed. The following opioids have special considerations in the elderly. Transdermal fentanyl should not be utilized in opioid naive patients as high drug concentrations within the patch can cause severe respiratory depression [11]. Morphine, codeine, and meperidine should be avoided in patients with renal dysfunction/failure as toxic metabolites can accumulate. Methadone, fentanyl, and sufentanil appear to be safe to use in patients with renal failure [12]. However, methadone has an unpredictable half-life and should be prescribed by providers with extensive experience and understanding of its pharmacokinetics. Oxymorphone, hydromorphone, and hydrocodone should be utilized with caution in hepatic and renal insufficiency [12].

Generally speaking, non-opioid medications are preferred to opioids for non-cancer pain due to side effects in older patients. The two most commonly used non-opioid medication for pain include NSAIDs and acetaminophen. Acetaminophen should be considered as a first line therapy in the treatment of persistent pain, particularly for nociceptive pain. It has a reasonable safety profile and can be very effective. The maximum daily dose of 4 g per 24 h should not be exceeded, but more often patients should be cautious about taking more than 3 g per 24 h [13]. The absolute contraindication to acetaminophen is liver failure. Lastly, acetaminophen is commonly found as a combination component of many medications, as such, all sources of acetaminophen should be taken into account.

NSAIDs are useful medications for nociceptive type pain. However, prolonged use of NSAIDs (for nociceptive pain) is not recommended in the elderly with chronic pain because of the increased risk of adverse events in this population. NSAIDs have been shown to adversely affect gastrointestinal, renal, and cardiac systems. As such, absolute contraindications to NSAIDs include heart failure, chronic kidney disease, and active peptic ulcer disease [14]. If NSAIDs are prescribed for older patients, using the lowest most effective dose and a defined, short course to mitigate the potential side effects is recommended [15].

For neuropathic pain, common medications used include anticonvulsants and antidepressants. Common side effects of anticonvulsants (i.e. gabapentin, pregabalin) include dizziness, weight gain, and somnolence. No dose adjustments for gabapentin and pregabalin are required in hepatic dysfunction, but doses need to be adjusted for renal dysfunction [16]. Tricyclic antidepressants (TCAs) are highly anticholinergic, which causes side effects of sedation, cognitive dysfunction, orthostatic hypotension, and urinary retention. Of the TCAs, amitriptyline causes the most anticholinergic effects, while nortriptyline and desipramine causes the least. Duloxetine is a serotonin, norepinephrine reuptake inhibitor which has also shown efficacy for neuropathic pain.

5 Additional Concerns

There are three main concerns regarding this patient population—evidence-based recommendations for pain treatments, the perceptions and biases surrounding chronic pain and its management, pain management education, and insurance coverage. Robust scientific evidence to guide one in managing pain in geriatric patients is limited. Due to stringent selection criteria in random controlled trials, complex elderly patients with multiple co-morbidities are frequently either excluded or inadequately represented. Second, pain is an under recognized and sub optimally treated symptom in the elderly as it seems to be underreported by the elderly and some health care providers fear geriatric patients will have adverse effects from therapies available to them. For pain management to be effective in the elderly, physicians and allied health care providers should be skilled in assessing pain, knowledgeable of the types of pain, and recognize the importance of a holistic, interdisciplinary team approach to pain management. Finally, insurance companies provide barriers to medical care for pharmacological and interventional therapies.

6 Conclusion and Future Directions

The elderly present with many challenges for pain practitioners, including comorbid medical conditions, polypharmacy, and declining physical and mental function. Current treatments or pain management therapies are largely based on the modulation of pain and with many new technologies entering the market (vibration with cold bracing, peripheral nerve stimulation, etc).

References

1. Andrade DC, Faria JW, Caramelli P, et al. The assessment and management of pain in the demented and non-demented elderly patient. Arq Neuropsiquiatr. 2011;69:387.
2. Denny DL, Guido GW. Under treatment of pain in older adults: an application of beneficence. Nurs Ethics. 2012;19(6):800–9.
3. Culberson JW, Ziska M. Prescription drug misuse/abuse in the elderly. Geriatrics. 2008;63:22.
4. Griffioen C, Willems EG, Husebo BS, Achterberg WP. Prevalence of the use of opioids for treatment of pain in persons with a cognitive impairment compared with cognitively intact persons: a systematic review. Curr Alzheimer Res. 2017;14:512.
5. Braddom RL. Physical medicine and rehabilitation. 3rd ed. Philadelphia: Saunders Elsevier; 2007. p. 1415–28.
6. Benedetti F, Arduino C, Costa S, et al. Loss of expectation-related mechanisms in Alzheimer's disease makes analgesic therapies less effective. Pain. 2006;121:133.
7. AGS Panel on Persistent Pain in Older Persons. The management of persistent pain in older persons. J Am Geriatr Soc. 2002;50:S205.

8. English KL, Paddon-Jones D. Protecting muscle mass and function in older adults during bed rest. Curr Opin Clin Nutr Metab Care. 2010;13(1):34–9. https://doi.org/10.1097/MCO.0b013e328333aa66.
9. Riva P, Wirth JH, Williams KD. The consequences of pain: the social and physical pain overlap on psychological responses. Eur J Soc Psychol. 2011;41:681–7. https://doi.org/10.1002/ejsp.837.
10. Fine PG, Mahajan G, McPherson ML. Long-acting opioids and short-acting opioids: appropriate use in chronic pain management. Pain Med. 2009;10(Suppl 2):S79–88.
11. Ortho-McNeil-Janssen Pharmaceuticals, Inc. Duragesic (transdermal fentanyl). Titusville: Ortho-McNeil-Janssen Pharmaceuticals; 2008.
12. Dean M. Opioids in renal failure and dialysis patients. J Pain Symptom Manag. 2004;28(5):497–504.
13. Kuehn BM. FDA focuses on drugs and liver damage: labeling and other changes for acetaminophen. JAMA. 2009;302:369.
14. American Geriatrics Society Panel on the Pharmacological Management of Persistent Pain in Older Persons. Pharmacological management of persistent pain in older persons. J Am Geriatr Soc. 2009;57(8):1331–46.
15. Scheiman JM, Hindley CE. Strategies to optimize treatment with NSAIDs in patients at risk for gastrointestinal and cardiovascular adverse events. Clin Ther. 2010;32:667.
16. Israni RK, Kasbekar N, Haynes K, Berns JS. Use of antiepileptic drugs in patients with kidney disease. Semin Dial. 2006;19(5):408–16.

Further Reading

Dagnino APA, Campos MM. Chronic pain in the elderly: mechanisms and perspectives. Front Hum Neurosci. 2022;3(16):736688. https://doi.org/10.3389/fnhum.2022.736688.

Special Considerations for Bedside Pain Management Interventions for Chronic Pain Patients

Abhishek Vaidya, Lahari Vudayagiri, Dmitri Souza, and Samer N. Narouze

Essential Concepts

- Bedside pain management interventions are beneficial for hospitalized patients with pre-existing chronic pain.
- These procedures are typically relatively easy to set up to perform.
- Bedside pain management procedures should be considered as a part of multimodal pain management in hospitalized patients.

1 Background

Chronic pain is an increasingly prevalent condition in the United States affecting up to 35% of the population [1]. Clinical evaluation, including a detailed history and physical exam, review of imaging studies, and verification of the underlying cause of chronic pain should always be prioritized. This is of particular importance in the perioperative period [2, 3]. Perioperative period is defined as the days immediately preceding, during, and post-operatively (up to 30 days) following surgical intervention [4].

Patients undergoing surgical intervention with a history of chronic pain commonly have increased anesthesia requirements as well as an increased need for

A. Vaidya · L. Vudayagiri
Department of General Surgery, Western Reserve Hospital, Cuyahoga Falls, OH, USA
e-mail: avaidya@westernreservehospital.org; lvudayagiri@westernreservehospital.org

D. Souza (✉) · S. N. Narouze
Center for Pain Medicine, Western Reserve Hospital, Cuyahoga Falls, OH, USA
e-mail: dsouza@westernreservehospital.org; snarouze@westernreservehospital.org

D. Souza et al. (eds.), *Bedside Pain Management Interventions*,
https://doi.org/10.1007/978-3-031-11188-4_19

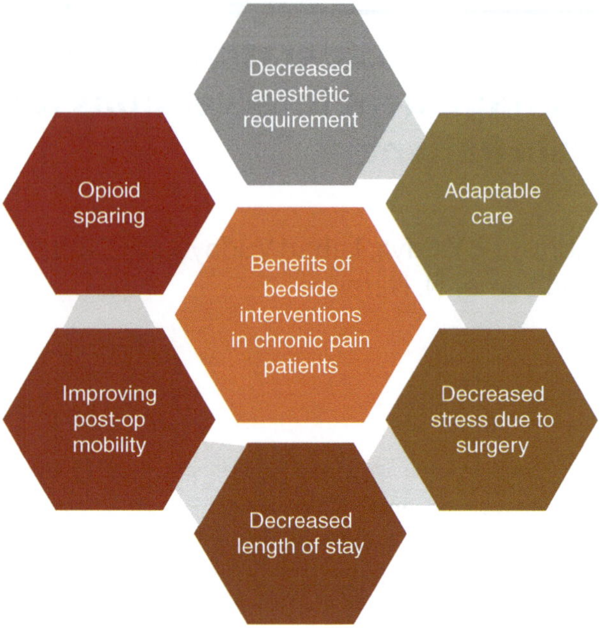

Fig. 1 Benefits of bedside pain management interventions for patients with pre-existing chronic pain

intra- and postoperative analgesia. Currently, the general understanding is that this acute on chronic pain is potentiated by central sensitization, opioid tolerance, and commonly undiagnosed opioid-induced hyperalgesia [5, 6]. As a result, pain control becomes a challenge due to concerns for respiratory depression, oversedation, and overdose of analgesics and antianxiety medicines [7, 8]. Bedside procedures for the management of chronic pain have proven to be efficacious in this regard. In the perioperative period, these procedures may provide additional pain relief as well as social and economic benefits presented in Fig. 1. Interventional bedside procedures include local nerve blocks, regional nerve blocks as well as epidural or spinal anesthesia.

2 Common Bedside Procedures

Bedside pain management interventions include a variety of strategies. Diagnostic or therapeutic blockade with local anesthetic, steroids, or other agents is the most common strategy. Bedside analgesia can also be achieved by indirect injection of local anesthetic to the affected site prior to or after the surgery [8–10]. The same modality is also regularly employed intraoperatively at incision sites. Another modality is spinal or epidural anesthesia. Anesthetic can be injected directly into the subarachnoid or epidural space. Bedside interventions for patients with chronic pain can also include myofascial release, manipulations, pain psychology interventions, transcutaneous neuromodulation, and other techniques described in this book [11, 12]. There are several reasons for bedside interventions be successful in chronic pain patients, including decreased anesthetic requirements, opioid sparing, improved mobility, avoiding polypharmacy, especially in the elderly, and many others (Fig. 1). However, there are certain considerations specific for the chronic pain patient population that needs to be taken into view prior to planning for bedside interventions [1, 13–16].

3 Special Considerations for Bedside Procedures in Chronic Pain Patients

Any procedural intervention requires consideration of the risk versus benefits of the procedure itself, and the best modality is one with the greatest benefit to the lowest risk to the patient. Risks of common bedside procedures include bleeding, infection, nerve injury, local anesthetic toxicity, and anaphylaxis. Hence, to minimize risk, the anatomy of the intervention site is carefully chosen, sterile procedures are enforced, and anesthetic dosing is carefully calculated [1]. Further considerations, specific for chronic pain patients, include the detailed history of the patient's chronic pain condition which may lead to deferral of some type of bedside procedures. Pre-existing neuropathy or nerve damage, any structural or functional damage, has to be documented prior to approaching any bedside interventional procedures [1, 17, 18].

Similar to the general inpatient population, contraindications are also an important factor when approaching bedside interventions for chronic pain patients. Sites with active infection, not unusual in hospitalized patients, or open or nonhealing wounds should not be chosen for nerve blocks, as well as for regional or spinal anesthesia. Furthermore, spinal or epidural anesthesia has an increased risk of respiratory depression if performed in the thoracic/cervical region as the phrenic nerve originates at a level of C3–C5. Due to invariable requests to increase the dose of opioids these types of procedures are to be carefully planned in terms of dosing and patient's consent. Patient refusal sometimes is seen in the chronic pain patient population and is also a contraindication to the bedside procedure. Patients with pain control devices such as stimulators or intrathecal pumps require special assessment, especially for regional and axial procedures. However, bedside interventions are not contraindicated in these patients [1, 19, 20].

4 Maximizing Outcomes

A multimodal approach to pain control, including bedside interventions, would typically help to maximize clinical outcomes [1]. During the perioperative period, it is crucial to managing the patient's expectations. Chronic pain patients should be informed of tolerance to opiates and possible opioid-induced hyperalgesia. It is important to manage chronic pain patients' anxiety during the perioperative period. Co-morbid conditions such as chronic kidney disease, diabetes, hypertension should also be optimized as these can inhibit the patient's recovery by complicating the healing process secondary to electrolyte abnormalities or hyperglycemia which inhibit wound healing [21, 22]. It is important to continue prescribing baseline antipsychotic and hypnotic medications chronic pain patients may use, unless contraindicated. Nicotine patches can also be used to decrease cravings in the perioperative for patients with tobacco use disorder and are routinely recommended. Appropriate conversion of oral opiates/opioids to intravenous formulations must be utilized to provide adequate coverage for pain control. Bedside pain management interventions can positively reflect on chronic pain patients' satisfaction with care provided for them [23–25].

5 Summary and Future Directions

Bedside pain management interventions for chronic pain patients can be exceptionally beneficial [1]. Pain relief can be achieved without a significant increase in the dose of opiates/opioids [26–28]. Multimodal pain management, including bedside interventions, would likely help to improve chronic pain patients' mobility, wound healing, and patient satisfaction. It is expected that the length of stay in the intensive care unit or hospital may be decreased as well. Furthermore, bedside pain management interventions may reflect on decreased risk of immediate intra- and postoperative adverse effects in chronic pain patients caused by anesthesia such as arrhythmia, altered mentation, nausea, and vomiting [29, 30]. The need for deep sedation and anesthesia requirements could be lessened as well. Consideration must always be used when performing any bedside interventional procedures for chronic pain patients, but the use of adequate sterile technique, careful evaluation of modality and site, ultrasound guidance, if indicated, and monitoring if indicated, can all decrease the risk of complications [1]. Bedside pain management interventions for chronic pain patients becoming increasingly popular in the perioperative period due to the evident improvement in outcomes and should be considered when applicable.

References

1. Souzdalnitski D, Halaszynski TM, Faclier G. Regional anesthesia and co-existing chronic pain. Curr Opin Anaesthesiol. 2010;23(5):662–70.
2. Souzdalnitski D, Bolinske T, Vadivelu N. Pain quality assessment scale: practical implications of factor analysis. Clin J Pain. 2009;25(5):453.
3. Cheng OT, Souzdalnitski D, Vrooman B, Cheng J. Evidence-based knee injections for the management of arthritis. Pain Med (United States). 2012;13(6):740–53.
4. Tubog TD. Overview of multimodal analgesia initiated in the perioperative setting. J Perioper Pract. 2021;31(5):191–8.
5. George S, Johns M. Review of nonopioid multimodal analgesia for surgical and trauma patients. Am J Health Syst Pharm. 2020;77(24):2052–63.
6. Pitchon DN, Dayan AC, Schwenk ES, Baratta JL, Viscusi ER. Updates on multimodal analgesia for orthopedic surgery. Anesthesiol Clin. 2018;36(3):361–73.
7. Wick EC, Grant MC, Wu CL. Postoperative multimodal analgesia pain management with nonopioid analgesics and techniques: a review. JAMA Surg. 2017;152(7):691–7.

8. Chen YYK, Boden KA, Schreiber KL. The role of regional anaesthesia and multimodal analgesia in the prevention of chronic postoperative pain: a narrative review. Anaesthesia. 2021;76(S1):8–17.
9. Ban VS, Bhoja R, McDonagh DL. Multimodal analgesia for craniotomy. Curr Opin Anaesthesiol. 2019;32(5):592–9.
10. Bruhn J, Scheffer GJ, van Geffen GJ. Clinical application of perioperative multimodal analgesia. Curr Opin Support Palliat Care. 2017;11(2):106–11.
11. Choi E, Nahm FS, Han WK, Lee PB, Jo J. Topical agents: a thoughtful choice for multimodal analgesia. Korean J Anesthesiol. 2020;73(5):384–93.
12. Carvalho B, Butwick AJ. Postcesarean delivery analgesia. Best Pract Res Clin Anaesthesiol. 2017;31(1):69–79.
13. Haskins SC, Bronshteyn Y, Perlas A, El-Boghdadly K, Zimmerman J, Silva M, et al. American Society of Regional Anesthesia and Pain Medicine expert panel recommendations on point-of-care ultrasound education and training for regional anesthesiologists and pain physicians—part I: clinical indications. Reg Anesth Pain Med. 2021;46(12):1031–47.
14. Haskins SC, Bronshteyn Y, Perlas A, El-Boghdadly K, Zimmerman J, Silva M, et al. American Society of Regional Anesthesia and Pain Medicine expert panel recommendations on point-of-care ultrasound education and training for regional anesthesiologists and pain physicians—part II: recommendations. Reg Anesth Pain Med. 2021;46(12):1048–60.
15. Narouze S, Souzdalnitski D. Ultrasound-guided percutaneous cervical and upper thoracic sympathetic chain neuromodulation for upper extremity complex regional pain syndrome. Ochsner J. 2017;17(2):199–203.
16. Souzdalnitski D, Vadivelu N, Chung KS. Low-dose ketamine as an adjunct to routine pain practice: are we ready yet? Pain Pract. 2009;9(5):405–6.
17. Smith N, Liew Z, Johnson S, Ellard DR, Underwood M, Kearney R. A systematic review of the methods and drugs used for performing suprascapular nerve block injections for the non-surgical management of chronic shoulder pain. Br J Pain. 2021;15(4):460–73.
18. Cogan CJ, Kandemir U. Role of peripheral nerve block in pain control for the management of acute traumatic orthopaedic injuries in the emergency department: diagnosis-based treatment guidelines. Injury. 2020;51(7):1422–5.
19. Charipova K, Gress K, Berger AA, Kassem H, Schwartz R, Herman J, et al. A comprehensive review and update of post-surgical cutaneous nerve entrapment. Curr Pain Headache Rep. 2021;25(2):1–8.
20. Taylor SS, Noor N, Urits I, Paladini A, Sadhu MS, Gibb C, et al. Complex regional pain syndrome: a comprehensive review. Pain Ther. 2021;10(2):875–92.
21. Beverly A, Kaye AD, Ljungqvist O, Urman RD. Essential elements of multimodal analgesia in enhanced recovery after surgery (ERAS) guidelines. Anesthesiol Clin. 2017;35(2):e115–43.
22. Joshi GP. Multimodal analgesia techniques and postoperative rehabilitation. Anesthesiol Clin N Am. 2005;23(1):185–202.
23. Agarwal D, Chahar P, Chmiela M, Sagir A, Kim A, Malik F, et al. Multimodal analgesia for perioperative management of patients presenting for spinal surgery. Curr Pharm Des. 2019;25(19):2123–32.
24. Helander EM, Menard BL, Harmon CM, Homra BK, Allain AV, Bordelon GJ, et al. Multimodal analgesia, current concepts, and acute pain considerations. Curr Pain Headache Rep. 2017;21(1):3.
25. Dancel R, Liles EA, Fiore D. Acute pain management in hospitalized children. Reviews on recent. Clin Trials. 2017;12(4):277–83.
26. Offodile AC, Sheckter CC, Tucker A, Watzker A, Ottino K, Zammert M, et al. Preoperative paravertebral blocks for the management of acute pain following mastectomy: a cost-effectiveness analysis. Breast Cancer Res Treat. 2017;165(3):477–84.
27. Scurrah A, Shiner CT, Stevens JA, Faux SG. Regional nerve blockade for early analgesic management of elderly patients with hip fracture—a narrative review. Anaesthesia. 2018;73(6):769–83.

28. Rathier MO, Baker WL. A review of recent clinical trials and guidelines on the prevention and management of delirium in hospitalized older patients. Hosp Pract (1995). 2011;39(4):96–106.
29. Qin L, You D, Zhao G, Li L, Zhao S. A comparison of analgesic techniques for total knee arthroplasty: a network meta-analysis. J Clin Anesth. 2021;1:71.
30. Berkowitz RA, McDonald TB. Post-operative pain management. Indian J Pediatr. 1997;64(3):351–67.

Further Reading

Rosenquist RW, Souzdalnitski D, Urman R. Chronic pain management for hospitalized patient. 1st ed. New York: Oxford University Press; 2016. p. 420.

Special Considerations for Bedside Pain Management Interventions for Morbidly Obese Individuals

Nicole Sarkisian, Dmitri Souza, and Samer N. Narouze

Essential Concepts

- There association between chronic pain and obesity is not coincidental, and the two are very much linked.
- Obesity is multifactorial. Various metabolic, biomechanical, genetic, environmental, cultural, social, and behavioral mechanisms play a role.
- With increased body mass index, more pressure is exerted on joints, causing more instability. In addition, the adipose tissue itself contributes to the pro-inflammatory state, and therefore, to persistent pain.
- Special attention to planning, conducting, and following up after bedside pain management intervention for obese individuals is essential. That includes a selection of the procedure, special attention to the aseptic practice, choice of imaging modality versus landmark technique, monitoring the patient during and after the procedure.

1 Overview

Obesity, as defined by World Health Organization (WHO), is a body mass index (BMI) that is greater than 30.0. This is a growing entity with greater than 500,000 million adults nationwide in this category and growing per year [1, 2]. Obese patients

N. Sarkisian
Department of Family Medicine, Western Reserve Hospital, Cuyahoga Falls, OH, USA

D. Souza (✉) · S. N. Narouze
Center for Pain Medicine, Western Reserve Hospital, Cuyahoga Falls, OH, USA
e-mail: dsouza@westernreservehospital.org

D. Souza et al. (eds.), *Bedside Pain Management Interventions*,
https://doi.org/10.1007/978-3-031-11188-4_20

often suffer from a combination of type 2 diabetes mellitus, hypertension, dyslipidemia, also known, when combined, as the "metabolic syndrome." These conditions as well as the metabolic syndrome are independent predictors of inpatient, and especially perioperative, morbidity and mortality [3]. There have been many studies that show that the association between chronic pain and obesity is not unexpected, and the two are very much linked [2]. With extra body mass, there is more pressure exerted on joints causing more instability. In addition, there is a body of evidence showing that with additional adipose tissue, the patient's state of inflammation evolves as well. The connection between pain and obesity includes many factors. There are genetic, environmental, metabolic, biomechanical, cultural, social, and behavioral mechanisms [2]. All these factors and the pathophysiology behind them make a wide range of interventions available for pain control. This chapter will elaborate on the specifics of bedside interventions for obese individuals [4].

2 Specifics of Bedside Interventions for Morbidly Obese Individuals

Several pharmacological and interventional pain management strategies have proven beneficial in morbidly obese hospitalized patients [2, 5]. Some studies specifically investigate interventional procedures to help alleviate the pain in the beast and morbidly obese individuals [2, 4]. Many interventional approaches in the obese population can also be seen in the general population. Examples of traditional approaches include peripheral nerve blocks, joint injections, tendon sheath, ligament injections, acupuncture, and invasive neuromodulation, including TENS and others. In this section, we will elaborate on available interventional modalities and the complications they can cause in the obese population [2, 6].

Epidural injections, despite recent criticism, remain one of the safest and highly effective techniques for treating acute radicular pain, which is common in morbidly obese patients. In the past, these procedures were commonly performed at the bedside, for example at the labor and delivery floor. However, with the wide availability of fluoroscopy, when possible, this procedure should not be routinely performed at the bedside, especially in morbidly obese individuals, except for the labor and delivery floor where axial procedures are still routinely performed at the bedside. It should be taken into consideration that the depth of the epidural space differs in obese patients compared with individuals with normal weight [2]. Other imaging techniques for bedside interventional procedures should be carefully chosen to ensure adequate imaging during the procedure because obesity creates challenges for seeing the target structure. This is especially important for ultrasound-guided procedures. For example, the success rate for lumbar facet injection was significantly lower in obese patients compared with normal-weight patients when ultrasonography was used for needle guidance [2, 4]. Some pain blocks, such as of the sciatic nerve in the gluteal area, can be performed faster with modifications to access the targeted structure better in obese patients [2]. Incautious use of corticosteroids for joint, tendon sheath, and ligamentous injections can compromise the safety of morbidly obese patients who commonly present with prediabetes or diabetes mellitus, and a history of significant weight gain from earlier corticosteroid injections.

Other treatment technologies are being developed. Platelet-rich plasma (PRP) is a blood-derived autologous concentrate of platelets. It is known to contain high levels of autologous growth factors, such as platelet-derived growth factors, fibroblastic growth factors, vascular endothelial growth factors, and others. The PRP can stimulate tissue healing via control of connective tissue regeneration and angiogenesis. There are reports of benefits of regenerative medicine technologies, specifically PRP therapy, in the treatment of knee pain associated with osteoarthritis in obese patients [2].

Joint, tendon sheaves, periarticular, and ligament injections are procedures that can be performed at the bedside in morbidly obese individuals to decrease musculoskeletal pain. Tendon sheaths injections also provide manipulation of that area to stimulate tissue changes through injury and regrowth. The concerns are very similar to epidural injections with imaging clarity and depth of injection. Other concerns in morbidly obese individuals include patient positioning during the bedside procedures and also potential for increased post-procedural pain. There are other concerns outlined in Fig. 1.

It is important to note that the inpatient care for morbidly obese individuals requires intensive collaboration of healthcare professionals including nurses, supporting staff, physicians, dietitians, physical and occupational therapy, and, on some occasions, psychology. These healthcare professionals should work to benefit the patient. Also, staff members may need additional training to assist with care for complex morbidly obese patients.

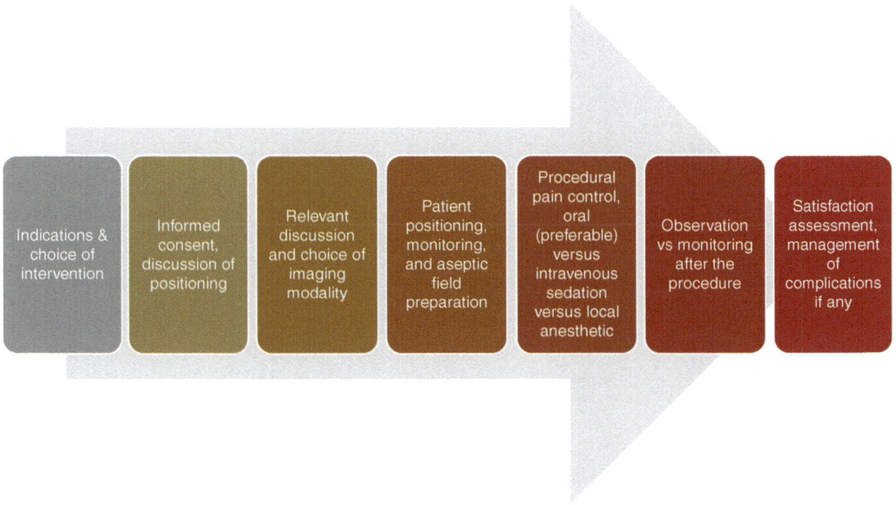

Fig. 1 Special considerations for bedside pain management interventions in morbidly obese individuals

3 Conclusion

Obesity and chronic pain are very much related. Bedside pain management interventions should be adjusted to adhere to the specifics of the obese patients' population. With the help of well-trained inpatient supporting staff, physicians, and multifaceted care, we can strengthen and build upon the comprehensive care of pain in obese patients that includes bedside interventions.

References

1. WHO Expert Consultation. Appropriate body-mass index for Asian populations and its implications for policy and intervention strategies. Lancet. 2004;363:157–63.
2. Narouze S, Souzdalnitski D. Obesity and chronic pain: systematic review of prevalence and implications for pain practice. Reg Anesth Pain Med. 2015;40:91–111.
3. Pouwels S, Buise MP, Twardowski P, Stepaniak PS, Proczko M. Obesity surgery and anesthesiology risks: a review of key concepts and related physiology. Obes Surg. 2019;29(8):2670–7.
4. Narouze S, Souzdalnitski D. Obesity and chronic pain: opportunities for better patient care. Pain Manag. 2015;5(4):217–9.
5. Belcaid I, Eipe N. Perioperative pain management in morbid obesity. Drugs. 2019;79(11):1163–75.
6. Souzdalnitski D, Halaszynski TM, Faclier G. Regional anesthesia and co-existing chronic pain. Curr Opin Anesthesiol. 2010;23(5):662–70.

Further Reading

Aronne LJ, Kumar RB. Obesity management: a clinical casebook. 1st ed. Cham: Springer Nature; 2019. p. 153.

Rosenquist RW, Souzdalnitski D, Urman R. Chronic pain management for hospitalized patient. 1st ed. New York: Oxford University Press; 2016. p. 420.

Special Considerations for Bedside Pain Management Interventions in the Emergency Department

Jessica E. Tullington, Grant Hubbard, and Rick Gemma

Essential Concepts

- Pain is the most common complaint in the emergency room and pain control is becoming a quality measure among emergency departments across the United States, and in other countries.
- Opiates and opioids, while still widely used, can cause a tolerance to the medication. These medications also have unpleasant and significant side effects, including respiratory depression, opioid-induced hyperalgesia, and addiction.
- Bedside nerve blocks, joint injections, and other interventional options for pain control are gaining popularity in the emergency department setting. They can be used in addition to other pain management modalities.
- Psychological interventions, acupuncture, and other complementary medicine modalities can be also utilized in the emergency setting to alleviate pain, though with varying efficacy.

1 Overview

Pain is the most common complaint in the emergency room with 70–80% of patients reporting pain on presentation. Inadequate pain management in the emergency room remains a worldwide problem [1]. Pain relief is often a patient's first priority when seen by a healthcare provider. There has been some progress in the

J. E. Tullington · G. Hubbard (✉) · R. Gemma
Department of General Surgery, Western Reserve Hospital, Cuyahoga Falls, OH, USA
e-mail: jtullington@westernreservehospital.org; ghubbard@westernreservehospital.org; rgemma@westernreservehospital.org

D. Souza et al. (eds.), *Bedside Pain Management Interventions*,
https://doi.org/10.1007/978-3-031-11188-4_21

treatment of pain: the timely administration of pain control has become a quality measure within emergency departments. Both the overuse of pharmacological agents and the inadequate treatment of pain remain significant problems in this setting. Achieving adequate pain relief for patients can be affected by multiple variables, related to both patient- and provider-specific factors. The inherent bias of healthcare providers can the decision to order pain medications, as well as the selection and timing of medications. Sources of potential bias include extreme ages, decreased cognitive function, language barriers, different belief systems, and a patient's unwillingness to ask for pain relief [2]. This chapter discusses additional interventional methods of pain control in the emergency department. These interventions serve as useful adjuncts to standard pain control regimens for providers seeing patients in an emergency room setting. These include bedside nerve blocks, joint injections, psychological interventions, acupuncture, and other complementary medicine modalities.

2 Historical Aspects

Opiate and opioid prescriptions escalated throughout the 2000's due to the chronic undertreatment of pain. The overprescription led to dependence, illegal prescription drug sales, and increase in overdose-related deaths. Opioid prescriptions have steadily decreased since 2011. However, the crisis is far from over, and has transiently worsened due to the COVID-19 pandemic. In the midst of this opioid crisis, adjunctive pain management strategies are gaining popularity. The increasing use, familiarity, and expertise of bedside ultrasound by clinicians has only broadened the options available to patients in the emergency room.

3 Bedside Interventional Pain Procedures

Peripheral Nerve Blocks

Peripheral nerve blocks work by inhibiting the perception of pain by the central cortex. The type of anesthetic, concentration, and volume used will affect the duration of action, onset, and potential side effects [3]. Nerve blocks also have a synergistic effect with opioids to increase their effectiveness. Lidocaine remains the most commonly used amide with a block duration of 80–90 min. Other options include mepivacaine (45–65 min), prilocaine (45–65 min), and articaine 90–120 min). Bupivacaine is the longest-acting anesthetic with a duration of 4–12 h for a block [3]. The most common nerve blocks are presented in Table 1.

Other nerve blocks, joint and periarticular injections are discussed elsewhere in this book.

Table 1 Commonly used peripheral nerve blocks [4–30]

Nerve block	Indications	Details	Additional comments
Femoral block	A femoral nerve block is very beneficial in femoral bone fractures, greatly reducing the need for opiates [4–6]	Patients are in a supine position. A 10–12 MHz linear transducer is placed transversely at the femoral crease, just distal to the inguinal ligament. The femoral vessels are located with the ultrasound transducer; the femoral nerve is located lateral to the vessels. The nerve is then centered on the ultrasound screen. The nerve will generally appear as a hyperechoic wedge or ovoid shape. Two fascial layers can be seen over the nerve, the superficial fascia lata, and the deeper fascia iliaca. The site is then prepped with chlorhexidine. A 20 gauge needle is then inserted about 1 cm lateral to the probe and advanced to the nerve in the plane of the transducer. A "pop" can typically be felt as you advance through the fascia. Twenty milliliters of anesthetic is then injected at about the 4 o'clock position	The ultrasound can visualize the complete encircling of the nerve [4]. A nerve stimulator can also be used to help identify the femoral nerve [5]
Interscalene brachial pexus block	Interscalene blocks are useful in shoulder injuries and dislocations as well as humerus injuries as C5–C7 nerve roots are targeted [7, 8]	The patient is supine with the head turned to the opposite side of the bed. A 10–12 MHz transducer is placed at the level of about C6 in a transverse fashion. The carotid artery and internal jugular veins are visualized and the probe is moved laterally to the anterior and middle scalene muscles [7]. Doppler imaging is utilized to avoid the vascular structures and the nerve roots are visualized. The area is prepped with chlorhexidine once the nerve roots are visualized. A 22 gauge needle is inserted into the skin about 1 cm lateral to the transducer. The needle can be visualized going through the middle scalene muscle and should be positioned between the C5–C6 or C6–C7 nerve roots	A "pop" may be felt as the needle is passed through the muscle. About 20 mL of anesthetic should be injected and visualized around the nerve roots on ultrasound [8–10]
Hematoma block	A hematoma block is a procedure where local anesthesia is injected directly into a fracture site. This block is typically only used on distal radius fractures, which is the most common upper extremity fracture [11]	A 7.5 MHz linear transducer is used to locate the fracture site. The fracture site is easiest to locate while holding the ultrasound transducer in the longitudinal orientation. The fracture is identified by the irregularity in the bone cortex. Once the fracture site is located the site is prepped with chlorhexidine. A 20 gauge needle attached to a syringe is then advanced into the fracture site under ultrasound visualization. It is usually easiest to get into the fracture site using a proximal to distal needle orientation. Blood can be aspirated once the fracture site is entered. Five to 15 mL of 1% lidocaine are then injected into the fracture site [12]. After about 15 min the analgesic takes effect and the bone can be manipulated	Tseng et al. showed hematoma blocks were as effective as procedural sedation in reducing radial fractures in both adult and pediatric populations [13]. There have been some studies showing its utilization in distal tibial or fibular fractures

(continued)

Table 1 (continued)

Nerve block	Indications	Details	Additional comments
Intercostal	Intercostal blocks can be used for thoracic radicular pain, such as herpetic neuralgia, as well as chest wall pain. Pain is a common complaint with rib fractures and is a cause of morbidity and mortality in these patients. The pain can cause a reduced respiratory effort leading to atelectasis and possible pneumonia [14]	The procedure can be performed with the patient in a lateral decubitus, prone, or sitting position. The use of fluoroscopic guidance is recommended but not necessary. The desired intercostal nerve is prepped with chlorhexidine just medial to the posterior axillary line. A 22 gauge needle is then advanced into the skin at the inferior edge of the rib. Once the needle hits the bone the needle is slowly and carefully walked inferiorly until the lower margin of the rib is identified. The needle is then advanced about 2 mm into the intercostal groove. Aspiration confirmed there is no blood or air and about 5 mL of anesthetic is injected into the space. There is collateral innervation, so it is recommended this be repeated for at least three adjacent segments to ensure adequate anesthesia [10]	The most common complication is iatrogenic pneumothorax; a post-procedural chest X-ray should be reviewed [15]
Occipital	Headaches are a common complaint in the emergency room. The goal is to rule out life threatening causes for headaches and to treat the primary pain. Greater occipital nerve block decreases sensory input to the trigeminal nucleus caudalis [16]	The patient is in a prone position with the head slightly flexed. A high frequency ultrasound probe oriented in the transverse direction is used to locate the greater occipital nerve. The nerve is found about 3 cm inferior and 1.5 cm lateral to the occipital protuberance. Chlorhexidine is used to prep the skin. Color flow Doppler is used to avoid injuring the greater occipital artery. The greater occipital nerve is found medial to the artery. Once the nerve is identified a 25 gauge needle attached to a syringe of local anesthetic is advanced into the skin just inferior to the probe and in line with the nerve. About 2–3 cc of anesthetic are injected around the greater occipital nerve. The ultrasound can visualize the nerve being encircled by the anesthetic. Multiple studies have been completed showing the efficacy of greater occipital nerve blocks for migraine headaches [16–18]	Most of the research into occipital nerve blocks include migraine headaches, however there has been some research into its use on other headache syndromes with some success [19]

Inferior alveolar block	The inferior alveolar nerve provides sensation to the ipsilateral mandible, lower lip, and chin. It is the most common block used in dental procedures, however it can be useful for patients presenting to the emergency room with dental pain [20, 21]	The patient is positioned in a supine and reclined (semisupine) position with the mouth open wide. The target area, which is the mucus membrane on the medial side of the mandibular ramus, is visualized. Visualize the intersection of the horizontal and vertical lines from the mandibular landmarks. Stretching the mucosa prior to injecting decreases local trauma. A 25 gauge needle is inserted at the intersection point from the opposite side of the mouth, parallel to the mandibular teeth and perpendicular to the ramus. The needle is slowly advanced until bone is contacted. At that point the needle is withdrawn about 1 mm and 1–2 mL of anesthesia is injected after aspiration confirms the needle is not located in the artery or vein [22]. Complications of alveolar blocks include hematoma formation or needle fracture. Occasionally facial paralysis can occur with injection of the anesthetic into the parotid gland, affecting the facial nerve. This is more common with the needle oriented more posterior [23]. Other rare complications reported include ptosis, extraocular muscle paralysis, aphonia, skin necrosis of the chin, and diplopia [22, 24–26]	Success of this block is typically related to the anesthetic being injected very close to the mandibular nerve as it goes through the foramen ovale [20]. Many studies have been completed discussing the location of the mandibular foramen [21]

(continued)

Table 1 (continued)

Nerve block	Indications	Details	Additional comments
Bier block	A Bier block is a technique of intravenous local anesthesia. It is useful in both upper and lower extremity injuries given they are distal to the elbow and knee [27, 28]	The technique essentially injects local anesthetics intravenously in an extremity that has been exsanguinated by gravity or compression with an Esmarch bandage and then is isolated from central circulation after exsanguination by a tourniquet. Typically 40 mL of 0.5% lidocaine without epinephrine is used for the block. Prior to starting the procedure the double tourniquet should be tested to ensure it functions properly. Patient should be supine. Two intravenous (IV) catheters should be placed, one in the injured extremity and one in an uninjured upper extremity. A kerlix bandage should be placed on the proximal extremity in the local where the tourniquet will be placed in order to protect the skin. The double tourniquet, or two single tourniquets, is then applied over the kerlix wrap. The extremity is then exsanguinated using the Esmarch bandage from proximal to distal, ending at the distal tourniquet band. The distal tourniquet band is then inflated, followed by the proximal tourniquet band; each cuff is inflated to 100 mmHg above the patient's systolic blood pressure. Lack of pulse can be confirmed with a pulse ox or a Doppler. The distal band can then be deflated. The exsanguination band is then removed. The local anesthetic is injected. It may take 10–15 min for the block to take effect. The extremity injury can then be addressed [29]. The tourniquet must remain inflated for a minimum of 20–25 min before deflating the cuff [27]. Deflating early can cause lidocaine toxicity and cardiovascular collapse. The tourniquet should be deflated in 10 s intervals to decrease peak levels of lidocaine. The patient should be on continuous monitoring from the start of the procedure to at least 10 min following deflation of the tourniquet	Bier block is contraindicated in Raynaud's disease, sickle cell disease, crush injuries, children under the age of 5, and with an unreliable tourniquet Epinephrine should never be added to the anesthetic due to risk of cardiac complications. There possibility of cardiovascular and central nervous system collapse, especially if the tourniquet is released before 20 min. A crash cart should always be in the room in case this happens. A second IV in an uninjured upper extremity allows for medication to be delivered. Other documented complications of the Bier block include seizures, potential nerve damage, compartment syndrome, thrombophlebitis, and skin discoloration [28, 29]

Acupuncture

Acupuncture can be used as a complementary or alternative treatment to opiates for pain management [30]. Acupuncture is partially mediated by endogenous opiate release [31, 32]. Inhibition of pain pathways by acupuncture as been visualized using functional magnetic resonance imaging [31]. More than 400 acupuncture points have been identified; most are located along the main meridians, which transport life energy according to Traditional Chinese Medicine [32]. There are 20 main meridians with 12 of these as "primary meridians" and correspond to internal organs [33].

The most common method of acupuncture involves penetrating the skin with thin, solid needles that are then stimulated either manually or electrically. Electroacupuncture involves attaching a battery-operated electronic device delivering energy through the needles. Electroacupuncture blocks pain by activating biochemicals. A frequency of 2–15 Hz has been shown to inhibit inflammatory and neuropathic pain [33].

Auricular acupuncture involves stimulating different points on the ear. Jan et al. performed a meta-analysis of auricular acupuncture on pain in the emergency room. The studies included pain complaints of migraines, hip fractures, low back pain, sore throats, biliary colic, and mixed pain. Battlefield acupuncture (BFA), which involves placing small semi-permanent needles into various points of the ear, was used in most of the studies. The advantage of BFA is that the needles can stay in for a few days. There was no clinical significant difference in pain with auricular acupuncture alone, however it was beneficial when added as an adjunct to pain medication. It may also be beneficial when narcotics are contraindicated, high abuse potential, or have unwanted side effects [34].

Grissa et al. found acupuncture to be more effective and have less side effects than IV morphine when used for acute pain [35]. Reinstein et al. found a decrease in anxiety as well as pain when utilized in the emergency room [36]. Acupuncture was measured in both studies by assessing pain and anxiety scores before and after treatment. Researchers found acupuncture was widely accepted by both practitioners as well as patients within the emergency room [37]. Arnold et al. completed a study that showed similar results in patients with acute, non-penetrating extremity injuries. Acupuncture did not increase emergency room length of stay [38].

Hypnotherapy, and Other Psychological Interventions in the Emergency Department

Hypnotherapy, or hypnosis, is a trance-like state that involves highly focused concentration, decreased peripheral awareness, and heightened suggestibility. Hypnosis has been demonstrated to decrease pain and anxiety with procedures, especially when added to local anesthetic. Studies have shown that mindfulness decreases thalamic amplification of pain signals via prefrontal cognitive control mechanisms [39].

Garland et al. studied whether a single session of hypnotic suggestion would decrease the intensity of acute pain in the hospital setting. The hypnotic suggestion consisted of a self-hypnosis session with a 15 min script instructing patients how to relax their body and ways to perceive pain as different sensations, such as coolness or warmth. There were 73 patients in the hypnosis group. They found patients reported a significant reduction in post-procedural pain. Patients also had decreased anxiety, unpleasant body sensations, and desire for opioids [40].

Other psychological and mind-body interventions can be a useful adjunct to pain management in the emergency room as well. They are described elsewhere in the book.

4 Conclusion

Pain remains the most common complaint in the emergency room. Despite health professionals' best efforts, patient satisfaction with pain control still remains low. Pain medication should be prescribed in a safe manner, aiming to decrease pain and anxiety while decreasing side effects and opioid exposure when possible. Bedside interventional procedures can be utilized in the emergency department to help control that pain. Acupuncture, psychological interventions, and other nonopioid treatment modalities can be used independently or in adjunct to opioid medications. The use of these and other bedside interventions can decrease pain and anxiety while improving patient experience in the emergency department.

References

1. Mills A, Shofer F, Chen E, Hollander J, Pines J. The association between emergency department crowding and analgesia administration in acute abdominal pain patients. Acad Emerg Med. 2009;16(7):603–8.
2. Heins A. Disparities in emergency department pain management. Acad Emerg Med. 2005;12(Supplement 1):158.
3. Becker D, Reed K. Local anesthetics: review of pharmacological considerations. Anesth Prog. 2012;59(2):90–102.
4. Nagel E, Gantioque R, Taira T. Utilizing ultrasound-guided femoral nerve blocks and fascia iliaca compartment blocks for proximal femur fractures in the emergency department. Adv Emerg Nurs J. 2019;41(2):135–44.
5. Mariano E, Loland V, Sandhu N, Bellars R, Bishop M, Afra R, et al. Ultrasound guidance versus electrical stimulation for femoral perineural catheter insertion. J Ultrasound Med. 2009;28(11):1453–60.
6. Newton-Brown E, Fitzgerald L, Mitra B. Audit improves emergency department triage, assessment, multi-modal analgesia and nerve block use in the management of pain in older people with neck of femur fracture. Aust Emerg Nurs J. 2014;17(4):176–83.
7. Blaivas M, Adhikari S, Lander L. A prospective comparison of procedural sedation and ultrasound-guided interscalene nerve block for shoulder reduction in the emergency department. Acad Emerg Med. 2011;18(9):922–7.
8. Lim M, Burt G, Rutter S. Use of three-dimensional animation for regional anaesthesia teaching: application to interscalene brachial plexus blockade. Br J Anaesth. 2005;94(3):372–7.
9. Stefanovich P. Pain procedures in clinical practice. 3rd ed. Amsterdam: Elsevier; 2000.

10. Zhang L, Singla A. Pain procedures in clinical practice. 3rd ed. Amsterdam: Elsevier; 2000.
11. Nellans K, Kowalski E, Chung K. The epidemiology of distal radius fractures. Hand Clin. 2012;28(2):113–25.
12. Gottlieb M, Cosby K. Ultrasound-guided hematoma block for distal radial and ulnar fractures. J Emerg Med. 2015;48(3):310–2.
13. Tseng P, Leu T, Chen Y, Chen Y. Hematoma block or procedural sedation and analgesia, which is the most effective method of anesthesia in reduction of displaced distal radius fracture? J Orthop Surg Res. 2018;13(1):62.
14. Truitt M, Murry J, Amos J, Lorenzo M, Mangram A, Dunn E, et al. Continuous intercostal nerve blockade for rib fractures: ready for primetime? J Trauma Injury Infect Crit Care. 2011;71(6):1548–52.
15. Finucane B. Complications of regional anesthesia. New York: Springer; 2007.
16. Ashkenazi A, Levin M. Greater occipital nerve block for migraine and other headaches: is it useful? Curr Pain Headache Rep. 2007;11(3):231–5.
17. Caputi C, Firetto V. Therapeutic blockade of greater occipital and supraorbital nerves in migraine patients. Headache J Head Face Pain. 1997;37(3):174–9.
18. Allen S, Mookadam F, Cha S, Freeman J, Starling A, Mookadam M. Greater occipital nerve block for acute treatment of migraine headache: a large retrospective cohort study. J Am Board Fam Med. 2018;31(2):211–8.
19. Ashkenazi A, Blumenfeld A, Napchan U, Narouze S, Grosberg B, Nett R, et al. Peripheral nerve blocks and trigger point injections in headache management—a systematic review and suggestions for future research. Headache J Head Face Pain. 2010;50(6):943–52.
20. Aggarwal V, Singla M, Miglani S, Kohli S. Comparative evaluation of mental incisal nerve block, inferior alveolar nerve block, and their combination on the anesthetic success rate in symptomatic mandibular premolars: a randomized double-blind clinical trial. J Endod. 2016;42(6):843–5.
21. Thangavelu K, Kannan R, Kumar N, Rethish E, Sabitha S, Sayeeganesh N. Significance of localization of mandibular foramen in an inferior alveolar nerve block. J Nat Sci Biol Med. 2012;3(2):156.
22. Khalil H. A basic review on the inferior alveolar nerve block techniques. Anesth Essays Res. 2014;8(1):3.
23. Chevalier V, Arbab-Chirani R, Tea S, Roux M. Facial palsy after inferior alveolar nerve block: case report and review of the literature. Int J Oral Maxillofac Surg. 2010;39(11):1139–42.
24. You T. Diplopia after inferior alveolar nerve block: case report and related physiology. J Dent Anesth Pain Med. 2015;15(2):93.
25. Aravena P, Valeria C, Nuñez N, Perez-Rojas F, Coronado C. Skin and mucosal ischemia as a complication after inferior alveolar nerve block. Dent Res J. 2016;13(6):560.
26. Surej Kumar L, Manuel S, Sudhesh A, Thaha K. Abducent nerve palsy following an inferior alveolar nerve block. J Maxillofac Oral Surg. 2010;9(1):106.
27. Gurich R, Langan J, Teasdall R, Tanner S, Sanders J. Tourniquet deflation prior to 20 minutes in upper extremity intravenous regional anesthesia. Hand. 2017;13(2):223–7.
28. Guay J. Adverse events associated with intravenous regional anesthesia (Bier block): a systematic review of complications. J Clin Anesth. 2009;21(8):585–94.
29. Löser B, Petzoldt M, Löser A, Bacon D, Goerig M. Intravenous regional anesthesia: a historical overview and clinical review. J Anesth Hist. 2019;5(3):99–108.
30. Pomeranz B, Chiu D. Naloxone blockade of acupuncture analgesia: endorphin implicated. Life Sci. 1976;19(11):1757–62.
31. Zhang R, Lao L, Ren K, Berman B. Mechanisms of acupuncture–electroacupuncture on persistent pain. Anesthesiology. 2014;120(2):482–503.
32. Wu M, Hsieh J, Xiong J, Yang C, Pan H, Chen Y, et al. Central nervous pathway for acupuncture stimulation: localization of processing with functional MR imaging of the brain—preliminary experience. Radiology. 1999;212(1):133–41.
33. Yang E, Li P, Nilius B, Li G. Ancient Chinese medicine and mechanistic evidence of acupuncture physiology. Pflügers Arch Eur J Physiol. 2011;462(5):645–53.

34. Deadman P, Al-Khafaji M, Baker K. A manual of acupuncture. East Sussex: Journal of Chinese Medical Publications; 2016.
35. Grissa M, Baccouche H, Boubaker H, Beltaief K, Bzeouich N, Fredj N, et al. Acupuncture vs intravenous morphine in the management of acute pain in the ED. Am J Emerg Med. 2016;34(11):2112–6.
36. Reinstein A, Erickson L, Griffin K, Rivard R, Kapsner C, Finch M, et al. Acceptability, adaptation, and clinical outcomes of acupuncture provided in the emergency department: a retrospective pilot study. Pain Med. 2016;18(1):169–78.
37. Arnold A, Ross B, Silka P. Efficacy and feasibility of acupuncture for patients in the ED with acute, nonpenetrating musculoskeletal injury of the extremities. Am J Emerg Med. 2009;27(3):280–4.
38. Jan A, Aldridge E, Rogers I, Visser E, Bulsara M, Niemtzow R. Does ear acupuncture have a role for pain relief in the emergency setting? A systematic review and meta-analysis. Med Acupunct. 2017;29(5):276–89.
39. Zeidan F, Vago D. Mindfulness meditation-based pain relief: a mechanistic account. Ann N Y Acad Sci. 2016;1373(1):114–27.
40. Garland E, Baker A, Larsen P, Riquino M, Priddy S, Thomas E, et al. Randomized controlled trial of brief mindfulness training and hypnotic suggestion for acute pain relief in the hospital setting. J Gen Intern Med. 2017;32(10):1106–13.

Further Reading

Duggan NM, Nagdev A, Hayes BD, Shokoohi H, Selame LA, Liteplo AS, Goldsmith AJ. Perineural dexamethasone as a peripheral nerve block adjuvant in the emergency department: a case series. J Emerg Med. 2021;61(5):574–80. https://doi.org/10.1016/j.jemermed.2021.03.032.

Special Considerations for Bedside Pain Management Interventions in the Intensive Care Unit

Brandon Roth, Deepak Agarwal, Gaurav Chauhan, and Pavan Tankha

Essential Concepts

- Pain is common in patients being treated in the intensive care unit
- Better pain control in the ICU is associated with better patient outcomes and satisfaction
- Interventions allow for decreased opioid administration, which has the added benefit of decreased opioid-related side effects

1 Overview

Patients who require intensive care treatment are either being managed for, or recovering from, failure of one or more organ systems. While the patient may be verbal, oftentimes they are not, and cannot readily communicate their feelings of pain. Identification and treatment of pain in the intensive care unit (ICU) is associated with better patient outcomes, decreased length of mechanical ventilation, hospital stay, and mortality [1–4]. Interventions that can be done at the bedside have an added advantage in that they are opioid-sparing and subsequently decrease opioid-related adverse effects.

B. Roth · D. Agarwal · G. Chauhan
Cleveland Clinic Foundation, Cleveland, OH, USA
e-mail: brandon.roth@paindoctor.com

P. Tankha (✉)
Cleveland Clinic Foundation, Cleveland, OH, USA

Comprehensive Pain Management, Cleveland Clinic, Cleveland, USA
e-mail: tankhap@ccf.org

D. Souza et al. (eds.), *Bedside Pain Management Interventions*,
https://doi.org/10.1007/978-3-031-11188-4_22

2 Bedside Pain Management Interventions for Trauma Patients in the Intensive Care Unit

Major joint surgery and traumatic injury entail massive nociceptive input via C afferents (blocked by opioids) and A-alpha and A-delta afferents (not blocked by opioids), leading to somatic pain and spasm of periarticular muscles [5]. Regional anesthesia is an excellent modality for pain relief in these patients. Regional nerve blocks have been reported to decrease the length of stay in intensive care units, improve patient comfort for transport, improve clinical workflow, facilitate neurological assessments, and significantly reduce the need for systemic analgesics [6, 7]. These blocks can be administered via a single-shot or a continuous peripheral nerve block catheter (CPNBC). The single-shot provides 12–18 h of analgesia, whereas CPNBC can be employed for days or weeks. Depending on drug concentration, the CPNBC can provide analgesia or anesthesia for the affected limb [8]. Capitalizing on the duality of CPNBC benefits as the traumatic injury evolves and continues as the patient requires repeated skin debridement, scar revisions, skin grafts, and/or fracture fixation.

In upper extremity trauma, varying techniques for brachial plexus block can be employed, injuries permitting. However, all variations of the brachial plexus block spare the medial aspect of the arm, which requires supplemental blockade of the intercostobrachial nerve. The interscalene approach is preferred for anesthesia or analgesia for shoulder etiologies [9]. This approach is associated with complications such as ipsilateral phrenic nerve blockade, spinal or epidural injection, vertebral artery injection leading to seizures, pneumothorax, hoarseness due to blockade of the recurrent laryngeal nerve, Horner's syndrome, and injury to the brachial plexus [10]. A phrenic nerve-sparing modification of the interscalene block, the superior trunk block, can provide similar analgesia in patients with diminished cardiopulmonary reserve [11]. The supraclavicular approach is preferred for trauma to the upper arm, elbow, forearm, and wrist to the fingertips. The complications of this technique include ipsilateral phrenic nerve blockade, Horner's syndrome and pneumothorax. An infraclavicular approach to the brachial plexus yields similar analgesic profile as a supraclavicular block. If the proximal brachial plexus is inaccessible, then an axillary approach can be employed. This approach can provide adequate analgesia to the elbow, forearm, and hand, but patient positioning requires the arm to be abducted, ideally up to 90°, which could be a limiting factor for some trauma patients. The phrenic nerve is not affected by infraclavicular or axillary approaches, so either can be performed bilaterally without compromising respiratory mechanics [9, 10].

Hip fracture is associated with significant morbidity and mortality, especially in the geriatric population. A recent systematic review of peripheral nerve blocks reported that femoral nerve blocks are effective for acute pain from a hip fracture [12]. Femoral nerve block also offers earlier ambulation, the ability to take deep breaths, and reduced incidence of delirium and should be included as a part of the primary treatment for patients with hip or femur fractures [12]. The fascia iliaca block, for hip and femoral shaft fractures, is technically easier to perform than

Table 1 Absolute and relative contraindications to bedside pain management interventions in the intensive care unit

Absolute	Relative
Infection at the potential puncture site Patient refusal	Sepsis Preexisting neurological deficits (i.e. preexisting nerve damage in targeted nerve or underlying demyelinating disease) Coagulopathy or other blood dyscrasias (may be absolute contraindication especially in certain neuraxial blocks) Structural deformities in the targeted region

femoral nerve block but may not offer the same degree of pain relief [12]. The sciatic nerve block, at the level of the popliteal fossa, in conjunction with a femoral nerve block, can reliably provide analgesia for below-knee amputations, knee replacement, foot, and ankle surgery. In patients with burns, severe trauma of the thigh, or where the proximal nerve blocks listed above cannot be performed, a psoas approach to the lumbar plexus can provide effective analgesia in the distributions of the femoral and obturator nerve [13]. Another alternative for analgesia in such scenarios are lumbar epidural catheters.

Rib fractures often result in splinting during either inhalation and/or exhalation, leading to an impairment of respiratory mechanics and increased risk of pneumonia [14]. Managing these patients exclusively on opioids runs the risk of sedation and respiratory compromise. An absolute contraindication to a regional anesthetic block is injury at the area of the procedure (Table 1).

If multiple ribs are fractured bilaterally, a thoracic epidural catheter can be threaded to the vertebral levels that corresponding dermatomal coverage is required. Challenges to this procedure include patient cooperation, positioning, and the technical skill required to place a thoracic epidural given the challenging anatomy. Additionally, the cardiac sympathetic accelerator fibers exit from the T1–T4 vertebral spaces and thus limit the ability to cover those dermatomes due to the risk of hemodynamic decline, especially in critically ill patients.

In patients with unilateral rib fractures, a thoracic paravertebral block (TPV) provide multi-level pain relief with a decreased chance of spinal cord injury, hypotension, nausea, and pruritus when compared to a neuraxial technique [14]. It can be performed in the lateral decubitus position with needle entry lateral to the spinous processes and near the level of the fracture with a coverage of 6–8 dermatomes in a cephalad–caudal direction [14]. It can be placed either with ultrasound guidance or using anatomic landmarks. However, due to the increased risk of pneumothorax, ultrasound guidance is recommended. TPV can be administered either as a single-shot or with a threaded catheter; dosing of local anesthetic and steroid can prolong relief. If bilateral blocks are performed, the dosing of local anesthetic should be monitored due to the increased risk of local anesthetic toxicity.

An erector spinae plane block (ESP) is performed laterally to the TPV, ventral the erector spinae muscles, but dorsal to the transverse processes, with or without ultrasound. The risk of pneumothorax is less likely as the needle does not have to travel beyond the transverse process, but it still displays spread to the epidural, paravertebral, and the lateral cutaneous intercostal nerve branches spread similar to the TPV [14, 15]. Multiple variations of these blocks exist including the retrolaminar block and mid-point transverse process to pleura block. These blocks and the ESP have a decreased risk of bleeding, and thus may be possible in patient with coagulopathies [15].

Intercostal nerve blocks (INT) can be performed at individual levels for isolated rib fractures and cover the blocked levels along with one level above and below. The benefit of this technique is that it can be performed anywhere between the midaxillary line and the paraspinal muscles, and thus can be performed in a supine patient [15]. Intravascular uptake of local anesthetic is high with INT, which results in a short block duration and potentially the need to repeat it, so local anesthetic dosing should be carefully monitored.

A serratus plane block (SP) is performed deeper to the serratus anterior muscle and superior to the intercostal muscles, and has been proven to be effective in reducing pain with coughing and has led to a decrease in oral morphine consumption [16]. It has the benefit of blocking the T2–T9 intercostal nerves anterior to the block, and results in less hypotension when compared to a thoracic epidural block [14]. It does convey the risk of pneumothorax, and thus ultrasound guidance should be used [15].

3 Bedside Pain Management Interventions for Patients After Cardiothoracic Surgery

Sternotomy and thoracotomy for cardiothoracic surgery pose unique challenges to regional analgesia in the ICU patient. The increased risk of bleeding in post sternotomy or percutaneous coronary intervention patients, who are often on dual anti platelet therapies or intravenous anticoagulants, has long made many anesthesiologists and intensivists cautious in their approach to these modalities. Therefore, they have relied often on intravenous patient-controlled analgesia with opioids, along with multimodal medication regimens, to help decrease the patient's discomfort, while weighing the risk of hypoxia and decreased sympathetic output. Regional anesthesia has the benefits of decreasing the patient's pain with a reduced risk of respiratory compromise, but the increased risk of hematoma formation. There has been a recent increase of alternative techniques for thoracic plane blocks, specifically due to their decreased risk of epidural hematoma. Sternotomies require either a neuraxial block or bilateral plane blocks, while ipsilateral plane blocks can be used for thoracotomies (Table 2).

Table 2 Bedside pain management interventions for patients after cardiothoracic surgery

Region	Procedure type
Sternotomy	Thoracic epidural, paravertebral, erector spinae, intercostal, pectoralis blocks
Thoracotomy	Epidural, paravertebral, erector spinae, intercostal, serratus anterior blocks

Continuous thoracic epidural blocks are effective for post cardiac or thoracic surgery pain control, and are considered the "gold standard." Typically, the catheter is inserted at the T6–T7 interlaminar level, and started post operatively, infusing a mixture of a local anesthetic such as ropivacaine and an opioid such as fentanyl [17]. Among the blocks we will discuss for both post sternotomy and post thoracotomy pain, this is the only technique that will require only one catheter for continuous, bilateral, pain relief. This "direct" neuraxial technique will also provide a more consistent somatic and sympathetic blockade when compared to the "indirect" techniques of the thoracic plane blocks which have inconsistent spread to the epidural space [18]. However, serious complications related to post-surgical heparin usage and coagulopathies, such as epidural hematoma, can occur and should be carefully monitored for [17, 18].

A thoracic paravertebral block (TPV) performed at the T6–T7 paravertebral level can provide adequate unilateral analgesia post operatively. Bilateral, continuous, TPV catheters used for cardiac surgery have been shown to result in shorter ICU stays, decreased urinary retention, and vomiting when compared to thoracic epidural analgesia [17]. A description of this procedure and the risks/benefits can be found in the section for rib fractures above.

Multiple variations of plane blocks have been described for chest wall procedures. Starting dorsal and moving ventrally, these blocks are the retrolaminar block (covering 2–4 epidural spaces) and erector spinae block (covering 3–5 epidural spaces), which is described above in relation to rib fractures.

A serratus plane block (SP) is performed deeper to the serratus anterior muscle and superior to the intercostal muscles. In post-thoracotomy patients, continuous bilateral SP blocks at the fourth or fifth ribs have been shown to result in similar visual analog scale scores when compared to those utilizing intravenous patient controlled opioid analgesia within the first 24 h [19]. It has the benefit of blocking the T2–T9 intercostal nerves anterior to the block, and results in less hypotension when compared to a thoracic epidural block [18]. It does run the risk of pneumothorax, and thus ultrasound guidance is recommended.

Ultrasound guided bilateral pectoralis nerve blocks have been proven to be effective in reducing the pain from a sternotomy, and have few complications. Due to the paucity of blood vessels as well as the location above the rib cage, both bleeding and pneumothorax risks are reduced. The "PECS" block has been shown to significantly reduce the duration of mechanical ventilation, pain at rest, and pain on coughing in patients with mid-sternotomies [20]. This block has two variations, PECS I, which only targets the fascial plane between the pectoralis major and minor muscles, and PECS II, which includes a serratus anterior plane block [18].

Of note, there exists contralateral innervation across the midline sternum that may result in an incomplete pain blockade with any of the unilateral blocks, and a bilateral block may be required for more thorough pain control [18] (Table 3).

Table 3 Bedside pain management interventions for trauma patients in the intensive care unit

Region	Procedure type
Upper extremity	
Shoulder	Interscalene, superior trunk block
Arm/elbow/hand	Supraclavicular, infraclavicular, axillary blocks
Hip	Lumbar plexus, femoral, fascia iliaca, lumbar epidural blocks
Lower extremity	Obturator, femoral, sciatic nerve, lumbar epidural blocks
Rib	Thoracic epidural, paravertebral, intercostal, serratus anterior blocks

4 Bedside Procedures for Patients After Abdominal Surgery

Abdominal procedures, whether open or laparoscopic, are rarely managed well exclusively with opioid medications [21]. Abdominal pain has two major components. One, somatic pain, which is described as a gnawing, aching or sharp sensation that is caused by the violation of skin, mucous membranes and muscles. The second—and major type of pain found in this patient population—visceral pain, is characterized as vague and non-localized.

Several techniques have shown efficacy for pain control and the reduction of opioid utilization in the post-operative setting. They can be performed before or after surgery, but the patient will likely benefit most if the block has been performed preoperatively [21]. Challenges to placing these blocks include coagulopathy or use of anticoagulants, positioning patients during catheter insertion, infections both active and potential, hemodynamic instability, and hypovolemia [22] (Table 4).

Abdominal wall blocks, which include the transversus abdominis plane (TAP) block, the rectus sheath (RS) block, and the quadratus lumborum (QL) block, are safely performed under ultrasound (US) guidance.

RS blocks are useful when surgical procedures are small, where small intra-abdominal incisions are utilized. The block provides analgesia to the 9th–11th intercostal nerves between the internal oblique and transversus abdominis muscles [21]. With larger abdominal incisions, TAP blocks may be preferable, as they have a larger area of coverage [23]. They have been used as "rescue procedures" following failed neuraxial analgesia on the ICU [24]. The QL block, which is a block performed more laterally relative to the TAP block, has the added benefit of providing visceral pain coverage secondary to injectate seeping into the paravertebral space. While its presence in the ICU literature is sparse, it is becoming much more prevalent in other area of the anesthesia literature [25, 26].

Neuraxial anesthesia, more specifically epidural anesthesia (EA) is another approach to the management of analgesia in critical patients having undergone abdominal surgery. It provides both somatic and visceral pain coverage, and is especially useful in controlling pain during movement (i.e. during respirations). In at least one major study, a metanalysis by Popping et al., there was a mortality benefit

Table 4 Bedside pain management interventions for patients after abdominal surgery

Region	Procedure type
Abdominal wall	Transversus abdominis plane, rectus sheath, quadratus lumborum, epidural blocks
Visceral	Quadratus lumborum, epidural

in patients having postoperative analgesia by epidural [27, 28]. EA also has the ability to favorably influence morbidity factors including the reduction of incidence in paralytic ileus, delirium, length of ICU stays, and duration of mechanical ventilation [29, 30].

5 Bedside Procedures for Patients with Pre-existing Chronic Pain Admitted to the Intensive Care Unit

It's estimated that 30% of the U.S. population suffers from chronic pain and those numbers increase with age [31]. Interventions to treat chronic pain as an outpatient are not always available in the intensive care unit. Reasons for this include patient physiologic disturbances (hemodynamic instability, renal insufficiency, hepatic failure), or patient positioning (the inability to properly position the patient to safely access pain generators). However, if the patient is able to communicate the type of pain and previous treatments, consider the following procedures after contraindications have been eliminated.

Trigger point injections or dry needling can target specific muscles that are in spasm. The use of ultrasound is encouraged if targets are in the thoracic or lower cervical region to avoid iatrogenic pneumothorax. Joint injections for shoulder, hip, or knee pain can also be done at bedside with or without the use of ultrasound guidance. Finally, if the pain generators are accessible, ultrasound guided facet or sacroiliac joint injections can also be performed.

6 Bedside Procedures for Patients Transitioned from Intensive Care to Palliative Care

In patients with disease involving the viscera, which is the case in cancers of the abdomen or pelvis, there are a number of interventions that have the potential to significantly decrease pain. The celiac plexus block is particularly useful in patients with upper abdominal malignancies (i.e. pancreatic cancer) that have moderate to severe pain despite medical management. It has the ability to reduce opioid requirements, while at the same time significantly reduce pain scores [32]. The procedure is safe with minimal complications in the majority of cases, though the sustainability of pain relief is variable [33–35]. Patients with pain from malignancies of lower abdominal or pelvic structures may benefits from superior hypogastric plexus or ganglion impar blocks [36]. These blocks can be performed at bedside with the assistance of ultrasound guidance.

7 Conclusion

Management of the critically ill patient is challenging and requires considerable skill in identifying and treating variables that will affect overall outcome. While potentially overlooked by other more pressing systemic complications, pain management has been shown to affect not only outcome, but a range of other variables including overall mortality. Understanding and putting into practice accessible bedside interventions can supplement existing pharmacological treatments and provide significant relief with fewer adverse effects.

References

1. Skrobik Y, Ahern S, Leblanc M, et al. Protocolized intensive care unit management of analgesia, sedation, and delirium improves analgesia and subsyndromal delirium rates. Anesth Analg. 2010;111:451–63.
2. Georgiou E, Hadjibalassi M, Lambrinou E, et al. The impact of pain assessment on critically ill patients' outcomes: a systematic review. Biomed Res Int. 2015;2015:503–830.
3. Payen JF, Bosson JL, Chanques G, et al. DOLOREA Investigators: Pain assessment is associated with decreased duration of mechanical ventilation in the intensive care unit: a post hoc analysis of the DOLOREA study. Anesthesiology. 2009;111:1308–16.
4. Robinson BR, Mueller EW, Henson K, et al. An analgesia-delirium-sedation protocol for critically ill trauma patients reduces ventilator days and hospital length of stay. J Trauma. 2008;65:517–26.
5. Mantyh PW. The neurobiology of skeletal pain. Eur J Neurosci. 2014;39(3):508–19.
6. Gadsden J, Warlick A. Regional anesthesia for the trauma patient: improving patient outcomes. Local Reg Anesth. 2015;12(8):45–55.
7. Capdevila M, Ramin S, Capdevila X. Regional anesthesia and analgesia after surgery in ICU. Curr Opin Crit Care. 2017;23(5):430–9.
8. Ilfeld BM. Continuous peripheral nerve blocks: an update of the published evidence and comparison with novel, alternative analgesic modalities. Anesth Analg. 2017;124:308–35.
9. De Tran QH, Clemente A, Doan J, Finlayson RJ. Brachial plexus blocks: a review of approaches and techniques. Can J Anesth. 2007;54(8):662–74.
10. Mian A, Chaudhry I, Huang R, Rizk E, Tubbs RS, Loukas M. Brachial plexus anesthesia: a review of the relevant anatomy, complications, and anatomical variations. Clin Anat. 2014;27(2):210–21.
11. Kang R, Jeong JS, Chin KJ, Yoo JC, Lee JH, Choi SJ, et al. Superior trunk block provides noninferior analgesia compared with interscalene brachial plexus block in arthroscopic shoulder surgery. Anesthesiology. 2019;131(6):1316–26.
12. Guay J, Parker MJ, Griffiths R, Kopp S. Peripheral nerve blocks for hip fractures: a Cochrane review. Anesth Analg. 2018;126(5):1695–704.
13. Murray JM, Derbyshire S, Shields MO. Lower limb blocks. Anaesthesia. 2010;65:57–66.
14. Ho AM, Ho AK, Mizubuti GB, Klar G, Karmakar MK. Regional analgesia for patients with traumatic rib fractures—a narrative review. J Trauma Acute Care Surg. 2019;88(1):e22–30.
15. Thiruvenkatarajan V, Eng HC, Adhikary SD. An update on regional analgesia for rib fractures. Curr Opin Anesthesiol. 2018;31(5):601.
16. Martinez T, et al. Serratus plane block is effective for pain control in patients with blunt chest trauma: a case series. Pain Pract. 2019;20:197–203.

17. El Shora HA, El Beleehy AA, Abdelwahab AA, Ali GA, Omran TE, Hassan EA, Arafat AA. Bilateral paravertebral block versus thoracic epidural analgesia for pain control post-cardiac surgery: a randomized controlled trial. Thorac Cardiovasc Surg. 68(05):410–6.
18. Chin K. Thoracic wall blocks: from paravertebral to retrolaminar to serratus to erector spinae and back again—a review of evidence. Best Pract Res Clin Anaesthesiol. 2019;33:67–77.
19. Reyad RM, et al. The impact of ultrasound-guided continuous serratus anterior plane block versus intravenous patient-controlled analgesia on the incidence and severity of post-thoracotomy pain syndrome: a randomized, controlled study. Eur J Pain. 2019;26:159.
20. Kumar KN, Kalyane RN, Singh NG, Nagaraja PS, Krishna M, Babu B, et al. Efficacy of bilateral pectoralis nerve block for ultrafast tracking and postoperative pain management in cardiac surgery. Ann Card Anaesth. 2018;21:338–43.
21. Hemmerling TM. Pain management in abdominal surgery. Langenbecks Arch Surg. 2018;403:791.
22. Park J-M, Kim JH. Assessment and treatment of pain in adult intensive care unit patients. Korean J Crit Care Med. 2014;29(3):147–59.
23. Ris F, Findley JM, Hompes R, Rashid A, Warwick J, Cunningham C, Jones O, Crabtree N, Lindsey I. Addition of transversus abdominis plane block to controlled analgesia for laparoscopic high anterior resection analgesia, reduces opioid requirement and expedites recovery of bowel function. Ann R Coll Surg Engl. 2014;96(8):579–85.
24. Niraj G, Kelkar A, Fox AJ. Application of the transversus abdominis plane block in the intensive care unit. Anaesth Intensive Care. 2009;37(4):650–2.
25. Jadon A, Mayur M, Asit KP, Neelam S. Postoperative analgesia by transmuscular quadratus lumborum block catheters. J Anesth Intensive Care Med. 2016;1(3):55562.
26. Mieszkowski MM, Zawazka EM, Tuyakov B, Mieszkoswka M, Zukowski M, Wasniewski T, Onichinowski D. Evaluation of effectiveness of the quadratus lumborum block type I using ropivacaine in postoperative analgesia after a cesarean section—a controlled clinical study. Ginekol Pol. 2018;89(2):89–96.
27. Hammerschlag JG, von Rhaden RP. Regional anaesthesia in the intensive care unit. In: Vizcaychipi M, Corredor C, editors. Key topics in management of the critically ill. Cham: Springer; 2016.
28. Pöpping DM, Elia N, Marret E, Remy C, Tramèr MR. Protective effects of epidural analgesia on pulmonary complications after abdominal and thoracic surgery: a meta-analysis. Arch Surg. 2008;143(10):990–9.
29. Venkataraju A, Narayanan M. Analgesia in intensive care: part 2. BJA Educ. 2016;16(12):397–404.
30. Ballantyne JC, Carr DB, de Ferranti S, et al. The comparative effects of postoperative analgesic therapies on pulmonary outcome. Anesth Analg. 1998;86:598–612.
31. Johannes CB, Le TK, Zhou X, Johnston JA, Dworkin RH. The prevalence of chronic pain in United States adults: results of an internet-based survey. J Pain. 2010;11:1230–9.
32. Jain PN, Shrikhande SV, Myatra SN, Sareen R. Neurolytic celiac plexus block: a better alternative to opioid treatment in upper abdominal malignancies: an Indian experience. J Pain Palliat Care Pharmacother. 2015;19(3):15–20.
33. Edelstein MR, Gabriel RT, Elbich JD, et al. Pain outcomes undergoing CT-guided celiac plexus neurolysis for intractable abdominal visceral pain. Am J Hosp Palliat Med. 2017;34(2):111–4.
34. Mercadante S, Catala E, Arcuri E, Casuccio A. Celiac plexus block for pancreatic cancer pain: factors influencing pain, symptoms and quality of life. J Pain Symptoms Manag. 2003;26(6):1140–7.
35. Zhong W, Yu Z, Zeng JX, Lun Y, Min XH, Yuan YH, Chen QK. Celiac plexus block for treatment of pain associated with pancreatic cancer: a meta-analysis. Pain Pract. 2014;14(1):43–51.
36. Chambers WA. Nerve blocks in palliative care. Br J Anesth. 2008;101(1):95–100.

Further Reading

Devlin JW, Skrobik Y, Gélinas C, Needham DM, Slooter AJC, Pandharipande PP, Watson PL, Weinhouse GL, Nunnally ME, Rochwerg B, Balas MC, van den Boogaard M, Bosma KJ, Brummel NE, Chanques G, Denehy L, Drouot X, Fraser GL, Harris JE, Joffe AM, Kho ME, Kress JP, Lanphere JA, McKinley S, Neufeld KJ, Pisani MA, Payen JF, Pun BT, Puntillo KA, Riker RR, Robinson BRH, Shehabi Y, Szumita PM, Winkelman C, Centofanti JE, Price C, Nikayin S, Misak CJ, Flood PD, Kiedrowski K, Alhazzani W. Clinical practice guidelines for the prevention and management of pain, agitation/sedation, delirium, immobility, and sleep disruption in adult patients in the ICU. Crit Care Med. 2018;46(9):e825–73. https://doi.org/10.1097/CCM.0000000000003299.

Part IV

Bedside Procedures for Head, Neck and Back Pain

Peripheral Nerve Blocks for the Management of Headache and Face Pain

Ryan J. Krogmann, Patrick J. Connell, Peter D. Weitzel, and Dmitri Souza

Essential Concepts

- Bedside peripheral nerve blocks are valuable diagnostic and therapeutic tools for the diagnosis and management of head and face pain syndromes
- Moreover, they can be beneficial as an abortive treatment for episodes of intractable headache.
- Targets of these nerve blocks include the supraorbital nerve, supratrochlear nerve, infraorbital nerve, inferior alveolar nerve, mental nerve, auriculotemporal nerve, greater auricular nerve, maxillary nerve, mandibular nerve, and glossopharyngeal nerve.
- High-quality studies are lacking. Well-designed studies are needed to ascertain the value of nerve blocks in refractory headache disorders.

R. J. Krogmann
Department of Otolaryngology, Western Reserve Hospital, Cuyahoga Falls, OH, USA
e-mail: rkrogmann@westernreservehospital.org

P. J. Connell
South Pointe Hospital, Cleveland Clinic Foundation, Cleveland, OH, USA
e-mail: connelp2@ccf.org

P. D. Weitzel
Mercy St.Vincent Hospital, Toledo, OH, USA
e-mail: pweitzel@mercy.com

D. Souza (✉)
Center for Pain Medicine, Western Reserve Hospital, Cuyahoga Falls, OH, USA
e-mail: dsouza@westernreservehospital.org

D. Souza et al. (eds.), *Bedside Pain Management Interventions*,
https://doi.org/10.1007/978-3-031-11188-4_23

- Due to the high vascularity of the face and the scalp, all nerve blocks render patients susceptible to local anesthetic toxicity. Subsequently, the local anesthetic dose should be cautiously calculated, especially if the plan is to perform the nerve block bilaterally. Vigilant monitoring must be established during the injection. The solution is injected slowly in increments. For the same reason, there is an increased risk of post-procedure ecchymosis and hematoma. Should this happen, manual pressure is applied to the area of the block. Applying ice packs for 15–20 min can reduce post-procedural pain and bleeding.

1 Overview

Bedside peripheral nerve blocks for head and neck pain can provide patient's with substantial relief of facial pain and headaches secondary to trauma, postherpetic neuralgia, other pain syndromes. In addition, these blocks may serve as diagnostic tests to localize the source of pain. In this chapter, we will discuss commonly used blocks, including supraorbital, infraorbital, and mental (Table 1).

Table 1 Peripheral nerve blocks for the management of headaches and facial pain[a]

Block type	Indications	Techniques
Supraorbital nerve, supratrochlear nerve	Diagnosis and treatment of supraorbital facial pain Supraorbital or supratrochlear entrapment neuropathies Herpes zoster Facial bone fractures Malignancy	Landmark technique Ultrasound-guided technique
Infraorbital nerve	Diagnosis and treatment of infraorbital facial pain Infraorbital entrapment neuropathies Herpes zoster Posttraumatic entrapment neuropathy Malignancy	Landmark technique Ultrasound-guided technique
Mental nerve	Diagnosis and treatment of facial pain Mental nerve entrapment neuropathies Herpes zoster Facial bone fractures Malignancy	Landmark technique (intraoral or extraoral) Ultrasound-guided technique

[a]Adapted with permission from From: Narouze SN (Ed.) Interventional Management of Head and Face Pain. Nerve Blocks and Beyond, 1st Ed. Springer Science+Business Media New York, 2014:17–27

2 Supraorbital Nerve Blocks

Indications and Contraindications

Supraorbital nerve block (SON) can be used in the diagnosis and treatment of facial pain in areas supplied by the supraorbital nerve secondary to supraorbital neuralgia, herpes zoster in the V1 distribution, facial bone fractures, facial malignancies, entrapment secondary to injury, or other causes. Similarly, a supratrochlear nerve block is a useful tool in the diagnosis and management of facial pain in areas supplied by the supratrochlear nerve whether due to entrapment neuropathy, facial bone fractures, or herpes zoster [1–3].

Common contraindications include infection at the injection site, intolerance or allergy to the injectate components, and patient refusal.

Clinical Anatomy

The supraorbital nerve originates from the frontal nerve, which is the largest branch of the ophthalmic division (V1) of the trigeminal nerve (Fig. 1). The frontal nerve exits the cranium through the superior orbital fissure to run in the roof of the orbit. The frontal nerve divides into a larger lateral branch, the supraorbital nerve, and a

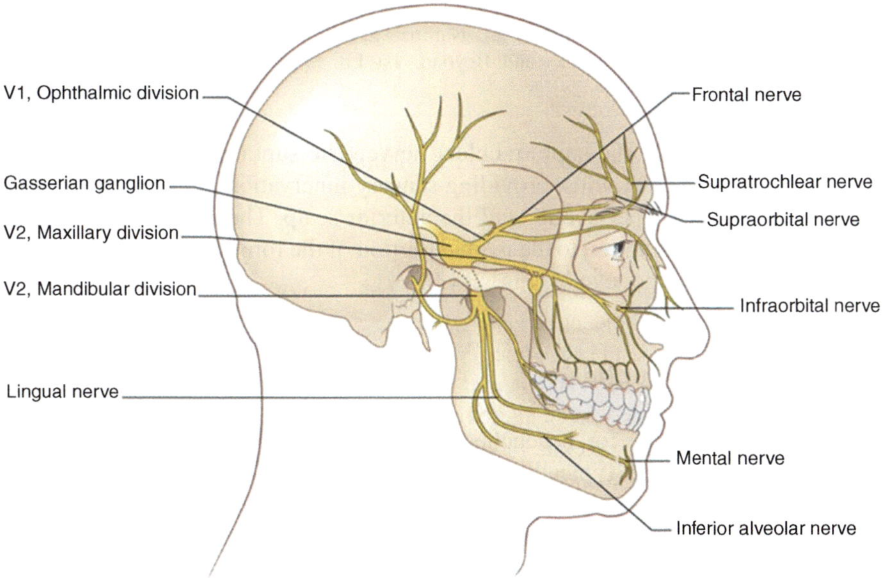

Fig. 1 Trigeminal nerve anatomy. (From: Narouze SN (Ed.) Interventional Management of Head and Face Pain. Nerve Blocks and Beyond, 1st Ed. Springer Science+Business Media New York, 2014:17–27)

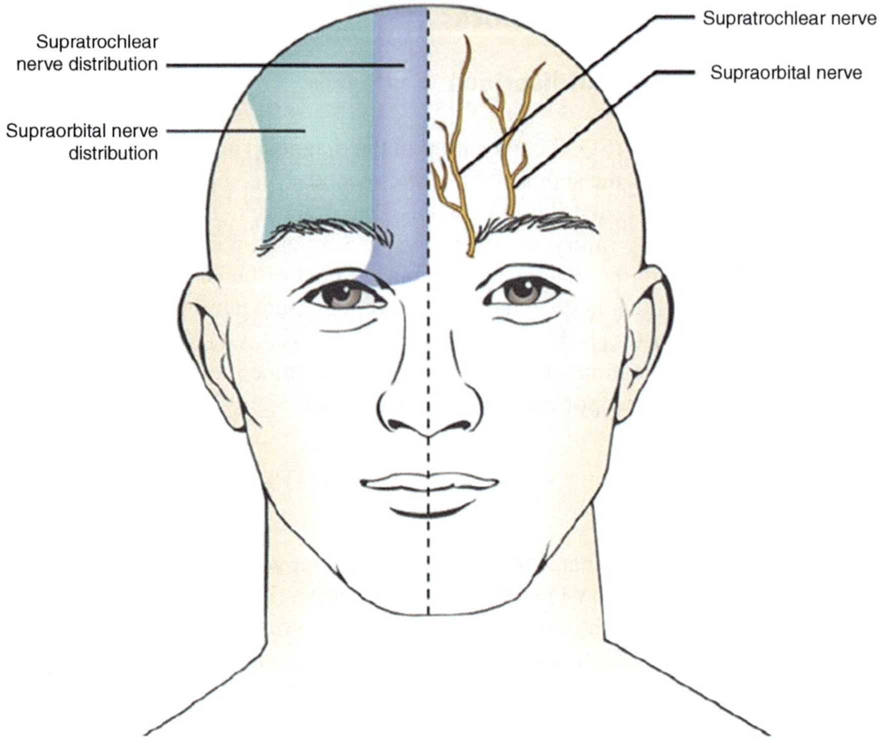

Fig. 2 Supraorbital nerve anatomy. (From: Narouze SN (Ed.) Interventional Management of Head and Face Pain. Nerve Blocks and Beyond, 1st Ed. Springer Science+Business Media New York, 2014:17–27)

smaller medial branch, the supratrochlear nerve. The supraorbital nerves give off nerve fibers to the vertex, thus, providing sensory innervation to the lateral portion of the forehead, the upper eyelid, and the anterior scalp. The supratrochlear nerve provides sensory innervation to the medial portion of the forehead, nasal bridge, and medial third of the upper eyelid (Fig. 2) [3].

Equipment and Supplies

Peripheral nerve blocks for headaches and facial pain can be conveniently performed at the bedside. Typically, a small syringe with a 25, 27 or 30-gauge, 0.5–1.5 in. needle is utilized to inject 0.5–3 ml of the anesthetic solution. The injectate usually consists of the local anesthetic lidocaine or bupivacaine, or a combination of the two, with or without a corticosteroid. We recommend using the non-particular steroid. The procedure does not typically require the use of specialized imaging guidance, but the use of real-time ultrasonography is very beneficial for appropriately directing the anesthetic accurately [7].

Techniques

Landmark Technique, Supraorbital Nerve Block

The patient is placed in the supine or seated position and is advised to report any paresthesia during the procedure along, the distribution of the nerve. The supraorbital notch is identified by palpation. The skin overlying the notch is prepped with an antiseptic solution. A 25-gauge, 1½-in. needle is introduced at the level of the notch and advanced medially 15° to avoid entering the foramen and avoid inducing paresthesia (Fig. 3). The needle is advanced until it approaches the periosteum. If the needle slips into the foramen, it should be withdrawn and redirected medially. After negative aspiration is confirmed, 0.5–3 ml of the solution is injected in a fanlike distribution. Meanwhile, a gauze sponge is gently applied on the upper eyelid and supraorbital tissues before, during, and after injecting the solution to prevent downward dissection of the solution in the loose areolar tissues of the upper eyelid [4, 5].

Ultrasound-Guided Technique, Supraorbital Nerve Block

The patient is placed in the supine or seated position. After prepping the skin with an antiseptic solution, a high-resolution linear probe is placed along the supraorbital

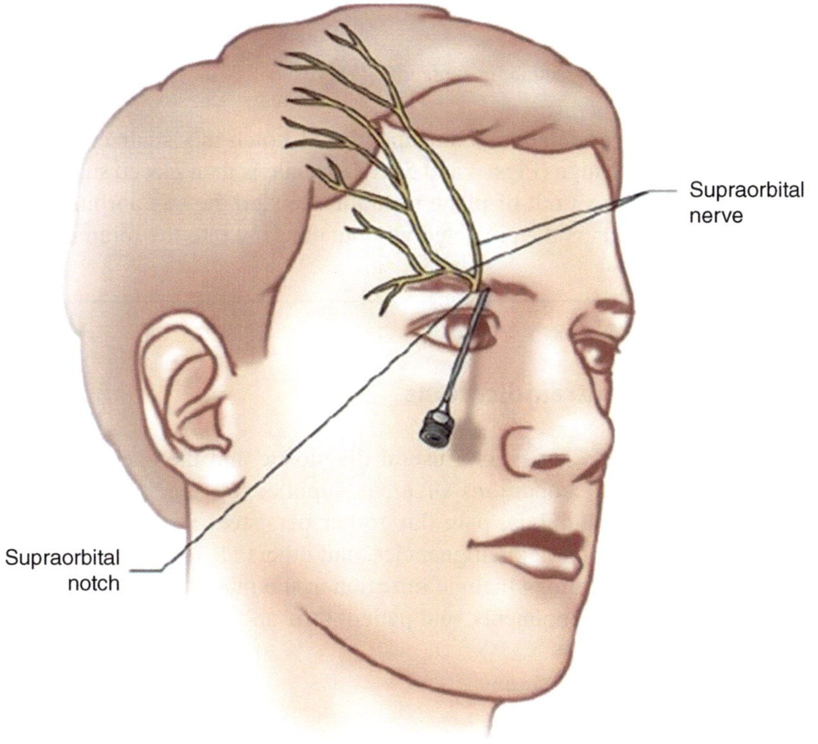

Fig. 3 Supraorbital nerve landmark injection. (From: Narouze SN (Ed.) Interventional Management of Head and Face Pain. Nerve Blocks and Beyond, 1st Ed. Springer Science+Business Media New York, 2014:17–27)

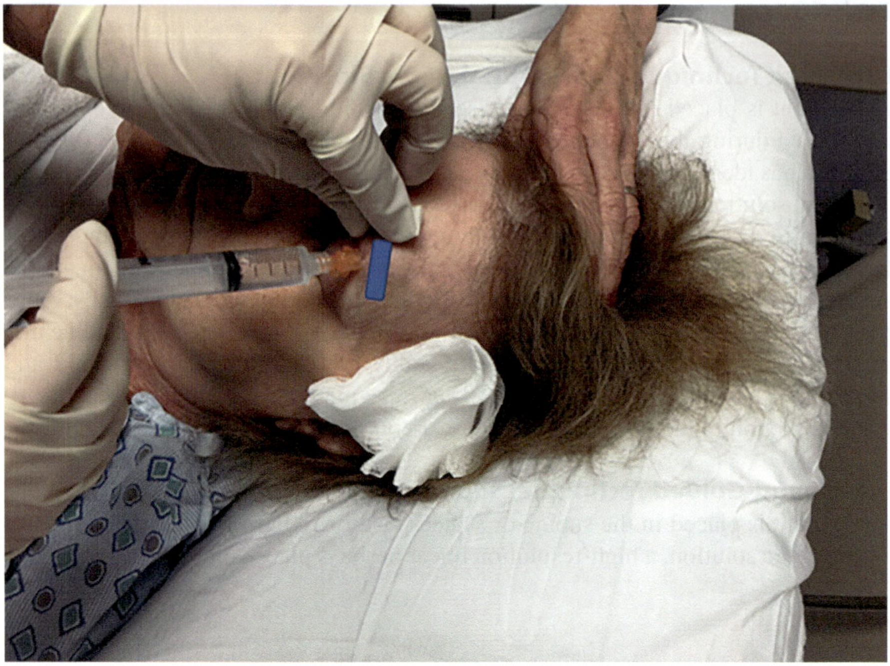

Fig. 4 Ultrasound image orientation for supraorbital nerve block

ridge in a transverse orientation. The supraorbital notch is visualized as a defect along the supraorbital ridge (Figs. 4 and 5). The needle is then placed superior to the probe and advanced in an out-of-plane technique toward the supraorbital foramen. 0.5–3 ml of the solution is then injected without entering into the foramen [6, 7].

3 Infraorbital Nerve Block

Indications and Contraindications

Infraorbital nerve block serves as a useful diagnostic and therapeutic tool in the management of painful conditions of areas supplied by the infraorbital nerve, including infraorbital neuralgia, pain due to her persistent in the V2 distribution, facial bone fractures, potential malignancies, and others [1, 2].

Common contraindications include infection at the injection site, intolerance or allergy to the injectate components, and patient refusal.

Clinical Anatomy

The infraorbital nerve originates from the maxillary nerve and enters the orbit through the inferior orbital fissure. It then courses along the floor of the orbit in the

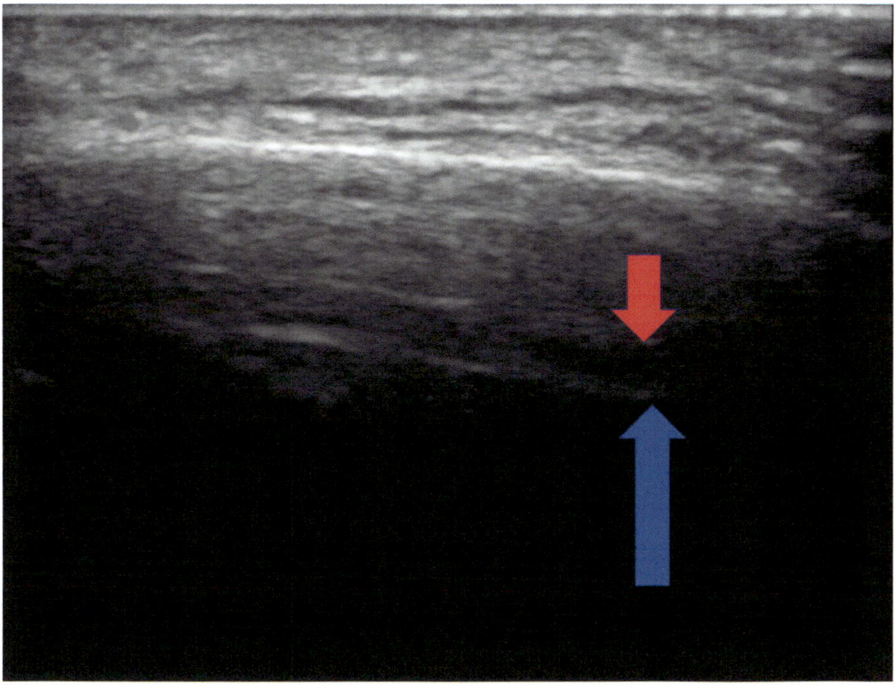

Fig. 5 Supraorbital nerve ultrasound-guided injection technique. The blue arrow indicates the supraorbital fissure, and the red arrow indicates the injection site

infraorbital groove. As the nerve exits the orbit through the infraorbital foramen, it gives off sensory branches to the lower eyelid, lateral nares, and upper lip. The superior alveolar nerve, a branch of the infraorbital nerve, innervates the upper incisor, canine, and the associated gingiva (Fig. 1).

Techniques

Landmark Technique, Infraorbital Nerve Block

The patient is placed in the supine or seated position and is advised to report any paresthesia during the procedure along the distribution of the nerve. The infraorbital foramen is identified by palpation. The skin overlying the notch is prepped with an antiseptic solution. A 25-gauge, 1½-in. needle is introduced at the level of the notch and is advanced medially 15° to avoid entering the foramen. The needle is advanced until it approaches the periosteum. If the needle slips accidentally into the foramen, it should be withdrawn and redirected medially. After negative aspiration is confirmed, 0.5–3 ml of the solution is injected in a fanlike distribution. Meanwhile, a gauze sponge should be used to apply gentle pressure on the lower eyelid and infraorbital tissues before, during, and after injecting the solution to prevent downward dissection of the solution into the loose areolar tissues of the eyelid [4, 5].

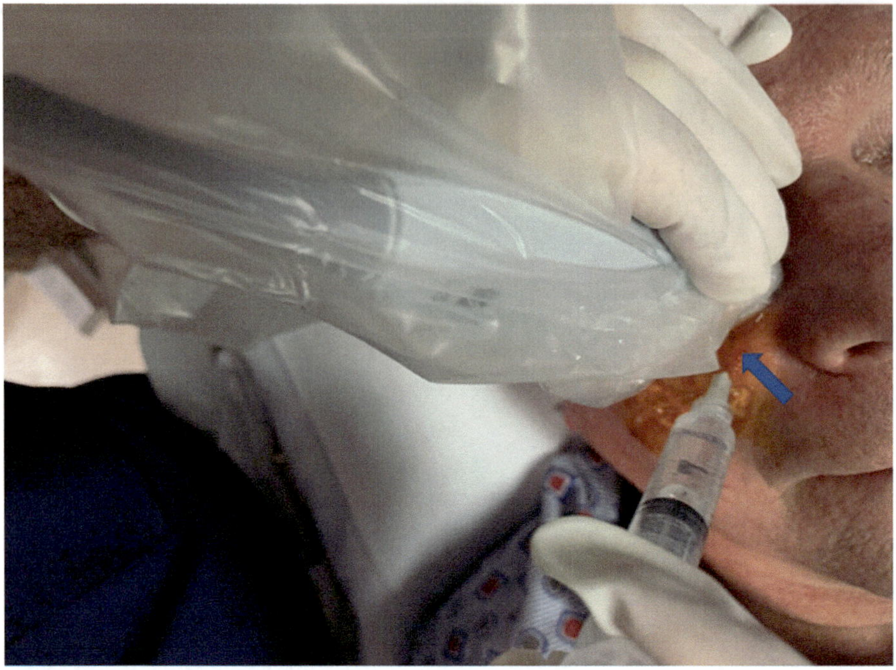

Fig. 6 Infraorbital nerve block, ultrasound-guided injection technique. The blue arrow indicates the injection site over the infraorbital fossa location

Ultrasound-Guided Technique, Infraorbital Nerve Block

The patient is placed in the supine or seated position. After prepping the skin with an antiseptic solution, a high-resolution linear probe is situated along the zygomatic bone in a transverse or oblique orientation. The infraorbital notch is visualized within the maxilla (Figs. 6 and 7). The needle is then placed inferior to the probe and advanced in an out-of-plane technique toward the infraorbital foramen. 0.5–3 ml of the solution is then injected to surround the nerve without entering into the foramen.

4 Mental Nerve Block

Indications and Contraindications

Mental nerve block serves as a useful diagnostic and therapeutic tool in the management of painful conditions of areas supplied by the mental nerve, including mental nerve neuralgia, pain due to herpes zoster in the V3 distribution, facial bone fractures, facial malignancies, and others [1, 2].

Common contraindications include infection at the injection site, intolerance or allergy to the injectate components, and patient refusal.

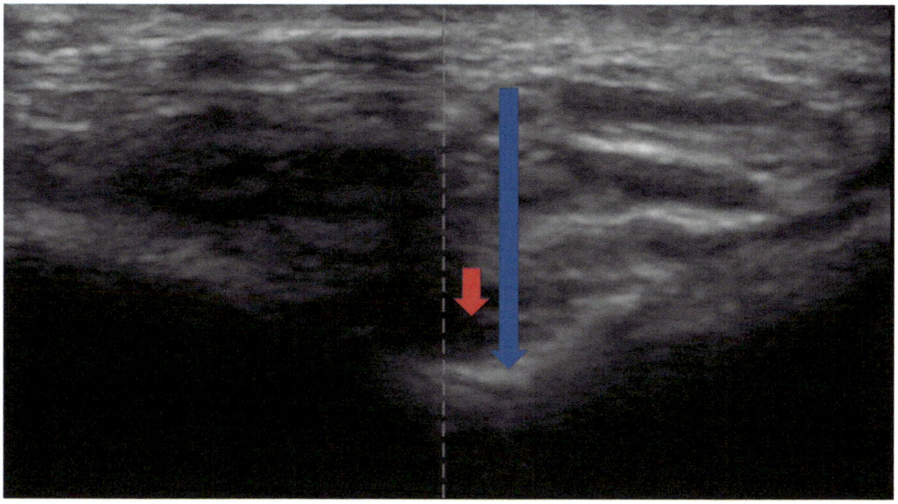

Fig. 7 Infraorbital nerve block, ultrasound-guided injection technique. The blue arrow points towards the infraorbital nerve in the intraorbital fossa. The dotted line demonstrated needle trajectory. The right arrow indicates injectate spread

Clinical Anatomy

The mental nerve originates from the mandibular nerve. The nerve emerges from the mandible through the mental foramen at the level of the second premolar; it then turns sharply and gives off sensory branches to the medial side of the chin (Fig. 1).

Technique

Extraoral Approach, Mental Nerve Block

The patient is placed in the supine or seated position and is advised to report any paresthesia along the distribution of the nerve. The mental notch is identified by palpation. The skin overlying the notch is prepped with an antiseptic solution. A 25-gauge, 1½-in. needle is introduced at the level of the foramen and advanced medially 15° to avoid entering the foramen (Fig. 8). The needle is advanced until it approaches the periosteum. If the needle slips accidentally into the foramen, it should be withdrawn and redirected medially. After negative aspiration is confirmed, 0.5–3 ml of the solution is injected in a fanlike distribution [4, 5].

Intraoral Approach, Mental Nerve Block

The patient is placed in the supine or seated position. The mental notch is identified by palpation. The lower lip is retracted down, and cotton balls soaked in 10%

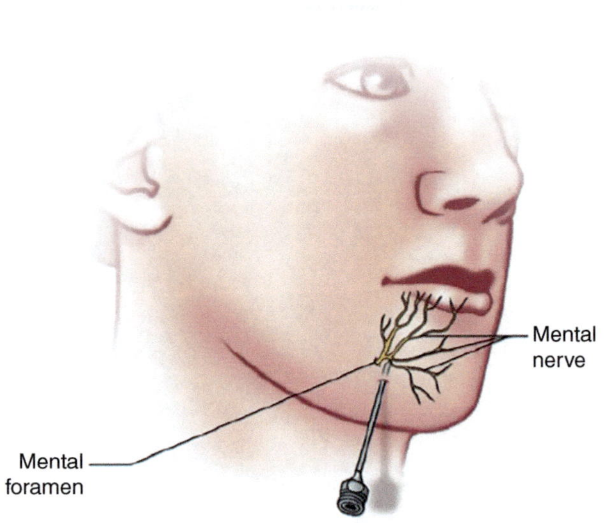

Fig. 8 Extraoral technique for mental nerve block. (From: Narouze SN (Ed.) Interventional Management of Head and Face Pain. Nerve Blocks and Beyond, 1st Ed. Springer Science+Business Media New York, 2014:17–27)

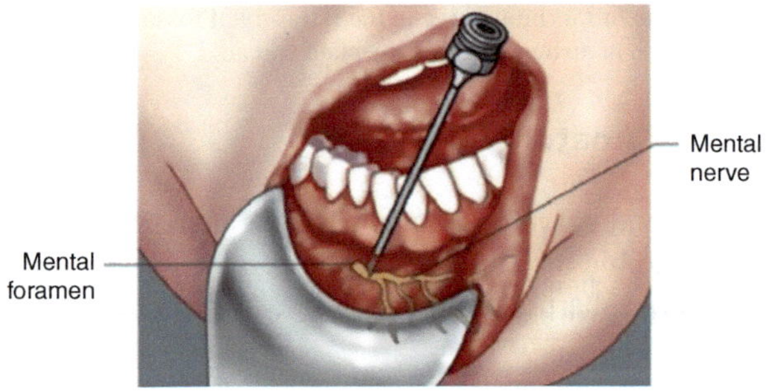

Fig. 9 Intraoral technique for mental nerve block.. (From: Narouze SN (Ed.) Interventional Management of Head and Face Pain. Nerve Blocks and Beyond, 1st Ed. Springer Science+Business Media New York, 2014:17–27)

cocaine solution or viscous 2% lidocaine are placed in the alveolar sulcus close to the mental notch for adequate topical anesthesia of the mucosa. A 25-gauge, 1½-in. needle is advanced toward the mental foramen, which may elicit paresthesia. However, there should be no paresthesia on injection. After negative aspiration is confirmed, 0.5–3 ml of the solution is injected in a fanlike manner (Fig. 9).

Ultrasound-Guided Approach, Mental Nerve Block

The patient is placed in the supine or seated position. After prepping the skin with an antiseptic solution, a high-resolution linear probe is situated along the lower border of the mandible in a transverse orientation. The mental foramen is visualized within the mandible (Figs. 10 and 11). The needle is then placed superior to the probe and advanced in an out-of-plane technique toward the mental foramen. One-half to 3 ml of the solution should be then injected without entering into the foramen [6, 7].

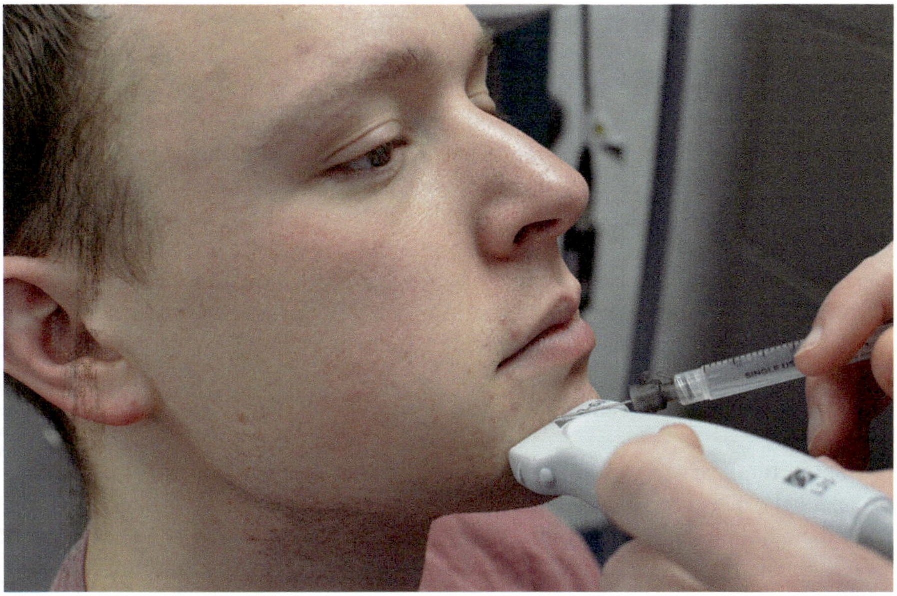

Fig. 10 Mental nerve block, ultrasound-guided injection technique. The figure demonstrates a proper orientation of the ultrasound probe and needle trajectory for mental nerve block

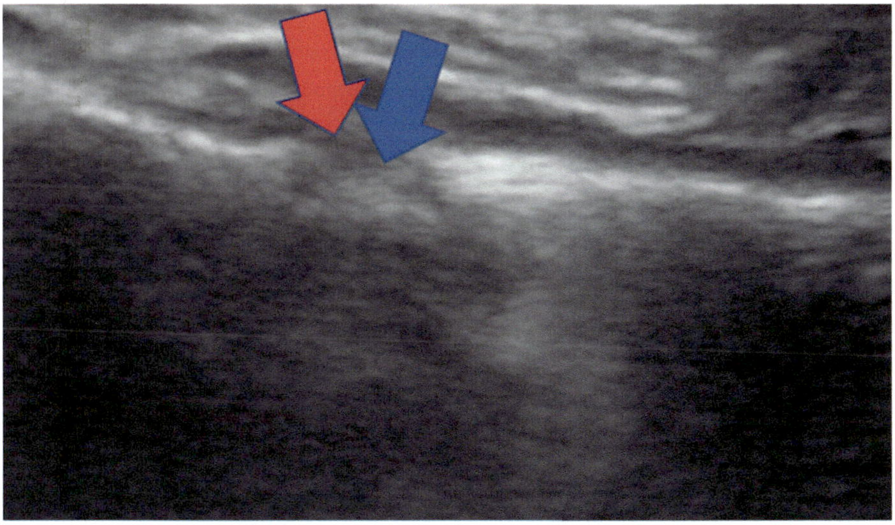

Fig. 11 Mental nerve block, ultrasound-guided technique. The blue arrow points towards the mental nerve fossa in the mandible. The right arrow indicates injectate spread

5 Potential Complications and Adverse Effects

Although generally well tolerated by patients, occasional adverse reactions and complications can occur which the clinician should be aware of when performing the bedside interventional procedures for the face and head pain.

Aside from the discomfort of pain or muscle spasms, adverse events are relatively rare. They include dizziness, lightheadedness, blurred vision, and slurred speech, which are signs of systemic absorption/toxicity. Patients may also report a metallic taste, perioral numbness, and tinnitus. Patients whom blocks are performed bilaterally are at more risk for adverse effects [4]. Other important complications and relevant considerations are presented in Table 2.

Clinical and Technical Pearls

- Supraorbital nerve and supratrochlear nerve blocks are usually performed simultaneously. This combination helps to alleviate pain induced by the herpes zoster of the ophthalmic division of the trigeminal nerve (V1) and its branches.
- Avoid placing the needle into the mental, infraorbital, and supraorbital foramina because injecting the solution into the bony canal can cause nerve damage as a result of entrapment neuropathy.
- The mental nerve block is vulnerable to blunt trauma due to the acute angle as it emerges out of the mental foramen.

Table 2 Additional potential Complications and Adverse Effects[a]

• Pressure should be applied to prevent hematoma production in patients with bleeding disorders or on anticoagulation
• Patients must be made aware of the potential for slightly unpleasant cosmetic disfigurement with local hair loss, hyperpigmentation, or cutaneous atrophy due to the corticosteroids utilized in the treatment. Local myotoxicity has been reported with bupivacaine
• Anaphylaxis can occur with the use of lidocaine or bupivacaine anesthetic, and blocks should not be performed if there has been a prior allergic reaction to the anesthetic
• Patients receiving frequent injections or perhaps using corticosteroids, either orally or as a result of other interventional procedures, are at risk for developing Cushing syndrome or adrenal insufficiency. Clinicians must be diligent in questioning patients specifically about the potential recent use of steroids as this medication history is often not reported by the patient
• Risks should be weighed against potential benefits when utilizing facial nerve blocks during pregnancy
• Meticulous attention should be paid to patients with bony defects (e.g., craniotomy, mastoidectomy, etc.) while per- forming greater auricular and occipital nerves blocks to avoid deep needle insertion through the bony defects which may result in serious CNS symptoms and coma

[a]Adapted with permission from Narouze SN (Ed.) Interventional Management of Head and Face Pain. Nerve Blocks and Beyond, 1st Ed. Springer Science+Business Media New York, 2014:17-27

References

1. Headache Classification Committee. The international classification of headache disorders, 2nd edition. Cephalalgia. 2004;24:1–160.
2. Blumenfeld A, Ashkenazi A, Napchan U, Bender SD, Klein BC, Berliner R, Ailani J, Schim J, Friedman DI, Charleston L 4th, Young WB, Robertson CE, Dodick DW, Silberstein SD, Robbins MS. Expert consensus recommendations for the performance of peripheral nerve blocks for headaches-a narrative review. Headache. 2013;53(3):437–46.
3. Evans RW, Pareja JA. Expert opinion: supraorbital neuralgia. Headache. 2009;49:278–81.
4. Tsui BCH, Dullane D, Funicane BT. Neural blockade for the surgery to the head and neck. Chronic pain. In: Cousins MJ, Carr DB, Horlocker TT, Bridenbaugh PO, editors. Cousins and Bridenbaugh's neural blockade in clinical anesthesia and pain medicine. 4th ed. Philadelphia: LWW; 2009. p. 486–91.
5. Levin M. Nerve blocks in the treatment of headache. Neurotherapeutics. 2010;7:197–203.
6. Spinner D, Kirschner JS. Accuracy of ultrasound-guided superficial trigeminal nerve blocks using methylene blue in cadavers. Pain Med. 2012;13(11):1469–73.
7. Tsui BC. Ultrasound imaging to localize foramina for superficial trigeminal nerve block. Can J Anaesth. 2009;56(9):704–6.

Further Reading

Narouze SN, editor. Interventional management of head and face pain. Nerve blocks and beyond. 1st ed. New York: Springer; 2014. p. 17–27.

Bedside Injections for Temporomandibular Pain

Dmitri Souza, Stephen McNulty, and Samer N. Narouze

Essential Concepts

- Temporomandibular joint (TMJ) disorders are a common cause of facial pain. They are prevalent but frequently undiagnosed. The differential diagnosis for TMJ pain is broad. TMJ disorders can be myofascial in nature, could be related to osteoarthritis, including structural changes such as disc displacement, other diagnoses should be excluded based on history, physical exam, and imaging studies if indicated. Dental source of jaw pain should be excluded.
- Initial management should be aimed at patient education and self-care. Short courses of pharmacologic treatment, oral splints, cold or hot packs, massage, osteopathic manipulative treatment, jaw exercises, and/or pain psychology should be considered for chronic TMJ disorders.
- Bedside interventions including intra-articular local anesthetic, steroid, and/or botulinum toxin injections to masseter muscles can be considered if other modalities failed.

1 Overview and Indications

Temporomandibular joint (TMJ) disorders or, more generally, temporomandibular disorders, are a common cause of facial pain affecting 4–12% of the general adult population [1, 2]. Temporomandibular disorder is a general term that

D. Souza (✉) · S. N. Narouze
Center for Pain Medicine, Western Reserve Hospital, Cuyahoga Falls, OH, USA
e-mail: dsouza@westernreservehospital.org; snarouze@westernreservehospital.org

S. McNulty
Internal Medicine, Western Reserve Hospital, Cuyahoga Falls, OH, USA
e-mail: smcnulty@westernreservehospital.org

D. Souza et al. (eds.), *Bedside Pain Management Interventions*,
https://doi.org/10.1007/978-3-031-11188-4_24

reflectsstructural, functional, or combined disorders associated with the temporomandibular joint or masseter muscles. While TMJ disorders are quite prevalent, they are frequently undiagnosed. The differential diagnosis for TMJ pain is broad. TMJ disorders can be myofascial in nature, could be related to osteoarthritis, including structural changes such as disc displacement; other diagnoses should be excluded based on history, physical exam, and imaging studies if indicated. Dental sources of jaw pain should be excluded as well [2, 3].

Etiology is commonly multifactorial such as genetic predisposition and aberrative oral habits like excessive gum chewing or bruxism. Various chronic pain disorders including fibromyalgia, diffuse myofascial pain dysfunction syndrome, or even comorbid psychiatric conditions may be contributory. There is a 2:1 female predominance [4, 5].

Bedside interventions including intra-articular local anesthetic, steroid, and/or botulinum toxin injections to masseter muscles can be considered if other modalities, including self-care orpharmacological management, have failed. Oral splints, cold or hot packs, massage, jaw exercises, osteopathic manipulative treatment, and/or pain psychology should be considered for chronic TMJ disorders. History of bruxism should prompt a referral to a dentist for an occlusal splint fitting [3–5].

Common contraindications include infection and the injection site, intolerance or allergy to injectate or its components, and patient refusal.

2 Clinical Anatomy

The temporomandibular joint (TMJ) is a synovial joint that articulates the glenoid fossa of the temporal bone and the condylar process of the mandible (Fig. 1). A unique feature of the TMJ is that the joint capsule contains an intra-articular disk [5]. This disc divides the TMJ into inferior and superior joint spaces. TMJ consists

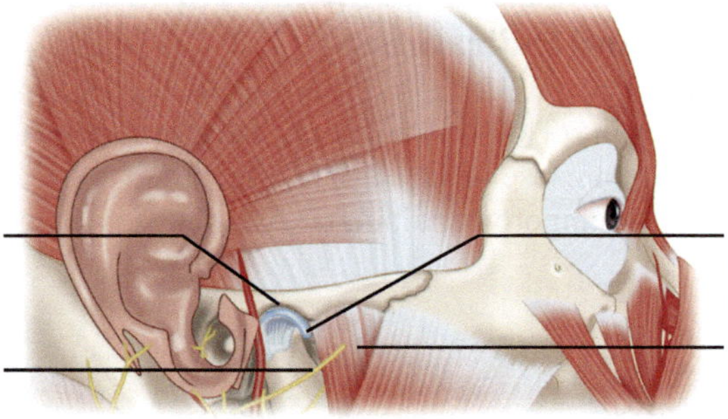

Fig. 1 Temporomandibular joint anatomy. (A) Synovial membrane of temporomandibular joint (colored green). (B) Articular disc of temporomandibular join. (C) Deep part of the masseter muscle. (D) Superior division of the Facial nerve

of fibrocartilage rather than hyaline cartilage which is typical in other joints. The inferior TMJ space is more susceptible to osteoarthritic changes. There is no clinically significant correlation between radiographic changes and TMJ and severity of temporomandibular disorder.

Common tasks, including talking or eating, are facilitated by the muscles of the cervical spine, head, and face (Fig. 1). The intra-articular disc is an important part of mouth opening that allows two sequential motions in the TMJ. Mouth opening is primarily provided by the movement of the lateral pterygoid; closure is controlled by the temporalis muscle, masseter muscles, and medial pterygoid muscle. Aberrant habits and patterns such as bruxism can predispose patients to myofascial symptoms [4–7].

3 Equipment and Supplies

TMJ injections can be conveniently performed at the bedside. Typically, a small syringe with a 25G 1 ½ in. needle is utilized to inject 0.5–3 ml of the anesthetic solution. The solution usually consists of local anesthetic, typically lidocaine with or without a corticosteroid. The procedure can be performed based on anatomic landmarks or with ultrasound guidance. The use of real-time ultrasonography is strongly recommended for appropriately navigating the needle and avoiding potential complications [4]. Botulinum toxin, 5–10 units per masseter or other muscles, can be utilized as well. Local anesthetic with or without corticosteroid can be prepared for injections into the temporalis, masseter, or other muscles to help with myofascial pain. There are reports of successful utilization of viscosupplementation into the TMJ [4–6]. Platelet-rich plasma (PRP) can be utilized as well if indicated [4, 7, 8]. The preparation of the PRP is outside of the scope of this chapter Auriculotemporal nerve block can be performed for TMJ or other temporomandibular disorders. Again, local anesthetic with or without corticosteroid can be injected around the nerve [9].

4 Techniques

The patient is placed in either a sitting or supine position and is advised to report any unusual sensations during the procedure. Sedation is not recommended. The TMJ is identified by palpation. The patient is asked to open and close the mouth for a better sense of joint anatomy. The skin overlying the TMJ is prepped with an antiseptic solution. A 25-gauge, 1½-inch needle is introduced "out-of-plane" under real-time visualization of the needle. (Fig. 2) The needle is advanced until it approaches the synovial membrane. Hydrolocalization of the needle tip can be utilized if needed. After aspiration, 0.5–3 ml of the solution is injected into the target joint,periarticular muscle, or around auriculotemporal nerve [4, 5].

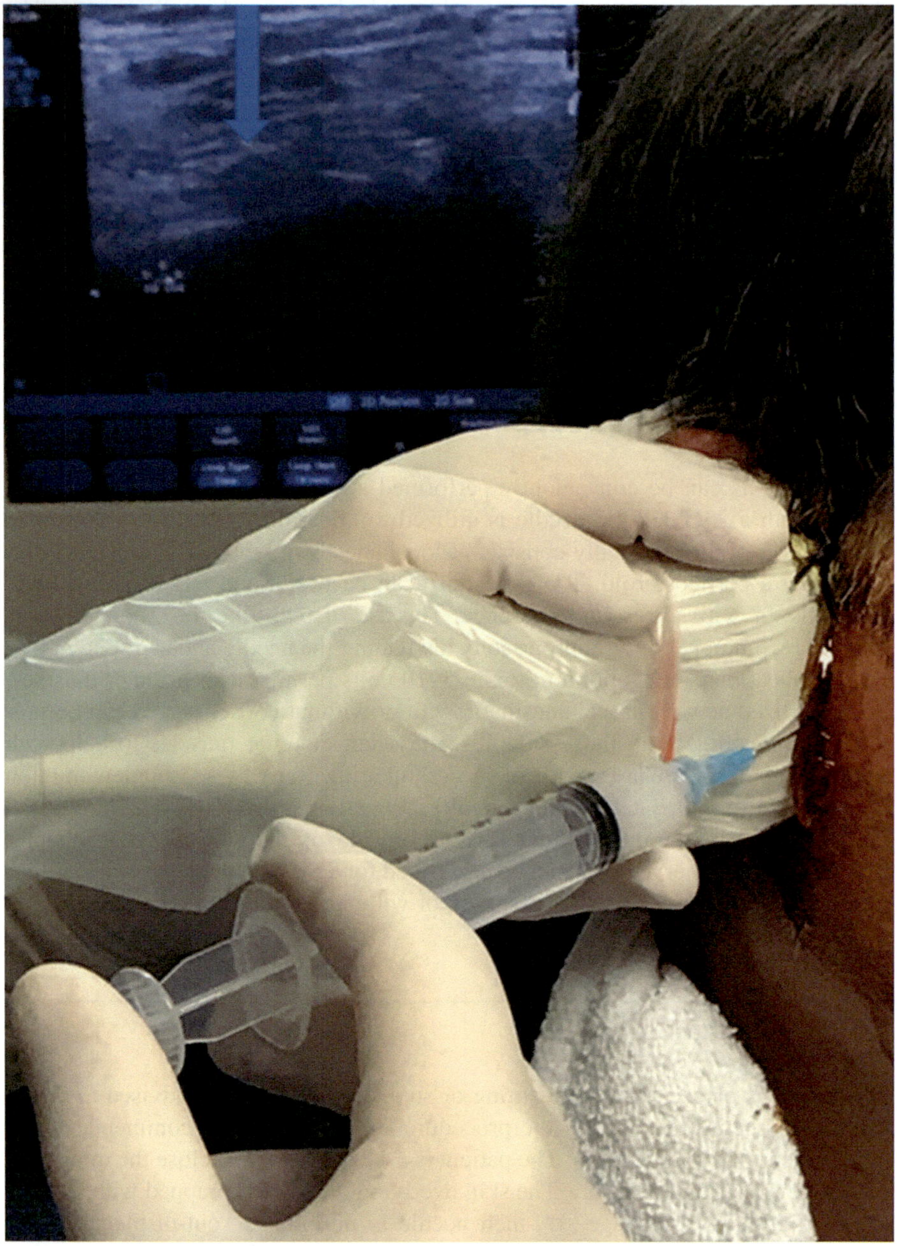

Fig. 2 Temporomandibular joint injection, needle trajectory. Blue arrow—temporomandibular joint

5 Potential Complications and Adverse Effects

Occasional adverse reactions and complications can occur which the clinician should be aware of when performing the bedside interventional procedures for temporomandibular joint pain and other temporomandibular disorders. Discomfort from pain on injection or muscle spasms may occur. But overall the adverse events are rare. They include dizziness, lightheadedness, blurred vision, and slurred speech, which are signs of systemic absorption/toxicity [4]. Patients may also report a metallic taste, perioral numbness, and tinnitus. All the symptoms may develop with the injection of the local anesthetic into the superficial temporal artery that is located in close proximity to the TMJ [4] (Fig. 3).

Ultrasonogram of this artery is presented in Fig. 4.

Particular formulations of steroids may contribute to the occlusion of small branches of this artery. Poor visualization of the artery or other technical concerns should prompt switching to non-particular steroid formulation. Patients on

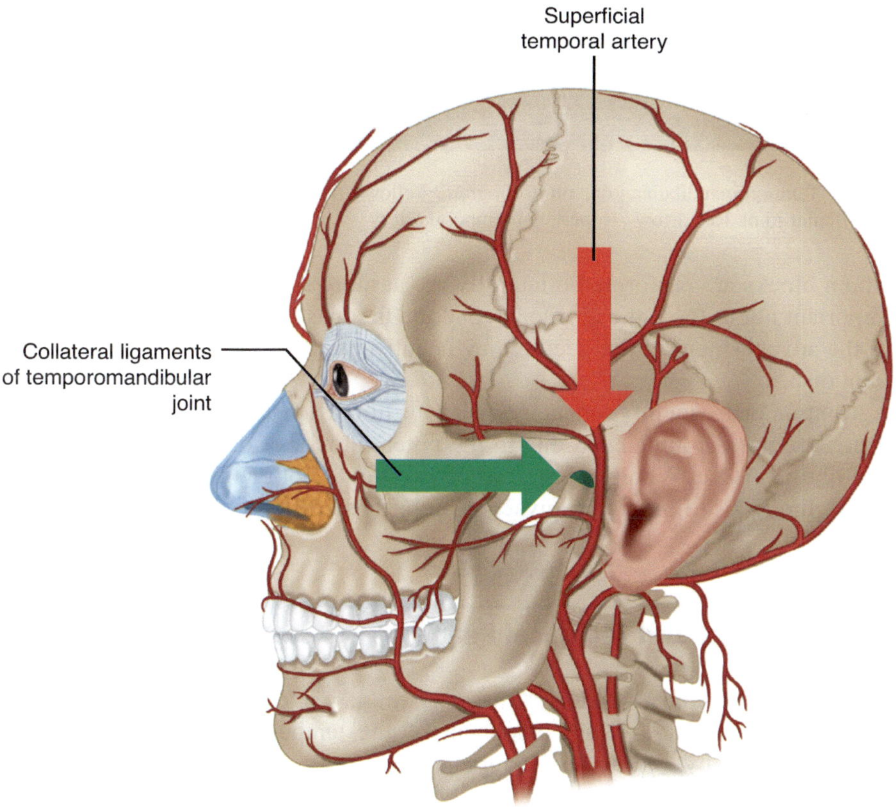

Fig. 3 Temporomandibular joint and superficial temporal artery. Green arrow—collateral ligaments of temporomandibular joint. Red arrow—superficial temporal artery

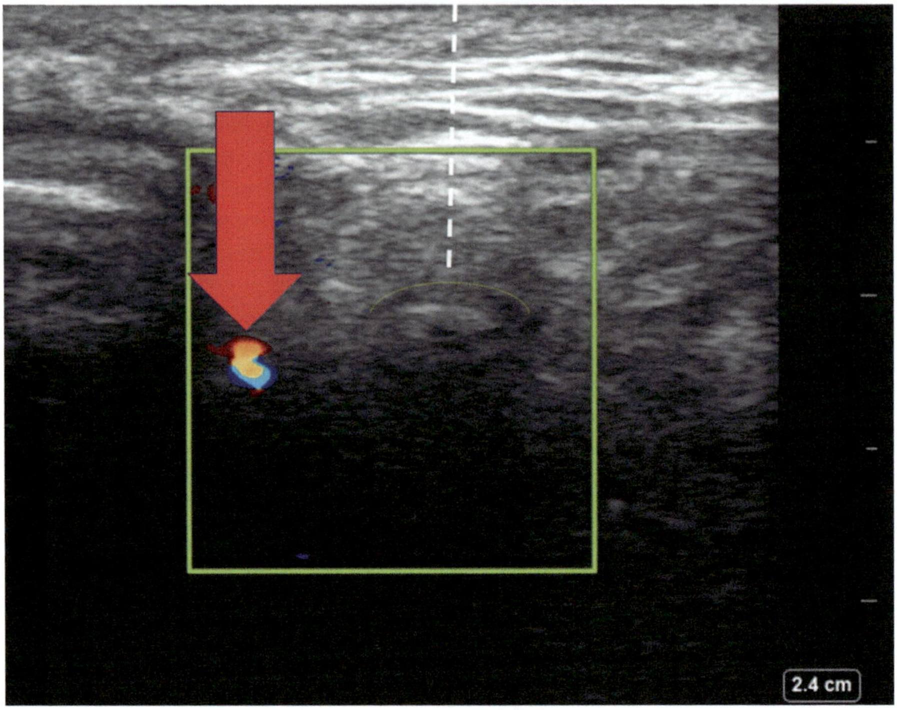

Fig. 4 Temporomandibular joint ultrasonogram. Yellow arc—synovial membrane of temporomandibular joint. Red arrow—superficial temporal artery

whom blocks are performed bilaterally are at more risk for adverse events. It is important not to force the needle beyond the first pass of the synovial membrane as the advancement of the needle may negatively affect the temporomandibular joint disc.

Routine or frequently repeated injections of corticosteroids for TMJ osteoarthritis are not recommended due to the potential risk of damage to the capsule and fibrous tissue. Whole autologous blood should not be injected into the TMJ due to the risk of fibrosis. Bupivacaine solutions can be toxic to the TMJ cartilage [4].

6 Clinical and Technical Pearls

- Temporomandibular joint and masseter muscle injections can be performed simultaneously if a joint component of the temporomandibular disorder is accompanied by a myofascial component.

- Avoid placing the needle beyond the first pass of the synovial membrane as it can cause temporomandibular joint disc damage.
- Be aware of the superficial temporal artery that is located in close proximity to the temporomandibular joint. Even a small amount of local anesthetic may produce toxicity if injected directly into this artery. In addition, particular corticosteroids, if used, can cause occlusion of the small branches.
- Blockade of the auriculotemporal nerve can be useful in the management of atypical facial pain secondary to temporomandibular joint dysfunction.

References

1. Ferneini EM. Temporomandibular joint disorders (TMD). J Oral Maxillofac Surg. 2021;79(10):2171–2.
2. Shrivastava M, Battaglino R, Ye L. A comprehensive review on biomarkers associated with painful temporomandibular disorders. Int J Oral Sci. 2021;13(1):23.
3. Lee E, Crowder HR, Tummala N, Goodman JF, Abbott J, Zapanta PE. Temporomandibular disorder treatment algorithm for otolaryngologists. Am J Otolaryngol. 2021;42(6):103155.
4. Grandhe R, Valeriano M, Souza D. Mechanical chronic jaw pain. In: Anitescu M, editor. Pain management review: a problem-based learning approach. 1st ed. Oxford University Press; 2018. p. 14–21.
5. Ahmad M, Schiffman EL. Temporomandibular joint disorders and orofacial pain. Dent Clin N Am. 2016;60(1):105–24.
6. Chen Y-W, Chiu Y-W, Chen C-Y, Chuang S-K. Botulinum toxin therapy for temporomandibular joint disorders: a systematic review of randomized controlled trials. Int J Oral Maxillofac Surg. 2015;44(8):1018–26. https://doi.org/10.1016/j.ijom.2015.04.003.
7. Kilic SC, Gungormus M, Sumbullu MA. Is Arthrocentesis plus platelet-rich plasma superior to arthrocentesis alone in the treatment of temporomandibular joint osteoarthritis? A randomized clinical trial. J Oral Maxillofac Surg. 2015;73(8):1473–83.
8. Giacomello M, Giacomello A, Mortellaro C, et al. Temporomandibular joint disorders treated with articular injection: the effectiveness of plasma rich in growth factors-Endoret. J Craniofac Surg. 2015;26(3):709–13.
9. Demirsoy MS, Erdil A, Tümer MK. Evaluation of the efficacy of auriculotemporal nerve block in temporomandibular disorders. J Oral Facial Pain Headache. 2021;35(4):326–31.

Further Reading

Gauer RL, Semidey MJ. Diagnosis and treatment of temporomandibular disorders. Am Fam Physician. 2015;91(6):378–86.

Greater Occipital Nerve Block

Dmitri Souza, Haroon Haque, and Nkiru Mills

Essential Concepts

- Greater occipital nerve block (GONB) provides blockade of nociceptive afferent fibers distributed over the upper neck, occipital region, vertex, sides of the head, as well as frontal area.
- Greater occipital nerve block may serve as an abortive treatment for intractable headache, tend to break intractable migraine headache cycle, but also may be helpful for acute occipital neuralgia, cluster headaches, and other common headache disorders
- Greater occipital nerve block typically provides rapid headache relief, that tends to last days to weeks and months.
- Greater occipital nerve block can be performed blindly at the level of the occipital ridge or with ultrasound guidance at the cervical level. The technical performance of the greater occipital nerve block is relatively simple, and typically well tolerated by patients.
- Greater occipital nerve block is remarkably safe if performed accurately.

1 Overview

Clinical experience suggests that greater occipital nerve block (GONB) can be utilized as a diagnostic and therapeutic tool for the abortive treatment of severe or intractable migraine headaches with status migrainosus [1]. It has been also

D. Souza (✉)
Center for Pain Medicine, Western Reserve Hospital, Cuyahoga Falls, OH, USA
e-mail: dsouza@westernreservehospital.org

H. Haque · N. Mills
Internal Medicine, Western Reserve Hospital, Cuyahoga Falls, OH, USA
e-mail: hhaque@westernreservehospital.org; nmills@westernreservehospital.org

D. Souza et al. (eds.), *Bedside Pain Management Interventions*,
https://doi.org/10.1007/978-3-031-11188-4_25

noted that it is helpful in the diagnosis and treatment of occipital neuralgia or entrapment neuropathy of the greater occipital nerve. There is a number of randomized control trials, as well as recent meta-analyses that support the efficacy of GONB for the treatment of severe and intractable migraine headaches [2, 3]. There is some evidence supporting the utilization of GONB in the treatment of exacerbation of cluster headaches, cervicogenic headaches, and some other primary and secondary headache disorders. There are reports indicating the efficacy of GONB in patients with posttraumatic headache, hemicrania continua, new daily persistent headache, post-dural puncture headache, and trigeminal neuralgia [4–7].

It is commonly noted in the literature that this procedure is remarkably safe if performed appropriately. It can be used in combination with oral and parenteral pharmacological treatment of severe or intractable headaches at the bedside. It can be combined with other treatment options, including biofeedback and other pain psychology interventions [8].

Greater occipital nerve block should be considered at the bedside for patients who are not responding to pharmacological treatment. Additionally, the patient with medication overuse headache may benefit from occipital nerve block to help the weaning process. It can be effectively used in patients with polypharmacy, in the geriatric population, and also may be considered, with the detailed assessment of risks versus benefits and consent, in pregnant women when the pharmacological options are limited [9].

2 Lndications and Contraindications

Indications for GONB include unilateral or bilateral occipital neuralgia. Ultrasound-guided technique for these injections is preferred. Greater occipital nerve block using a landmark technique would be of limited to no value for this particular indication. The same relates to various other entrapment neuropathies of the greater occipital nerve. The landmark technique or ultrasound-guided technique can be utilized for status migrainosus or severe/intractable migraine headaches in hospitalized patients when pharmacological treatment and other noninvasive techniques are either contraindicated or ineffective. Other indications include cluster headaches, cervicogenic headaches, posttraumatic headaches, hemicrania continua, new daily persistent headache, post-dural puncture headache, trigeminal neuralgia, and medication overuse headache [1, 4, 7, 9].

Common contraindications include infections at the injection site, allergy or intolerance to injectate or its components, patient refusal. Skull defects after craniotomy or mastoidectomy are contraindications to blind greater occipital nerve injection. Greater occipital nerve block can be performed in these patients using an ultrasound-guided technique.

3 Clinical Anatomy

The greater occipital nerve (GON) is the largest of three occipital nerves. The lesser occipital nerve (LON) runs laterally, and the third occipital nerve (TON) runs medially to the GON (Fig. 1) [10].

The GON originates from the dorsal primary ramus of the second cervical nerve. It is located between the inferior oblique muscle and semispinalis capitis. As the GON travels upward, it penetrates the *m. semispinalis capitis*, and then the *m. trapezius*. These are the common sites of GON entrapment. The GON then runs cephalad. It can be detected approximately 2 cm laterally to the superior nuchal line. Then GON runs laterally to the vertex and medially to the occipital artery (OA) (Fig. 1) [11].

The LON mainly consists of branches of the superficial cervical plexus and it has contributions from the C2 and C3 ventral rami. The LON travels upward and laterally, on the posterior border of the sternocleidomastoid muscle. It provides sensory innervation of the scalp laterally to the GON distribution, up to the posterior part of the ear.

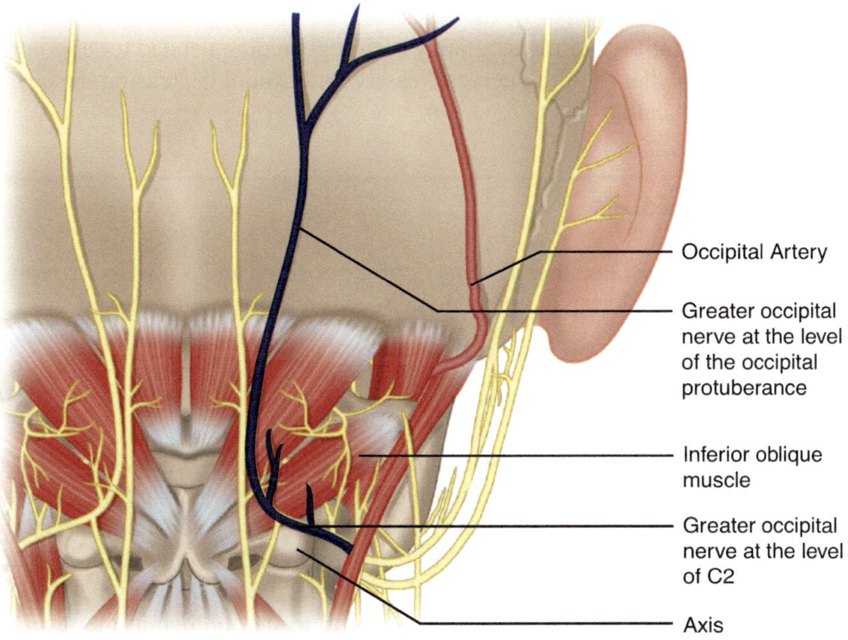

Fig. 1 Greater occipital nerve (GON) anatomy

The TON is a branch of the third cervical nerve and typically connects to the GON from below and medially. It is responsible for providing sensations to the back of the scalp and the lower occipital region.

4 Equipment and Supplies

A greater occipital nerve block can be conveniently performed at the bedside. Typically, a small syringe with a 25–30G 1.5 in. needle is utilized to inject 3–5 ml of the anesthetic solution. The injectate usually consists of the local anesthetic, either lidocaine 1% or bupivacaine 0.5%, with or without a corticosteroid. We recommend utilizing the non-particular corticosteroid to avoid embolization of small vessels. Methylprednisolone (20–125 mg, half-life 18–36 h), or Dexamethasone (1–5 mg, half-life 36–54 h) can be mixed with the anesthetic solution. Adding a corticosteroid to the local anesthetic showed to prolong the therapeutic effect of regional nerve blockade. However, the utilization of corticosteroids for the GONB remains controversial [12].

The procedure can be performed based on anatomic landmarks or with ultrasound guidance.

The use of real-time ultrasonography is strongly recommended for appropriately directing the needle, avoiding nerves, vessels, and overall decreasing the chance of potential complications [11].

5 Techniques

The patient is placed in either a sitting or prone position and is advised to report any unusual sensations during the procedure. Sedation is not recommended.

Anatomic Landmark Technique

In the past, prior to the widespread of ultrasonography, GON blocks were performed exclusively with the landmarks technique [13]. When using a landmark technique, a patient should be placed in a sitting or prone position. The occipital artery should be palpated on the back of the head at or slightly caudal to the superior occipital protuberance about 3–4 cm lateral to the midline. The GON is typically located medial to the artery approximately 2 cm lateral to the midline at the level of the occipital protuberance (Fig. 2).

Palpating this area would commonly be accompanied by occipital tenderness, or even headache, which may help to guide the blockade. The GON blockade can be performed on both sides depending on the patient's symptoms. It is important to avoid injecting into the occipital artery during the injection. It is recommended, therefore, to palpate the artery before making skin wheal with the local anesthetic. In addition, the injection should be performed medially to the pulsation of the occipital artery (Figs. 1 and 2) [10, 11].

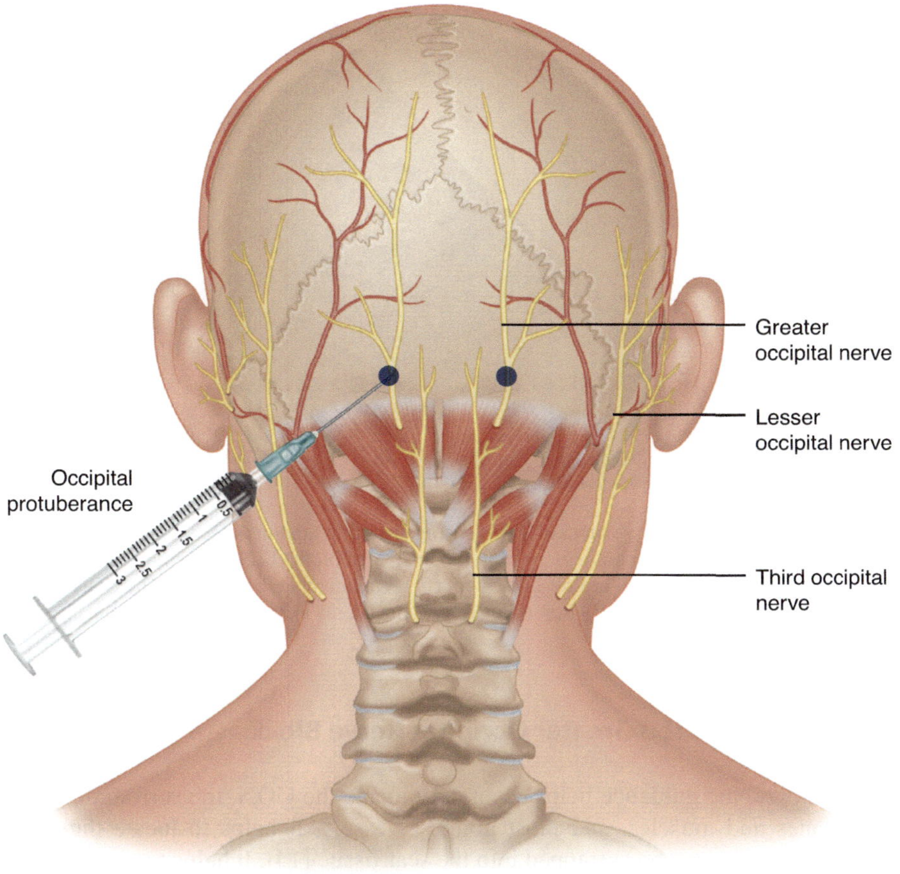

Fig. 2 Landmark injection schematics. Needs redrawing. OP—occipital protuberance. GON—greater occipital nerve. TON—third occipital nerve. LON—lesser occipital nerve. Blue circle—target area

When performing this injection based on the anatomic landmarks, there increase in the volume of local anesthetic up to 10 ml may be required in order to achieve clinical success. This is because of the variations in the course of the GON.

With the anatomic landmark technique, the needle is advanced until the patient reports paresthesia or the bony periosteum is encountered. To avoid injection into the periosteum, the needle needs to be then slightly withdrawn (Fig. 3). The aspiration should be performed, and if negative, the local anesthetic can be injected in the located tender point. Additional injections can be performed in a fanlike manner. These additional injections would contribute to field block and will likely improve the chance of a successful blockade. Blockade of the TON or LON branches is expected with a field block as these nerves are located in close proximity to the GON.

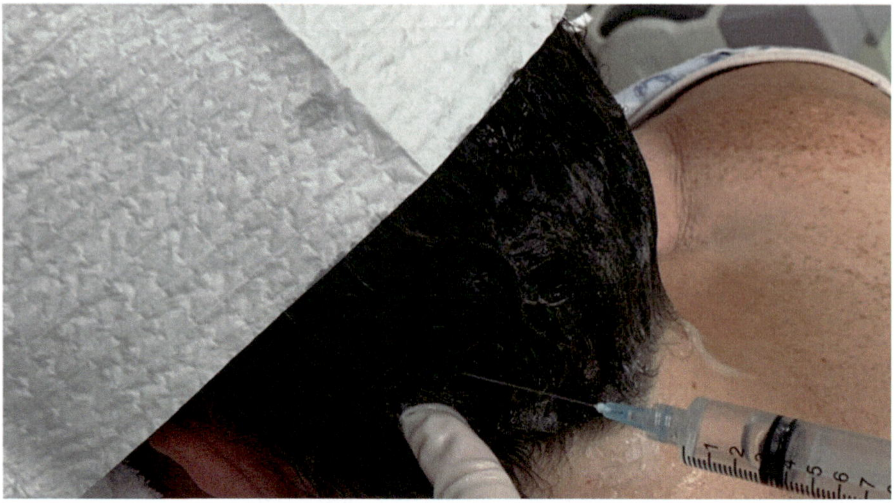

Fig. 3 Greater occipital nerve block (GONB) using anatomic landmark technique. The patient is in a sitting position. The occipital artery should be palpated on the back of the head at or slightly caudal to the superior occipital protuberance about 3–4 cm lateral to the midline. The GON is typically located medial to the artery approximately 2 cm lateral to the midline at the level of the occipital protuberance

Ultrasound-Guided Greater Occipital Nerve Block

Ultrasonographic guidance helps accurately locate the GON, the surrounding fascial planes and muscles, and most notably, vessels. It helps to locate the areas where the nerve may be entrapped into the scar tissue [14]. It helps to visualize the size of the nerve. The increased cross-section of the GON correlates with neuritis secondary to entrapment in the muscles or fascia or other reasons. The ultrasound guidance also provides real-time visualization of the tip of the needle as it is advanced towards the target, as well as the observation and direction of the injection itself. It has been shown that ultrasound-guided GON blocks may have better outcomes, and, potentially safer interventions. Ultrasound-guided GON block can be performed at the same location as the traditional landmark technique or lower, at the C2 level, where the GON is located just above the inferior oblique capitis muscle (Figs. 1 and 4).

The GON block typically provides rapid, within 15–30 min, pain relief that typically lasts days to months.

Either in-plane or out-of-plane techniques can be utilized. The needle should not be advanced if tip of the needle cannot be seen. After aspiration 0.5–3 ml of the solution is injected into the joint, or another target, including muscles surrounding the GON (Figs. 4 and 5).

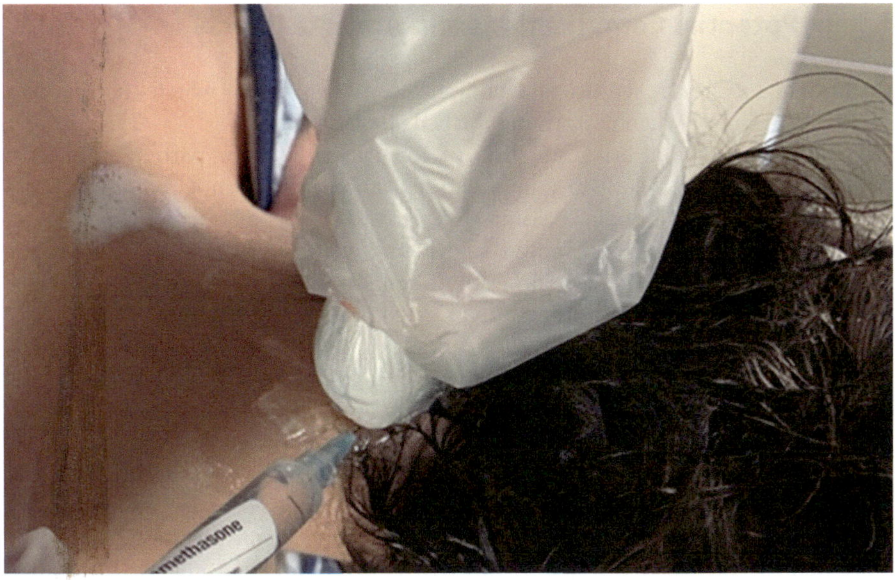

Fig. 4 Orientation of the probe for the GONB with ultrasound guidance. Please pay attention to the orientation and tilt of the ultrasound transducer

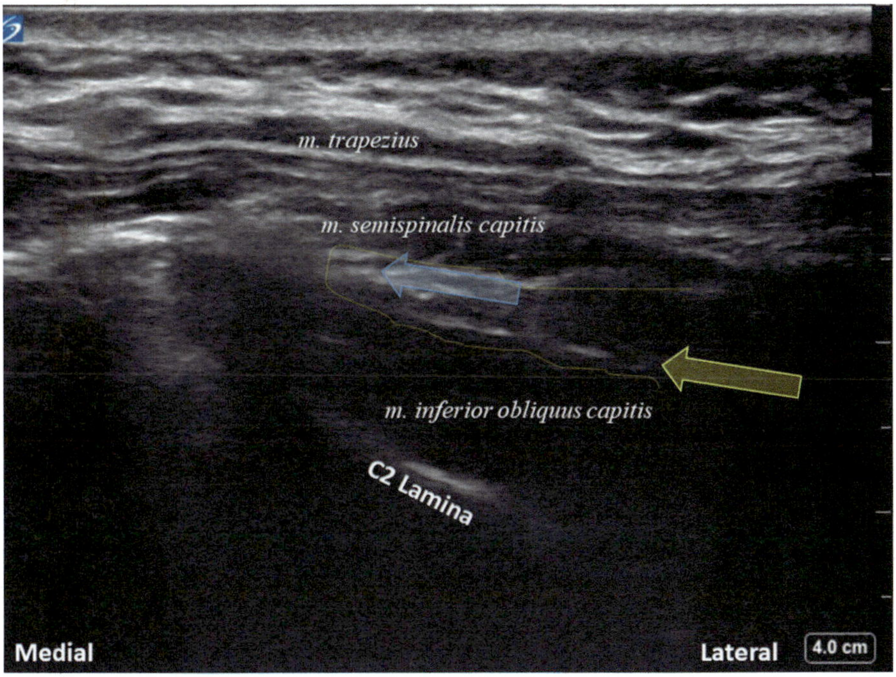

Fig. 5 Ultrasonographic image of the GONB. The injectate spread (Blue Line) can be seen just around the third occipital nerve (blue arrow) and the GON (yellow arrow) in the fascial plane between the inferior oblique muscle and semispinalis capitis muscle

6 Potential Complications and Adverse Effects

Occasional adverse reactions and complications can occur which the clinician should be aware of when performing the bedside GONB.

Inadvertent intra-arterial injection of local anesthetic or particulate steroid (triamcinolone) can result in complications including and not limited to scalp necrosis, hair loss, and hair discoloration. However, this may happen even without intra-arterial injection. Lipodystrophy may occur with this type of injection and the possibility of this potential complication should be discussed with the patient in detail prior to the procedure [13, 15]. Patients receiving frequent injections or perhaps using corticosteroids, either orally or as a result of other interventional procedures, are at risk for developing Cushing syndrome or adrenal insufficiency. Clinicians must be diligent in questioning patients specifically about the potential recent use of steroids as this medication history is often not reported by the patient.

In patients with a history of craniotomy, mastoidectomy, or other procedures that may result in bony defects, it is important to avoid deep needle insertion through the bony defects; this may result in serious CNS symptoms and coma. Ultrasound-guided GONB injections and longer monitoring times should be preferable for these patients.

Risks should be weighed against potential benefits when utilizing the GONB during pregnancy.

Anaphylaxis can occur with the use of lidocaine or bupivacaine anesthetic, and blocks should not be performed if there has been a prior allergic reaction to the anesthetic.

Clinical and Technical Pearls

- Hydrolocalization of the tip or needle tip bevel rotation can be performed the tip of the needle is inadequately visualized. The needle should not be advanced without proper visualization of the tip.
- Wiggling the needle for the purpose of better visualization is not recommended as it can be quite painful for the patient.
- Patients must be made aware of the potential for slightly unpleasant cosmetic disfigurement with local hair loss, hyperpigmentation, or cutaneous atrophy due to the corticosteroids utilized in the treatment. Local myotoxicity has been reported with bupivacaine.
- The GONB can be performed for patients on antiplatelet or anticoagulation therapy. The procedure requires a detailed discussion on risk and benefits and alternative options. Pressure should be applied to prevent hematoma production in patients with bleeding disorders or on anticoagulation.

References

1. Inan LE, Inan N, Unal-Artik HA, Atac C, Babaoglu G. Greater occipital nerve block in migraine prophylaxis: narrative review. Cephalalgia. 2019;39(7):908–20. https://doi.org/10.1177/0333102418821669.
2. Tang Y, Kang J, Zhang Y, Zhang X. Influence of greater occipital nerve block on pain severity in migraine patients: a systematic review and meta-analysis. Am J Emerg Med. 2017;35(11):1750–4. https://doi.org/10.1016/j.ajem.2017.08.027.
3. Zhang H, Yang X, Lin Y, Chen L, Ye H. The efficacy of greater occipital nerve block for the treatment of migraine: a systematic review and meta-analysis. Clin Neurol Neurosurg. 2018;165:129–33. https://doi.org/10.1016/j.clineuro.2017.12.026.
4. Lambru G, Abu Bakar N, Stahlhut L, McCulloch S, Miller S, Shanahan P, et al. Greater occipital nerve blocks in chronic cluster headache: a prospective open-label study. Eur J Neurol. 2014;21(2):338–43. https://doi.org/10.1111/ene.12321.
5. Kinfe TM, Schuss P, Vatter H. Occipital nerve block prior to occipital nerve stimulation for refractory chronic migraine and chronic cluster headache: myth or prediction? Cephalalgia. 2015;35(4):359–62. https://doi.org/10.1177/0333102414541685.
6. Gaul C, Roguski J, Dresler T, Abbas H, Totzeck A, Gorlinger K, et al. Efficacy and safety of a single occipital nerve blockade in episodic and chronic cluster headache: a prospective observational study. Cephalalgia. 2017;37(9):873–80. https://doi.org/10.1177/0333102416654886.
7. Busch V, Jakob W, Juergens T, Schulte-Mattler W, Kaube H, May A. Occipital nerve blockade in chronic cluster headache patients and functional connectivity between trigeminal and occipital nerves. Cephalalgia. 2007;27(11):1206–14. https://doi.org/10.1111/j.1468-2982.2007.01424.x.
8. Voigt CL, Murphy MO. Occipital nerve blocks in the treatment of headaches: safety and efficacy. J Emerg Med. 2015;48(1):115–29. https://doi.org/10.1016/j.jemermed.2014.09.007.
9. Young WB. Blocking the greater occipital nerve: utility in headache management. Curr Pain Headache Rep. 2010;14(5):404–8. https://doi.org/10.1007/s11916-010-0130-x.
10. Mosser SW, Guyuron B, Janis JE, Rohrich RJ. The anatomy of the greater occipital nerve: implications for the etiology of migraine headaches. Plast Reconstr Surg. 2004;113(2):693–700. https://doi.org/10.1097/01.PRS.0000101502.22727.5D.
11. el Sekily NM, Zedan IH. Surgical anatomy of greater occipital nerve and its relation to occipital artery. Alexandria J Med. 2015;51:199–206.
12. Ashkenazi A, Blumenfeld A, Napchan U, Narouze S, Grosberg B, Nett R, et al. Peripheral nerve blocks and trigger point injections in headache management - a systematic review and suggestions for future research. Headache. 2010;50(6):943–52.
13. Greengrass RA, Narouze S, Bendtsen TF, Hadzic A. Cervical plexus and greater occipital nerve blocks: controversies and technique update. Reg Anesth Pain Med. 2019;44(6):623–6.
14. Narouze S. Occipital neuralgia diagnosis and treatment: the role of ultrasound. Headache. 2016;56(4):801–7.
15. Narouze S, Peng PWH. Ultrasound-guided interventional procedures in pain medicine: a review of anatomy, sonoanatomy, and procedures: part ii: axial structures. Reg Anesth Pain Med. 2010;35(4):386–96.

Further Reading

Narouze S, editor. Interventional head and face pain management: nerve blocks and beyond. 1st ed. New York: Springer; 2014. p. 29–34.

Narouze S, Souzdalnitski D. Occipital nerve entrapment within the semispinalis capitis muscle diagnosed with ultrasound. Cephalalgia. 2013;33(16):1358–9.

Tepper SJ, Stillman MJ. Cluster headache: potential options for medically refractory patients (when all else fails). Headache. 2013;53(7):1183–90.

Intranasal Block

Kris Ferguson, Tyler Weeks, Antoun Nader,
and Dmitri Souza

Essential Concepts

- Intranasal block is a safe and efficient bedside block to treat a variety of common and uncommon headache and pain conditions
- The mechanism of action is thought to be blunting of the trigeminovascular reflex
- Pain relief is often rapid with a variable duration of pain relief.
- Repeated blocks have a cumulative effect which can prolong the duration of pain relief
- It is important to note that the current understanding is that intranasal local anesthetic injection, commonly referred to in the past as one of the variants of the sphenopalatine ganglion (SPG) block, is not a true SPG block.

1 Overview

Intranasal block is a relatively simple and beneficial interventional procedure. The intranasal block gained popularity after it that was discovered over a century ago [1, 2].

K. Ferguson
Langlade Hospital Pain Clinic, Antigo, WI, USA

T. Weeks
ENT, Western Reserve Hospital, Cuyahoga Falls, OH, USA

A. Nader
Department of Anesthesiology, Northwestern Memorial Hospital, Northwestern University, Feinberg School of Medicine, Chicago, IL, USA

D. Souza (✉)
Center for Pain Medicine, Western Reserve Hospital, Cuyahoga Falls, OH, USA
e-mail: dsouza@westernreservehospital.org

D. Souza et al. (eds.), *Bedside Pain Management Interventions*,
https://doi.org/10.1007/978-3-031-11188-4_26

The traditional thought was that the intranasal block is the true sphenopalatine ganglion (SPG) block. [2–4] It was noted that the SPG plays a substantial role in various pain syndromes involving the head, neck, and face [5]. The SPG is a conduit for sensory, sympathetic, and parasympathetic fibers. Blocking the SPG was thought to minimize the trigeminovascular reflex providing pain relief [6–8]. The traditional thought is that it can be effectively used at the bedside for patients with severe or intractable migraines, some of the trigeminal autonomic cephalalgias, tension headaches, post-dural puncture headaches, and some other types of headaches [9].

It is important to note that the current understanding is that intranasal local anesthetic injection, commonly referred to in the past as one of the variants of the sphenopalatine ganglion (SPG) block, is not a true SPG block [1, 2]. In fact, intranasal local anesthetic application as SPG block is probably "groundless and unfounded, as simply we do not have a clinical biomarker to validate an effective SPG block." [2] There are too many assumptions to consider the intranasal application as SPG block including (1) assumption that most of the nasally applied local anesthetic will not be swallowed; (2) that the remaining solution can passively diffuse through the nasal mucosa and the sphenopalatine foramen, and (3) that the SPG lies directly under the nasal mucosa [2]. Postulated mechanisms of actions of intranasal block include the placebo effect, trigeminal autonomic reflex modulation, topical anesthesia of trigeminal (ethmoidal) nerves, activation of descending inhibitory pathways, possibly systemic local anesthetic effect, and possibly actual sphenopalatine ganglion block [10]. While the nomenclature changes, an intranasal block continues to serve as a safe and efficient technique that can often provide rapid relief for a disabling headache which is typically well-tolerated [6, 8, 9]. Some of the authors suggested that this blood can be self-administered [11].

2 Indications and Contraindications

Commonly accepted indications include acute migraine, acute and chronic cluster headache, herpes zoster involving the ophthalmic nerve, other trigeminal autonomic cephalalgia's, trigeminal neuralgia, persistent idiopathic facial pain, other facial neuralgias, and post-dural puncture headache [7, 9, 12, 13]. There are also case reports supporting efficacy in head trauma, fibromyalgia, post-traumatic headache, intractable migraines, tear secretion, nicotine addiction, post-traumatic pseudo-cerebrospinal fluid rhinorrhea, head and neck cancer pain, hyperhidrosis, eye pain due to herpes keratitis [2].

Common contraindications include local infection or severe systemic infection, intolerance or allergy to injectate or its components, bleeding disorders or uncontrolled iatrogenic anticoagulation state, and skull fracture. Skull fracture would make the insertion of a stylet or cotton-tipped applicator unsafe.

3 Clinical Anatomy

The sphenopalatine ganglion is also known as the pterygopalatine ganglion or Meckel's ganglion and sits in a small triangular-shaped structure close to the sphenopalatine foramen posterior to the middle turbinate and maxillary sinus [7, 14] (Fig. 1). It is situated in the pterygopalatine fossa that is located between the maxillary, sphenoid, and palatine bones. The sphenopalatine ganglion is the largest peripheral parasympathetic ganglion. The SPG ganglion contains the largest collection of neurons outside the brain. While it is predominantly a parasympathetic ganglion, it also transports sensory and sympathetic fibers. The parasympathetic fibers, in contrast to the parasympathetic fibers, pass through the ganglion without synapsing.

It has connections to the trigeminal and facial nerves, the sympathetic and parasympathetic systems as well as somatosensory nerves. Stimulation of the SPG may result in the release of acetylcholine, vasoactive intestinal peptide, and nitric oxide in dural blood vessels. This may increase plasma protein extravasation with resultant neurogenic inflammation and activation of trigeminal nociceptors contributing to pain and triggering headaches (Fig. 1).

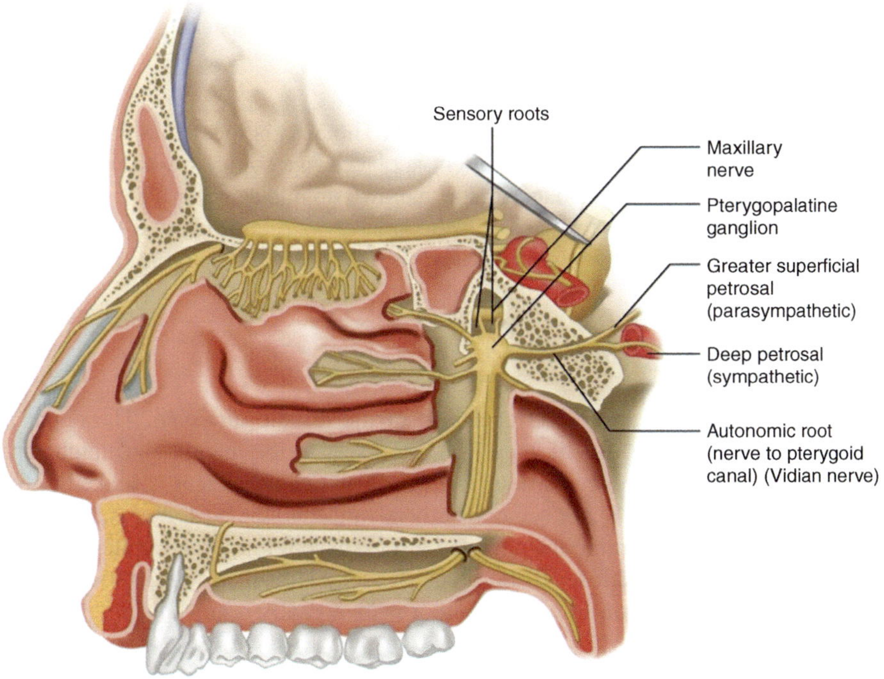

Fig. 1 Sphenopalatine ganglion neuroanatomy. The pterygopalatine fossa is located between the maxillary, sphenoid, and palatine bones. The sphenopalatine ganglion, located in this fossa, is the largest peripheral parasympathetic ganglion. While it is predominantly a parasympathetic ganglion, it also transports sensory and sympathetic fibers. The parasympathetic fibers, in contrast to the parasympathetic fibers, pass through the ganglion without synapsing. (Adapted with permission from Narouze S. (Ed.) Interventional head and face pain management: Nerve blocks and beyond. 1st Ed. Springer Science + Business Media New York; 2014:47–52)

Table 1 Required supplies for intranasal local anesthetic block

Syringe	3 mL
Applicator	Cotton tip Sphenocath Allevio Tx360 or other
Anesthetic	0.5% bupivacaine or 1–8% lidocaine

4 Equipment and Supplies

An intranasal local anesthetic block can be conveniently performed at the bedside. The intranasal local anesthetic block can be performed at the bedside by two different methods. Either 0.5% bupivacaine or 1–4% and rarely 8% lidocaine can be used for either procedure. A cotton tip applicator or a catheter is used to apply the anesthetic depending on which method is used (Table 1).

5 Techniques

Intranasal Block, Drip Method

This is one of the safest and simplest methods. The SPG is located in the posterior aspect of the middle turbinate. The patient is placed in a supine position with their head extended. 1–2 mL of local anesthetic is drawn up into a syringe. The anesthetic is dripped into the nostril ipsilateral to the side of pain and directed towards the middle turbinate. If the block is successful, pain relief should be rapid (Fig. 2).

Intranasal Block, Q-Tip Method

The SPG is located in the posterior aspect of the middle turbinate. The depth is estimated by measuring the distance from the nares to the mandibular notch. The patient is placed in a supine position. The cotton-tipped applicator is soaked in the local anesthetic. The applicator is then gently advanced to the posterior aspect of the middle turbinate ipsilateral to the pain and left in place for several minutes to allow the local anesthetic to diffuse. If the block is successful, pain relief should occur within minutes. The cotton-tipped applicator is then gently removed (Fig. 3).

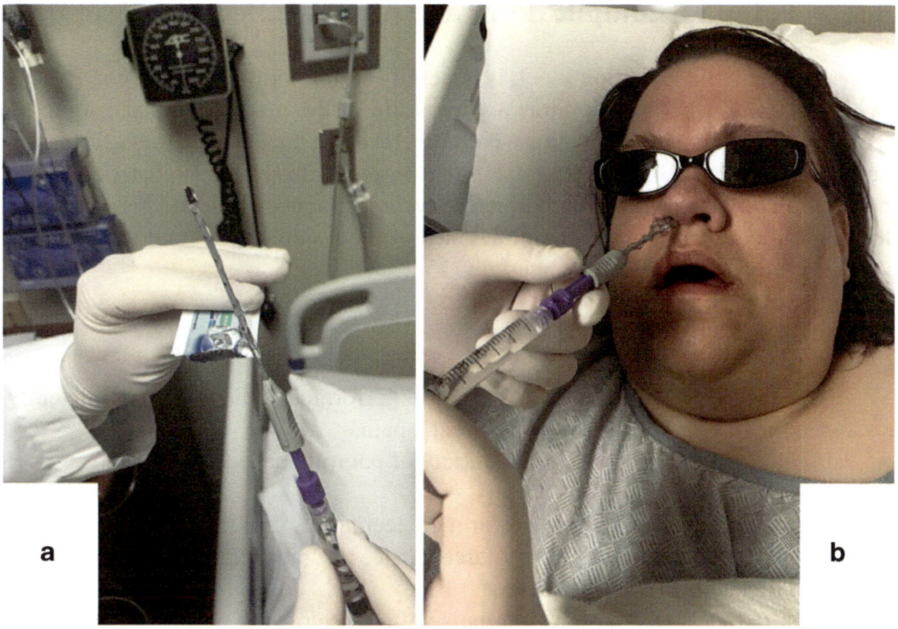

Fig. 2 Intranasal local anesthetic block at the bedside. Drip method. Local anesthetic is dripped into the patient's nose, directed towards the middle turbinate

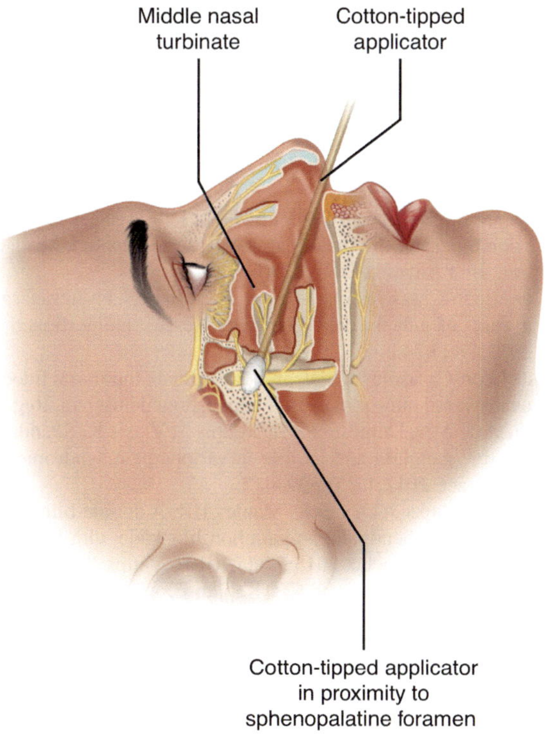

Fig. 3 Intranasal local anesthetic block at the bedside. Q-tip method. A cotton-tipped applicator with local anesthetic is directed towards the posterior aspect of the middle turbinate. Nasal mucosa separates intranasal space from the pterygopalatine fossa. The exception could be sphenopalatine foramen

6 Potential Complications and Adverse Effects

The sphenopalatine ganglion block is generally well tolerated by patients. Patients may complain of mild discomfort and pressure in the nose when performing the technique. Potential complications include epistaxis, facial hematoma, infection, nerve damage, no pain relief, worse pain, proptosis from retrobulbar hematoma, perforation of the nasal wall and orbit, bradycardia, tachycardia, allergic reaction to local anesthetic, corticosteroids intolerance of their side effects, and numbness of the upper teeth, hard palate, or pharynx [15].

Clinical and Technical Pearls

- The intranasal local anesthetic block be performed unilaterally or bilaterally depending on the location of the patient's pain.
- Pain relief is typically rapid for a variety of painful headache conditions as well as neuralgias
- There are a variety of ways to perform the technique: drip method, cotton-tipped applicator, or commercially available devices. Unique patient characteristics should dictate the method chosen.
- Repeating blocks can have a cumulative effect prolonging pain relief

References

1. Waldman SD. Sphenopalatine ganglion block—80 years later. Reg Anesth. 1993;18(5):274–6.
2. Narouze S. Topical intranasal lidocaine is not a sphenopalatine ganglion block. Reg Anesth Pain Med. 2021;46(3):276–9.
3. Giaccari LG, Aurilio C, Coppolino F, Pace MC, Passavanti MB, Pota V, et al. Peripheral nerve blocks for postdural puncture headache: a new solution for an old problem? In Vivo. 2021;35(6):3019–29.
4. Jespersen MS, Jaeger P, Ægidius KL, Fabritius ML, Duch P, Rye I, et al. Sphenopalatine ganglion block for the treatment of postdural puncture headache: a randomised, blinded, clinical trial. Br J Anaesth. 2020;124(6):739–47.
5. de Leon-Casasola O, Matson BL, Juarez F. Intranasal lidocaine sphenopalatine block: a case of unanswered questions versus unquestioned answers. Reg Anesth Pain Med. 2022;47(1):74.2–75.
6. de Leon-Casasola O, Matson BL, Juarez F. Intranasal lidocaine sphenopalatine block: a case of unanswered questions versus unquestioned answers. Reg Anesth Pain Med. 2022;47(1):74–5.
7. Piagkou MN, Demesticha T, Troupis T, Vlasis K, Skandalakis P, Makri A, et al. The pterygopalatine ganglion and its role in various pain syndromes: from anatomy to clinical practice. Pain Pract. 2012;12(5):399–412.
8. Cady R, Saper J, Dexter K, Manley HR. A double-blind, placebo-controlled study of repetitive transnasal sphenopalatine ganglion blockade with tx360((R)) as acute treatment for chronic migraine. Headache. 2015;55(1):101–16. https://doi.org/10.1111/head.12458.
9. Robbins MS, Robertson CE, Kaplan E, Ailani J, Charleston L, Kuruvilla D, et al. The sphenopalatine ganglion: anatomy, pathophysiology, and therapeutic targeting in headache. Headache. 2016;56:240–58.

10. Narouze S. Intranasal local anesthetic application: possible mechanisms of action. Reg Anesth Pain Med. 2022;47(1):75–6. https://doi.org/10.1136/rapm-2021-102964.
11. Rocha-Romero A, Roychoudhury P, Cordero RB, Mendoza ML. Self-applied sphenopalatine ganglion block for postdural puncture headache: four case reports. Braz J Anesthesiol. 2020;70(5):561–4.
12. Mojica J, Mo B, Ng A. Correction to: sphenopalatine ganglion block in the management of chronic headaches. Curr Pain Headache Rep. 2017;21(12):53.
13. Araújo R, Pinho S, Xavier J, Cabido H, Cavaleiro C, MacHado H. Sphenopalatine ganglion block followed by an epidural blood patch for postdural puncture headache management in postpartum patients: is it a confounder? Reg Anesth Pain Med. 2019;44.
14. Anugerah A, Nguyen K, Nader A. Technical considerations for approaches to the ultrasound-guided maxillary nerve block via the pterygopalatine fossa: a literature review. Reg Anesth Pain Med. 2020;45(4):301–5.
15. Kaufman AG, Dunbar SA, Cain CF, Cherukuri S, Ferrante FM. Sphenopalatine ganglion block for the treatment of myofascial pain of the head and neck. Reg Anesth. 1995;20(2).

Further Reading

Narouze S, editor. Interventional head and face pain management: nerve blocks and beyond. 1st ed. New York: Springer; 2014. p. 47–52.

Botulinum Toxin Injections for Chronic Migraine and Cervical Dystonia

Alexander Feoktistov

Essential Concepts

OnabotulinumtoxinA injections for treatment of chronic migraine and cervical dystonia are safe and effective and can be performed at the bedside or in the office.

Landmark approach is utilized in the chronic migraine paradigm, while ultrasound or EMG guidance is required during cervical dystonia treatment.

Understanding muscle anatomy and physiology is critical to achieving the best therapeutic results and safety outcomes.

1 OnabotulinumtoxinA Injections for Chronic Migraine and Cervical Dystonia

Overview

According to migraine prevalence and burden study [1], migraine headache affects nearly 12% of the United States population. Not only do migraine headaches affect patients in different age groups, but it especially impacts our most productive years. It has been estimated that migraine headaches affect 7.4% of males between ages 30 and 39 and an astounding 24.4% of females in the same age group. In addition to migraine's impressive prevalence, over 50% of all patients with migraine report significant impairment and/or requirement for bed rest during migraine attacks. According to the most recent 2016, Global Burden of Disease report migraine is the leading cause of years lived with disability among patients between ages 15 and 49 [2].

A. Feoktistov (✉)
Synergy Integrative Headache Center, Northfield, IL, USA
e-mail: drfeoktistov@synergyheadache.com

D. Souza et al. (eds.), *Bedside Pain Management Interventions*,
https://doi.org/10.1007/978-3-031-11188-4_27

Cervical dystonia is a less prevalent neurological condition affecting between 28 and 183 cases per million of the population. Cervical dystonia presents with various clinical features making diagnosis very challenging in some cases. Considering clinical variability, it is a common belief that cervical dystonia is a significantly underdiagnosed condition [3]. It has been estimated that approximately 5 years pass from the time of cervical dystonia onset to actual diagnosis [4].

OnabotulinumtoxinA injections (although different in their methodology) represent safe and effective treatment options for chronic migraine and cervical dystonia.

Clinical Presentation and Indications

Migraine presentation differs from patient to patient and in general presents as moderate or severe headache lasting between 4 and 72 h, usually affecting one side of the head and being described as a throbbing pain. The headache is associated with photo and phonophobia, nausea and occasional vomiting. Up to 30% of patients with migraine headaches may experience an aura (Table 1) [5].

Chronic migraine should be considered in those patients experiencing at least 15 headache days per month (for at least 3 months), with each headache episode lasting at least 4 h/day and at least 8 of those 15 headaches being considered migraines (ie meeting migraine diagnostic criteria described above). Chronic migraine may occur with or without acute medication overuse (Table 2) [5]. OnabotulinumtoxinA is indicated for any patient with chronic migraine who had previously failed at least 1 or 2 established preventative medications [6].

Cervical dystonia presentation varies dramatically between patients. The most common symptoms are neck posture change, neck pain, and tremor. Depending on specific neck posture there are 4 major types of cervical dystonia: torticollis (the most common type, affecting 82% of patients and associated with cervical rotation), laterocollis (affecting 42% of patients and associated with flexion of the neck to one side), anterocollis (affecting up to 25% of patients and associated with forward flexion of the neck), and retrocollis (affecting 29% of patients and associated with posterior neck extension). It also appears that the majority of the patients may present

Table 1 Migraine diagnostic criteria

A. At least five attacks fulfilling criteria B–D
B. Headache attacks lasting 4–72 h
C. Headache has at least two of the following characteristics:
1. Unilateral location
2. Pulsating quality
3. Moderate or severe pain intensity
4. Aggravation by or causing avoidance of routine physical activity (e.g. walking or climbing stairs)
D. During headache at least one of the following:
1. Nausea and/or vomiting
2. Photophobia and phonophobia
E. Not better accounted for by another ICHD-3 diagnosis

Table 2 Chronic migraine diagnostic criteria

1. Headaches on more than 15 days/month for more than 3 months
2. In a patient with history of at least 5 prior migraine attacks, with/without aura
3. On 8 days/months, for more than 3 months, headache fulfills criteria for one or more of the following:
(a) At least 2 of the following:
• Unilateral
• Pulsating
• Moderate or severe pain
• Aggravated by physical activity
AND at least 1 of the following:
• Nausea and/or vomiting
• Photophobia and phonophobia
(b) At least one of the following reversible aura symptoms: Visual, sensory, speech/language, motor, brainstem, retinal: AND at least 2 of the characteristics of aura
(c) Relieved with triptans or ergot derivative
4. Not better accounted for by any ICH D3 diagnosis
5. With or without medication overuse

with a combination of different postures which further complicates the diagnosis [7]. OnabotulinumtoxinA injections are indicated for any patients with diagnosed cervical dystonia.

Clinical Anatomy

When injecting onabotulinumtoxinA for chronic migraine, following the chronic migraine paradigm [8, 9] with a focus on symmetrical injections and 7 different muscle groups. Frontal injections involve injecting of the medication into frontalis muscle (which proximally attaches to the epicranial aponeurosis and distally to the skin of the forehead and eyebrows and functions as eyebrow elevator which produces horizontal frontal wrinkles), bilateral corrugator muscles (which attach medially to the nasal–frontal bone and laterally to the skin of the eyebrow and functionally they are considered to be an eyebrow depressors that pull eyebrows toward each other and downwards producing vertical wrinkles between the brows) and procerus muscle (which originates distally from the fascia covering the lower part of the nasal bone and attaches proximally to the skin over the lower part of the forehead between the eyebrows and functionally it pulls the eyebrows down creating horizontal wrinkles over the bridge of the nose). Lateral injections of the head consist of temporalis muscle injection which is located in the temporal fossa and attaches distally to the coronoid process of the mandible. The temporalis muscle is a muscle of mastication and it produces clenching of the teeth. Posterior injections of the head and neck consist of injections of the occipitalis muscles bilaterally (which originate distally at the nuchal line and insert proximally into the epicranial aponeurosis), cervical paraspinal muscle group (which consists of splenius capitis and semispinalis capitis muscles which stabilize cervical spine and allow for movement of the head and neck) and trapezius muscle (especially medial portion of it which stabilizes the neck and provides extension of the head and neck posteriorly and flexion ipsilaterally) [10].

When injecting onabotulinumtoxinA for cervical dystonia treatment we are focusing on cervical muscles only. Although multiple cervical muscles might be involved in cervical dystonia presentation the following muscles have been approved for onabotulinumtoxinA injections:

1. Sternocleidomastoid muscle: attaches superiorly to the mastoid process and inferiorly to the manubrium and middle one-third of the clavicle. When activated unilaterally it flexes the head ipsilaterally and rotates the head to the opposite side or extends the head and pulls the neck backward when activated bilaterally. It is located on the side of the neck and can be easily localized with a contralateral rotation of the head.
2. Splenius capitis muscle: attaches superiorly to the mastoid process and inferiorly to the spinous processes of C7 - T3. When activated unilaterally it rotates and bends the head to the same side or extends the head posteriorly when activated bilaterally. It can be localized immediately anterior to the trapezius muscle and posterior to the sternocleidomastoid muscle in the proximal part of the neck.
3. Splenius cervices muscle: attaches superiorly to the transverse processes of C1-C3 and inferiorly to the spinous processes of T3-T6. When activated unilaterally it rotates the upper neck and flexes it to the same side or when activated bilaterally, it produces posterior extension of the neck). It can be localized anterior and deep to the trapezius muscle, inferior and parallel to the splenius capitis muscle and medial to the levator scapula muscle.
4. Semispinalis capitis muscle: attaches superiorly to the medial aspect of the nuchal lines and inferiorly to the transverse processes of the lower cervical and upper thoracic vertebrae and it provides posterior extension of the head. It is located approximately 3 cm below the occipital protuberance and approximately 3 cm lateral from the midline at a depth of 3–4 cm.
5. Scalenus anterior/medius/posterior muscles: attach superiorly to the transverse processes of C2-C7 and inferiorly to the first and second ribs and it produces ipsilateral bending of the neck if activated unilaterally and, if activated bilaterally, produces forward flexion of the neck. It can be localized approximately 2 fingerbreadths anterior to the superior edge of the trapezius and 2 fingerbreadths above the clavicle.
6. Trapezius muscle: attaches superiorly to medial one-third of the superior nuchal line and the occipital protuberance and inferiorly to the lateral one-third of the clavicle, acromion, scapular spine as well as to the spinous processes of the thoracic and lower cervical vertebrae. It contributes to the head rotation to the opposite side and bending of the neck to the same side when activated unilaterally, and if activated bilaterally it produces posterior neck extension. It can be localized approximately 3 cm below the nuchal line.
7. Longissimus capitis and cervicis muscles: attaches superiorly to the mastoid process and transverse processes of C2-C6 and inferiorly to the transverse process of the lower cervical and upper thoracic vertebrae. When activated

unilaterally it produces rotation and bending of the head and neck to the same side and when activated bilaterally it extends the head and neck posteriorly. It is located approximately 3 fingerbreadths lateral from the midline at the proximal part of the neck (approximately 3 cm below the mastoid process or lower border of the skull).

8. Levator scapula muscle: attaches superiorly to the transverse processes of C1-C4 and inferiorly to the medial scapular border. When activated unilaterally it rotates and bends the neck to the same side or, when activated bilaterally, extends the neck posteriorly. It can be localized anterior to the superior edge of the trapezius muscle at the angle of the neck [10].

Equipment and Supplies for Chronic Migraine Injections

Typically, several 1 mL syringes with 30-gauge, half an inch needles will be required to perform this procedure. 200 units of onabotulinumtoxinA should be diluted in 4 mL of preservative-free normal saline to achieve 5 units of onabotulinumtoxinA in every 0.1 mL of the solution which will allow for accurate and simple injection protocol. This procedure does not require any imaging or EMG guidance and should be safely performed using a landmark approach only [8, 9].

2 OnabotulinumtoxinA Injections for Chronic Migraine, Landmark Technique

Chronic migraine injection protocol consists of 31 injection across 7 muscle groups. Each injection site contains 5 units of onabotulinumtoxinA, thus the total dose injected during a single treatment equals 155 units. The patient should be positioned comfortably in a supine or sitting position. We recommend to start the procedure with frontal injections and gradually move on to other sites bilaterally and finish the procedure with trapezius muscle injections. Make sure that the injection sites are cleaned with alcohol or other approved solution prior to injection and blood aspiration is performed prior to each injection. Although all injections are considered to be intramuscular, it is recommended to inject medication in to the most superficial aspect of the muscle to avoid contact with periosteum or excessive muscle weakness. Start the procedure with corrugator muscle injection. Ask the patient to furrow the eyebrow so that you could palpate and pinch the corrugator muscle between the thumb and index finger of your left hand and while holding syringe in your right hand insert the needle at a 90 degree angle into the belly of the corrugator muscle (approximately 1.5 cm above the medial inferior edge of the superior orbital rim) without touching periosteum. Aspirate and if there is no blood return gently inject 0.1 cc (5 units of onabotulinumtoxinA) into the corrugator muscle belly. Repeat the same procedure on the opposite side. Procerus muscle is injected in a similar fashion approximately midway between the 2 corrugator injections. The rest of the injections will be performed pointing needle upward at a

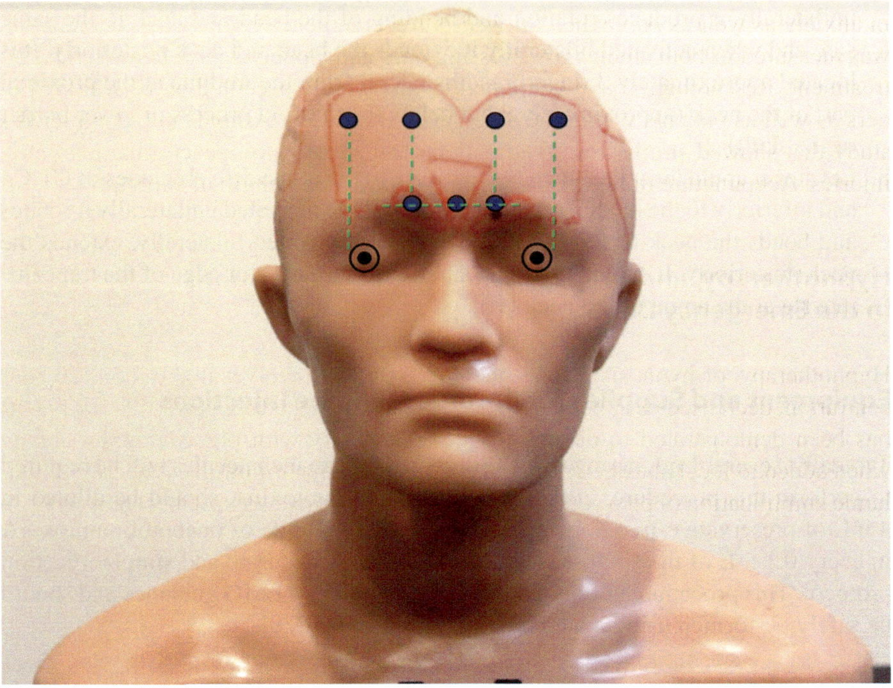

Fig. 1 Frontal injections. Examples of procerus, corrugator and frontalis muscle injections are marked with blue dots. Green lines indicate corresponding anatomical landmarks for injections localization

45-degree angle (once again, without touching the periosteum) (Fig. 1). Next, proceed to frontalis muscle injection. Visually draw a vertical line extending from the corrugator muscle injection and inject a medial portion of the frontalis muscle at the upper one-third of the forehead. Lateral frontalis muscle injection site is also located at the upper one-third of the forehead at the level of the imaginary vertical line passing through the lateral limbus of the cornea.

When injecting temporalis muscle start with locating the patient's tragus of the ear and move finger vertically about 3 cm above the tragus for the first injection site. Continue to move your finger along the same vertical line approximately 1.5 cm to 3 cm above the first injection to inject the second temporalis muscle site. The third injection site is located midway between the first and second injection sites and 1.5 cm anteriorly (yet staying within the hairline). The fourth injection site of the temporalis muscle is located about 1.5 cm posterior to the second injection site (at the same horizontal level) and approximately above the helix of the ear (Fig. 2).

For the first occipitalis muscle injection first, locate external occipital protuberance and drawing an imaginary line from the inion to the ipsilateral mastoid

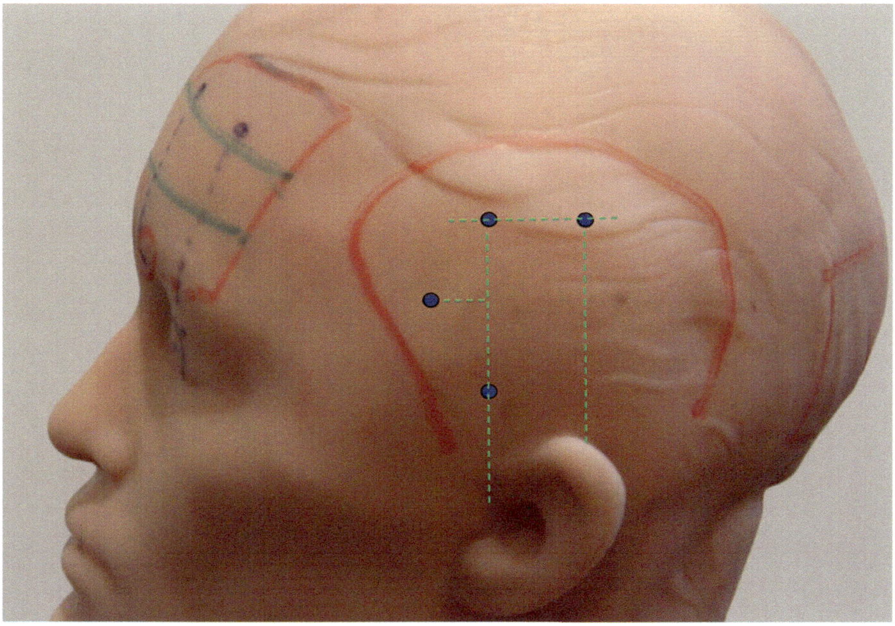

Fig. 2 Temporal injections. Examples of temporal muscle injections are marked with blue dots. Green lines indicate corresponding anatomical landmarks for injections localization

process. The first injection site is located in the midway of that line approximately at the level of the superior nuchal ridge. The second occipitalis muscle injection is located 1 fingerbreadth laterally, diagonally and superiorly to the first occipitalis muscle injection. The third injection of the occipitalis muscle is located 1 fingerbreadth medially, diagonal and superiorly to the first occipitalis muscle injection. Repeat the same procedure on the opposite side.

Upper cervical paraspinal muscle injections are located within the hairline. The first injection site is located 3 cm inferior to the lower border of the occipital protuberance and 1 cm laterally from the midline. The second injection is located 1.5 cm laterally, diagonally and superiorly from the first injection site (Fig. 3).

For trapezius muscle injection, first, divide the upper portion of the trapezius muscle in half from the necklace line to the acromioclavicular joint. Inject 0.1 cc of the solution to the most superficial layer of the trapezius muscle (at the superior edge of the muscle) at this level (first injection site). The second injection site is located at the superior edge of the trapezius muscle halfway between the first injection in the acromioclavicular joint. The third injection is once again located at the superior edge of the trapezius muscle halfway between the first injection in the necklace line or corner of the neck (Fig. 4).

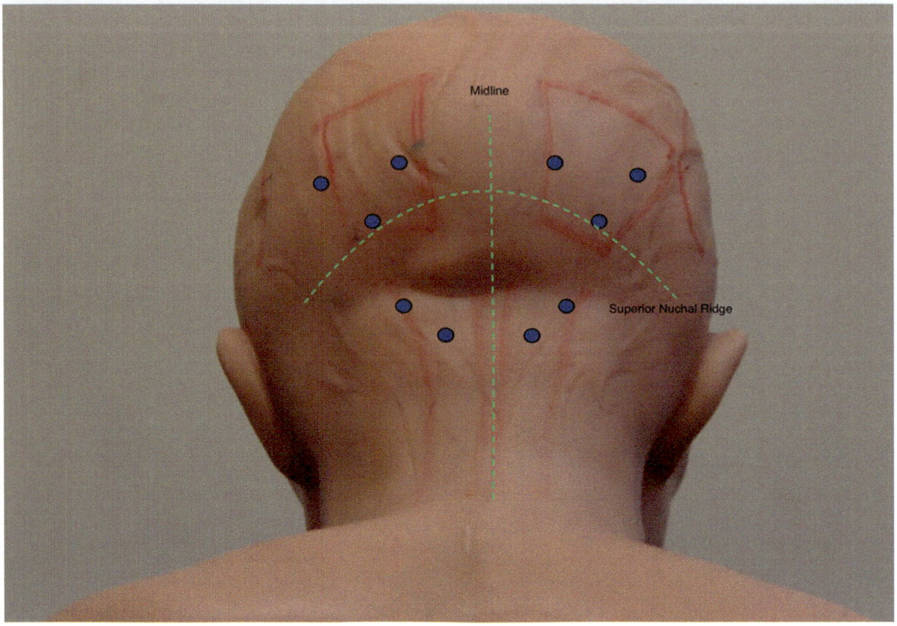

Fig. 3 Occipital and upper cervical injections. Examples of occipital and proximal paraspinal cervical muscle injections are marked with blue dots. Green lines indicate corresponding anatomical landmarks for injections localization

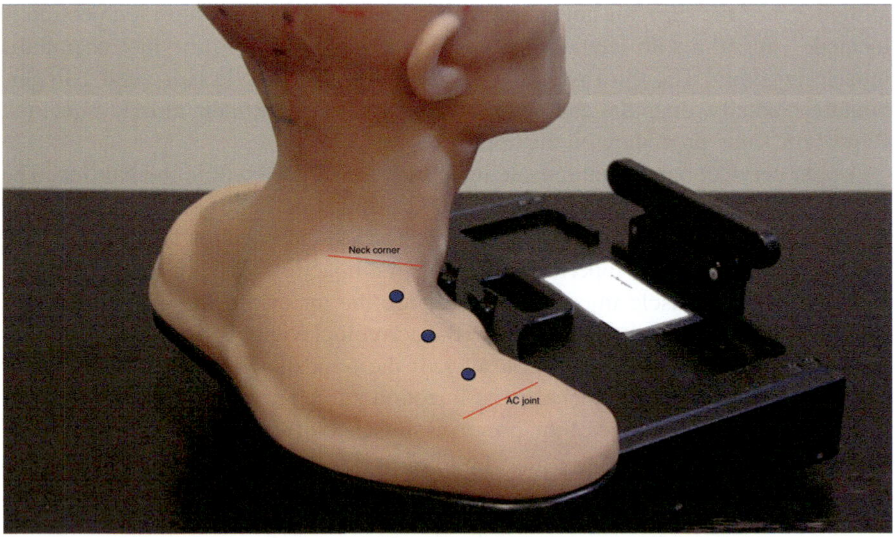

Fig. 4 Shoulder injections. Examples of trapezius muscle injections are marked with blue dots. Green lines indicate corresponding anatomical landmarks for injections localization

Table 3 Adverse reactions as observed during PRREMPT clinical trials

Adverse reaction	OnabotulinumtoxinA (%)	Placebo (%)
Headache	5	3
Facial paresis	2	0
Eyelid ptosis	4	<1
Bronchitis	3	2
Neck pain	9	3
Muscular weakness	4	<1
Myalgia	3	1
Injection site pain	3	2

Potential Complications and Adverse Events

This procedure is generally well tolerated by patients. The most common adverse events observed during PREEMPT clinical trials and as seen in clinical practice include neck pain, headache, muscle weakness, eyelid ptosis and injection site pain (Table 3) [6].

Clinical and Technical Pearls

- The patient should be informed of the possibility of temporary frontal muscle weakness preventing eyebrow frowning and forehead wrinkling
- Always keep in mind that injection should be administered into the most superficial layer of the muscle
- Discontinuation of anticoagulation is not required for this procedure

Equipment and Supplies for Cervical Dystonia Injections

Typically, several 1 mL syringes with 25-gauge needles, one and half-inch needles will be required to perform this procedure. Considering that dose/units injected during cervical dystonia treatment are significantly higher than during chronic migraine protocol and depending on the dose planned to be injected you may dilute 200 units of onabotulinumtoxinA in 4 mL of preservative-free normal saline to achieve 5 units of onabotulinumtoxinA in each 0.1 mL of the solution, or in 2 mL of preservative-free normal saline to achieve concentration of 10 units per 0.1 mL or even in 1 mL of preservative-free normal saline to achieve concentration of 20 units per 0.1 mL. This procedure requires either an ultrasound and EMG guidance to help identify specific muscles.

3 OnabotulinumtoxinA Injections for Cervical Dystonia, Ultrasound/EMG Guided Technique

There is no standard or universal injection protocol for cervical dystonia and every patient should be injected differently depending on their particular clinical presentation and response to therapy. It is important to recognize that injection protocol may need to be adjusted from time to time. First, determine what type of dystonia your patient is presenting with. Then determine which muscles are contributing to the patient's posture/symptoms. Finally, decide what dose to inject. Each muscle may be injected at one or more sites. In general, avoid injecting more than 50 units of onabotulinumtoxinA per site. The total dose of onabotulinumtoxinA should not exceed 400 units in the 3 months interval. You may need to use either an ultrasound or EMG guidance to better localize these muscles (Figs. 5 and 6).

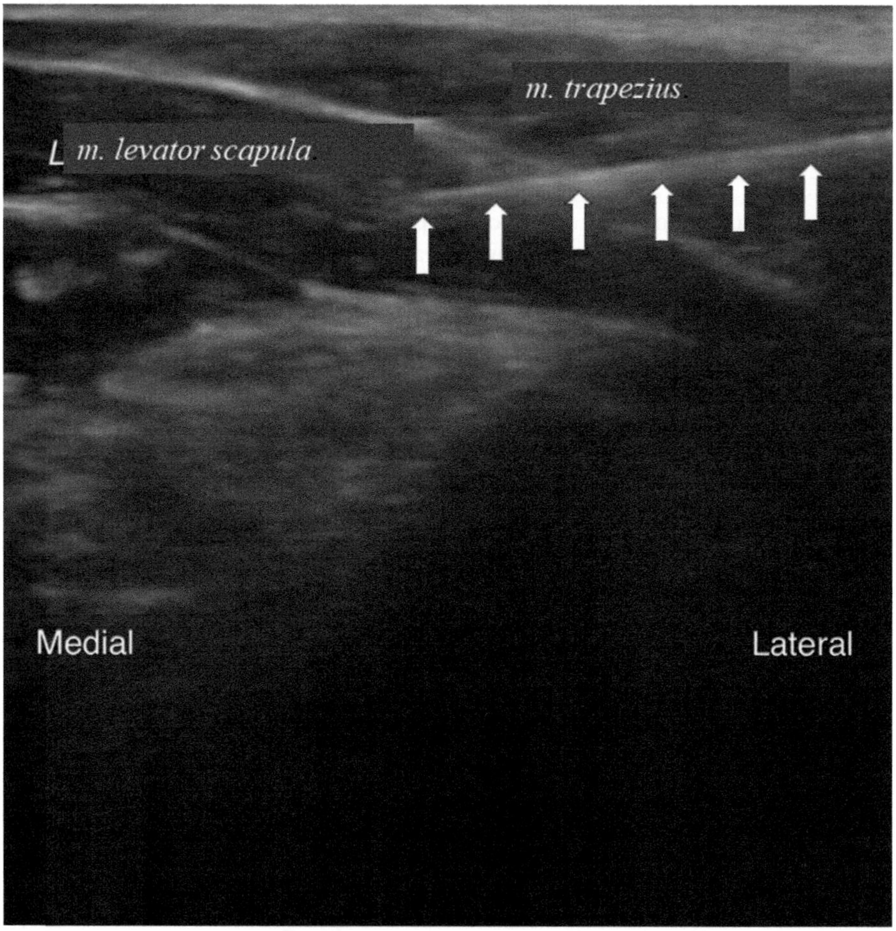

Fig. 5 Ultrasonogram of *m. levator scapula* injection. Example of *m. levator scapula* injection for the treatment of cervical dystonia using ultrasound guidance. White arrows point towards the needle shaft

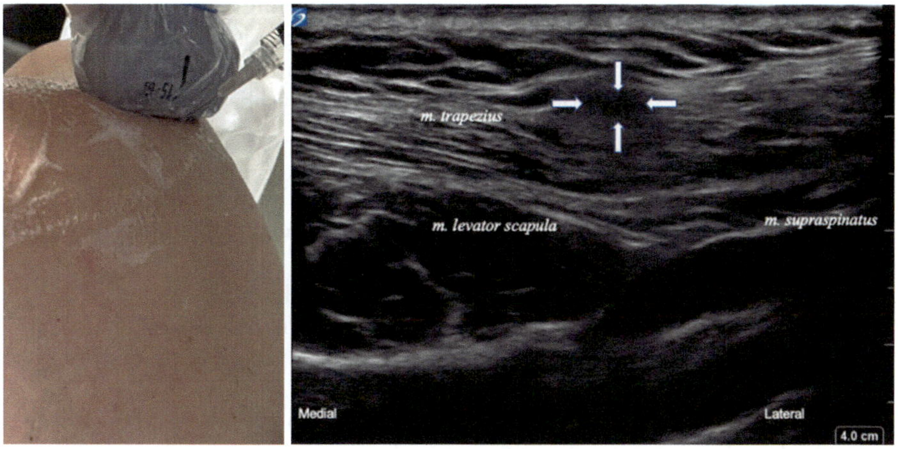

Fig. 6 Trapezius injections. Example of onabotulinumtoxinA injection into trapezius muscle for cervical dystonia. Please note the spread of the injectate in this muscle marked with white arrows. Ultrasound guidance helps precisely deposit the injectate, and also helps to avoid potential complications, including intravascular injections and pneumothorax. (Image - courtesy of Dmitri Souza, MD, PhD)

In the treatment of torticollis, you should be focusing on injection of the following muscles: ipsilaterally to torticollis (rotation), we should target splenius capitis (15–100 units), splenius services (20–60 units), levator scapula (20–100 units) and longissimus muscles (30–100 units). Contralateral to torticollis we should target sternocleidomastoid (15–100 units), trapezius (20–100 units) and scalenus anterior (20–30 units) muscles.

The following muscles are involved and should be targeted in the treatment of laterocollis: levator scapulae (20–100 units), upper trapezius muscle (20–100 units), scalenus anterior/medius/posterior complex (15–50 units), splenius capitis (15–100 units), and longissimus capitis and cervices (30–100 units). Anterocollis involves sternocleidomastoid muscle (15–100 units) and scalenus anterior/medius (15–50 units) bilaterally. And finally, retrocollis involves levator scapulae (20–100 units), upper trapezius muscle (20–100 units), longissimus capitis and longissimus services muscles (30–100 units), splenius capitis (15–100 units), splenius cervices (20–60 units), and semispinalis capitis muscles (30–100 units) bilaterally [11].

Potential Complications and Adverse Events

This procedure is generally well tolerated by patients. The adverse events that may occur include dysphagia (especially after sternocleidomastoid muscle injection), neck pain, headache, muscle weakness, injection site pain. Hypersensitivity reactions have been described when using onabotulinumtoxinA. This reaction included anaphylaxis, soft-tissue edema, serum sickness, and dyspnea. If any of these reactions occur, discontinue onabotulinumtoxinA injections and implement appropriate medical therapy. Extra care should be taken when treating individuals with preexisting neuromuscular disorders such as myasthenia gravis, amyotrophic lateral sclerosis, or Lambert-Eaton syndrome as they may be at increased risk of generalized muscle weakness, diplopia, proptosis, severe dysphagia, and respiratory compromise.

Clinical and Technical Pearls

Schedule a follow-up appointment for 2–6 weeks after each procedure to re-evaluate the patient's response to treatment and adverse events.

Adjust treatment protocol including dose and injected muscles as needed.

Start at a lower (yet therapeutic) dose and gradually increase dose/add new muscles to the injection protocol to reduce the risk of adverse events and improve efficacy.

Do not exceed 400 units of onabotulinumtoxinA (even if a patient is being treated for multiple indications) in a 3 months interval.

References

1. Lipton RB, Bigal ME, Diamond M, Freitag F, Reed ML, Stewart WF. Migraine prevalence, disease burden, and the need for preventive therapy. Neurology. 2007;68(5):343–9.
2. Vos T, Abajobir AA, Abbafati C, Abbas KM, Abate KH, Abd-Allah F, et al. Global, regional, and national incidence, prevalence, and years lived with disability for 328 diseases and injuries for 195 countries, 1990-2016: a systematic analysis for the global burden of disease study 2016. Lancet. 2017;390(10100):1211–59.
3. Defazio G, Jankovic J, Giel JL, Papapetropoulos S. Descriptive epidemiology of cervical dystonia. Tremor Other Hyperkinet Mov (N Y). 2013;3.
4. Charles PD, Adler CH, Stacy M, Comella C, Jankovic J, Manack Adams A, et al. Cervical dystonia and pain: characteristics and treatment patterns from CD PROBE (cervical dystonia patient registry for observation of onabotulinumtoxinA efficacy). J Neurol. 2014;261(7):1309–19.
5. Olesen J, Bes A, Kunkel R, Lance JW, Nappi G, Pfaffenrath V, et al. The international classification of headache disorders, 3rd edition (beta version). Cephalalgia. 2013;33(9):629–808.
6. Aurora SK, Dodick DW, Turkel CC, Degryse RE, Silberstein SD, Lipton RB, et al. OnabotulinumtoxinA for treatment of chronic migraine: results from the double-blind, randomized, placebo-controlled phase of the PREEMPT 1 trial. Cephalalgia. 2010;30(7):793–803.
7. Jankovic J, Leder S, Warner D, Schwartz K. Cervical dystonia. Neurology. 1991;41(7):1088–91.
8. Mathew NT, Frishberg BM, Gawel M, Dimitrova R, Gibson J, Turkel C, et al. Botulinum toxin type A (BOTOX®) for the prophylactic treatment of chronic daily headache: a randomized, double-blind, placebo-controlled trial. Headache. 2005;45(4):293–307.
9. Silberstein SD, Stark SR, Lucas SM, Christie SN, Degryse RE, Turkel CC. Botulinum toxin type a for the prophylactic treatment of chronic daily headache: a randomized, double-blind, placebo-controlled trial. Mayo Clin Proc. 2005;80(9):1126–37.
10. Standring S, Borley NR, Gray H. In: Standring S, editor. Gray's anatomy. 40th ed. Churchill Livingstone/Elsevier; 2008. 1551 p.
11. Stacy M. In: Stacy M, editor. Handbook of dystonia. CRC Press; 2012. 440 p.

Further Reading

Blumenfeld AM, Stark RJ, Freeman MC, Orejudos A, Manack AA. Long-term study of the efficacy and safety of OnabotulinumtoxinA for the prevention of chronic migraine: COMPEL study. J Headache Pain. 2018;19(1):13.

Rodrigues FB, Duarte GS, Marques RE, et al. Botulinum toxin type A therapy for cervical dystonia. Cochrane Database Syst Rev. 2020;11(11):CD003633.

Noninvasive Vagus Nerve Stimulation and Electrotherapy for Headaches

Alexander Feoktistov

Essential Concepts

- Transcutaneous supraorbital nerve stimulation, noninvasive vagus nerve stimulation, and remote electrical neuromodulation devices provide noninvasive and nonpharmacological therapeutic options for patients with migraine and cluster headaches.
- These noninvasive neuromodulation devices could be safely used in office, at the bedside, or at home by patients.
- These clinically proven and drug-free methods of pain management should be utilized as additional treatment options for patients with migraine and cluster headaches.

1 Noninvasive Vagus Nerve Stimulation and Electrotherapy for Headaches

Overview

There are multiple classes of preventative and acute medications that are available to our patients with migraine and cluster headaches. Yet, as many as two-thirds of patients with migraine headaches, who are candidates for prophylactic therapy do not use them [1]. It has also been estimated that over 70% of patients discontinue preventative medication after 6 months of therapy. The most common reasons for that are lack of efficacy and side effects [2]. Clinically, we also encountered situations when drug interactions represent may pose a major concern. There are also

A. Feoktistov (✉)
Synergy Integrative Headache Center, Northfield, IL, USA
e-mail: drfeoktistov@synergyheadache.com

D. Souza et al. (eds.), *Bedside Pain Management Interventions*,
https://doi.org/10.1007/978-3-031-11188-4_28

patients who prefer nonpharmacological treatment modalities. With recent technological advances, we now have noninvasive and nonpharmacological treatment modalities that could be helpful in these situations.

Indications and Contraindications

All patients with migraine or cluster headaches (both chronic and episodic forms) require effective and reliable acute/abortive therapeutic options. All noninvasive neuromodulation devices can be safely utilized in conjunction with more traditional pharmacological interventions. In general, we recommend use of neuromodulation devices in patients with contraindications to triptans and ergotamine-containing medications, in patients who experience side effects from their current acute or prophylactic therapy, or in those who are unsatisfied with therapeutic outcomes. Another group of patients that may benefit from nonpharmacological acute or prophylactic treatment options are patients with medication overuse headache or patients with an acute medication overuse who are at risk of developing medication overuse headache. Also considering the remarkable safety profile of these neuromodulation devices it is hard to find a patient who may not benefit from at least a trial of such therapeutic intervention. That being said, it is important to recognize that these devices have not been studied and therefore safety and efficacy have not been established in the pediatric population, adolescents or pregnant/nursing patients.

Clinical Anatomy

The vagus nerve (tenth cranial nerve) is the largest cranial nerve and it contains both afferent and efferent fibers. It enters the central nervous system via the trigeminal nuclear caudalis in the brainstem and proceeds further into the periaqueductal gray and raphe nucleus [3]. In the neck area, the vagus nerve travels within the sheath of the carotid artery and can be found at an average depth of 1.3–1.5 cm in the anterior cervical triangle (where we would normally palpate carotid pulse) [4]. Stimulation of the vagus nerve has been shown to reduce central excitability via the reduction of glutamate in the trigeminal nucleus caudalis, suppression of spontaneous neuronal firing in the trigeminal cervical complex, as well as suppression of cortical spreading depression susceptibility [5, 6].

The trigeminal nerve is the main sensory nerve in the head and face. Its anatomy has been well described. It appears that external trigeminal nerve stimulation reduces hypometabolism in the areas of the brain involved in central pain control (orbitofrontal and rostral anterior cingulate areas) [7].

Nonpainful remote electrical stimulation that is applied to the distant from the headache area (upper arm) has been shown to activate the descending antinociceptive pathway via the conditioned pain modulation effect [8].

Equipment and Supplies

All neuromodulation techniques described here are noninvasive and require no anesthesia or guidance. Noninvasive vagus nerve stimulation requires a hand-held stimulator marketed under the name GammaCore (Fig. 1). The GammaCore device, depending on the stimulation pattern, can be utilized as an acute therapeutic option for migraine treatment and/or as an acute or prophylactic option for cluster headache treatment.

An external trigeminal nerve stimulator, marketed under brand name Cefaly, can also be utilized as an acute or preventative migraine therapy. Currently, there is a single Cefaly device available that provides both acute and prophylactic stimulation.

Finally, the remote electrical stimulation device marketed under the brand name Nerivio is approved for acute treatment of migraine headaches and is controlled via smartphone app (Fig. 2).

Stimulation Technique and Protocol

When using noninvasive vagus nerve stimulation, the patient should be instructed to palpate the carotid pulse on the anterolateral area of the neck (which represents the correct treatment/stimulation location) at the earliest sign of pain. The patient should then apply a small amount of supplied gel to the stimulation surface of the device, turn the device on, and position it vertically along the pathway of the vagus nerve/carotid artery. Stimulation should be adjusted gradually by the patient until he/she experiences a slight pull or twitching at the corner of the lip. This muscular

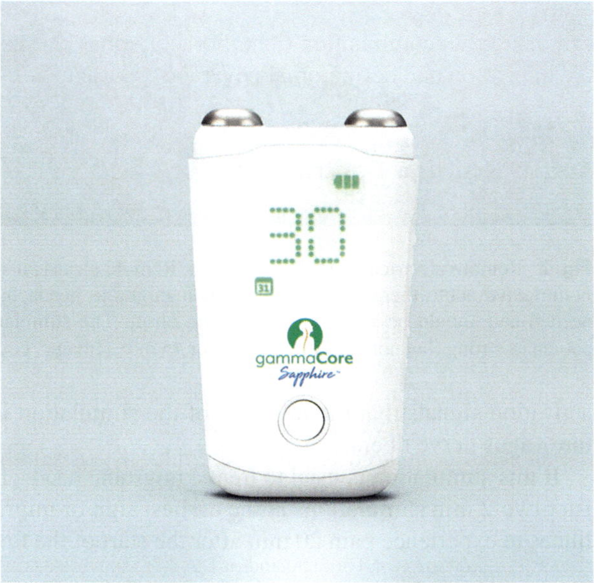

Fig. 1 Noninvasive vagus nerve stimulator. Noninvasive vagus nerve stimulation provides safe, effective and easy to use treatment of migraine headache. This particular treatment modality offers both acute and prophylactic stimulations. Image reprinted with permission from ElectroCure

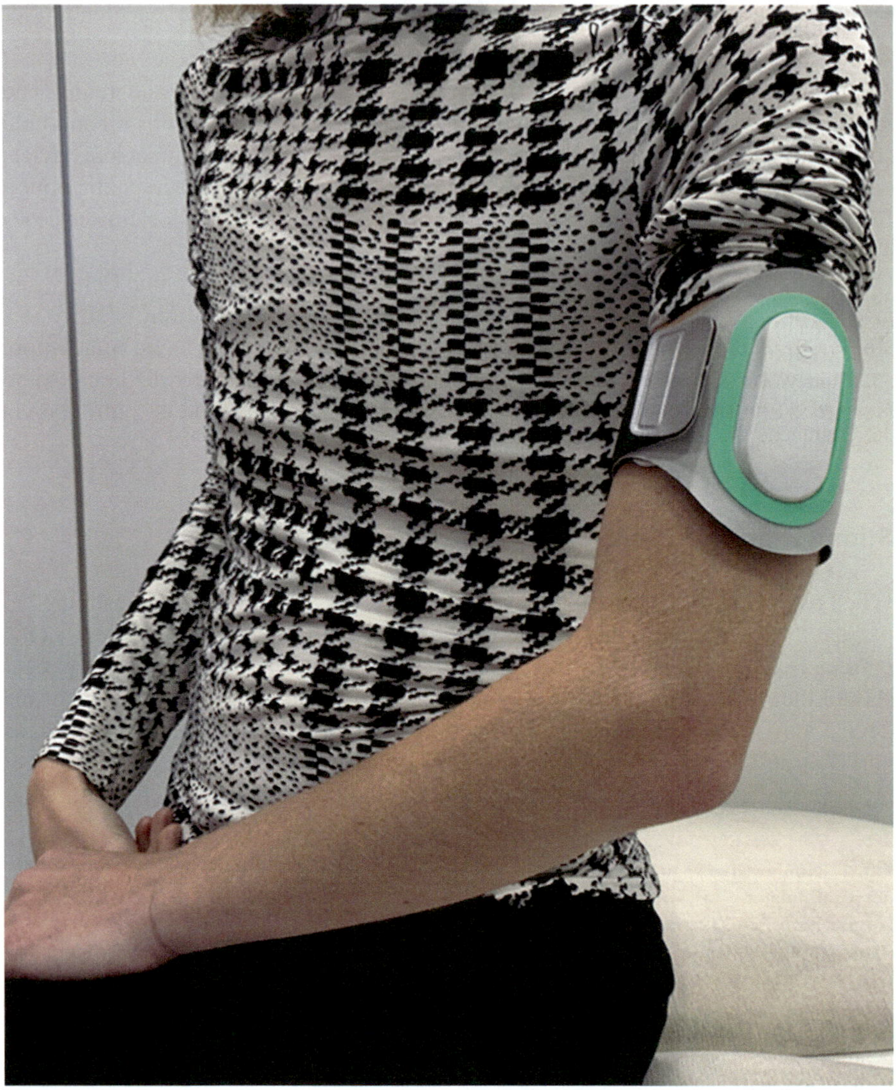

Fig. 2 Remote electrical stimulation device. Remote electrical stimulation device provides novel noninvasive acute therapy for patients with migraine headache. The stimulation is applied as needed and should be initiated at migraine onset. The stimulation should be perceived by the patient as strong (but not painful) and last for 45 min. (Image - courtesy of Dmitri Souza MD, PhD)

activation signals that the intensity of the stimulation is significant enough to capture vagus nerve fibers.

If this stimulation is used to treat a migraine headache the patient should administer two 2 min stimulations at the earliest sign of migraine pain. If the patient continues to experience pain 20 min after the start of the first treatment, the patient may administer 2 more stimulations. The patient may administer the third additional treatment (consisting of two 2 min stimulations) if pain persists 2 h after the start of treatment 1 [9].

If noninvasive vagus nerve stimulation is being used to acutely treat episodic cluster headache the patient should administer treatment consisting of three 2 min stimulations at the onset of the cluster headache attack. If pain persists, the patient may administer the second treatment (consisting of three 2 min stimulations) 3 min after completion of the first treatment. The patient may treat up to 4 attacks for a total of 24 stimulations per day [10–12].

For cluster headache prophylaxis the patient should administer the first treatment (consisting of three 2 min stimulations) within 1 h of waking. A second treatment should be administered at least 7–10 h after the first treatment.

When using external trigeminal nerve stimulation (Cefaly) as an acute treatment for migraine headache, patients should apply an adhesive electrode to the lower frontal area (between eyebrows) at the onset of a migraine attack. Next the patient should attach the stimulator to the electrode and activate the stimulator by pressing the button and administer 1-hour of high-frequency stimulation. If the stimulator is used prophylactically, the patient should apply the adhesive electrode and stimulator in a similar way and activate preventive stimulation consisting of a 20-minute low-frequency session.

When using a remote electrical stimulation device (Nerivio) advise patients to initiate stimulation within 60 min of migraine onset. The patient should apply the device to the upper arm and secure it with the supplied supporting armband. Using a smartphone app, the patient should gradually increase treatment intensity to the level that feels strong, yet not painful. Treatment should continue for 45 min [8].

Potential Complications and Adverse Events

Overall, all noninvasive neuromodulation treatment modalities have been found to be safe and well-tolerated. The most common device-related adverse events with noninvasive vagus nerve stimulation were application site erythema and discomfort and perioral myokymia during treatment.

The most common side effects noticed with external trigeminal nerve stimulations were intolerance to the paresthesia in the forehead, sensation of fatigue/sedation during and shortly after the treatment, and headache.

The most common adverse reactions related to remote electrical neuromodulation devices were muscle spasms, arm pain, a sensation of warmth and/or numbness at the application site, and redness.

Clinical and Technical Pearls

- When using noninvasive vagus nerve stimulation patients should apply the conductive gel before each stimulation.

- Noninvasive vagus nerve stimulation could be administered on the same side of the neck or the patient may switch sides if desired.
- Inform the patient of the risk of uncomfortable paresthesias in the distribution of the supraorbital and supratrochlear nerves during external trigeminal nerve stimulation.
- Advise patients that external trigeminal nerve stimulation should be applied daily for at least 2 months to achieve a consistent reduction in migraine frequency.
- Advise patients to initiate remote electrical neuromodulation treatment within 60 min from the migraine onset.

References

1. Lipton RB, Bigal ME, Diamond M, Freitag F, Reed ML, Stewart WF. Migraine prevalence, disease burden, and the need for preventive therapy. Neurology. 2007;68(5):343–9.
2. Hepp Z, Dodick DW, Varon SF, Gillard P, Hansen RN, Devine EB. Adherence to oral migraine-preventive medications among patients with chronic migraine. Cephalalgia. 2015;35(6):478–88.
3. Yuan H, Silberstein SD. Vagus nerve and vagus nerve stimulation, a comprehensive review: part i. Headache. 2016;56(1):71–8.
4. Frangos E, Komisaruk BR. Access to vagal projections via cutaneous electrical stimulation of the neck: fMRI evidence in healthy humans. Brain Stimul. 2017;10(1):19–27. https://doi.org/10.1016/j.brs.2016.10.008.
5. Akerman S, Simon B, Romero-Reyes M. Vagus nerve stimulation suppresses acute noxious activation of trigeminocervical neurons in animal models of primary headache. Neurobiol Dis. 2017;102:96–104. https://doi.org/10.1016/j.nbd.2017.03.004.
6. Nonis R, D'Ostilio K, Schoenen J, Magis D. Evidence of activation of vagal afferents by non-invasive vagus nerve stimulation: an electrophysiological study in healthy volunteers. Cephalalgia. 2017;37(13):1285–93.
7. Magis D, D'Ostilio K, Thibaut A, De Pasqua V, Gerard P, Hustinx R, et al. Cerebral metabolism before and after external trigeminal nerve stimulation in episodic migraine. Cephalalgia. 2017;37(9):881–91.
8. Yarnitsky D, Dodick DW, Grosberg BM, Burstein R, Ironi A, Harris D, et al. Remote electrical neuromodulation (REN) relieves acute migraine: a randomized, double-blind, placebo-controlled, multicenter trial. Headache. 2019;59(8):1240–52. https://doi.org/10.1111/head.13551.
9. Yarnitsky D, Volokh L, Ironi A, Weller B, Shor M, Shifrin A, et al. Nonpainful remote electrical stimulation alleviates episodic migraine pain. Neurology. 2017;88(13):1250–5. https://doi.org/10.1212/WNL.0000000000003760.
10. Silberstein SD, Mechtler LL, Kudrow DB, Calhoun AH, McClure C, Saper JR, et al. Non–invasive vagus nerve stimulation for the ACute treatment of cluster headache: findings from the randomized, double-blind, sham-controlled ACT1 Study. Headache. 2016;56(8):1317–32.
11. De Coo IF, Marin J, Silberstein SD, Friedman DI, Gaul C, Tyagi A, et al. Non-invasive vagus nerve stimulation for acute treatment of episodic and chronic cluster headache: pooled analysis of data from two randomized, double-blind, sham-controlled clinical trials. Cephalalgia. Conference: 18th congress of the international headache society, IHC 2017. Canada, 2017;37(1 Supplement 1):175–176. https://www.cochranelibrary.com/central/doi/10.1002/central/CN-01470041/full
12. Goadsby PJ, de Coo IF, Silver N, Tyagi A, Ahmed F, Gaul C, et al. Non-invasive vagus nerve stimulation for the acute treatment of episodic and chronic cluster headache: a randomized, double-blind, sham-controlled ACT2 study. Cephalalgia. 2018;38(5):959–69.

Further Reading

Diener HC, Goadsby PJ, Ashina M, et al. Non-invasive vagus nerve stimulation (nVNS) for the preventive treatment of episodic migraine: the multicentre, double-blind, randomised, sham-controlled PREMIUM trial. Cephalalgia. 2019;39(12):1475–87.

Evers S. Non-invasive neurostimulation methods for acute and preventive migraine treatment-A narrative review. J Clin Med. 2021;10(15):3302.

Superficial Cervical Plexus Nerve Block

Awnik K. Sarkar, Colleen McKenna O'Connor, and Robert B. Goldstein

Essential Concepts

- Superficial cervical plexus block is a simple and relatively safe technique to treat chronic cervicalgia, atypical cervicogenic headaches, post herpetic neuralgia, and persistent postoperative neck pain.
- Deep cervical plexus blocks have had a key role historically in perioperative analgesic and anesthetic techniques but due to the risk of inadvertant epidural, intrathecal, and vertebral artery injection, as well as Local Anesthetic Systemic Toxicity (LAST), it has fallen out of favor. SCPB is often as sufficient for lateral neck analgesia or anesthesia.
- Adverse effects of cervical plexus block include phrenic nerve palsy, Horner's Syndrome, voice hoarseness, and LAST.
- Pain relief can last anywhere from several hours to several months depending on the medication used, correct needle placement, and specific patient conditions.

A. K. Sarkar (✉)
University of Virginia, Charlottesville, VA, USA

C. M. O'Connor
Department of Anesthesiology and Perioperative Medicine, Tufts Medical Center, Boston, MA, USA

R. B. Goldstein
Anesthesiology, University of Virginia, Charlottesville, VA, USA
e-mail: RBG7A@hscmail.mcc.virginia.edu

D. Souza et al. (eds.), *Bedside Pain Management Interventions*,
https://doi.org/10.1007/978-3-031-11188-4_29

1 Superficial Cervical Plexus Block

Overview

The cervical plexus contributes to both sensory and motor innervation; most notably it gives rise to the phrenic nerve and provides sensory innervation to the lateral neck, ear, and upper chest [1]. Cervical plexus nerve blocks are a relatively easy and safe procedure that can be performed at the bedside to help with a variety of conditions. The two subtypes of cervical plexus blocks can be categorized into superficial and deep. Deep Cervical plexus block is not indicated typically for chronic pain management due to the risk of severe side effects outweighing the benefit. Superficial cervical block is more common for treatment of chronic pain. These blocks can be diagnostic or therapeutic and can have benefit for as much as 10–77 days [2].

Indications and Contraindications

Since the cervical plexus provides sensory innervation to a large area, there are several indications for cervical plexus blocks.

These indications include:

- Cervicogenic headaches.
- Cervicothoracic myofascial pain syndrome.
- Post Herpetic Neuralgia [3].
- Post-operative or post-radiation pain in cervical region [4].
- Referred Somatic Pain from Cervical Spine.
- Atypical face pain.
- Pain around the ear.

Contraindications to cervical plexus block include allergy or intolerance to injectate, including local anesthetics or steroids, patient refusal, and systemic or local infection. Relative contraindications include poor pulmonary status, anatomic distortion. Coagulopathy, including iatrogenic, and platelet dysfunction, including iatrogenic, are not contraindications for the ultrasound-guided superficial cervical plexus block. However, risks and benefits should be weighted, and thoroughly discussed with the patient (Table 1).

Clinical Anatomy

The anterior rami of C1-C4 coalesce together to make up the cervical plexus. This consortium of neural tissue lies anterior to the scalenus medius and levator scapulae muscles and deep to the sternocleidomastoid (SCM). Innervation may be compared from deep to superficial branch coverage. Deep branches innervate the SCM, trapezius, levator scapulae, scalenus medius, and also connect with CN XI(Spinal

Table 1 Cervical plexus nerve blocks

Procedure	Indications	Techniques	Contraindications
Superficial cervical plexus nerve block	Cervicogenic headaches Cervicothoracic myofascial pain syndrome Postherpetic neuralgia Post-operative or post-radiation pain in the cervical region (Valls) [4] Somatic referred cervical spine pain	Landmark technique Ultrasound-guided	*Absolute*: Patient refusal Systemic/site infection Allergy to local anesthetic *Relative*: Poor pulmonary status Anatomic distortion
Deep cervical plexus nerve block	Perioperative analgesia or anesthesia for neck procedures (CEA, neck dissection, thyroid surgery, etc.)	Landmark technique Ultrasound-guided	*Absolute*: Patient refusal Systemic/site infection Coagulopathy Allergy to local anesthetic *Relative*: Poor pulmonary status Anatomic distortion TP fracture

Accessory Nerve). The superficial branches innervate cutaneous structures over the lateral cranium and neck with contribution from anterior cutaneous, occipital, supraclavicular, and greater auricular nerves (Fig. 1) [5].

Equipment and Supplies

Both deep and superficial nerve blocks are easily performed at bedside. Supplies needed depend on indication and goal for the block. The most common local anesthetics used for the blocks are ropivacaine and bupivacaine. Different supplies are needed for superficial and deep blocks (Table 2).

Cervical Plexus Block, Landmark Technique

Approach can be anterior, lateral, or posterior; most common is anterolateral. Patient is positioned in Supine or Back up position at 30–45 degrees.

- Deep block: 3 separate injections at level of transverse process of C2–4, can use bony landmarks or ultrasound guidance. Due to the risk:benefit ratio being low, this procedure is not reasonably indicated for bedside chronic pain management. As such will not discuss procedure specifics in depth.

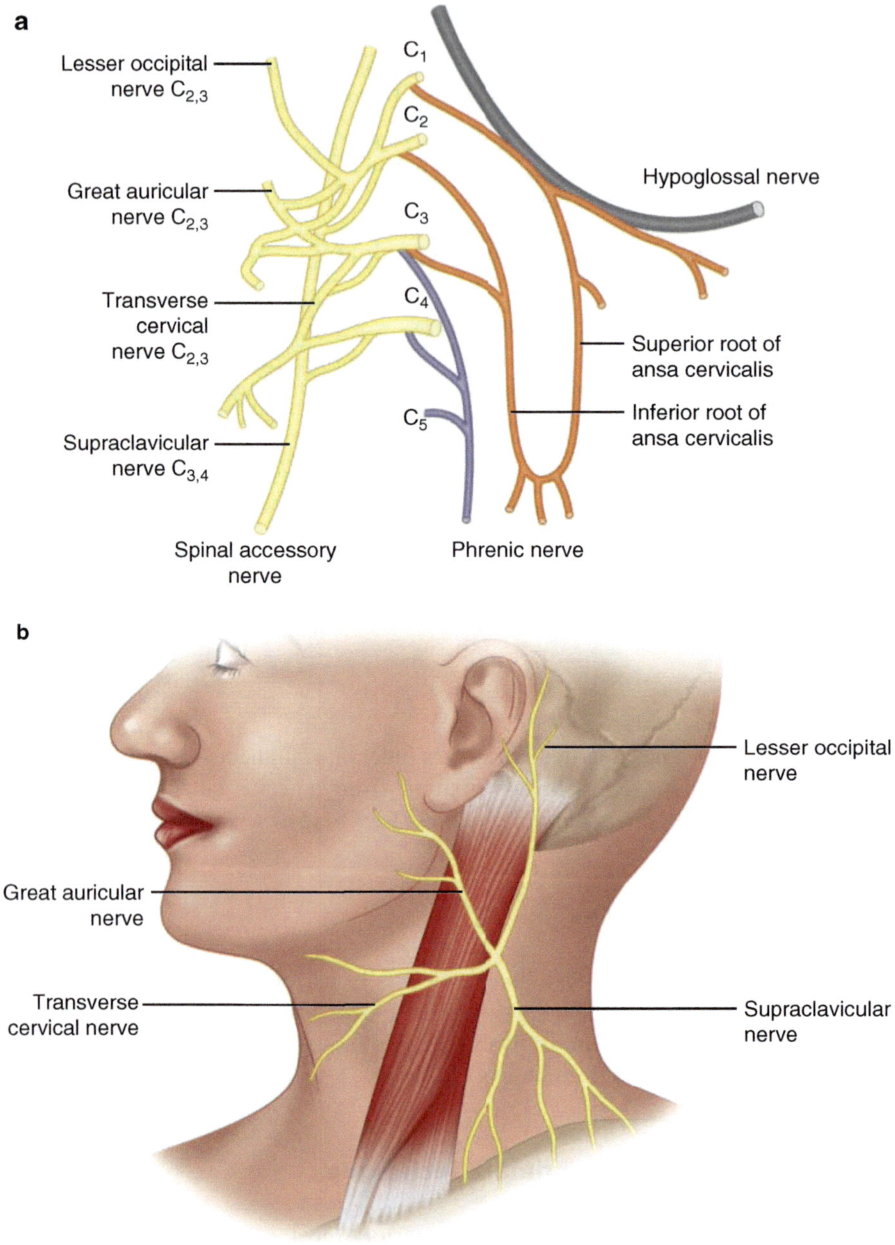

Fig. 1 Cervical plexus anatomy, as labeled. (**a**) Yellow depicts cervical nerve roots forming superficial cervical plexus. Orange lines illustrate cervical nerve roots forming deep cervical plexus. (**b**) Peripheral nerves (marked yellow) which comprise superficial cervical plexus

Table 2 Required supplies for cervical plexus nerve blocks

Syringe	5 or 10 ml
Needle	25, 27, 30 gauge; ½–1 in for superficial; 22 gauge, 3.5 inch spinal needle for deep
Anesthetic	0.125% ropivacaine, 0.25% bupivacaine 1–2% lidocaine
Corticosteroid choices for adjuncts	Triamcinolone –10–20 mg (t1/2 life: 18–36 h) Methylprednisolone 40–80 mg (t1/2 life: 18–36 h) Dexamethasone 2–4 mg (t1/2 life: 36–54 h)

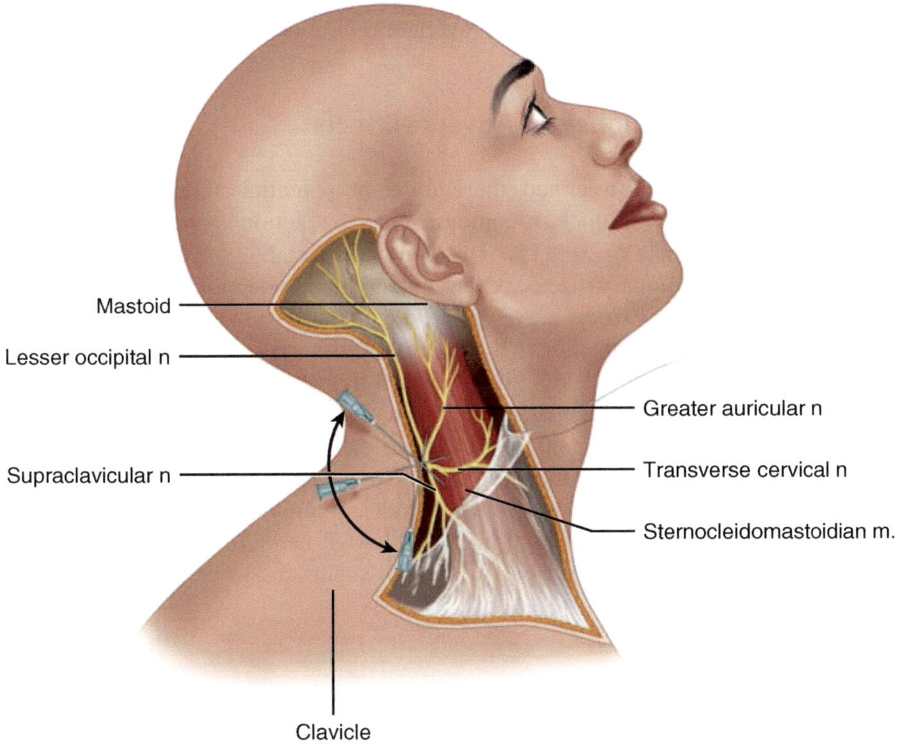

Fig. 2 Needle trajectory shown at the insertion site of mid-body of the sternocleidomastoid muscle for superficial cervical plexus block

- Superficial block: performed at midpoint between mastoid process and sternal notch at the posterior edge of SCM. The needle is placed at 45 degrees to the skin at the midpoint of the posterior border of the SCM pointed towards the midline (trachea). The needle is inserted 0.5–1.0 cm. Medication is administered at this point. The needle is retracted to the dermis and the needle is angled 30 degrees caudally from neutral position and inserted 0.5–1 cm and again medication is deposited here. The needle is finally retracted to the dermis and angled 30 degrees cranially from neutral and advanced 0.5-1 cm and medication is deposited here (Fig. 2).

Ultrasound Technique

Linear transducer positioned transversely over mid-body of the SCMs Posterior Border. Patient positioned in supine position back up at 30–45 degrees with head turned to the contralateral side of the procedure. Superficial Cervical Plexus might be seen deep or lateral to the posterior border of the SCM as hyperechoic nodules, although this is not always visualized. The goal is to place the needle tip deep to SCM next to the cervical plexus and deposit medication here. If superficial plexus cervical plexus is not seen on ultrasound imaging then medication may be deposited slightly deep to the lateral border of the SCM and superficial to the deep cervical fascia which is located superficial to prevertebral fascia (Figs. 3 and 4).

Potential Complications and Adverse Effects

Although generally well tolerated, there are some potential complications associated with cervical plexus block. A common adverse reaction is phrenic nerve palsy which has an incidence of 61% [5]. This can be especially concerning in patients with underlying pulmonary disease. Other potential complications include Horner's Syndrome, spinal accessory nerve palsy, hematoma formation, infection, and adverse reactions to medications. If corticosteroids are used, there is a risk for adverse cosmetic effects including hair loss and hyperpigmentation and associated metabolic disturbances of exogenous corticosteroid administration. Caution should be used in patients with prior surgical incisions as anatomy may be distorted. Rare but severe adverse events are most typically associated with Deep Cervical Plexus block and not SCPB. These severe events include epidural/intrathecal injection, brachial plexus block, vertebral arterial injection, LAST, nerve root injury, and paralysis. Due to risk of phrenic nerve palsy, bilateral superficial or deep cervical plexus block is not advised.

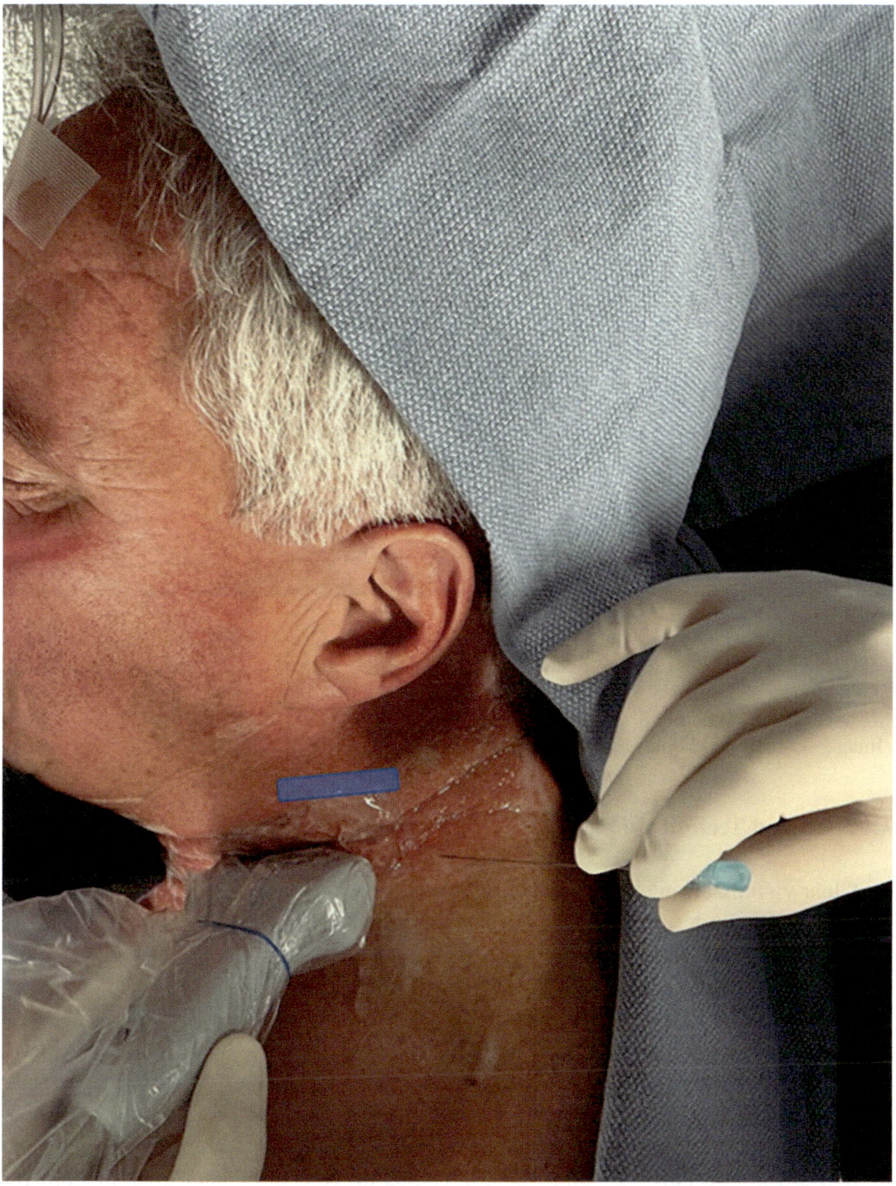

Fig. 3 Superficial cervical plexus block, ultrasound probe orientation. An ultrasound probe should be placed on the mid-body of the sternocleidomastoid muscle. (Image—courtesy of Dmitri Souza MD, PhD)

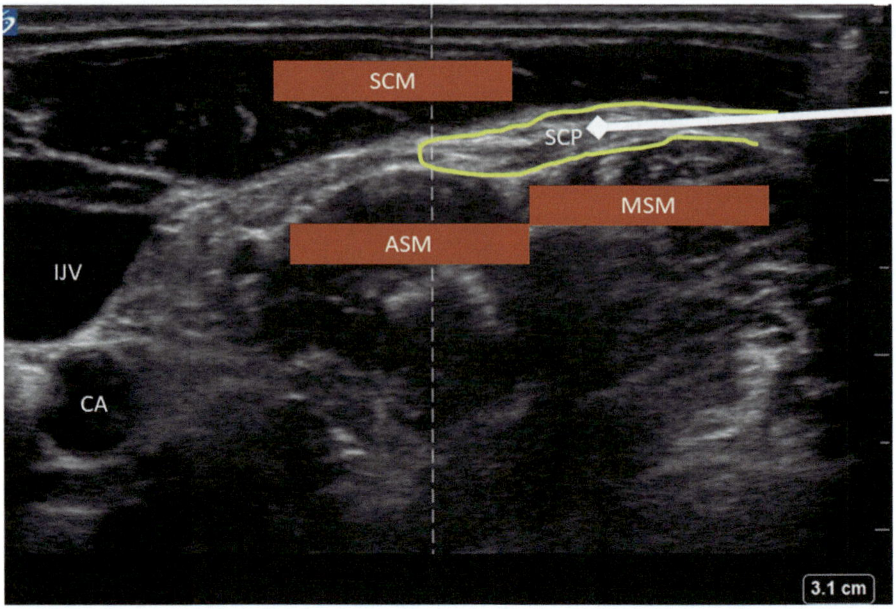

Fig. 4 A needle trajectory (white uninterrupted line) outlined from lateral to medial approach. The yellow area demarcates the superficial cervical plexus and the area of final medication deposition. SCP—Superficial Cervical Plexus. SCM—Sternocleidomastoid muscle. ASM—Anterior Scalene Muscle. MSM—Middle Scalene Muscle. CA—Carotid Artery. IJV—Internal Jugular Vein. (Image—courtesy of Dmitri Souza MD, PhD)

Clinical and Technical Pearls

- Clear visualization under ultrasound is not necessary as SCP is not always clearly discernible under SCM [6].
- Reliable anesthesia may be achieved in the distribution of the Superficial Cervical Plexus with deposition of 10 cc of local anesthetic deep to superficial fascial layer of SCM [6].
- The ease at which the procedure may be completed by even novice operators either via anatomical based or US guided technique, makes this an effective and efficient method of Pain Management at the bedside.
- Deep Cervical Plexus block has fallen out of favor for perioperative analgesic and anesthetic purposes and essentially has no role in bedside intervention for chronic pain management due to risk of neuraxial injection, vertebral artery injection, and LAST.

References

1. Thawale R, Alva S, Niraj G. Ultrasound-guided intermediate cervical plexus block with depot steroids in the management of refractory neck pain secondary to cervicothoracic myofascial pain syndrome. A A Pract. 2019;13(12):446–9.

2. Goldberg M, Schwartzman R, Domsky R, Sabia M, Torjman M. Deep cervical plexus block for the treatment of Cervicogenic headache. Pain Physician. 2008;11:849–54.
3. Shin HY, Kim DS, Kim SS. Superficial cervical plexus block for management of herpes zoster neuralgia in the C3 dermatome: a case report. J Med Case Rep. 2014;8:59.
4. Valls JMO, Soto E, Martínez MF, Nebreda C, Tornero CT. Cervical plexus as anatomical target for the treatment of postoperative cervical neuropathic pain. J Pain Res. 2019;12:1217–21.
5. Kim J-S, Ko JS, Bang S, Kim H, Lee SY. Cervical plexus block. Korean J Anesthesiol. 2018;71:274–88.
6. Cervical plexus block. www.NYSORA.com Assessed 12 Mar 2022.

Further Reading

Opperer M, Kaufmann R, Meissnitzer M, Enzmann FK, Dinges C, Hitzl W, Nawratil J, Koköfer A. Depth of cervical plexus block and phrenic nerve blockade: a randomized trial. Reg Anesth Pain Med. 2022;47(4):205–11. https://doi.org/10.1136/rapm-2021-102851.

Cervical Medial Branch Block

Jacob R. Caylor, Sopyda Yin, and Imanuel R. Lerman

Essential Concepts

- Facet joint pain is responsible for the majority of chronic axial neck pain.
- Cervical Medial Branch blocks (MBB) are an effective diagnostic and therapeutic tool in treating chronic facet-mediated neck pain.
- The mechanism of action is a result of blockade of nociceptive afferent fibers in the medial branches supplying the zygapophyseal joints
- The duration of therapeutic benefit with neurotomy may last weeks to months.

1 Ultrasound-Guided Cervical Medial Branch Block

Overview

Particularly prevalent amongst women, cervicogenic headache and chronic axial neck pain are morbid conditions potentially sharing a common nociceptive etiology: the cervical zygapophyseal or facet joints [1]. In patients with chronic neck pain unresponsive to conservative therapy, diagnostic medial branch block (MBB) or intraarticular injection of local anesthetic may offer temporary relief, indicative of facet-mediated nociceptive origin. Responding patients may then undergo therapeutic radiofrequency neurotomy of the medial branches supplying the joint for

J. R. Caylor
Northwest Pain Care, Spokane, WA, USA

S. Yin · I. R. Lerman (✉)
Department of Anesthesiology, University of California San Diego, La Jolla, CA, USA
e-mail: ilerman@health.ucsd.edu

D. Souza et al. (eds.), *Bedside Pain Management Interventions*,
https://doi.org/10.1007/978-3-031-11188-4_30

more sustained benefit. Notably, the prevalence of facet joint pain origin is 36–67% in patients with axial neck pain, 70% in cervicogenic headache and 30–60% in trauma-related chronic neck pain [2–4]. Moreover, as a single diagnostic cervical MBB has a false positive rate of up to 38%, a second confirmatory block is often performed prior to therapeutic intervention [5]. While historically these procedures were done under fluoroscopy, the advantages of ultrasound-guided diagnostic cervical MBB has recently become clear due to real-time visualization, decreased procedure time and improved safety profile [6]

Indications and Contraindications

Chronic neck pain can be categorized as radicular or axial, and has multiple etiologies originating from either the anterior or posterior spinal structures, in addition to the paraspinous musculature. As diarthrodial synovial joints, the facet or zygapophyseal joints are susceptible to a similar degenerative process seen in larger joints, including osteophyte formation, osteosclerosis and degeneration of the synovial components [7]. Both the fibrous joint capsule and synovial joint are known to be independent pain generators [8]. Critically interdependent with the intervertebral disc in sharing the axial load and maintaining cervical stability, facet joint osteoarthritis is largely seen in concert with anterior disc degeneration and may represent disease progression [9]. Though inciting injuries such as trauma or whiplash may play a role in the pathogenesis of facet-mediated pain, independent risk factors for facet osteoarthritis remain to be elucidated [7]. Largely a diagnosis of exclusion, facet joint mediated pain is highly prevalent, and workup is based on ruling out serious pathology including disc disease, spinal stenosis and occult fracture. In patients with normal cervical spine imaging, axial pain and point tenderness, it is reasonable to recommend diagnostic MBB to rule in/out pain contribution from facet joints. Moreover, it is also appropriate to consider MBB and third occipital nerve block in patients who fit diagnostic criteria for cervicogenic headache (Table 1) [10]. Therapeutic MBB using radiofrequency neurotomy is indicated in patients who have

Table 1 ICHD-3 diagnostic criteria for cervicogenic headache [10]

A. Any headache fulfilling criterion C
B. Clinical and/or imaging evidence of a disorder or lesion within the cervical spine or soft tissues of the neck, known to be able to cause headache
C. Evidence of causation demonstrated by at least two of the following: 1. Headache has developed in temporal relation to the onset of the cervical disorder or appearance of the lesion 2. Headache has significantly improved or resolved in parallel with improvement in or resolution of the cervical disorder or lesion 3. Cervical range of motion is reduced and headache is made significantly worse by provocative maneuvers 4. Headache is abolished following diagnostic blockade of a cervical structure or its nerve supply
D. Not better accounted for by another ICHD-3 diagnosis

responded positively to diagnostic blocks and in those who experienced prior benefit with therapeutic MBB previously. Radiofrequency neurotomy for patients with cervical facet joint pain may have extended benefit these pain syndromes are unlikely to recover with conservative therapies [11]. While medial branch blocks or facet joint injections can be performed with ultrasound guidance at the bedside, radiofrequency ablation procedures are conventionally performed with fluoroscopy.

Common contraindications to medial branch blocks and facet joint injections include infection at the planned injection site, pathological or iatrogenic coagulopathy, patient being on antiplatelet therapy, severe systemic disease, and patient refusal.

Clinical Anatomy

Critical to mechanical stability and movement, the zygapophyseal or facet joints in addition to the vertebral bodies comprise the load-bearing structures of the cervical spine and are susceptible to pathology including degenerative osteoarthritis and traumatic injury [7]. Bounded by a lubricating synovium and a fibro-ligamentous capsule, the facet joints are formed by the articulation of superior and inferior processes from the vertebrae and are known pain generators (Fig. 1). progressing caudad from C2, the angle of articulation in these diarthrodial joints starts relatively horizontal and becomes more vertically and posterolaterally oriented [12, 13].

Innervation to the facet joints is provided by the terminal articular branches of the cervical dorsal rami. As the dorsal rami course posteriorly over the root of the transverse process, they give off the medial and lateral branches. In general, the medial branches wrap around the waist of the articular pillars and give off articular branches supplying the facet joint above and below the spinal level (Fig. 1) [14, 15]. In as much, each facet joint receives dual innervation: articular branches above and below the joint both contribute sensory information and thus must be targeted during interventions. As a common target for interventional procedures regarding facetogenic pain, medial branches exhibit course variability for C3, C6 and C7 [14, 15] and redundant branches in C4, C5 and C6 [16]. Notably, the medial branch of C7 courses dorsally near the peak of the C7 articular pillar. While the C3-C6 medial branches have a similar course, the C2–3 facet joint has unique anatomy and innervation. For example, though the C3–4 joint receives its cephalad innervation from the deep medial branch of C3, the C2–3 facet joint is innervated by articular branches of the third occipital nerve (TON) (Fig. 1). The superficial medial branch of C3, the TON is larger in caliber and gives off articular branches as it courses across the facet joint [14, 15]. Understanding the variability in medial branch anatomy is key to providing reliable diagnostic and therapeutic interventions.

Equipment and Supplies

The necessary materials for cervical MBB include skin disinfectant solution, a syringe with needle, local anesthetic and a high frequency ultrasound probe. While

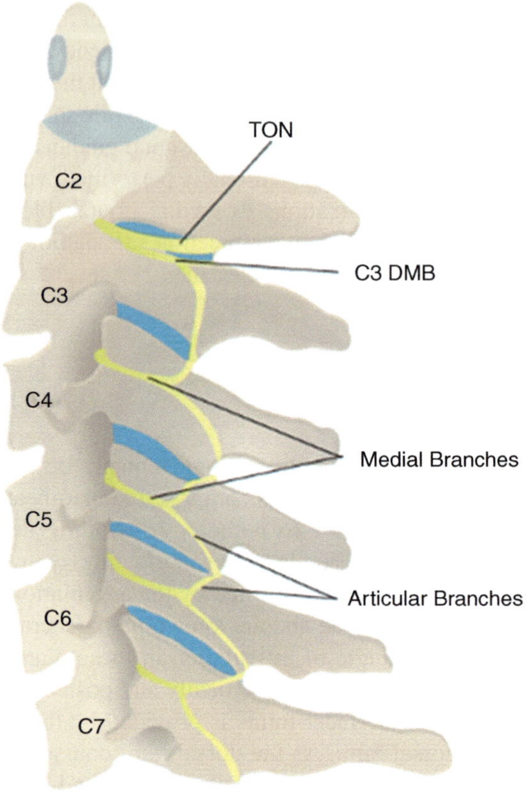

Fig. 1 Lateral view of the cervical spine demonstrating innervation of the facet joints. The third occipital nerve (TON) and C3 deep medial branch (DMB) course posteriorly over the C2/3 facet joint. While the courses of the TON, C4 and C5 medial branches are conserved, C3 DMB, C6 and C7 medial branches exhibit marked course variability

Table 2 Required supplies for cervical medial branch blocks

Syringe	3 or 5 ml
Needle	25, 27, 30 gauge ½–1 in.
Anesthetic	0.25–0.5% bupivacaine 1–2% lidocaine Lidocaine/bupivacaine combination: 1:1–1:3 ratio
Ultrasound	12–4 mHz high frequency linear transducer Sterile ultrasound gel and probe cover
Other	Sterile gloves and skin disinfectant

other supplies are routinely used in pain procedures, an ultrasonography machine capable of color flow doppler in addition to a high frequency probe is required in order to adequately visualize relevant blood vessels, nerves and osseous landmarks (Table 2).

Cervical Medial Branch Block, Long Axis (Coronal) Technique

The long axis technique is primarily used for blocking the medial branches supplying C2–6 facet joints. With the patient in the lateral decubitus position and head

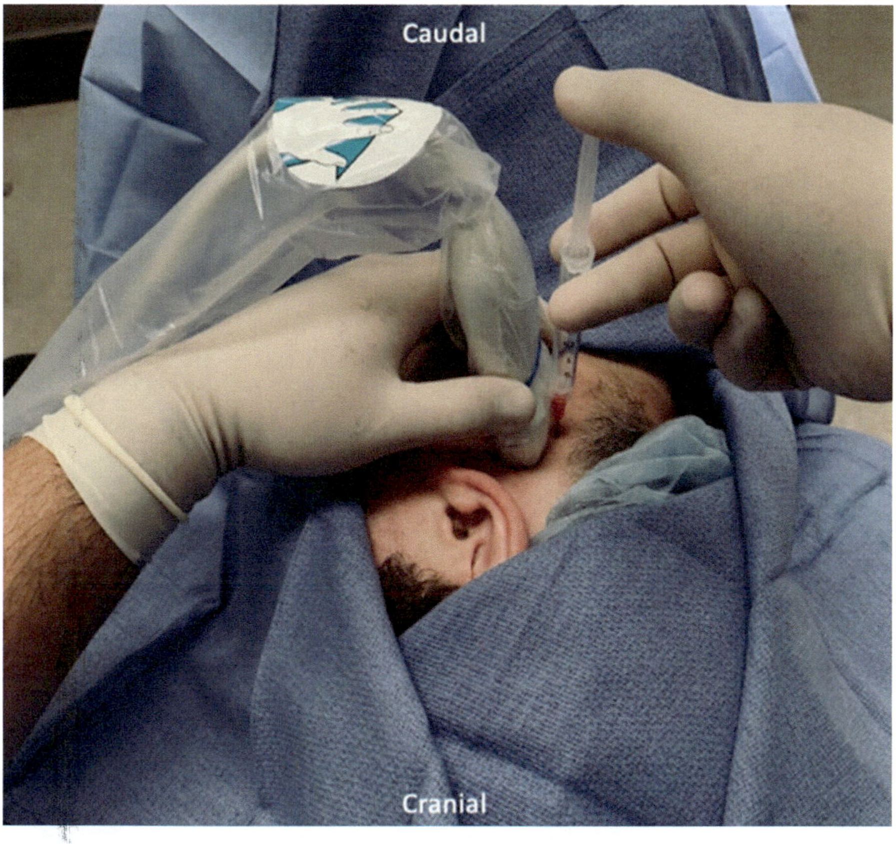

Fig. 2 Patient positioning for ultrasound-guided medial branch block with the probe in the long-axis plane. The patient is placed in the left lateral decubitus position, with the head supported neutrally. After scout images are obtained, the patient is then prepped and draped in the usual sterile fashion

supported neutrally, the neck is prepped and draped in the usual sterile fashion (Fig. 2). The ultrasound probe is oriented coronally over the neck, identifying the mastoid bone cranially and transverse process of C1 caudally. Slight rotation or angulation of the probe should bring the image into view (Fig. 3). The probe is then shifted caudad until the transverse process of C2 comes into view. The vertebral artery can now be identified as a pulsing hypoechoic structure, which can be confirmed with color flow doppler (Fig. 4). Centered over the TP of C2, the probe is then shifted dorsally and translated slightly caudad until the C2–3 facet joint is located (Fig. 5). At this point the TON can be viewed as it crosses the C2–3 facet joint, demarcated as a beaded hyperechoic structure with thin hypoechoic rim. The TON can be blocked at this level using an in-plane approach, or the transducer can be further translated caudad to identify the C3 deep medial branch, taking care to note the anatomy, orientation and identify vessels in the case of uncertainty using color doppler ultrasonography (Fig. 6). The probe is then translated caudad in the coronal plane and shifted dorsally until the articular pillars and associated medial

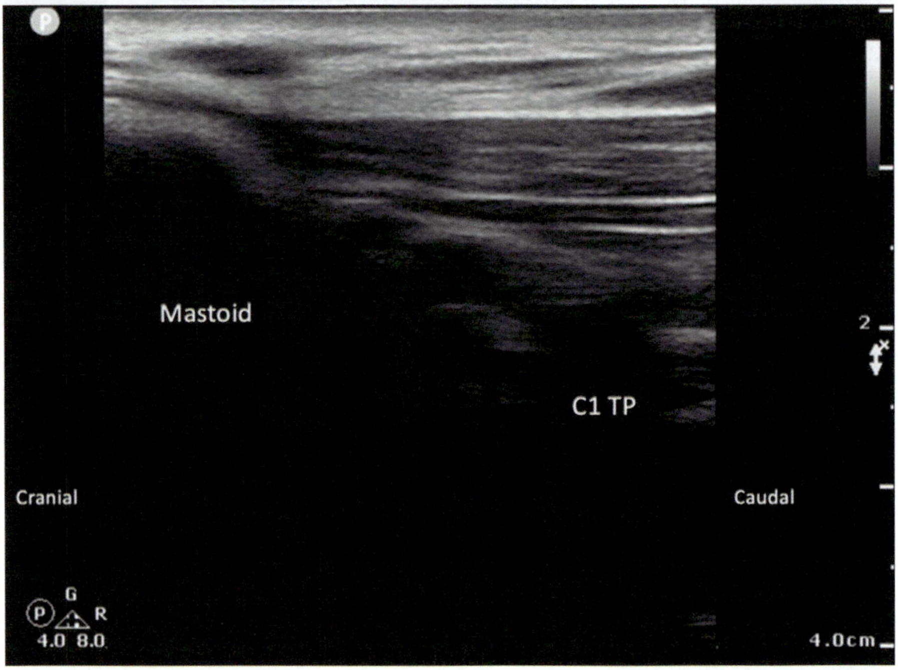

Fig. 3 Ultrasound coronal view of the mastoid process and transverse process of C1 (C1 TP)

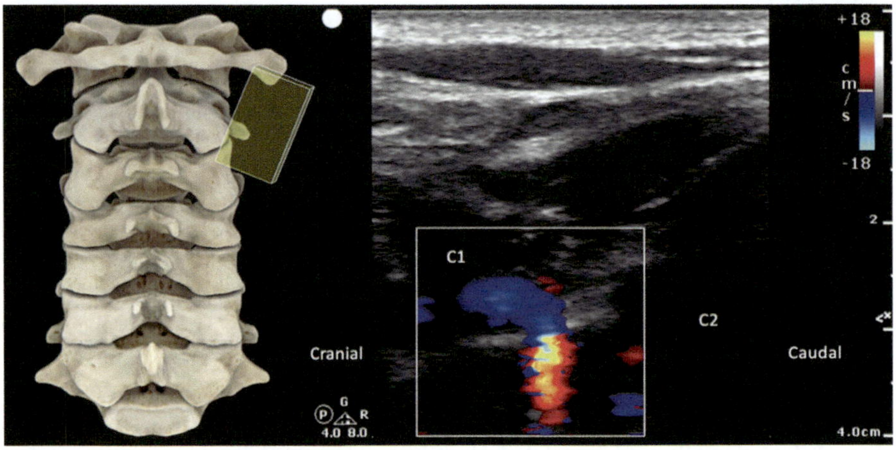

Fig. 4 Ultrasound coronal view with color flow doppler demonstrating the vertebral artery arising from the transverse foramen of C2 and entering the transverse foramen of C1

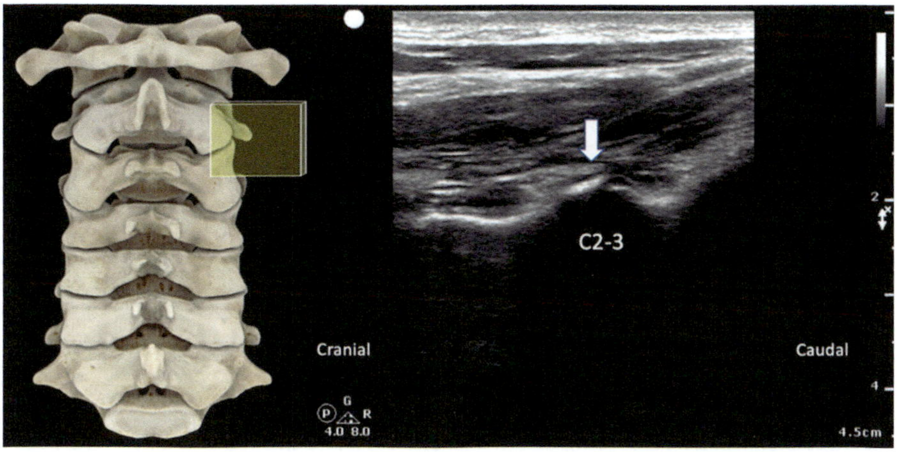

Fig. 5 Ultrasound coronal view of the C2–3 facet joint with the third occipital nerve noted by the block arrow

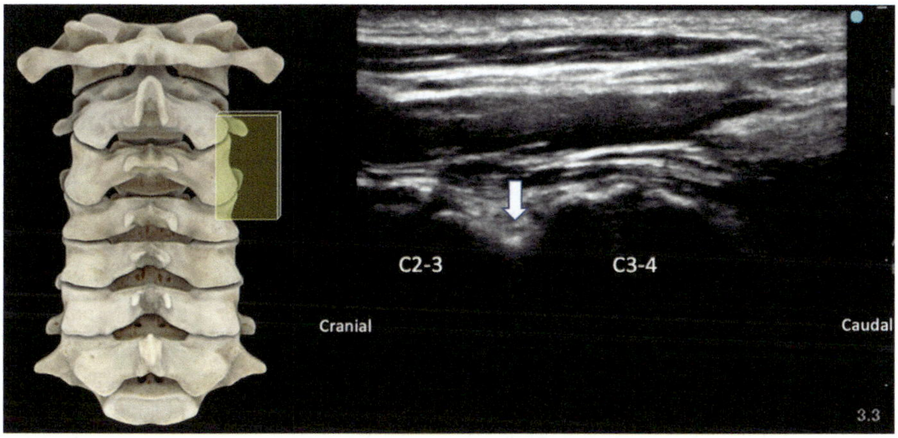

Fig. 6 Ultrasound coronal view of the C2–3 and C3–4 facet joint with the C3 deep medial branch denoted by the block arrow

branch nerves come into view (Fig. 7). As the probe is translated caudad, keeping the facet joints in view, an alteration in trajectory following the cervical lordosis is likely necessary to keep the facet joints in view. Further translation in the longitudinal plane will reveal the medial branches of C4 at the waist of the articular pillar and the C3–4 facet joint (Fig. 7). Particularly inflamed nerves may appear larger than non-affected nerves by ultrasound. Ultrasound-guided C7 medial branch block is difficult in the longitudinal technique; therefore, the transverse technique is described in the following section.

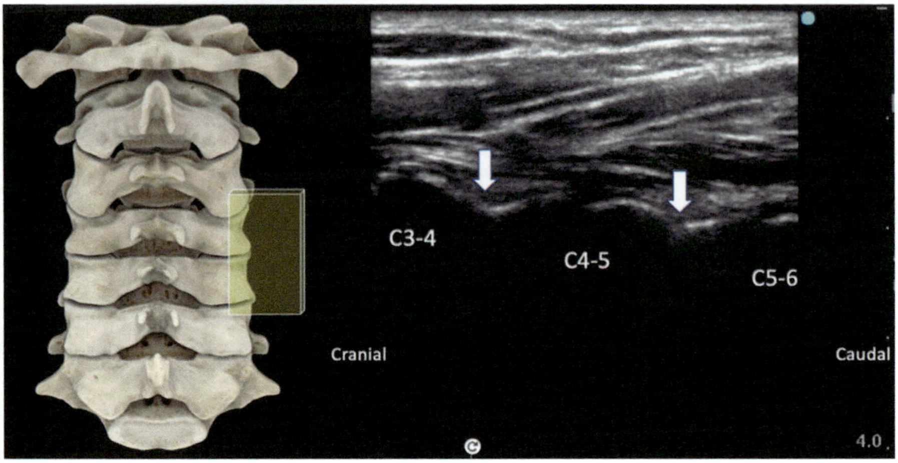

Fig. 7 Ultrasound coronal view of the C3–4, C4–5 and C5–6 facet joints. The associated medial branches are denoted by the block arrows

Cervical Medial Branch Block, Transverse Technique

For patients in whom the long axis approach is ill-suited due to needle entry site or probe handling, the transverse technique for MBB offers another option; this is frequently used in the MBB of C7 due to obstruction by the thoracic cage, though it is also routinely used in C5 and C6 MBB. With the patient prepped and draped in the previously described position, the probe is oriented in the transverse plane on the lateral neck (Fig. 8). Level confirmation can be completed by scanning coronal plane and then rotating the probe 90 degrees to the transverse position. The probe is translated cephalad and caudally until C6 is identified by its prominent anterior tubercle and classic "snail shell" shape of the articular process (Fig. 9). Translating the probe slightly caudad leads to flattening of the "snail shell" and is the site of C6 MBB (Fig. 10). C7 can by identified by translating the probe caudad. Alternatively, the C7 superior articular pillar can be identified by first locating the broad transverse process of T1 in the transverse plane (Fig. 11). Scanning cephalad, the more anterior, singular and narrow transverse process of C7 comes into view (Fig. 12). Further translating the probe cephalad yields the superior articular process of C7 (Fig. 13). With the needle insertion posterior to the probe, an in-plane ultrasound-guidance is used to direct the needle between the periosteum of the C7 superior articular pillar and the semispinalis capitus muscle, where local anesthetic is deposited.

Potential Complications and Adverse Effects

Potential complications are rare, but include ineffective procedure, patient discomfort, intravascular injection, intrathecal injection and nerve injury. Anesthesia or dysesthesia in the nerve-associated dermatome is possible, though in one study none of the participants found theses sensory changes troublesome [11].

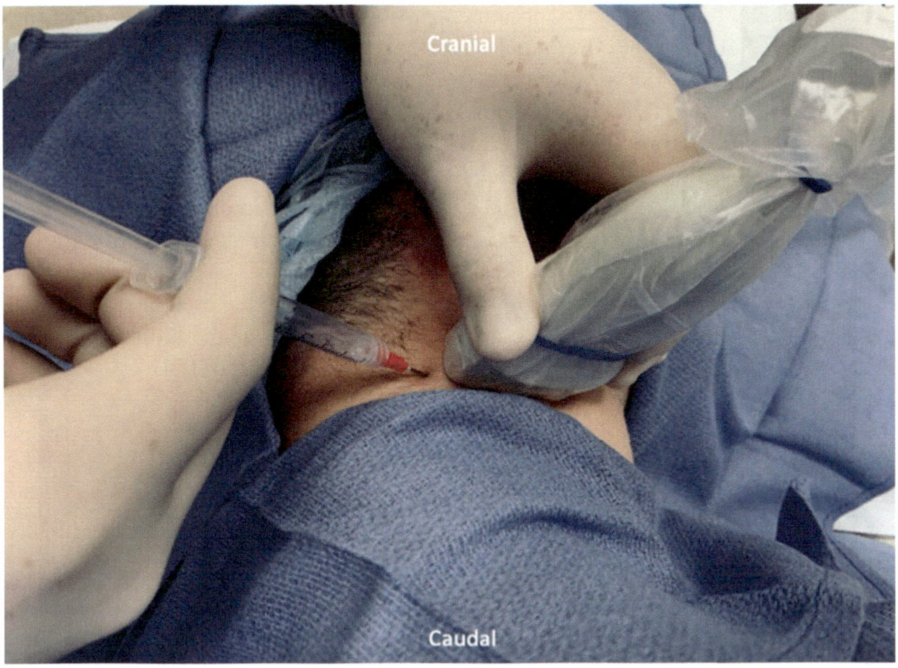

Fig. 8 Patient positioning for ultrasound-guided medial branch block with the probe oriented in the transverse plane. The patient is placed in the left lateral decubitus position, with the head supported neutrally. After scout images are obtained (pictured above), the patient is then prepped and draped in the usual sterile fashion

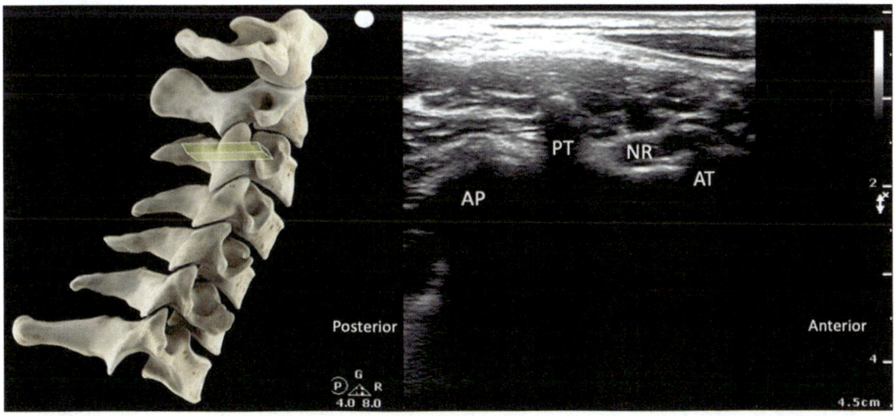

Fig. 9 Ultrasound transverse view of C6, including the prominent anterior tubercle (AT), nerve root (NR) and posterior tubercle (PT). Here the articular process (AP) has a characteristic "snail shell" appearance

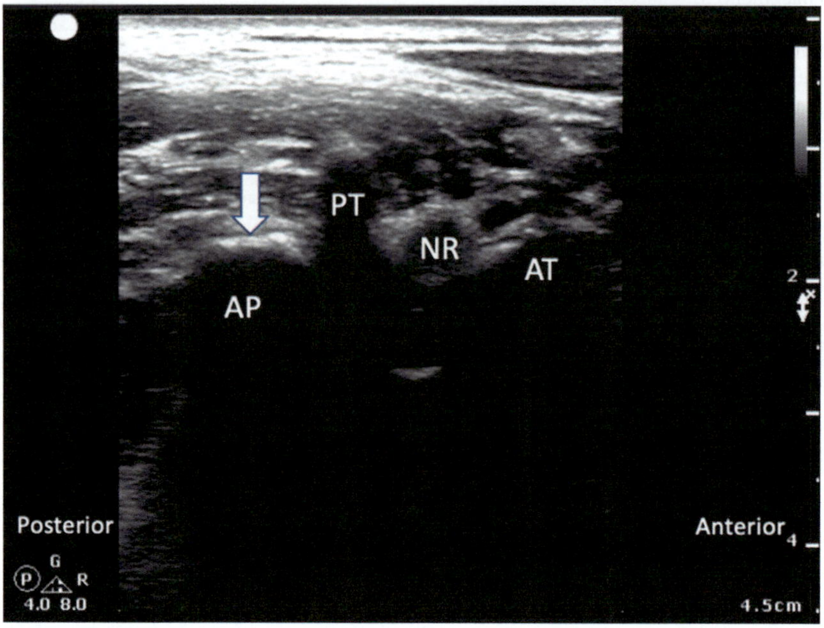

Fig. 10 Ultrasound transverse view of C6, including the prominent anterior tubercle (AT), nerve root (NR) and posterior tubercle (PT). Scanning caudad from the prior view, the "snail shell" has flatted and become the articular pillar (AP). The block arrow noting the osseous flattening marks the articular pillar and is the block target with C6 medial branch block

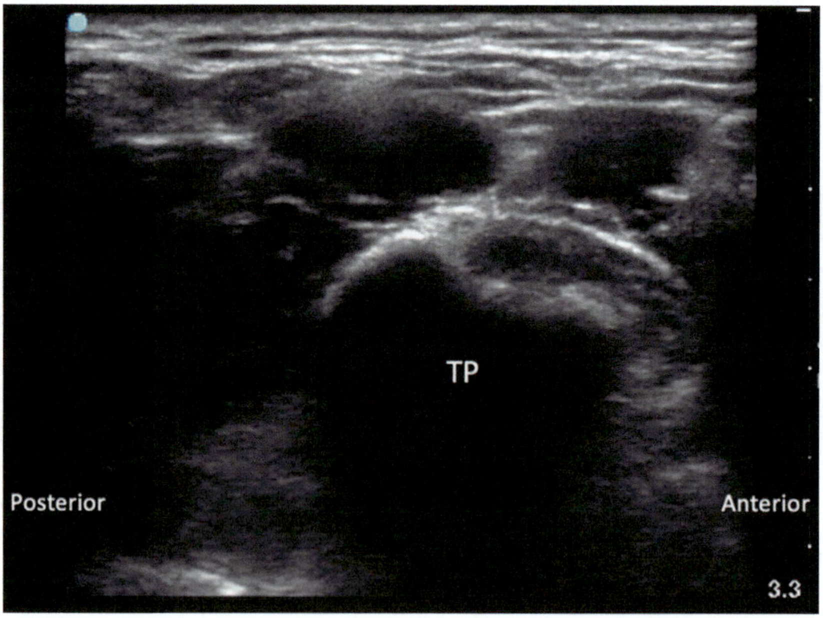

Fig. 11 Ultrasound transverse view at T1. The transverse process (TP) of T1 is notably broader and flatter than the TP of the cervical vertebrae. Scanning cephalad slowly will yield the narrow TP of C7 anteriorly (pictured in Fig. 12)

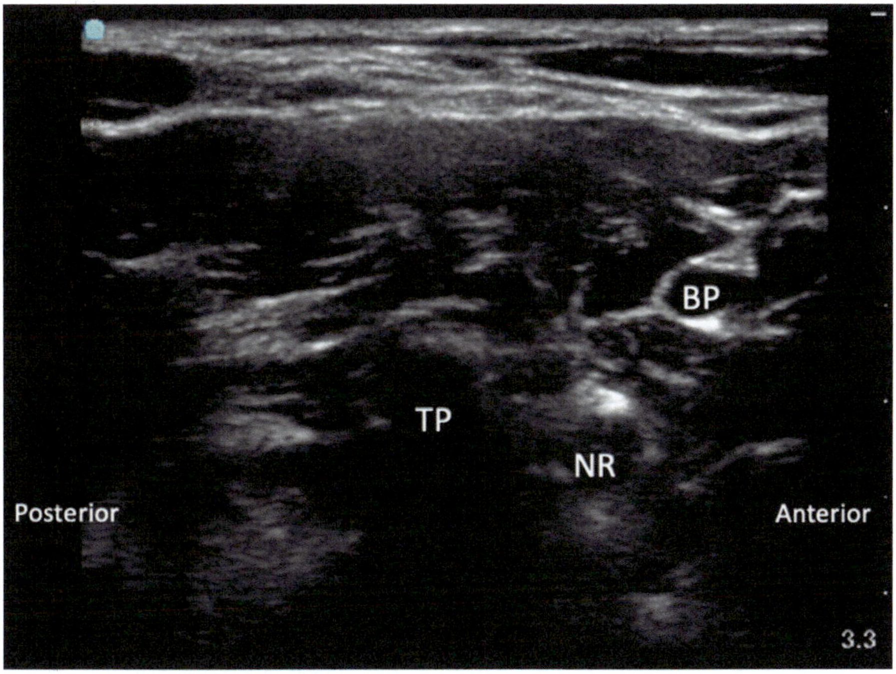

Fig. 12 Ultrasound Transverse view of the C7 transverse process, C7 nerve root (NR), and brachial plexus (BP). Scanning slightly cephalad will yield the view for C7 Medial branch block

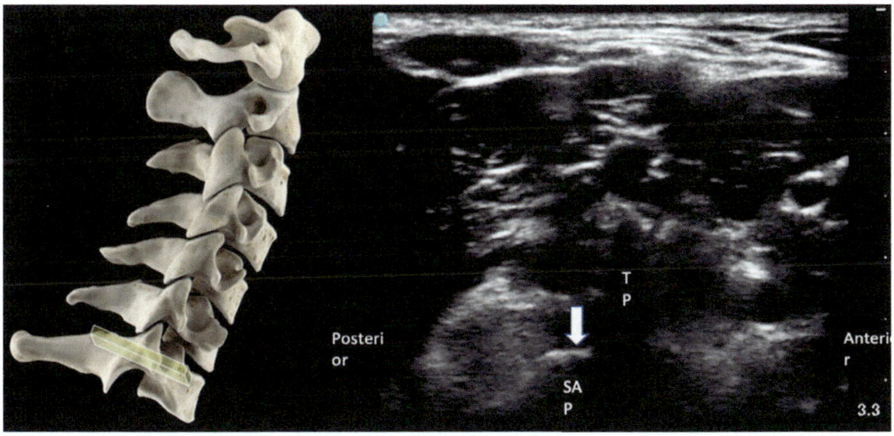

Fig. 13 Ultrasound Transverse view of the C7 transverse process and superior aspect of the articular pillar (SAP), where the C7 medial branch most likely courses. The block arrow notes the location for C7 medial branch block

Clinical and Technical Pearls

- Cervical medial branch blocks are usually performed unilaterally at multiple levels and offer a diagnostic and therapeutic approach to chronic neck pain
- Currently, ultrasound-guided cervical medial branch blocks are limited to diagnostic procedures, while radiofrequency neurotomy utilizes a fluoroscopic approach
- Ultrasonographic identification of anatomy including osseous landmarks, nerves and blood vessels improves safety and efficiency
- Careful surveillance of the anatomy and needle trajectory planning should be observed prior to performing the procedure.
- Technical proficiency with an in-plane approach should be demonstrated prior to performing the procedure, as complete needle tip visualization is required for safety and block efficacy.

References

1. Hogg-Johnson S, van der Velde G, Carroll LJ, et al. The burden and determinants of neck pain in the general population: results of the bone and joint decade 2000–2010 task force on neck pain and its associated disorders. Spine (Phila Pa 1976). 2008;33(4 Suppl):S39–51.
2. Boswell MV, Manchikanti L, Kaye AD, et al. A best-evidence systematic appraisal of the diagnostic accuracy and utility of facet (zygapophysial) joint injections in chronic spinal pain. Pain Physician. 2015;18(4):E497–533.
3. Gellhorn AC. Cervical facet-mediated pain. Phys Med Rehabil Clin N Am. 2011;22(3):447–58.
4. Mehnert MJ, Freedman MK. Update on the role of z-joint injection and radiofrequency neurotomy for cervicogenic headache. PM R. 2013;5(3):221–7.
5. Barnsley L, Lord S, Wallis B, Bogduk N. False-positive rates of cervical zygapophysial joint blocks. Clin J Pain. 1993;9(2):124–30.
6. Finlayson RJ, Etheridge J-PB, Tiyaprasertkul W, Nelems B, Tran DQH. A randomized comparison between ultrasound-and fluoroscopy-guided c7 medial branch block. Reg Anesth Pain Med. 2015;40(1):52–7.
7. Gellhorn AC, Katz JN, Suri P. Osteoarthritis of the spine: the facet joints. Nat Rev Rheumatol. 2013;9(4):216.
8. Kallakuri S, Singh A, Chen C, Cavanaugh JM. Demonstration of substance P, calcitonin gene-related peptide, and protein gene product 9.5 containing nerve fibers in human cervical facet joint capsules. Spine. 2004;29(11):1182–6.
9. Suri P, Miyakoshi A, Hunter DJ, et al. Does lumbar spinal degeneration begin with the anterior structures? A study of the observed epidemiology in a community-based population. BMC Musculoskelet Disord. 2011;12(1):202.
10. Headache Classification Committee of the International Headache S. HIS. The international classification of headache disorders. Cephalalgia. 2018;38(1):110.
11. Lord SM, Barnsley L, Wallis BJ, McDonald GJ, Bogduk N. Percutaneous radio-frequency neurotomy for chronic cervical zygapophyseal-joint pain. N Engl J Med. 1996;335(23):1721–6.
12. Jaumard NV, Welch WC, Winkelstein BA. Spinal facet joint biomechanics and mechanotransduction in normal, injury and degenerative conditions. J Biomech Eng. 2011;133(7):071010.
13. Yoganandan N, Knowles SA, Maiman DJ, Pintar FA. Anatomic study of the morphology of human cervical facet joint. Spine (Phila Pa 1976). 2003;28(20):2317–23.
14. Bogduk N. The clinical anatomy of the cervical dorsal rami. Spine. 1982;7(4):319–30.

15. Lord SM, McDonald GJ, Bogduk N. Percutaneous radiofrequency neurotomy of the cervical medial branches: a validated treatment for cervical zygapophysial joint pain. Neurosurg Q. 1998;8(4):288–308.
16. Kweon TD, Kim JY, Lee HY, Kim MH, Lee Y-W. Anatomical analysis of medial branches of dorsal rami of cervical nerves for radiofrequency thermocoagulation. Reg Anesth Pain Med. 2014;39(6):465–71.

Further Reading

Li J, Szabova A. Ultrasound-guided nerve blocks in the head and neck for chronic pain management: the anatomy, sonoanatomy, and procedure. Pain Physician. 2021;24(8):533–48.

Stellate Ganglion Block

Anna C. Irwin and Christian Renwick

Essentials Concepts

- Stellate Ganglion Block (SGB) is a cervical sympathetic chain block that may be accomplished by infiltration of a local anesthetic into the region of the sympathetic ganglia
- Primarily used to treat CRPS, but can be used for angina, phantom limb pain, vascular insufficiency, hyperhidrosis, Raynaud's syndrome, anxiety, posttraumatic stress disorder, atypical face pain, as well as a variety of other pain and non-pain related conditions.
- With ongoing efforts to improve the safety of the procedure, the techniques for SGB have evolved over time, from the use of a landmark-based technique to fluoroscopy, and, over the last decade, to an ultrasound-guided approach which enables it to be performed safely at the bedside.

1 Stellate Ganglion Block

Overview

Stellate Ganglion Blocks (SGB) have been used for almost a century to treat a variety of conditions. The block was initially described by Leriche for angina and then refined by Findley and Patzer. Also known as a cervicothoracic block, it is primarily used to treat complex regional pain syndrome (CRPS but can be used for angina,

A. C. Irwin (✉)
Pain Medicine and Anesthesiology, University of Virginia, Charlottesville, VA, USA
e-mail: ai5a@virginia.edu

C. Renwick
University of Virginia, Charlottesville, VA, USA
e-mail: CMR4KB@hscmail.mcc.virginia.edu

D. Souza et al. (eds.), *Bedside Pain Management Interventions*,
https://doi.org/10.1007/978-3-031-11188-4_31

phantom limb pain, vascular insufficiency, hyperhidrosis, Raynaud's syndrome, anxiety, atypical face pain, as well as a variety of other pain and non-pain related conditions. It helped, for example, to reduce the number of hot flushes and nightly awakenings suffered by breast cancer survivors and women experiencing extreme menopause [1]. There is also emerging evidence for stellate ganglion blocks in the treatment of depression and post-traumatic stress disorder [2, 3] as well as refractory ventricular tachycardia [4]. Techniques for performing SGB include the use of a landmark-based technique, fluoroscopy, and, over the last decade, an ultrasound-guided approach enabling the procedure to be performed at the bedside.

Indications and Contraindications

Common indications include CRPS, type I and type II, hyperhidrosis, angina, cardiac arrhythmias, Raynaud's syndrome, vascular insufficiency, frostbite, posttraumatic stress disorder, postherpetic neuralgia, atypical face pain, vascular headaches, phantom pain, anxiety, depression, and other conditions.

Common contraindications include injection at the planned injection site, moderate to severe systemic infection, coagulopathy, including iatrogenic, platelet dysfunction, including iatrogenic, cardiac conduction block, glaucoma, and patient refusal (Table 1).

Clinical Anatomy

The cervical sympathetic trunk contains three interconnected ganglia: the superior, middle, and inferior ganglion. In 80% of the population, the stellate is formed by the fusion of the inferior cervical ganglion and first thoracic ganglion. If not fused, the inferior ganglion is referred to as the stellate ganglion [5, 6] (Fig. 1).

It is approximately 2.5 cm in length, 1 cm in width, and 0.5 cm in thickness. The stellate ganglion lies lateral to the longus colli muscle, medial to the scalene muscles, and anterior to the transverse process and prevertebral fascia. The vertebral

Table 1 Common indications and contraindications for stellate ganglion block

Indications	Contraindications
Complex regional pain syndrome type I or type II	Patient refusal
Phantom pain	Local or systemic infection
Angina	Coagulopathy or platelet dysfunction
Cardiac arrhythmias	Glaucoma
Frostbite	Cardiac conduction block
Accidental arterial injection of medications	
Post-traumatic stress disorder	
Post herpetic neuralgia	
Atypical face pain	
Vascular headaches	
Hyperhidrosis	
Raynaud's phenomena, or disease	

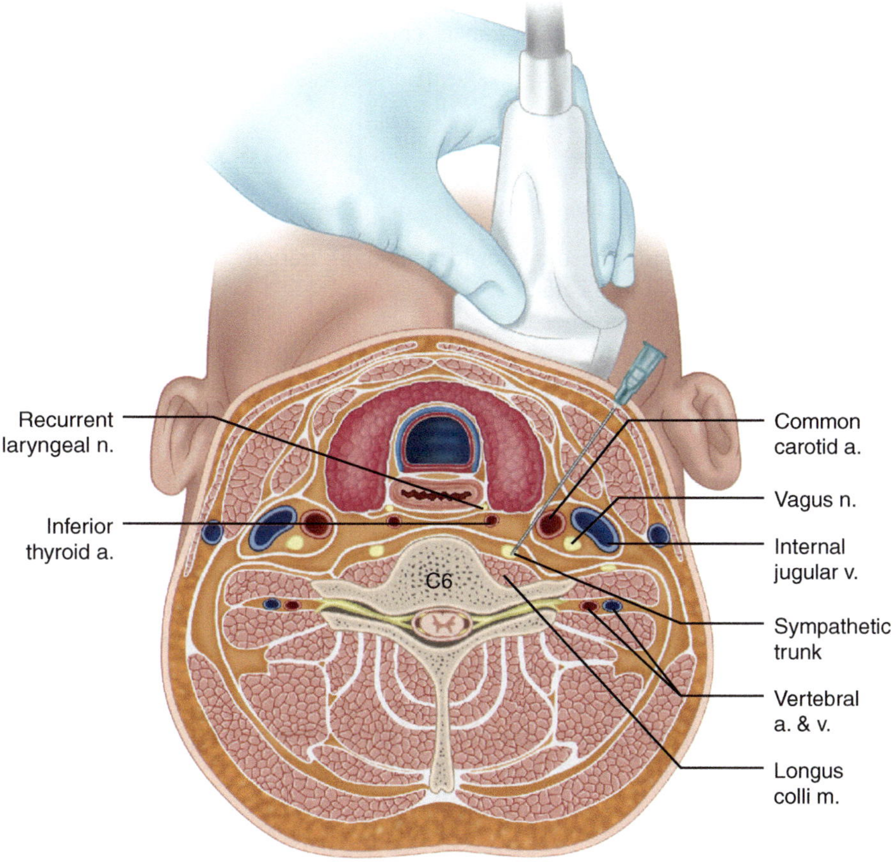

Fig. 1 Cross-sectional anatomy of stellate ganglion block as labeled

artery which arises from the subclavian artery lies anterior to the ganglion at C7 then enters the vertebral foramen posterior to the anterior tubercle of C6 (Chassaignac's Tubercle) in 90% of the population. In the other 10% the artery enters at C5 or higher [7]. The cervical ganglia receive preganglionic fibers from the lateral gray column of the spinal cord and myelinated preganglionic fibers from the anterolateral horn of the spinal cord. Nerve fibers from the upper thoracic spinal cord come from the ventral spinal root and join the spinal nerves at the start of the ventral rami. These nerve fibers leave the spinal nerve through white rami communicans, which may then enter corresponding thoracic ganglia and travel cephalad into the neck. Innervation for the head and neck arise predominantly from T1 to T3, while innervation of the upper extremities originates predominantly from T2 toT6. The fibers travel cephalad through the sympathetic trunk into the cervicothoracic ganglion where they synapse. After they synapse, the postganglionic fibers either travel to the head and neck or to the brachial plexus to innervate the arm. These postganglionic fibers control sudomotor and vasoconstriction of the face and neck. When the fibers are blocked, ptosis, miosis, enophthalmos occur as well as abolition of face and neck sweat [8].

Equipment and Supplies

- Informed Consent
- Syringe with 27-gauge needle—for local skin infiltration
- 5–10 ml Syringe—for injectate
- 22- or 25-gauge, 3.5-inch needle
- Skin temperature monitor
- Ultrasound Linear High-Frequency Probe
- Appropriate equipment and medications for medical resuscitation

For safety reasons, an intravenous line should be inserted before the procedure. All patients should be monitored by electrocardiography, noninvasive blood pressure measurement, and pulse oximetry during and for 30 min after the block. With the ongoing efforts to improve the safety of this procedure, the techniques for SGB have evolved. There are a variety of techniques described to perform this block. Imagine guidance has appeared to improve success but practicality and modalities continue to be debated. CT guidance, for instance, has a high success rate however it is often impractical to use and exposes patients and physicians to high doses of radiation and cannot be utilized at the bedside. There continues to be a variable success rate with this block regardless of the employed technique.

Landmark Technique

The patient is positioned supine with neck slightly extended and mouth opened slightly to relax neck musculature. In a blind technique, the physician is taught to palpate Chassaignac's tubercle. This is located roughly 3 cm cephalad to the sternoclavicular joint at the medial border of the sternocleidomastoid muscle [7]. The physician's non-dominant hand retracts the carotid artery and SCM laterally. The needle is inserted and advanced until contacting bone which is either Chassaignac's tubercle or the junction between the tubercle and C6 vertebral body. The needle is then withdrawn 2–4 mm to position the needle outside of the longus colli muscle. Aspiration should be performed before injecting any local anesthetic and a dose of 0.5–1 ml should be slowly injected to look for signs of intravascular injection. If aspiration is negative, 5–8 ml of bupivacaine or lidocaine can be injected in small increments. This technique can produce unreliable results and can be associated with a variety of complications such as intravascular injection, hematomas, esophageal injury, and damage to the recurrent laryngeal nerve [9]. Narouze et al.

further emphasized the risks of a blind approach pointing out that blind injection at the C6 level on the left side may cause inadvertent esophageal puncture or may traverse the thyroid [10]. It is generally no longer recommended to perform a blind technique.

Stellate Ganglion Block, Ultrasound Technique

Ultrasound allows direct visualization of vessels and soft tissues and should theoretically minimize damage to these structures. Clear imaging of the muscles, fascia, blood vessels, viscera, and bony landmarks allows for increased safety and efficacy. Various ultrasound techniques exist to perform this block. Improper placement of the needle can also occur despite confirmatory tests. If the needle is placed in the longus colli muscle, the result will be an ineffective block [11]. Thus, success rate may vary.

Anterior Approach at C6

The patient is supine with the neck slightly extended and slightly rotated to the contralateral side, increasing the distance between the carotid artery and trachea. The ultrasound probe is placed at the level of the cricoid cartilage, transversely just lateral to the trachea on the ipsilateral side. The C6 transverse process is identified by the prominent anterior tubercle. Scanning caudally will visualize the C7 transverse process which has no tubercle. Pressure can be applied with the ultrasound transducer, reducing the distance between the skin and tubercle and depressing the dome of the lung to reduce risk of pneumothorax. A quick scan caudally will help confirm that the inferior thyroid artery is not in the path of the needle. The ganglion may be visualized; however, if not, the goal is to use an in-plane approach to deposit the medication in the fascial plane anterior to the longus colli. Injection of 1–2 ml is typically performed to verify filling of the fascial plane, then a total volume of 3–5 ml can be injected [12, 13]. (Fig. 2).

Anterior Approach at C7

Ultrasound can also be utilized by scanning downward from C6. C7 has only a vestigial tubercle that is not readily palpable or easily visualized on ultrasound, thus identifying C6 and proceeding caudally to C7 may be helpful. At C7, the risk of vertebral artery injury and pneumothorax are generally considered higher. In addition, the risk of esophageal puncture appears higher. In one study it was reported that when performed on the left, the esophagus was located along the needle path in 39 out of 60 cases at C7 vs 22 out of 60 cases at C6 [14]. The benefits of a C7 approach include that of being closer to the ganglion so a smaller volume of local is needed. We typically inject around 3 cc of local anesthetic. This is often useful if there was a failed block at C6 (Fig. 3).

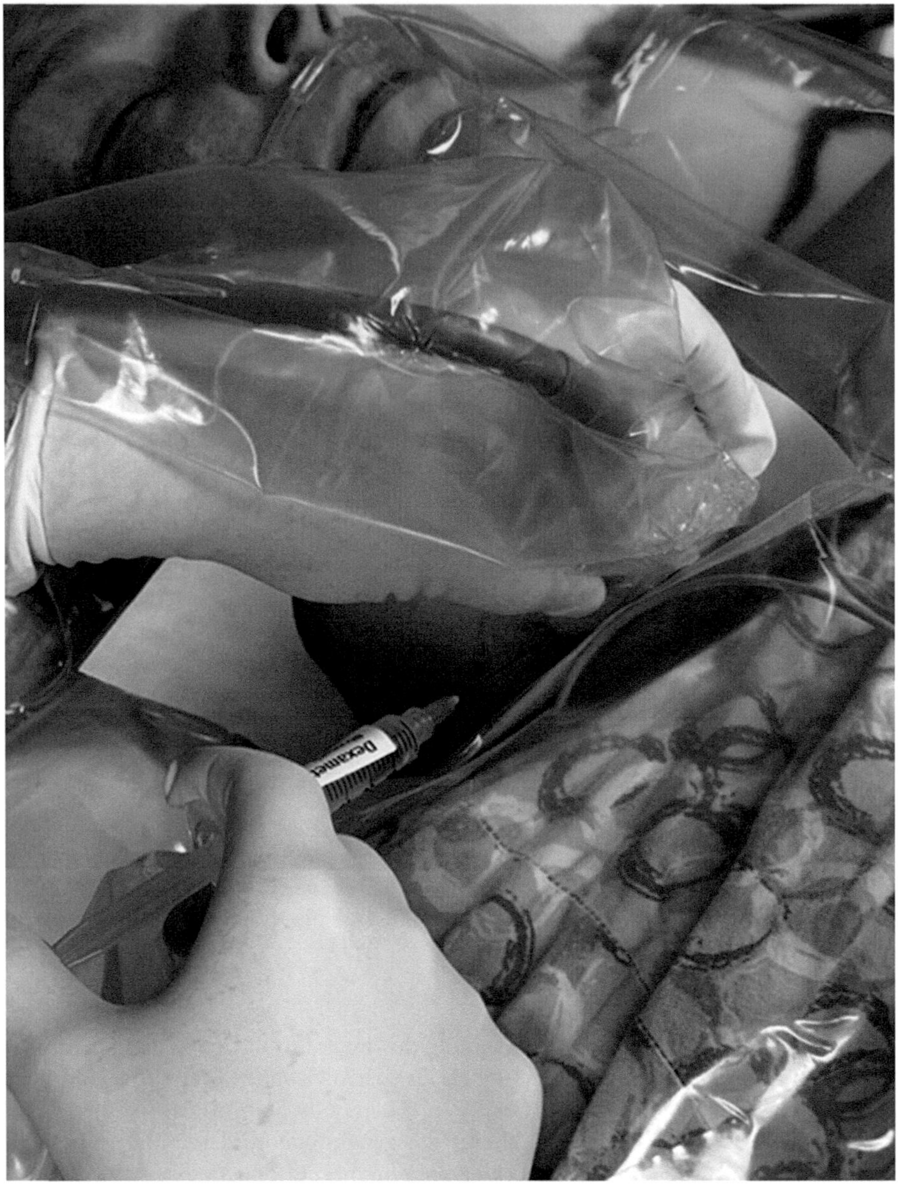

Fig. 2 Right stellate ganglion block: needle and ultrasound transducer positioning. This procedure can be performed with a needle advanced using in plane or out of plane technique. The image demonstrates in plane technique. (Image–courtesy of Dmitri Souza, MD, PhD)

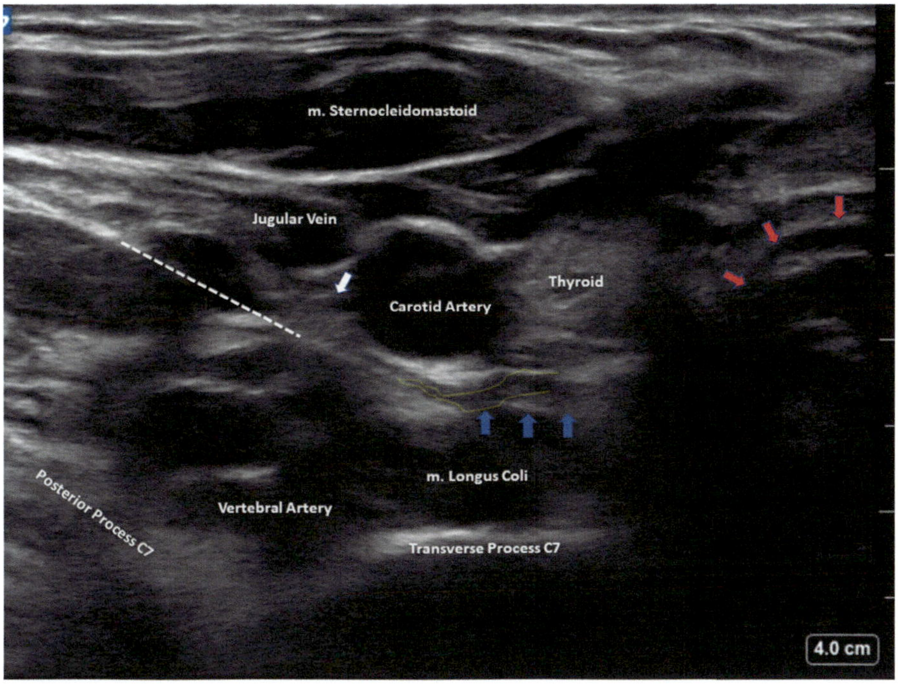

Fig. 3 Ultrasonogram of stellate ganglion block at C7 level, is labeled. Red arrows point towards the trachea. Blue arrows points towards prevertebral fascia and injectate spread. White arrow points towards valgus nerve. Dashed line highlights needle trajectory. (Image–courtesy of Dmitri Souza, MD, PhD)

Response from the Block

There are some expected changes that result from a stellate ganglion block. These changes last the duration of the local anesthetic (4–6 h). Changes include Horner's syndrome (ptosis, miosis, anhidrosis), a bloodshot eye on the injected side, nasal congestion on the injected side (Guttman's sign), and a temperature increase on the injected side. Hoarseness may also be noticed. The presence of Horner's syndrome signifies a sympathetic block of the head and neck but does not verify an upper extremity block. Temperature increase in the ipsilateral extremity is the easiest clinical sign to confirm a sympathetic block. Various changes in temperature have been considered significant in a successful sympathetic blockade. The magnitude of temperature increase is dependent on the starting temperature because skin temperature will nearly approximate core body temperature. Patients whose baseline skin temperatures are lower because of vasoconstriction (late-stage CRPS) will experience a larger increase in temperature than in a vasodilated patient (early stage CRPS) [15]. (Fig. 4).

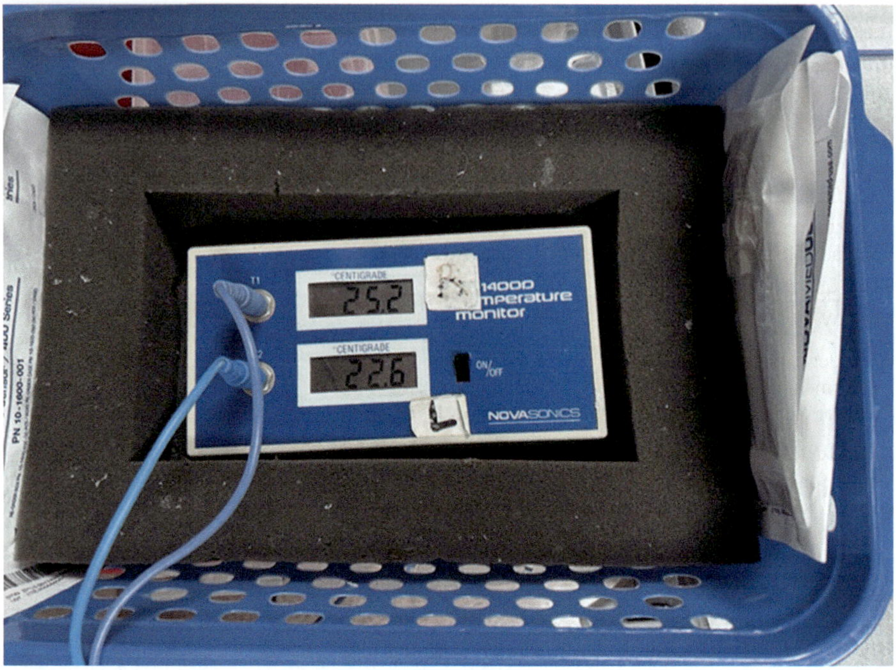

Fig. 4 Change in temperature between right and left thumb after correctly performed stellate ganglion block. (Image–courtesy of Dmitri Souza, MD, PhD)

Potential Complications and Adverse Effects

Although infrequent, risks from the procedure include seizure (if the medication is incidentally injected into a blood vessel), pneumothorax, brachial plexus block, high spinal or epidural block, that may result in cardiorespiratory arrest, allergy to, or intolerance of the injectate, including local anesthetics or corticosteroids, nerve damage. Bruising or soreness at the injection site may occur. Respiratory compromise secondary to an incidental phrenic nerve block, or compression of the trachea by intervention-induced hematoma, are extremely rare [16]. Most experts agree that the chance of complication can be decreased dramatically with an ultrasound-guided approach, primarily because of direct visualization of the target structure in the needle tip during the procedure (Table 2).

Table 2 Stellate ganglion block. Potential complications

Bleeding/hematoma
Pneumothorax/hemothorax
Vertebral artery injury
Esophageal trauma
Recurrent laryngeal nerve injury
Tracheal trauma
Phrenic nerve injury
Brachial plexus injury

Clinical and Technical Pearls

- The success rate of the stellate ganglion block is variable. The rate is so variable because it may be difficult to evaluate the success of the block, and improper placement of the needle can also occur despite confirmatory tests.
- The success or failure of either landmark-based technique or fluoroscopic-guided injection depends on the thickness of the longus coli muscle, and on the anatomic location of the cervical sympathetic trunk. The endpoint for injection in the ultrasound-guided technique is the pre-vertebral fascia, and not contact with bone as with fluoroscopic and blind techniques.
- An interesting application for stellate ganglion block has been described in literature where a right sided stellate ganglion block is performed and appears to improve symptoms of PTSD. It appears that this procedure performed on the right side has the ability to confer greater benefit than the left.

References

1. Hansen HC, Trescot AM, Manchikanti L. Stellate ganglion block. In: Manchikanti L, Singh V, editors. Interventional techniques in chronic non-spinal pain. Paducah: ASIPP Publishing; 2009. p. 115–40.
2. Rae Olmsted KL, Bartoszek M, Mulvaney S, McLean B, Turabi A, Young R, Kim E, Vandermaas-Peeler R, Morgan JK, Constantinescu O, Kane S, Nguyen C, Hirsch S, Munoz B, Wallace D, Croxford J, Lynch JH, White R, Walters BB. Effect of stellate ganglion block treatment on posttraumatic stress disorder symptoms: a randomized clinical trial. JAMA Psychiatry. 2020;77(2):130–8. https://doi.org/10.1001/jamapsychiatry.2019.3474; Erratum in: JAMA Psychiatry. 2020 Jan 2;: Erratum in: JAMA Psychiat 2020 Sep 1;77(9):982.
3. Li Y, Loshak H. Stellate ganglion block for the treatment of post-traumatic stress disorder, depression, and anxiety. Ottawa, ON: Canadian Agency for Drugs and Technologies in Health; 2021.
4. Narasimhan B, Tandri H. Stellate block in refractory ventricular tachycardia: the calm after the storm. Circ Arrhythm Electrophysiol. 2019;12(9):e007707. https://doi.org/10.1161/CIRCEP.119.007707; Epub 2019 Sep 13
5. Elias M. Cervical sympathetic and stellate ganglion blocks. Pain Physician. 2000;3(3):294–304. https://www.painphysicianjournal.com/linkout?issn=1533-3159&vol=3&page=294
6. Marples IL, Atkin RE. Stellate ganglion block. Pain Rev. 2001;8:3–11.

7. Mehrotra M, Singh P. Neuroanatomy, stellate ganglion [monograph online]. StatPearls Publishing LLC; 2019 [cited 2019 November 24]. NCBI.
8. Deer TR, Leong MS, Buvanendran A, Gordin V, Kim PS, Panchal SJ, et al. Comprehensive treatment of chronic pain by medical, interventional, and integrative approaches. New York: Springer; 2013.
9. Benzon H, Raja SN, Fishman SM, Liu SS, Cohen SP. Essentials of pain medicine. Elsevier; 2017.
10. Narouze S, Vydyanathan A, Patel N. Ultrasound-guided stellate ganglion block successfully prevented esophageal puncture. Pain Physician. 2007;10:747–52. https://www.painphysicianjournal.com/linkout?issn=1533-3159&vol=10&page=747
11. Ates Y, Asik I, Ozgencil E, et al. Evaluation of the longus colli muscle in relation to the stellate ganglion block. Reg Anesth Pain Med. 2009;34(3):219–23.
12. Narouze SN. Ultrasound-guided stellate ganglion block: safety and efficacy. Curr Pain Headache Rep. 2014;18(6):424. https://doi.org/10.1007/s11916-014-0424-5.
13. Raj PP. Stellate ganglion block. In: Waldman W, editor. Interventional pain management. Philadelphia: Saunders; 1996.
14. Siegenthaler A, Mlekusch S, Schliessbach J, Curatolo M, Eichenberger U. Ultrasound imaging to estimate risk of esophageal and vascular puncture after conventional stellate ganglion block. Reg Anesth Pain Med. 2012;37(2):224–7.
15. Stevens RA, Stotz A, Kao TC, Powar M, Burgess S, Kleinman B. The relative increase in skin temperature after stellate ganglion block is predictive of a complete sympathectomy of the hand. Reg Anesth Pain Med. 1998;23(3):266–70. https://doi.org/10.1016/s1098-7339(98)90053-0.
16. Goel V, Patwardhan AM, Ibrahim M, Howe CL, Schultz DM, Shankar H. Complications associated with stellate ganglion nerve block: a systematic review. Reg Anesth Pain Med. 2019;rapm-2018-100127. https://doi.org/10.1136/rapm-2018-100127; Epub ahead of print.

Further Reading

Baek J, Kim BS, Yu H, Kim H, Lim C, Song SO. Comparison of ultrasound-guided stellate ganglion block at 6th and 7th cervical vertebrae using the lateral paracarotid out-of-plane approach for sympathetic blockade in the upper extremity. Yeungnam Univ J Med. 2018;35(2):199–204. https://doi.org/10.12701/yujm.2018.35.2.199; Epub 2018 Dec 31.

Ghai A, Kaushik T, Kundu ZS, Wadhera S, Wadhera R. Evaluation of new approach to ultrasound guided stellate ganglion block. Saudi J Anaesth. 2016;10(2):161–7. https://doi.org/10.4103/1658-354X.168815.

Trigger Point Injections

Matthew Riley, Janki Patel, and Lynn Kohan

Essential Concepts

- Trigger point injections are effective in treating myofascial trigger points that cause persistent pain and limited range of motion.
- Goals for trigger point injections include rapid pain relief and increased range of motion of the affected muscles.
- Trigger point injections are easy to perform in clinic and are generally well tolerated by patients
- Pain relief from these injections is rapid and can last days, weeks, and even months

1 Overview

Myofascial trigger points are taut bands of skeletal muscle fibers that result in persistent pain and limited range of motion of the affected muscles [1]. In addition to pharmacotherapy and other non-invasive treatment options for this type of pain, trigger point injections offer an additional treatment modality. Trigger point injections are generally low risk and well tolerated injections performed at the bedside. These injections usually contain local anesthetics that may or may not be supplemented with steroids. They can be administered by simple palpation or under ultrasound guidance. These injections are generally safe and have few side effects or complications.

M. Riley · J. Patel · L. Kohan (✉)
Department of Anesthesiology, University of Virginia Health System, Charlottesville, VA, USA
e-mail: MDR5Gx@hscmail.mcc.virginia.edu; JP9VT@hscmail.mcc.virginia.edu; LRK9G@hscmail.mcc.virginia.edu

D. Souza et al. (eds.), *Bedside Pain Management Interventions*,
https://doi.org/10.1007/978-3-031-11188-4_32

2 Indications and Contraindications

Candidates for trigger point injections are commonly patients with myofascial pain syndrome. These patients often have points of tenderness that are caused by sudden or repetitive strain on skeletal muscles. Active trigger points often result in pain, stiffness, and decreased range of motion. Paresthesias may also occur. Many patients with myofascial pain also have fibromyalgia. It is important to distinguish between the two, as trigger point injections may worsen fibromyalgia symptoms. Fibromyalgia symptoms typically include diffuse pain and tenderness in soft muscles with normal mobility [2]. Contraindications for this procedure include trigger points that cannot be safely accessed by the needle, infection of the overlying skin, poorly controlled systemic illnesses that can delay healing or predispose to infection, bleeding disorders, and patient refusal [1, 2].

3 Clinical Anatomy

Trigger points are described as "knots" or tight bands of muscle fibers found in the bodies of skeletal muscles. The most commonly involved muscles are the trapezius, splenii, cervical and lumbar paraspinal, quadratus lumborum, and sternocleidomastoid [3, 4]. Involvement of the trapezius muscle commonly results in headaches, shoulder, neck and arm pain [3]. Characteristic physical findings and ultrasound characteristics are outlined in Table 1 [5].

Table 1 Myofascial Trigger Point Characterization Using US examination and Diagnostic Criteria. (Reprinted with permission from Kumbhare D, et al. Ultrasound-guided interventional procedures: myofascial trigger points with structures literature review. Regional Anesthesia and Pain Medicine 2017; 42: 407-412)

MTrP characterization	
Physical characteristics	US examination
A taut band	Spherical/Elliptically shaped or a bandlike area (Bmode)
Local tenderness upon palpation	Hypoechoic—appearing as darker gray areas (Bmode)
Local pain heightens with use	Stiffer—reduced vibration amplitude (Elastography)
Pain recognition	High peak systolic velocity and low diastolic peak systolic velocity than normal muscle tissue (Doppler)
Referred pain	Retrograde diastolic flow (Doppler)
Local twitch response (LTR)	Blood volume at MTrP increased (Doppler)
Restricted range of motion	Increased outflow resistance/vasoconstriction (Doppler)
Reproducible pain pattern	
Weakness without atrophy	

The column on the left outlines the clinical and physical characteristics of myofascial pain syndrome and MTrPs. The column on the right shows the features of US imaging and what different US modes may display

4 Equipment and Supplies

- 5 or 10 cc syringe
- 18 g blunt needle for withdrawing medication
- Medication of choice: commonly—0.25% or 0.5% Bupivacaine; 1% or 2% lidocaine
- 25–27 g Hypodermic needles. Length of 5/8″ to 1–1/4″
- Alcohol swabs or chlorhexidine swab
- Skin marker
- 2 × 2 or 4 × 4 gauze
- Band-aids
- Personal protective equipment—gloves and goggles
- Patient monitoring devices for blood pressure and pulse oximetry should be considered

5 Procedure

Have the patient identify the areas where they experience the most severe pain. To identify trigger points, palpate within the area for tightened knots/bands of muscle fiber. Palpation of the trigger point is usually painful and will often cause of the patient to wince, cry out, or withdraw. This is referred to as "jump sign" [6]. Once identified, mark the trigger point(s) with a skin marker.

Before performing the injections consider placing monitoring devices on the patient. Put on your gloves and eye protection. To perform the injection, start by using an alcohol swab or chlorhexidine swab to clean the site. Advance the needle perpendicular to the skin to a depth adequate to engage the trigger point within the muscle fiber; the patient may demonstrate a local twitch response (LTR) once the needle has been inserted into the trigger point. Aspirate to reduce risk of intravascular injection. Inject 1–2 cc of the chosen medication. Withdraw the needle and hold pressure with gauze over site if bleeding. Repeat at the next identified trigger point.

Another common procedure for trigger point release is called "dry needling." Dry needling and trigger point injection are similar; however, dry needling uses smaller gauge needles to elicit a LTR without injecting a substance. A practitioner will insert the needle into the identified trigger point to elicit a LTR (Fig. 1).

One technique consists of rapidly advancing and withdrawing the needle through various positions within the trigger point to elicit as many LTRs as possible [7].

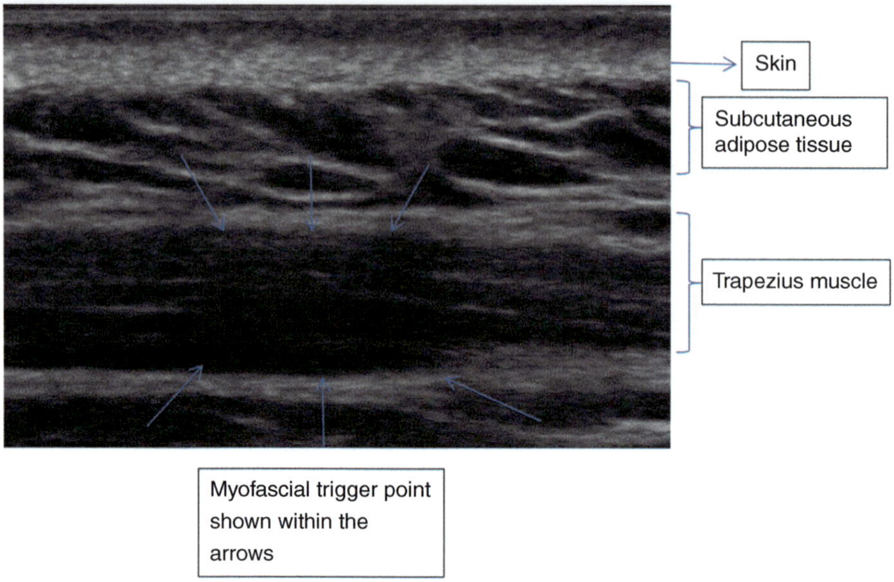

Fig. 1 Dry Needling Technique. Dry Needling. A series of images are shown in which the myofascial trigger point is identified, the needle is inserted in the myofascial trigger point using a swift tap, the muscle and surrounding fascia are probed with an up and down motion of the needle in a clockwise direction, and the needle is left in place for 1–2 min for full therapeutic benefit. (Reprinted with permission from Shah J. et al. Myofascial Trigger Points Then and Now: A Historical and Scientific Perspective. PMR 2015; 7 (7): 746–761)

6 Ultrasound Technique

While the use of palpation is a popular modality to locate trigger points, there are other developing techniques utilizing ultrasound technology for identification and injection of trigger points. The most popular technology currently being studied is standard 2-dimensional ultrasound and vibration sonoelastography [5, 6]. Trigger points visualized under 2-dimensional ultrasound have been described as elliptical, round or band-like hypoechoic foci within the muscle fiber [5] (Figs. 2 and 3).

When utilizing ultrasound, from superficial to deep, the images depict skin, subcutaneous tissue, fascia, then skeletal muscle [5]. The transducer should be aligned longitudinally along the course of the muscle fibers. Speckling might be apparent, which appears as small irregular white regions within the muscle fiber which may represent fascia, aponeuroses, or intramuscular adipose [5]. The ultrasound guided trigger point injection technique involves first palpating the area of tenderness. One should then scan the impacted muscle group to identify the trigger point via ultrasound. The trigger point should appear as a spherical or elliptical shaped object or band that is hypoechoic on B-mode of the ultrasound [5]. The clinician should then insert the needle using sterile technique at approximately a 30-degree angle and

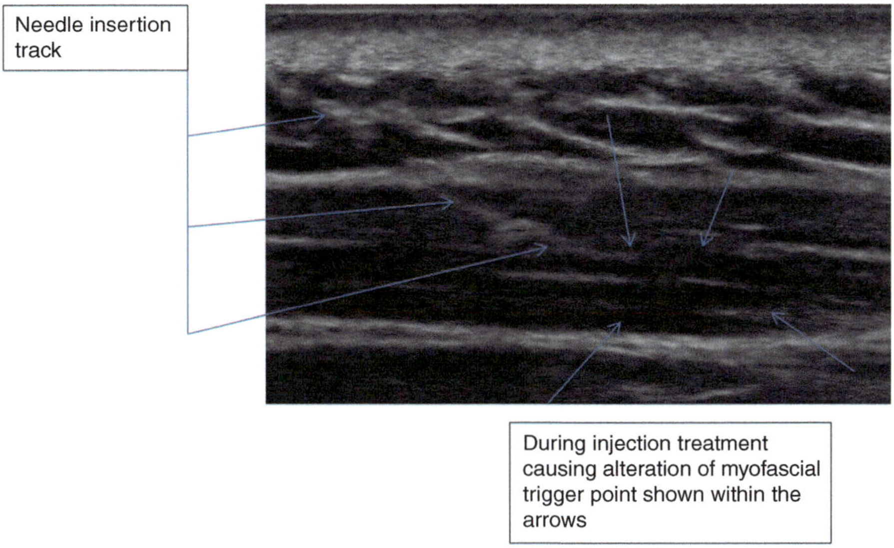

Fig. 2 Ultrasound Image of myofascial trigger point. (Reprinted with permission from Kumbhare D, et al. Ultrasound-guided interventional procedures: myofascial trigger points with structures literature review. Regional Anesthesia and Pain Medicine 2017; 42: 407–412)

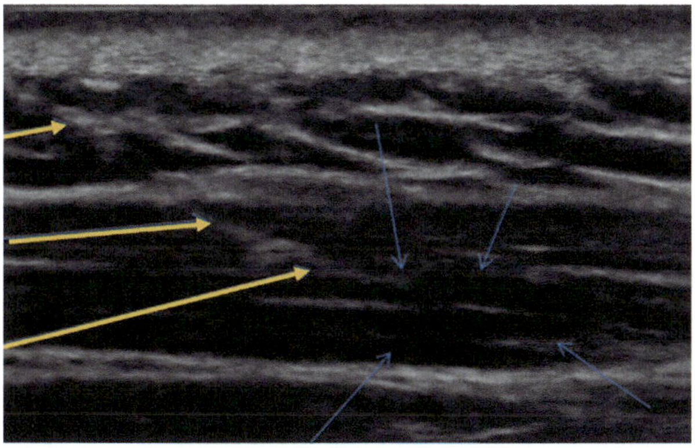

Fig. 3 US image demonstrating injection of the myofascial trigger point with the needle insertion track and alteration of the trigger point during injection. (Reprinted with permission from Kumbhare D, et al. Ultrasound-guided interventional procedures: myofascial trigger points with structures literature review. Regional Anesthesia and Pain Medicine 2017; 42: 407–412)

visualize the needle going into the trigger point. The injectate can then be delivered or dry needling can be employed. The physician should also look for the LTR. The physician may use the ultrasound to see if there is a change in the ultrasound appearance of the trigger point [5]. The needle should be withdrawn and a Band-aid applied if warranted.

Vibration sonoelastography uses ultrasound and a vibrational source to measure relative stiffness or viscosity of tissue and trigger points are thought to be stiffer, with reduced vibrational amplitude, when compared to surround muscle [5]. Unfortunately, there is not yet a consensus on the ultrasound findings for trigger points and further research is required [5, 6].

The use of ultrasound during trigger point injection could provide advantages. During needling or injection of the trigger point, the LTR can be viewed in real time. There is some evidence ultrasound use could be superior at detecting LTR at trigger point injections within deeper tissue [5], which is significant as evidence suggests that needling or injection that elicits LTR gives the most benefit [5]. Secondly, there is potentially increased safety using ultrasound to guide needling or injection to the appropriate location and avoid injections in unintended surrounding tissue.

7 Potential Complications and Adverse Effects

Trigger point injections are generally well tolerated by patients. However, adverse reactions and complications can occur on occasion. These include increased pain, infection, swelling, and bleeding at the injection site, intravascular injection, vasovagal reaction, possible pleural puncture, and if local anesthetic is injected, Local Anesthetic Systemic Toxicity is possible [2].

Clinical and Technical Pearls.

- Be mindful of needle advancement in the thoracic region to reduced risk of pleural puncture and possible pneumothorax
- Steady the hand holding the syringe and needle by bracing it against the patient to reduce risk of unwanted needle motion if patient were to jump or move during insertion and injection
- After initial insertion subcutaneously, some practitioners advance the needle multiple times, without exiting the skin, in different directions through the identified trigger point to maximize stimulation of the local twitch response.
- There is currently no evidence showing an advantage of relieving myofascial trigger point pain between specific injection techniques or even an advantage of injecting medication, sometimes referred to as "wet needling," compared to the technique of dry needleing [2, 8–10].
- There is no evidence showing an advantage in pain relief when comparing one medication to another, including additive such as steroids [2, 8].

References

1. Fowler GC. Pfenninger & Fowlers procedures for primary care. Philadelphia, PA: Elsevier; 2014.
2. Nicol AL, Crooks M, Hsu E, Ferrente MF. Myofascial pain syndrome. In: Essentials of pain medicine. Philadelphia, PA: Elseiver; 2018. p. 207–12.

3. Robbins MS, Kuruvilla D, Blumenfeld A, Charleston L, Sorrell M, Robertson CE, et al. Trigger point injections for headache disorders: expert consensus methodology and narrative review. Headache. 2014;54(9):1441–59.
4. Rivers EW, Benzon HT, Khan F, Asenjo JF. Practical management of pain. Philadelphia, PA: Elsevier Mosby; 2014.
5. Kumbhare D, Singh D, Rathbone HA, Gunn M, Grosman-Rimon L, Vadasz B, et al. Ultrasound-guided interventional procedures. Reg Anesth Pain Med. 2017;42(3):407–12.
6. Finlayson RJ. Ultrasound guidance for trigger point injections. Reg Anesth Pain Med. 2017;42(3):279–80.
7. Singh V, Trescot A, Nishio I. Injections for chronic pain. Phys Med Rehabil Clin N Am. 2015;26:249–61. https://doi.org/10.1016/j.pmr.2015.01.004.
8. Desai MJ, Saini V, Saini S. Myofascial pain syndrome: a treatment review. Pain Ther. 2013;2:21–36. https://doi.org/10.1007/s40122-013-0006-y.
9. Scott NA, Guo B, Barton PM, Gerwin RD. Trigger point injections for chronic non-malignant musculoskeletal pain: a systematic review. Pain Med. 2009;10(1):54–69.
10. Soares A, Andriolo RB, Atallah ÁN, da Silva EMK. Botulinum toxin for myofascial pain syndromes in adults. Cochrane Database Syst Rev. 2014;2014(7):CD007533. https://doi.org/10.1002/14651858.CD007533.pub3.

Further Reading

Money S. Pathophysiology of trigger points in myofascial pain syndrome. J Pain Palliat Care Pharmacother. 2017;31(2):158–9.

Bedside Ligamentous Injections

Paul K. Cheng and Tariq M. Malik

Essential Concepts

- One key cause of axial spine pain is ligamentous pain which is often caused by defects in ligament healing or ligament laxity
- Many ligaments in the spine can be targets for ultrasound-guided injections including the supraspinous and interspinous ligament in the cervical, thoracic and lumbar spine areas as well as the iliolumbar ligament and the ligaments around the sacroiliac area such as the sacrotuberous ligament, sacrospinous ligament, posterior sacroiliac ligaments, dorsal sacroiliac ligament, and interosseous sacroiliac ligament
- Common injectates include corticosteroids. Biologics or prolotherapy have been described as well.
- More research needs to be done to further evaluate outcomes and standardize the technique

1 Bedside Ligamentous Injections

Overview

Musculoskeletal disorders are the most common source of chronic pain experienced by American adults and the single most common reason for patients to visit their physicians [1]. Among the many types of musculoskeletal pain, lumbar and cervical spine-related pain stand out as the two most common types for which adult patients seek medical intervention [1]. One key cause of axial spine pain that is oftentimes overlooked is ligamentous pain [2]. There are many ligaments connecting vertebral bodies together and each can be a source of pain. The true incidence is unknown and

P. K. Cheng · T. M. Malik (✉)
University of California Davis Medical Center, Walnut Creek, CA, USA
e-mail: pkcheng@ucla.edu; TMuslim@dacc.uchicago.edu

D. Souza et al. (eds.), *Bedside Pain Management Interventions*,
https://doi.org/10.1007/978-3-031-11188-4_33

there are no pathognomonic clinical features or any magnetic resonance imaging findings that can definitively identify a ligament as source of pain. Diagnosis is often clinical and based on circumstantial evidence, with patients complaining of vague localized pain with or without any radiation pattern. That being said, the diagnosis of ligament-based pain can often be confirmed with a significant beneficial response to a low volume injection of local anesthetic-containing medication into the ligament itself.

2 Indications and Contraindications

Ligamentous pain occurs when a physiologic demand overwhelms structural integrity of the ligament and causes acute injury such as a tear of the ligament [3]. Normal ligament healing involves retraction of the disrupted ends of the ligament and formation of a hematoma, which is subsequently resorbed and replaced with a heavy cellular infiltrate [3]. Within this process, increased blood flow to the area brings fibroblasts that form a dense, cellular, and collagenous connective tissue matrix to bridge the torn ligament ends. As time progresses the collagenous material aligns, however, the collagen ratios remain abnormal to the point that cross-linking, innervation, fibril diameters, and vascularity all remain altered [3]. Long-term ligament injury and related chronic pain are generally due to instability persisting after routine ligament healing or failures in the steps of acute ligament healing. Chronic ligamentous pain may also have a significant inflammatory component [4].

The literature involving ligamentous pain is quite sparse however research shows distinct areas that can contribute significantly to chronic spine pain. The supraspinous and interspinous ligaments can lead to axial pain in the cervical, thoracic, and lumbar spine while atypical pain in the low back and buttock can stem from the iliolumbar ligaments [5]. Additionally, some case reports discuss ligamentous pain to be a key component of Baastrup's disease, a condition otherwise known as "kissing spine disease" [2, 6], where the spinous processes of adjacent vertebrae come in contact with one another.

The incidence of Baastrup's disease is thought to be 6.2–22.1% based on autopsy studies and though much debate exists as to where the pain originates, many theories point towards ligamentous pain or bursitis around the interspinous ligament which is compressed in this disease state. Case reports and studies accordingly demonstrate pain relief with corticosteroid injections into the interspinous ligament for patients with Baastrup's disease [2, 3, 6].

Ligamentous pain is the most common indication for ligamentous injection. The injection can be diagnostic (typically with local anesthetic only) or therapeutic (typically with local anesthetic and corticosteroid).

Contraindications for ligament injections include infection cellulitis/abscess over the site of injection, allergy to or intolerance to the injectate, including local anesthetic, corticosteroid, biologic agent, or concentrated glucose that is used for prolotherapy. Another absolute contraindication is patient refusal. Coagulopathy, including iatrogenic, and platelet dysfunction, including iatrogenic, are not contraindications to ligament injections [7].

3 Clinical Anatomy

Throughout the cervical, thoracic, lumbar, and sacral portion of the spine there exist many different ligamentous structures which stabilize the spine and join adjacent vertebral segments (see Figs. 1 and 2) [8].

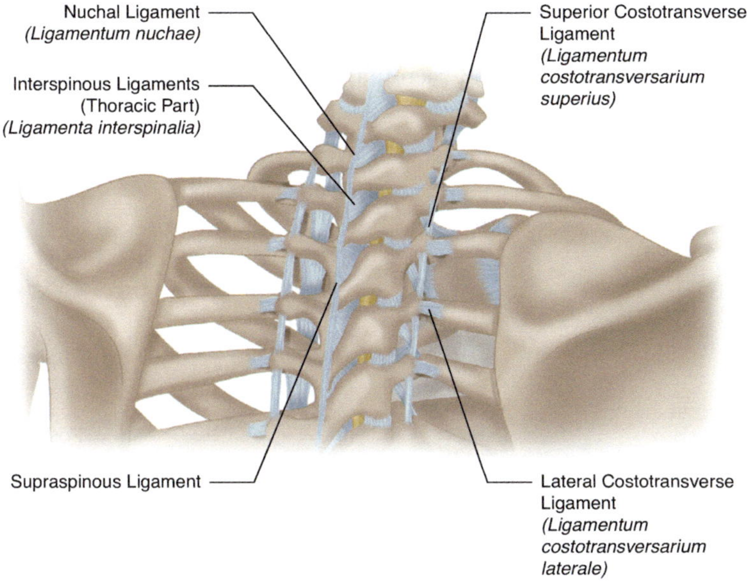

Fig. 1 Ligaments of the cervical and thoracic spine, as labeled

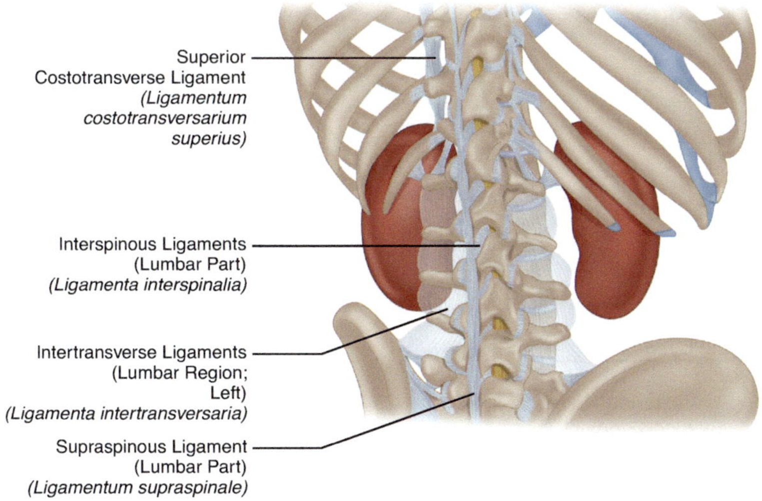

Fig. 2 Ligaments of the lumbar spine, as labeled

Running vertically along the anterior and posterior surfaces of the vertebral bodies, the anterior and posterior longitudinal ligaments re-enforce the alignment of the vertebral bodies and intervertebral discs. The triangularly shaped ligamentum flavum lines the posterior aspect of the spinal canal while the interspinous ligament and supraspinous ligament, two key targets for interventional procedures, connect adjacent spinous processes [8]. Lower down in the lumbar spine, the iliolumbar ligaments connect the iliac crest to the transverse process of L4 and L5. Further down in the sacrum, multiple ligaments exist which stabilize the sacroiliac area including the sacrotuberous ligament, sacrospinous ligament, posterior sacroiliac ligaments, dorsal sacroiliac ligament, and interosseous sacroiliac ligament (Fig. 3).

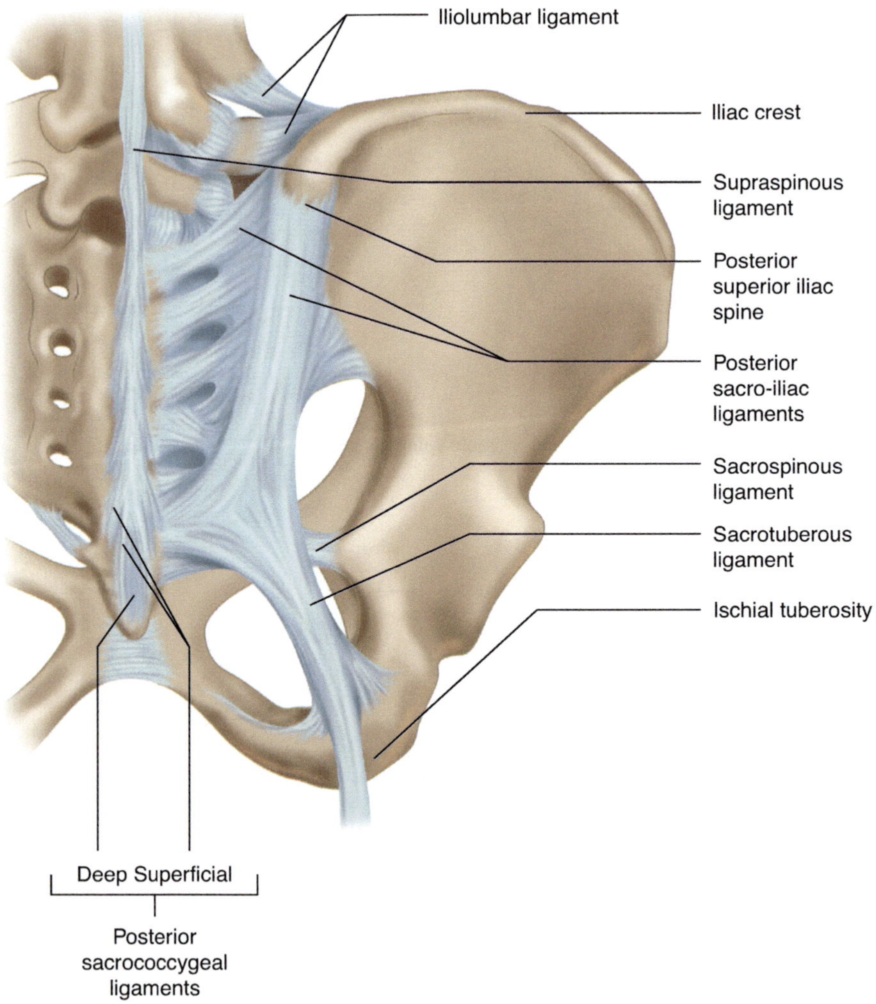

Fig. 3 Ligaments of the sacrum and pelvis, as labeled

Table 1 Equipment and supplies

Antiseptic		4% chlorhexidine or 10% povidone-iodine (Betadine)
Ultrasound probe		5–20 MHz linear probe, with sterile cover and sterile gel
Syringes		5–10 ml
Needle		22–25 gauge 1.5–3.5 in.
Injectate for hydrolocalization or hydrodissection		Normal saline or local anesthetic
Injectate	Local anesthetics	0.25–0.5% bupivacaine 0.5% Ropivacaine 1–2% lidocaine
	Corticosteroids	Triamcinolone 10–40 mg Dexamethasone 4–10 mg Methylprednisolone 80–120 mg

4 Equipment and Supplies

Ligamentous injections can be easily performed at the bedside. An antiseptic solution, typically 4% chlorhexidine, 22–25 Gauge 1.5–3.5-inch needle, 5–10 ml syringe for injectate, mask, and sterile gloves should be typically prepared for this procedure. Local anesthetic with or without corticosteroids is typically prepared for this injection as well. Other types of injectates will be discussed further in the chapter. Normal saline or local anesthetic can be utilized for ultrasound guidance during hydrolocalization. An ultrasound unit with a high-frequency linear transducer will be typically needed (Table 1).

5 Ligamentous Injections, Landmark, and Ultrasound-Guided Techniques

Ligamentous injections are usually reserved for patients that have chronic pain which persists despite a 4–8 week trial of conservative measures [7]. Usually involving corticosteroids mixed with local anesthetics, these injections can alternatively involve injection of sclerosing or regenerative substances.

These injections can be performed based on the landmark techniques, however, ultrasound guidance is recommended for these procedures as studies show that non-image guided injections are frequently placed outside the target area of treatment, and ultrasound (US) can help visualize various structures including the ligaments themselves and the surrounding muscles, tendons, and nerve tissue, vessels, and lungs allowing for a safer injection technique [7].

Ultrasound-Guided Interspinous and Supraspinous Injection

The supraspinous and interspinous ligament injection can be done throughout the cervical, thoracic, and lumbar spine however we will use the lumbar spine to demonstrate the basic technique. With the patient in seated or prone position with some flexion of the lumbar spine, use the low frequency curvilinear transducer in both the midline longitudinal orientation (see Fig. 5) and the transverse orientation (see Fig. 6) to visualize the supraspinous and interspinous ligaments. In the longitudinal midline view (see Fig. 5), the first hyperechoic line visualized is the thoracolumbar fascia and deep to this line, the spinous processes appear as a set of hyperechoic peaks. The supraspinous ligament connects the tips of spinous processes together while the interspinous ligament connects the bodies of adjacent spinous processes. These ligaments are visible in the ultrasound image as hyperechoic structures made of parallel fibrils [5]. In the midline transverse view (see Fig. 6), each individual spinous process appears as a convex hyperechoic line with posterior acoustic shadowing [5]. Cranial and caudal tilt can be used to optimize the image by moving the transducer until its angle is parallel to the corresponding spinous process and interspace. On either side and deep to the spinous process, the laminae of the vertebrae produce two horizontal hyperechoic lines with posterior acoustic shadowing and lateral to each lamina exists the facet. Though it is harder to visualize, the facet joint has a distinctive hypoechoic zone, which is the joint capsule, sandwiched between two hyperechoic bony structures [5]. Laying in the convexities of the spine formed by the lamina are the paraspinal muscles, which can be inadvertently injected if the transducer shifts away from the midline. The deep and most hyperechoic mass is the multifidus muscle while the more-superficial mass is the erector spinae muscle group, consisting of the iliocostalis, longissimus, and spinalis [5]. Interestingly, the epidural space and spinal canal may be visible in this view if the interspinous space is sufficiently wide [5].

Using an out-of-plane technique in either the longitudinal or transverse views, or toggling between the two, introduce a needle into the supraspinous or interspinous ligament. Once the needle tip is confirmed to be located into the body of the ligament, inject the solution of choice carefully under direct visualization. As ligaments are generally dense structures, significant feedback or resistance while injecting should be expected.

The technique described above can be applied to the cervical and thoracic spine as well with some key considerations (see Fig. 4).

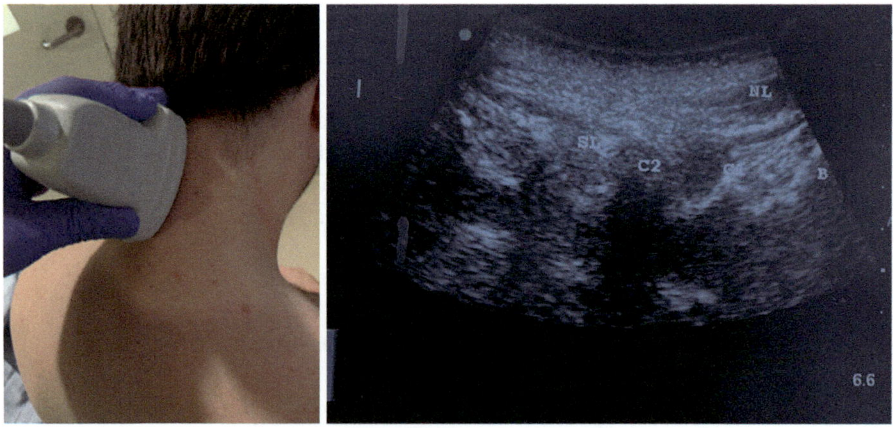

Fig. 4 Longitudinal ultrasound view of the cervical spine. Visualized are the C1 and C2 spinous processes as well as the supraspinous ligament (SL), nuchal line (NL), and the base of the skull (B)

In the cervical spine, either the low-frequency or high-frequency probe can be used for relatively thin patients. The linear high-frequency probe can provide greater resolution as the cervical vertebrae and associated ligaments are located more superficial than in the lumbar region. In the thoracic spine, the spinous processes take a sharper caudal angulation so a strong tilt on the US transducer for the transverse view is required to match that angle and better visualize the ligamentous structures.

Ultrasound-Guided Iliolumbar and Sacral Ligament Injections

Another target or ligamentous injection is the iliolumbar ligament, which connects the transverse process of L4 and L5 to the posterior portion of the iliac crest [5, 9]. With the patient in prone or seated position with some flexion of the lumbar spine, use the low frequency curvilinear transducer in the midline longitudinal and transverse orientation and with the technique described above, identify the L4 and L5 spinous processes. Then in the transverse orientation, move the transducer superior and lateral until the transverse process, which appears as a hyperechoic bony structure more superficially-located than the lamina, and the edge of the iliac crest are visualized (see Fig. 5).

The iliolumbar ligament is the narrow hyperechoic band connecting the transverse processes and iliac crest, deep to the erector spinae muscles, and it can be injected using either in-plane or out-of-plane technique [5].

The final areas for ligamentous injection are the sacral area ligaments which include the sacrotuberous ligament, sacrospinous ligament, posterior sacroiliac ligaments, dorsal sacroiliac ligament, and interosseous sacroiliac ligament (see Figs. 3 and 6).

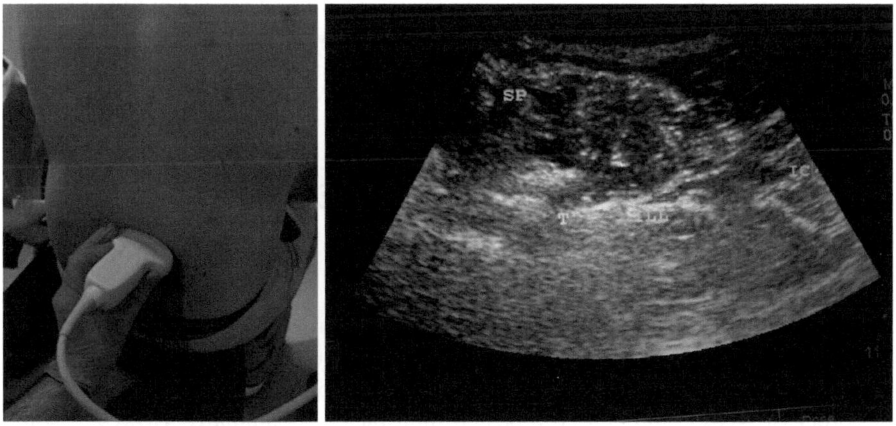

Fig. 5 Transverse ultrasound view of the iliolumbar ligament (ILL). Also visualized are the transverse process (T) and the iliac crest (IC) which serve as attachment points for the iliolumbar ligament and the spinous process (SP) of the associated lumbar vertebra

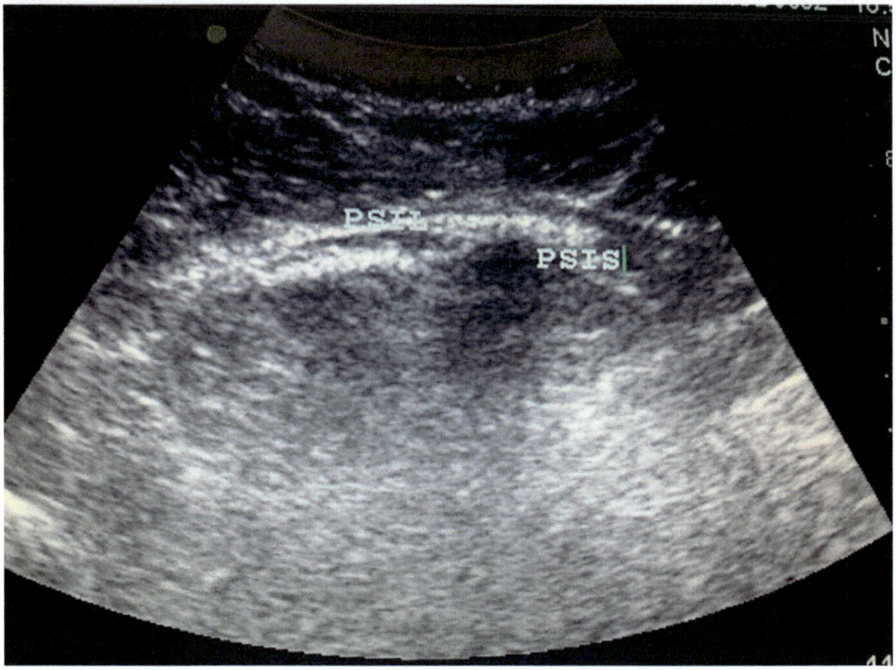

Fig. 6 Ultrasound image of the posterior longitudinal ligament (PSIL). The probe is oriented along the course of the PSIL, which is visualized attaching to the posterior superior iliac spine (PSIS)

With the patient in seated or prone position, orient the linear transducer, or curvilinear transducer for patients with larger habitus, along the course of each ligament. Just like the other ligaments described previously, the ligaments around the sacrum appear as hyperechoic bands with made of parallel fibrils. Advance a needle in the in-plane or out-of-plane technique into the body of the ligament structure and inject under direct visualization, making sure to keep superficial to the cortex of the sacrum, which will appear as a thin hyperechoic line with acoustic shadowing [5].

6 Ligamentous Injections, Various Injectates

Corticosteroids

Corticosteroids are widely used to treat the inflammatory component of chronic ligamentous pain [3, 4]. Often mixed with local anesthetics such as bupivacaine or lidocaine, the corticosteroids provide significant short-term analgesia, usually on the order of weeks, and can be repeated multiple times annually. However, some research suggests adverse effects of corticosteroids on ligament function as they can inhibit collagen synthesis and potentially weaken the ligaments of the spine in the long term [3, 6].

Prolotherapy

Prolotherapy consists of injecting an irritant or sclerotic solution into a soft tissue structure to produce a low-grade inflammatory reaction that initiates healing of the damaged tissue through stimulation of fibroblastic proliferation and collagen growth [1, 3, 10]. In its application for pain treatment, prolotherapy is thought to treat ligament laxity which is the source of chronic ligamentous pain and lead to rehabilitation of the incompetent structure [3].

Two main types of prolotherapy solution are described—hypertonic dextrose solutions and sclerosing agents. Hypertonic dextrose solutions act by dehydrating cells at the injection site leading to local tissue trauma which attracts granulocytes and macrophages to initiate the inflammatory process. Concentrations higher than 10% are used since less-concentrated solutions do not incite an inflammatory reaction [1]. Sclerosing agents, such as glycerin and phenol, are direct chemical irritants that initiate a controlled acute inflammatory response [1, 10]. Of the two, sclerosing agents are the best-studied prolotherapy agents [3].

Dating back to the 1930s, prolotherapy has been increasing in popularity over the past few decades. It has been studied for many applications of chronic musculoskeletal pain including spine pain with prolotherapy injections directed towards the supraspinous and interspinous ligament as well as the sacroiliac area ligaments [1, 3, 10]. It is important to note, however, that research differs considerably in the recommended treatment protocol, particularly the solution injected and the total number and frequency of injections [10]. The most commonly injected agent is hypertonic dextrose with volumes ranging from 1–30 ml injected a total of 1–10 times. The frequency ranges on the order of once weekly to once monthly [10]. Additionally, some protocols also describe additional steps to the prolotherapy treatment including needling of the soft tissue prior to injection of the chosen solution. Finally, adverse events are not uncommon for this procedure and include temporary increase in pain or stiffness in the target area, headache, nausea, diarrhea, vertigo, and cough [10].

Platelet-Rich Plasma

An increasingly popular modality, platelet-rich plasma (PRP) injections, have been used since 1987 for regeneration and augmentation of wound healing [3]. PRP consists of plasma containing high concentrations of platelets which is centrifuged from autologous blood obtained via venipuncture immediately prior to injection. Platelets contain a large number of key signal proteins, growth factors, chemokines, cytokines, and other bioactive factors that initiate and regulate the inflammatory cascade [3, 4] They are thought to stimulate proliferation and differentiation of mesenchymal stem cells at the injury site, such as within a ligament of the spine, and thereby cause structural healing of the ligament [3]. PRP injections are particularly useful for anatomic structures that typically receive less blood flow including ligaments, tendons, and intervertebral discs. Currently the research on PRP is more geared towards treatment of tendinopathy but there is some early evidence for use of PRP to treat ligamentous injury. That being said, much of the research involves ligaments of the knee and not the spine [3, 4].

Potential Complications

Reported adverse reactions include pain and ecchymosis at the injection site, inflammatory flare reaction, infection, vasovagal reaction, intolerance of the injectate, anaphylaxis, subcutaneous tissue atrophy from local anesthetics, or steroids, skin depigmentation, vascular dementia, pneumothorax, and nerve damage [7, 8].

Conclusion

Though the literature on this technique is in its infancy, ultrasound-guided ligamentous injection in the spine can be a useful modality through which physicians can address a significant subsect of axial back pain. It holds potential for pain relief as well as regeneration of key anatomic structures which stabilize the spine. Key target sites for intervention include the interspinous, supraspinous, and iliolumbar ligaments as well as the ligaments surrounding the sacrum. More research is needed to fully elucidate the outcomes for this type of injection and determine best practices and standard technique for this promising procedure.

References

1. Hauser RA, Lackner JB, Steilen-Matias D, Harris DK. A systematic review of dextrose Prolotherapy for chronic musculoskeletal pain. Clin Med Insights Arthritis Musculoskelet Disord. 2016;9:139–59.
2. Mitra R, Ghazi U, Kirpalani D, Cheng I. Interspinous ligament steroid injections for the management of Baastrup's disease: a case report. Arch Phys Med Rehabil. 2007;88(10):1353–6.
3. Mautner K, Blazuk J. Where do injectable stem cell treatments apply in treatment of muscle, tendon, and ligament injuries? PM R. 2015;7(4 Suppl):S33–40.
4. Paoloni J, De Vos RJ, Hamilton B, Murrell GA, Orchard J. Platelet-rich plasma treatment for ligament and tendon injuries. Clin J Sport Med. 2011;21(1):37–45.
5. Darrieutort-Laffite C, Hamel O, Glémarec J, Maugars Y, Le Goff B. Ultrasonography of the lumbar spine: sonoanatomy and practical applications. Joint Bone Spine. 2014;81(2):130–6.
6. Okada K, Ohtori S, Inoue G, Orita S, Eguchi Y, Nakamura J, et al. Interspinous ligament lidocaine and steroid injections for the Management of Baastrup's disease: a case series. Asian Spine J. 2014;8(3):260–6.
7. Inês LP, da Silva JA. Soft tissue injections. Best Pract Res Clin Rheumatol. 2005;19(3):503–27.
8. Morton D, Albertine K, Foreman B. Chapter 1 Back anatomy. The big picture: gross anatomy. 2nd ed. New York: McGraw-Hill; 2019.
9. Valat JP, Rozenberg S. Local corticosteroid injections for low back pain and sciatica. Joint Bone Spine. 2008;75(4):403–7.

10. Dagenais S, Haldeman S, Wooley JR. Intraligamentous injection of sclerosing solutions (prolotherapy) for spinal pain: a critical review of the literature. Spine J. 2005;5(3):310–28.

Further Reading

Liu W, Xie X, Wu J. Platelet-rich plasma promotes spinal ligament healing after injury. Clin Lab. 2020;66(7). https://doi.org/10.7754/Clin.Lab.2019.191154.

Paravertebral Blocks

Brian L. Hom, Scott Masson, and Ankit Maheshwari

Essential Concepts

- The paravertebral block is a bedside pain intervention that involves injecting local anesthetic in the paravertebral space to treat acute and chronic pain originating from the chest or abdomen.
- Paravertebral blocks can be performed in the thoracic or lumbar region of the spine.
- Paravertebral blocks may be performed using a traditional landmark technique. However, the ultrasound technique has several advantages including greater precision and therefore, less complications.
- Complications are relatively low. Most common complications may include hypotension, vascular puncture, pleural puncture, pneumothorax, injection of local anesthetic into intravascular, epidural, or intrathecal space.

1 Paravertebral Blocks

Overview

The paravertebral block is a technique that was first performed in the early 1900s for thoracic surgeries but fell out of favor from the 1950s to 1970s. The technique is primarily used as an adjunct therapy for pain but has been used as a sole anesthetic in certain cases. The technique is easily performed at the bedside with either traditional (landmark based) or ultrasound technique. Lumbar paravertebral blocks are similar to thoracic paravertebral blocks, but are less commonly used in clinical practice. There are anatomic differences in the lumbar and thoracic paravertebral spaces which affect the procedural technique. Lumbar and thoracic paravertebral blocks

B. L. Hom (✉) · S. Masson · A. Maheshwari
University Hospitals/Case Western Reserve University, Cleveland, OH, USA

D. Souza et al. (eds.), *Bedside Pain Management Interventions*,
https://doi.org/10.1007/978-3-031-11188-4_34

can be used in combination (i.e., thoracolumbar paravertebral block) depending on the indication and dermatomal coverage requirements.

Indications and Contraindications

Paravertebral blocks may be used for a variety of procedures as described in Table 1 below.

The most common use of the thoracic paravertebral block is for postoperative analgesia for breast surgery, thoracic surgery, rib fractures, and nephrectomy. Thoracic paravertebral blocks (TPVB) may be preferred over thoracic epidurals when minimization of hypotension is desired. Unilateral paravertebral technique preserves respiratory and sympathetic function on the contralateral side and reduces hypotension compared to thoracic epidural [1]. Lumbar paravertebral blocks are typically used in combination with TPVB (T10 through L2) for surgical anesthesia

Table 1 Indications for Thoracic and/or Lumbar Paravertebral Blocks[2]

Anesthesia
Breast surgery
Heniorrhaphy (thoracolumbar anesthesia)
Chest wound exploration
Adjunct therapy for pain regimen post operatively
Thoracotomy
Thoracoabdominal esophageal surgery
Video-assisted thoracoscopic surgery
Renal surgery
Breast surgery
Cholecystectomy
Liver resection
Appendectomy
Cardiac surgery
Chronic pain management
Benign and malignant neuralgia
Cancer pain
Complex regional pain syndrome
Other
Postherpetic neuralgia
Thoracoabdominal neuralgia
Pleuritic chest pain
Rib fractures
Hyperhydrosis
Liver capsule pain after blunt abdominal trauma

Table 2 Contraindications to Paravertebral Blocks [2, 3]

Absolute contraindications
Infection at injection site
Allergy to local anesthetic
Empyema
Neoplastic mass occupying paravertebral space
Patient refusal
Relative contraindications
Coagulopathy
Bleeding disorder
Patient taking anticoagulation medication
Abnormal thoracic anatomy (i.e., kyphosis)

during inguinal herniorrhaphy. It may be beneficial as rescue block in patients with severe pain after total hip replacement. It may also be used for diagnostic purposes during evaluation of groin or genital pain, such as nerve entrapment syndrome after inguinal herniorrhaphy. Contraindications for paravertebral blocks are similar for thoracic and lumbar paravertebral blocks as listed in Table 2.

Clinical Anatomy

The thoracic paravertebral space (TPS) is a wedged shaped, extra-pleural, potential space located on bilateral sides of the spinal column. It is defined posteriorly by the superior costotransverse ligament, anterolaterally by parietal pleura, medially by the vertebra and intervertebral foramen, and inferiorly and superiorly by the heads of the ribs [2]. The TPS contains adipose tissue and within it contains the intercostal (spinal) nerve, dorsal ramus, intercostal vessels, gray rami communicantes, and anteriorly, the sympathetic chain. The spinal nerves are bundled, but lie freely in the adipose tissue, making them susceptible to local anesthetic solutions (Fig. 1).

The lumbar paravertebral space (LPS) borders include the psoas major muscle anterolaterally, vertebral bodies and intervertebral discs medially, and the transverse process and ligaments connecting adjacent transverse processes posteriorly [3]. The LPS is primarily occupied by the psoas major muscle. The psoas muscle is separated by a thin fascia into two parts near the vertebral body. The target of the injection is within this fascial layer, which is where the spinal nerve roots lie in conjunction with the ascending lumbar veins. A lumbar paravertebral block produces ipsilateral dermatomal anesthesia by direct effect on lumbar spinal nerves and medial extension into epidural space by the intervertebral foramen.

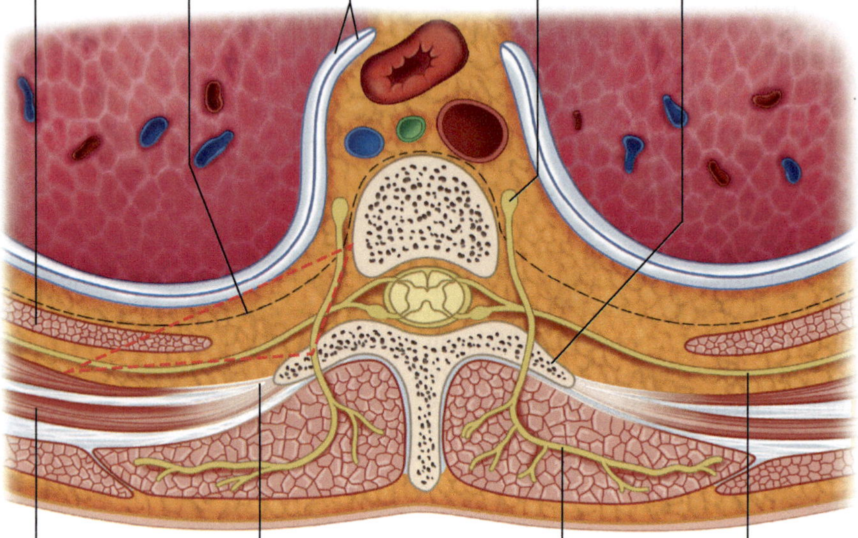

Fig. 1 Horizontal Cross section of Thoracic Paravertebral Space· as labeled

Equipment and Supplies

Thoracic and lumbar paravertebral blocks are easily performed at the bedside. Standard monitors including ECG, pulse oximeter, and blood pressure cuff should be used to monitor the patient throughout the block. Mild sedation, with either a benzodiazepine or opioid, while not preferable, could potentially be employed for patient comfort. The sedation would require appropriate monitoring.

Materials required to perform paravertebral blocks include an ultrasound with a linear or curvilinear transducer, Tuohy needles, and local anesthetic solution. Anesthetic solution should be chosen based on duration of analgesia desired from the blockade. Commonly used local anesthetics include 2% lidocaine, 0.5–0.75% ropivacaine, and 0.5% bupivacaine. About 20 mL of the chosen anesthetic will be required to perform either the single injection or multiple injection technique (Table 3).

Table 3 Required supplies for Paravertebral Blocks

Syringe	10 mL syringe
Needle	25 gauge needle for skin infiltration with short acting local anesthetic 18–20 gauge echogenic Tuohy needle
Anesthetic	0.25–0.5% bupivacaine ± epinephrine 1–2% lidocaine 0.5–0.75% Ropivacaine

2 Paravertebral Block, Landmark Technique

Paravertebral blocks are typically performed in the sitting position, due to better visualization of surface anatomy. The spine should be curved into a kyphotic position. They may also be performed prone or lateral as well. Palpate the superior and inferior border of the scapula. The superior border of the scapula approximates to T3 and the inferior border approximates the T7 vertebrae. Palpation of the spinous processes from these landmarks to the target level is best to determine entry site in a cranial/caudad direction. After identifying the cranial/caudal level in question, skin markings are made about 2.5 cm lateral to midline. A 18–20 gauge Tuohy needle is inserted perpendicular to skin and advanced until contact is made with the transverse process. Afterwards, withdraw the needle and direct it caudally approximately 1 cm. Loss of resistance may be felt after the needle penetrates the costotransverse ligament. Aspirate the needle and make sure there is no CSF, blood, or air. If negative aspiration, inject local anesthetic in 3–5 mL aliquots with aspiration in between until the target volume of 15–20 mL is administered [3, 4]. The depth of the transverse process is difficult to assess with the landmark technique.

- Similar to thoracic paravertebral blocks, lumbar paravertebral blocks can be performed in the sitting, lateral, or prone position. The iliac crest corresponds to the L3-L4 interspace. Skin markings are made 2.5 cm lateral to midline at the levels to be blocked. An 18–20 gauge Tuohy needle is used. The most common method is a fixed distance technique where the needle is advanced by a predetermined distance of about 1.5–2.0 cm beyond the transverse process. The block needle is inserted perpendicular to skin until transverse process is contacted. Depth of the transverse process varies by patient body type. After the transverse process is contacted, note the depth on the needle and advance 1.5–2.0 cm beyond the previously marked depth. Withdraw the needle to subcutaneous tissue and reinsert either 10–15 degrees superior or inferior so that it slides off the edge of the transverse process. Aspirate and monitor for blood or CSF. Inject local anesthetic after negative aspiration. Target volume at this level is similar to TPVB, approximately 10–15 mL. While paravertebral block can be performed utilizing the landmark-based technique, ultrasound-guided technique would be a preferable option for this procedure.

3 Ultrasound Technique

The ultrasound technique has several advantages over the traditional technique. It allows precision through visualization of the needle and reduction in complications. Identify spinous processes C7 to T7. Orient the ultrasound transducer with linear array in the parasagittal plane adjacent to the spine. Identify the transverse process, head of the rib, costotransverse ligament and pleura. The bright white line at the bottom of the image indicates the pleura. (Figs. 2 and 3) Between the pleura and transverse processes is the paravertebral space. The paravertebral space may be approached in the parasagittal plane caudal to cephalad or lateral to medial in the transverse plane [2].

- Insert the needle at a 45-degree angle. Note the approximate distance of paravertebral space on ultrasound to guide depth of needle insertion. Insert the needle until it reaches the transverse process. Redirect the needle through the costotransverse ligament into the paravertebral space. Visualize the needle in plane to avoid advancement into the pleura. Inject local anesthetic and observe downward displacement of the pleura. A single injection or multiple injection technique may be used, depending on the extent of the block. In the multiple injection technique, injections occur in alternate levels (T2/4/6 or T3/5/7). Multiple injection technique produces more reliable radiographic and clinical distribution compared to a single injection technique [5]. However, single shot technique may be

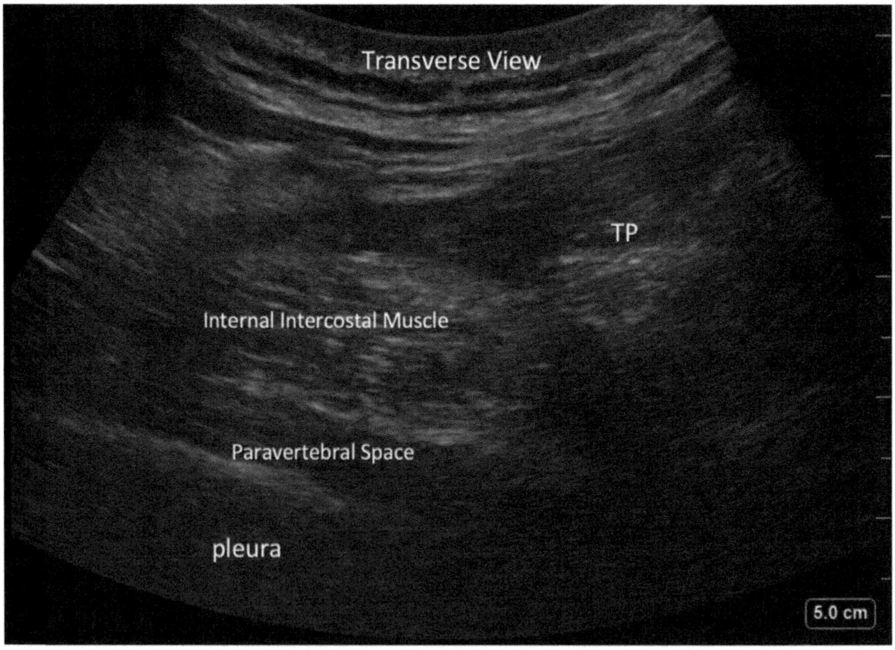

Fig. 2 Transverse view of paravertebral space. Ultrasonogram, as labeled TP-transverse process

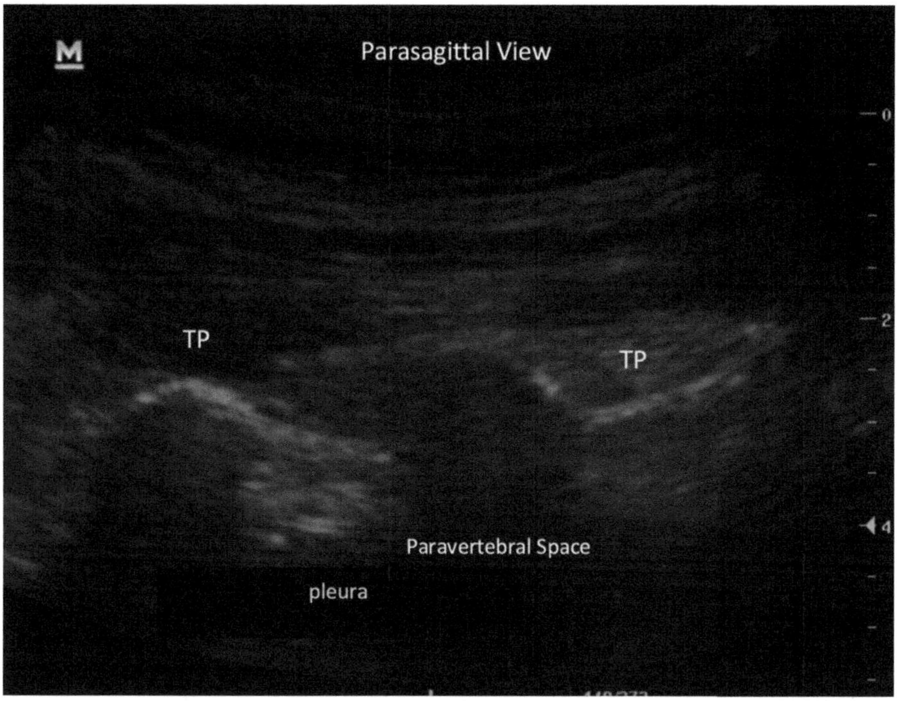

Fig. 3 Ultrasound parasagittal view of the paravertebral space, as labeled TP-transverse process

sufficient for postoperative analgesia or chronic pain. Inject 3–5 mL at each level for multiple injection technique. For the single injection technique, a larger volume of local anesthetic may be injected. Inject 15–20 mL in 5 mL increments with aspiration between injections. The sensory distribution will typically cover four to five dermatomes this volume. Visualize the spread of local anesthetic caudad and cephalad on ultrasound.

4 Potential Complications and Adverse Effects

Overall, complications are relatively low. They vary from 2.6% to 5% [4, 6]. The most common complications include hypotension (4.6%), vascular puncture (3.8%), pleural puncture (1.1%), and pneumothorax (0.5%). Paravertebral blocks are reported to have fewer minor complications such as hypotension, nausea, vomiting, and urinary retention without a difference in mortality or length of stay than thoracic epidurals [1]. Failure of paravertebral blocks in adults is estimated at 10.1% [7]. Hypotension is rare in euvolemic patients if the block is performed unilaterally because sympathetic function is preserved on the contralateral side. However, paravertebral blocks should still be used in caution in patients who are hemodynamically unstable because there is some risk of hypovolemia.

Pleural puncture is a potentially serious complication of thoracic paravertebral blocks. Signs that suggest pleural puncture may be significant loss of resistance after the needle enters the chest cavity, cough, sharp chest or shoulder pain, or sudden hyperventilation. Air cannot be aspirated through the needle unless the lung is also punctured or there is air in the pleural cavity. Pneumothorax may be delayed in onset and an early chest radiograph may not detect it. Systemic local anesthetic toxicity can occur due to inadvertent intravascular injection or from using large dose of local anesthetic. Dosage should be adjusted in elderly and frail patients. An epinephrine containing local anesthetic solution may be useful for early recognition of intravascular injection and reduce absorption of local anesthetic into the systemic circulation. Inadvertent epidural, subdural, or intrathecal injection and spinal anesthesia can occur. This is more likely when the needle is directed medially. Aspiration test should be performed before injection. Local anesthetic can spread cephalad to the stellate ganglion or to the preganglionic fibers of the first few segments of thoracic spinal cord. Bilateral Horner's syndrome has been reported likely due to epidural spread or prevertebral spread to contralateral stellate ganglion.

Contraindications for lumbar paravertebral block is similar to thoracic paravertebral blocks. Perform with caution in patients on anticoagulation due to risk of psoas hematoma with lumbar plexopathy. It is possible to inject local anesthetic into intravascular, epidural, or intrathecal spaces during LPVB, especially if the needle is directed medially. Monitor to ensure needle is perpendicular to skin. Intraperitoneal injection or visceral injury (kidney) could occur if there was significant technical error. Motor weakness may develop if L2 spinal nerve is blocked (femoral nerve L2-L4), resulting in quadriceps weakness.

Clinical and Technical Pearls

- Awareness of needle tip location is essential to avoid pleural puncture or entry into the intervertebral foramen.
- Anterior displacement of parietal pleura indicates correct needle tip location in all ultrasound guided TVPB techniques
- Injecting saline can be useful to help assess proper needle tip location when anatomy on ultrasound is unclear
- Signs of pleural puncture may be significant loss of resistance after the needle enters the chest cavity, cough, sharp chest or shoulder pain, or sudden hyperventilation

References

1. Yeung JH, Gates S, Naidu BV, Wilson MJ, Gao smith F. Paravertebral block versus thoracic epidural for patients undergoing thoracotomy. Cochrane Database Syst Rev. 2016;2:CD009121.
2. Butterworth JF, Mackey DC, Wasnick JD. Morgan & Mickhails clinical anesthesiology. New York: McGraw-Hill Education; 2018.
3. New York School of Regional Anesthesia. Thoracic and lumbar paravertebral block-landmarks and nerve stimulator technique. NYSORA website. 2019. https://www.nysora.com/

regional-anesthesia-for-specific-surgical-procedures/abdomen/thoracic-lumbar-paravertebral-block/. Accessed 15 Oct 2019.
4. Ng SC, Chazapis M, West S. Regional anaesthesia tutorial 376: ultrasound-guided paravertebral block. World Federation of Societies of Anaesthesiologists (WFSA). https://www.wfsahq.org/components/com_virtual_library/media/fa1ae6b5c25ab584b61583890f28655f-atow-376-00-01.pdf. Accessed 3 Apr 2018.
5. Harmon D, Barrett J. Paravertebral block. https://aneskey.com/paravertebral-block-2/ 28 July 2016. Accessed 15 Oct 2019.
6. Coveney E, Weltz CR, Greengrass R, et al. Use of paravertebral block anesthesia in the surgical management of breast cancer: experience in 156 cases. Ann Surg. 1998;227(4):496–501.
7. Lonnqvist PA, MacKenzie J, Soni AK, Conacher ID. Paravertebral blockade. Failure rate and complications. Anaesthesia. 1995;50(9):813–5.

Further Reading

Helander EM, Webb MP, Kendrick J, Montet T, Kaye AJ, Cornett EM, Kaye AD. PECS, serratus plane, erector spinae, and paravertebral blocks: a comprehensive review. Best Pract Res Clin Anaesthesiol. 2019;33(4):573–81. https://doi.org/10.1016/j.bpa.2019.07.003; Epub 2019 Jul 17.

Interfascial Plane Blocks

Serkan Tulgar and Hesham Elsharkawy

Essential Concepts

- Interfascial plane blocks are a recently described ultrasound-technique with expanding indications for acute on chronic pain.
- The target for interfasical plane blocks are peripheral nerves that typically travel in the interfascial plane.
- Ultrasonography allows for direct visualization during the procedure resulting in a lower complication rate.

1 Overview

Interfascial plane blocks (IPB) were first defined as blind techniques used for post-operative analgesia but have since transformed into ultrasound-guided(USG) techniques that are safe and easy to perform [1, 2]. "Fascia" is an anatomical term that defines a spectrum of undifferentiated mesenchymal tissues that act like a packing material wrapped around organs and tissues of the body. Fascia has mechanical properties and also serves as an exoskeleton. It plays an important role in venous return, perception of movement and position of the body via proprioceptors, and transmission of muscle force. Importantly, it plays a role in the pathophysiology of pain because of its rich innervation. There are two types of fascia: superficial and deep. Superficial fascia can be seen as a cutaneous muscle layer found in mammals. The fascia serves as part of the exteroceptive system that responds to stimuli from

S. Tulgar
Department of Anesthesiology and Reanimation, Faculty of Medicine, Samsun Training and Research Hospital, Samsun University, Samsun, Turkey

H. Elsharkawy (✉)
Department of Anesthesiology, Pain and Healing Center, MetroHealth, Case Western Reserve University, Cleveland, OH, USA

D. Souza et al. (eds.), *Bedside Pain Management Interventions*,
https://doi.org/10.1007/978-3-031-11188-4_35

outside the body. This feature relates to the ample amount of nerve fibers that adhere to the fascia on bony prominences and at various ligamentous folds.

Additionally, muscles give fascial insertions into the deep fascia that cause the deep fascia to stretch upon contraction [3]. Deep fascia surrounds all muscles, ligaments, and aponeuroses and is typically named according to the anatomic location of its respective muscle group. After separating from the nerve roots, nerves generally course between the fasciae of two muscles. Interfascialplane nerve blocks do not target nerves directly as peripheral nerves blocks do. These blocks work only if enough volume of local anesthetic (LA) is injected into the interfascial space. These procedures lead to the relaxation of muscles in the case of nerve entrapment syndromes. Aside from neuropathic pain, other types of pain, such as myofascial pain, can also be relieved by IPB. Hydrodissection performed as a part of the block can also lead to relief of myofascial pain due to the effect of the IPB on fascial adhesions [4]. Other mechanisms include the spread of local anesthetics proximally and distally along the peripheral nerves, sympathetic blockade, neuraxial spread, systemic LA absorption, and placebo effect.

Domingo et al. [5] reported the anatomical-histological features and clinical success of (LA) application between the trapezius muscle and the levator scapula or rhomboid major muscles for the treatment of myofascial pain. This report was the first to present ultrasound-guided IPB for chronic pain. After that, IPB was reported to relieve chronic pain associated with various painful head, neck, and back conditions. Shortly after discovering the clinical value of USG IPB, these procedures become a common way to help patients with acute and chronic pain. Ultrasound-guided interfascial plane blocks were recently described and continue to evolve. As with some other procedures, clinicians don't have a complete consensus regarding the technique, volume, content, and application level [6–9]. Erector spinae plane block (ESPB) is a commonly performed IPB. This block will be discussed in detail below. The other IPBs will be presented briefly due to the limited scope of this chapter. More about IPBs can be found in the "additional reading" section at the end of this chapter.

2 Erector Spinae Plane Block

Anatomy

Erector spinae muscles (ESM) are a group of muscles that keep the body erect and are formed by the spinalis (multifidus), longissimus, and iliocostalis muscles in the cervical, thoracic and lumbar areas. Deep to the ESM is an interfascial plane between the transverse vertebral process and the ESM, in which the application of LA is termed an erector spinae plane block (ESPB). Although ESPB application is defined as applying LA in the interfascial plane between the ESM muscle and the transverse process, the target of the needle is not the transverse process. Injecting just under the ESM muscle between the intertransverse ligament and the ESM muscle is acceptable, assuming that the craniocaudal spread can be verified sonographically. ESPB targets the branches of both the dorsal and ventral rami of the spinal nerves. While the dorsal rami of spinal nerves give rise to lateral and medial branches in the thoracic vertebral levels, they give rise to the lateral, medial, and intermediate branches at the lumbar level [10]. If the goal is to block only the dorsal ramus for analgesic purposes, injected LA volume should be less than with typical ESPB for postoperative analgesia. The concern is the possibility of the remote spread, including craniocaudal, with the large volume of local anesthetic. It can also spread into the ventral rami and neuroaxis [11–13].

The greater occipital nerve is formed by the dorsal ramus of the second cervical spinal nerve (C2) with variable contributions from the C1, C3, and C4 nerve roots. The dorsal ramus of the C3 forms the third occipital nerve. The lesser occipital nerve originates from the lateral branch of the ventral ramus of C2 and sometimes branches from C3. Theoretically, the ESP in the upper cervical area can block the dorsal and ventral rami that form the occipital nerves. Further research of the ESPB for head and neck pain would be beneficial.

Indications and Contraindications

The erector spinae plane block can be performed at various vertebral levels. Myofascial pain and tension headaches that are not responding to conventional treatment modalities are potential indications for cervical and upper thoracic ESPB [14–16]. These blocks have also been used for low back pain [17]. These procedures also have been used for cluneal nerve entrapment and lumbosacral radiculopathies [18–20]. IPB can be used in the lumbosacral region with high volumes of local anesthetic. In our opinion, the IPB can be used when transforaminal epidural injections are challenging. The spread of LA has been confirmed with MRI-demonstrating ipsilateral and contralateral epidural spread [21].

The interfascial plane block is contraindicated in patients with local or systemic infection, allergy, or intolerance to injectate's components. The patient's refusal is an absolute contraindication as well. Anticoagulation, including iatrogenic and platelet dysfunction, including iatrogenic, are typically not contraindications for these procedures. However, a careful review of the case should be performed, followed by a detailed discussion with the patient.

Equipment

Although a blind ESPB has been reported, the USG ESPB is safer and should be preferred. A high-frequency linear ultrasound transducer for the thoracic levels and low-frequency curvilinear transducers for the lumbar and sacral regions may be used. A 1.5–3.5 inch needle, 10–20 mL syringe, LA solution (0.25–0.5% bupivacaine, 0.2% ropivacaine, or 1–2% lidocaine) with or without corticosteroid are typically used. The same types of injectate are recommended for other IPBs.

Technique

The level of the block must be carefully considered to match the indication. Indications and application levels are shown in Table 1, and the probe and needle positioning and the ultrasonograms are presented in Fig. 1.

The USG transducer is placed 2.5–3 cm lateral of the spinous process in the thoracic level, 4–6 cm lateral to the spinous process in the lumbar levels in the lateral parasagittal plane in order to visualize the transverse process. After identifying the transverse process and ESM superficial to the transverse processes, LA is administered between the transverse process and the ESM. The needle may be advanced using in-plane or out-of-plane techniques. While many authors suggest cephalad to caudal in-plane approach, the out-of-plane technique may be used.

Table 1 Samples of published cases in erector spinae plane block for head, neck and back pain

Reference	Indication	Level of the injection	Medications	Comments
Ueshima and Otaka [16]	Tension headache - two patients	Thoracic (T4)	15 mL of 0.25% levobupivacaine, bilaterally	Null
Tulgar et al. [14]	Lower cervical and interscapular myofascial pain, one patient	Thoracic (T3)	Bilaterally, (10 mL 0.5% bupivacaine, 5 mL 2% lidocaine and 8 mL isotonic NaCl and 40 mg/2 mL methylprednisolone)	8w followup, NRS:0/10
Piraccini et al. [15]	Myofascial pain in the right dorsal paravertebral region from T4 to T11	Thoracic (T8)	Levobupivacaine 45 mg and triamcinolone 40 mg within 15 mL of normal saline	We weekly repeated the injection 2 more times. The NRS decreased to 2 and the patient was able to start a satisfactory physiotherapy and return to the previous work
Schwarts et al. [22]	Discogenic low back pain L3-L4, L4-L5, L5-S1 One patient	Lumbar (L4?)	The total injectate consisted of, 30 mL of 0.2% ropivacaine was mixed with 5 mg of preservative free dexamethasone. (bilaterally)	80 percent pain relief over a 6-week period
Piraccini et al. [19]	L5 radicular pain -one patient	Sacral (S2)	15 mL of solution containing ropivacaine 30 mg and triamcinolone 40 mg	NRS:0 after injection and <4 for first 7 days
Celik et al. [21]	L3–4 and L4–5 discopatie -one patient	Lumbar (L4)	20 mL bupivacaine, 10 mL lidocaine, 8.6 mL saline, 40 mg/mL methylprednisolone 1 mL, and 0.4 mL gadobutrol	NRS ≤3/10 8w after injection, MRI demonstrated contrast in epidural area

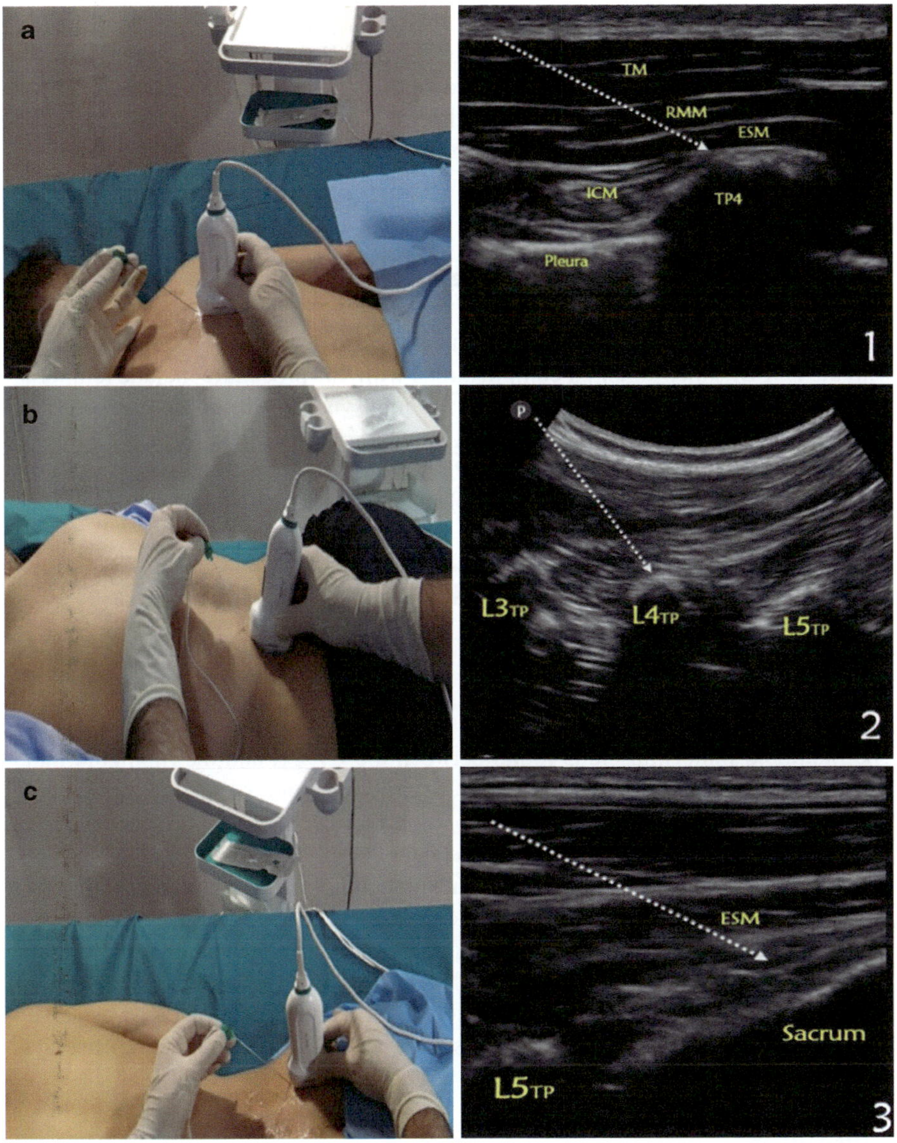

Fig. 1 Probe and needle positioning for erector spinae plane blocks (ESPB) at different vertebral levels. (**a**) Thoracic ESPB with ultrasonogram on the right. (**b**) Lumbar ESPB with ultrasonogram on the right. (**c**) Sacral ESPB with ultrasonogram on the right. *TM* trapezius muscle. *RMM* rhomboid major muscle. *ESM* erector spinae muscles. *ICM* intercostal muscles. *T* thoracic vertebrae. *L* lumbar vertebrae. Arrows: needle directions and injection targets

Tulgar and Aksu described additional, other than parasagittal approaches [7]. In Tulgar's approach, some of the LA during lumbar ESPB is injected deep to, and into the intertransverse ligament. In Aksu's approach, the transverse scan (Shamrock technique) is used with the patient in the lateral position for lumbar ESPB. In sacral ESPB, the transducer is placed on the sacrum on the transverse or sagittal plane, and the LA is injected between the intermediate sacral crest and ESM and ligaments.

Potential Complications and Adverse Effects

Pneumothorax, motor weakness, minor and advanced LA toxicity have been reported with the ESPB. Other potential complications with this procedure include temporary dizziness, disorientation, priapism, and Harlequin syndrome resulting from the T2–3 inadvertent sympathetic block [7, 23]. No nerve injury has been reported. Although bleeding was not described with the ESPB, special attention should be exercised in patients with coagulation problems, antiplatelet and anticoagulant use.

3 Rhomboid Block (RB) and Rhomboid: Sub Serratus Plane Block (RSS)

Anatomy

The rhomboid minor muscle is found between the C7-T1, and the rhomboid major muscle is located between the T2–5 spinous processes and the medial aspect of the scapula. In some cases, it can be seen as a single blended muscle instead. Local anesthetic, injected into the fascial plane between the rhomboid muscles and the intercostal muscles over the ribs, blocks the lateral cutaneous branches of intercostal nerves. It also blocks the dorsal rami via dorsolateral LA spread [8, 24]. Dermatomal coverage is generally limited to T2-T7. The application of LA between the serratus and intercostal muscles below the scapula at the 7th–8th rib level is termed "sub-serratus block." When combined with rhomboid block, it is called "rhomboid intercostal- sub-serratus plane block." It typically provides good T2 to T10–11 dermatome coverage.

Indications

The rhomboid block was first described in a letter to the editor with a case presentation of a patient with multiple rib fractures that improved after the rhomboid block [25]. The authors of the case report also presented a cadaver dissection. Later on, a case series was published with the description of RS. Rhomboid block and RSS were utilized in thoracic and abdominal surgeries and myofascial pain syndromes [4, 8, 26]. Contraindications are the same as for the ESPB.

Equipment and Technique

Similar equipment are used in RISS and ESPB. The in-plane cephalad to caudal approach have been described (Fig. 2).

The transducer is placed adjacent to the medial edge of the scapula at the T5–6 level, and LA is injected between the rhomboid muscle and the rib. At the T7–8 level, the transducer is positioned obliquely at the lower corner of the scapula. When LA is applied between the serratus muscle and the rib, it is defined as the subserratus component of the RSS. The volume may be lower when compared to ESPB. 10–15 mL of LA could be used depending on the targetted dermatomes. We consider this procedure a safe and effective technique for treating myofascial pain in the interscapular area. The potential complications and adverse effects are the same as with ESBP.

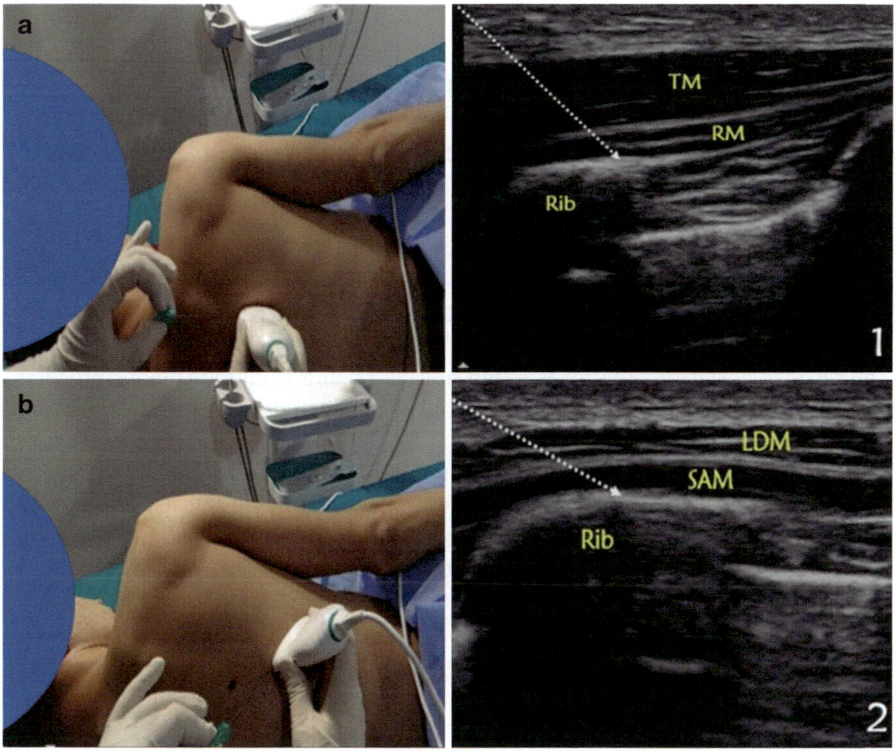

Fig. 2 Probe and needle positioning for rhomboid and subserratus blocks. (**a**) Probe and needle positioning for the rhomboid block with ultrasonogram on the right. (**b**) Probe and needle positioning for subserratus block. *TM* trapezius muscle. *RM* rhomboid major muscle. *LDM* latissimus dorsi muscle. *SAM* serratus anterior muscle. Arrows: needle directions and targets for the injection

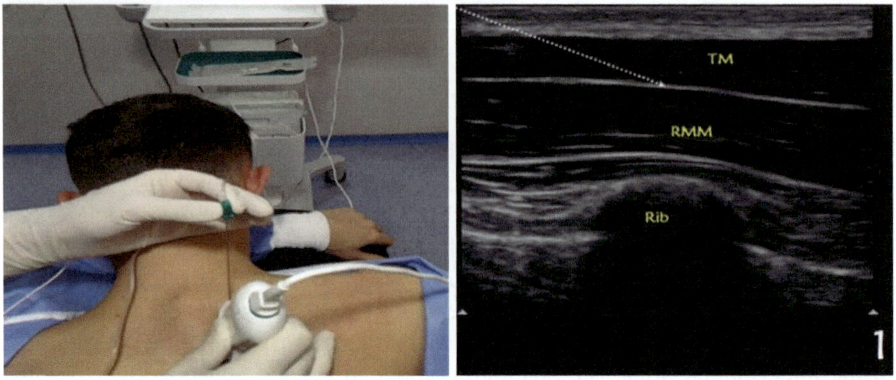

Fig. 3 Probe and needle positioning for trapezius muscle plane block. Probe and needle positioning for trapezius muscle plane block (on the left) with ultrasonogram on the right. *TM* trapezius muscle. *RM* rhomboid muscle. Arrow: needle directions and targets for the injection

4 Trapezius Muscle Plane Block

This block was the first ultrasound-guided intrafascial plane block reported [5]. Indications include relevant myofascial pain syndromes, especially associated with adhesions. (Fig. 3).

5 Serratus Posterior superior Muscle Plane block

The serrates posterior superior is a thin muscle arising from the spinous processes of the C7-T2 that inserts laterally to the 2nd - 5th rib angles. This muscle is a common source of myofascial pain [27].

The linear transducer is placed on the upper border of the scapula in the sagittal position, and the 1st - 3rd ribs are to be visualized. Following visualization of the trapezius, rhomboid major and serratus posterior superior muscles, LA is injected between the rhomboid muscle and serratus posterior superior muscle. This block can be applied using the in-plane or out-of-plane techniques using 15 mL of LA (Fig. 4).

This block can be used in myofascial pain of the interscapular area, the lateral branches of the dorsal ramus of the upper thoracic nerves, and presumably the dorsal scapular nerve are blocked [28].

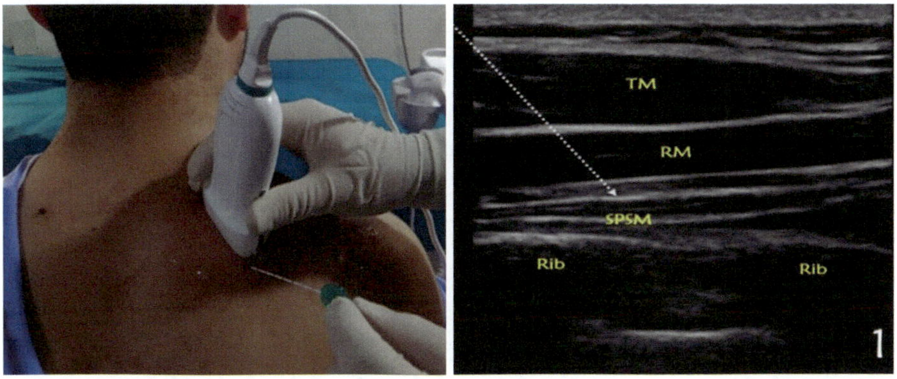

Fig. 4 Probe and needle positioning for serratus posterior superior muscle plane block. Probe and needle positioning for serratus posterior superior muscle plane block (on the left) with ultrasonogram on the right. *TM* trapezius muscle. *RM* rhomboid muscle. *SPSM* serratus posterior superior muscle. Arrow: needle directions and targets for the injection

6 Thoracolumbar Interfascial Plane Block

Thoracolumbar interfascial plane block (TLIP) was first described by Hand et al. [29]. In this block, LA is applied between the multifidus and longissimus muscles, blocking the thoracolumbar nerves' dorsal ramus. This technique was later modified by Ahiskalioglu et al. They recommended spreading LA between the longissimus and iliocostalis muscles which was shown to produce similar clinical effects [30, 31]. The authors suggest that modified TLIP is easier to perform and has less risk for neuraxial puncture.

Equipment and Technique

A linear probe is typically used for ultrasound guidance, and the depth and acquisition are adjusted for optimal image quality. The first step is to visualize the spinous process at the L3 level. Then, the probe is slid in a lateral direction to visualize the multifidus, longissimus, and iliocostalis muscles. A needle should be inserted between the longissimus and iliocostalis muscles' planes after advancing the needle at a 15° angle in a medial to lateral direction for modified TLIP block (Fig. 5). We recommend using the in-plane technique. This block can be an effective tool for managing chronic lower back pain [32].

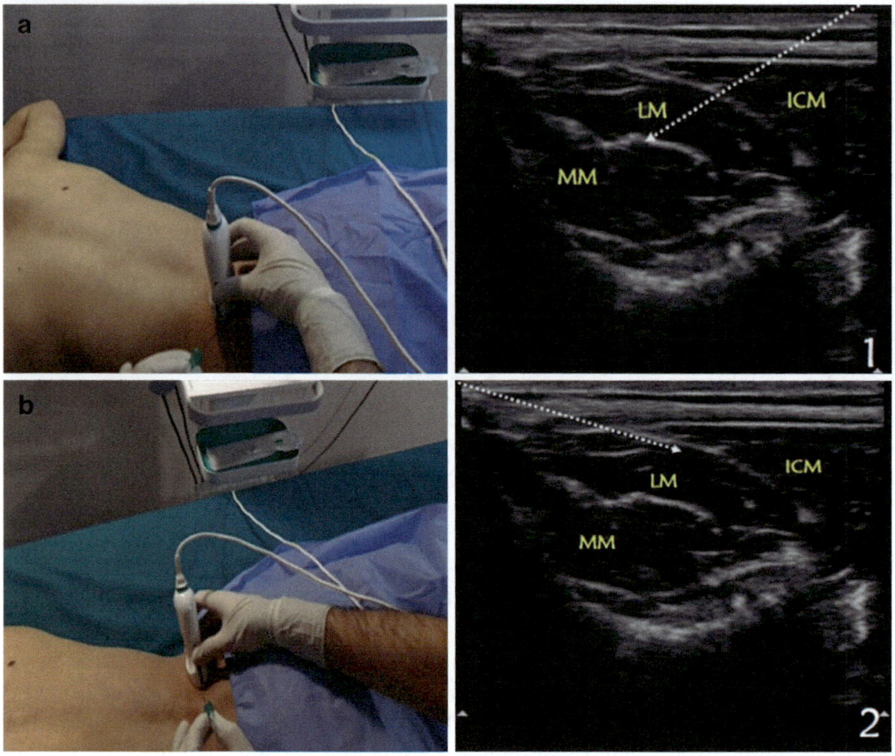

Fig. 5 Probe and needle positioning for thoracolumbar interfascial plane block (TLIP). (**a**) Probe and needle positioning for the thoracolumbar interfascial plane block with ultrasonogram on the right. (**b**) Probe and needle positioning for the modified thoracolumbar interfascial plane block with ultrasonogram on the right. *MM* multifidus muscle. *LM* latissimus muscle. *ICM* iliocostalis muscles. Arrows: needle directions and injection targets

7 Lumbosacral Interfascial Plane block

Superior cluneal nerve (SCN) entrapment in thoracolumbar fascia and other low back interfascial planes are frequently overlooked causes of low back pain (LBP). The superior cluneal nerve originates from the dorsal branches of T12-L3 nerve roots. The incidence of SCN entrapment is 1.6–14% of causes of LBP [31]. The true incidence of SCN entrapment is unknown, probably because it is frequently mistakenly associated with other pathologies [33]. While lumbosacral interfascial plane block was previously performed based on the anatomic landmarks, the USG procedure has recently been reported [34]. Although this technique was reported as an accessory block for hip surgery, it is thought to be effective in chronic back pain without radiculopathy[35]. The subfascial position between the erector spinae muscle and the posterior layer of the thoracolumbar fascia under the lattissimus dorsi muscle is injected with 10 mL of LA to target their SCN (Fig. 6) [34]

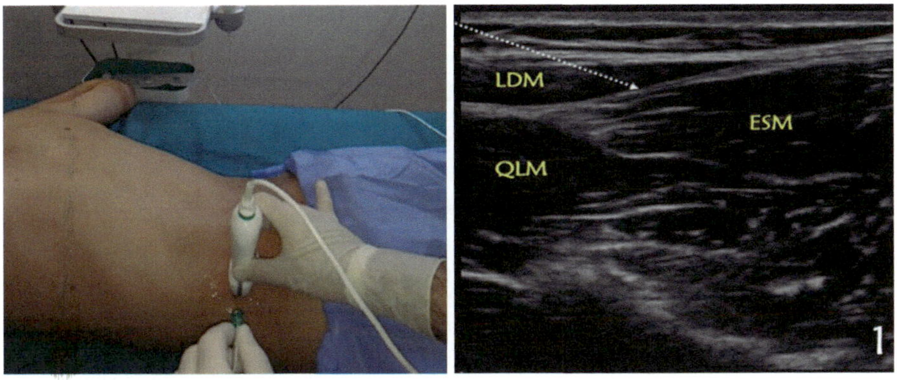

Fig. 6 Probe and needle positioning for lumbosacral interfascial block plane block on the left with ultrasonogram on the right. The superior cluneal nerve is running in this plane. *LDM* latissimus dorsi muscle. *ESM* erector spinae muscles. *QLM* quadratus lumborum muscle

8 Future Directions

Ultrasound-guided IPBs are effective and safe techniques that can be used alone or as a component of multimodal bedside management of acute or chronic pain (Table 2). In addition to the techniques mentioned above, it is very likely that new interfascial plane blocks will be identified in the near future. Local anesthetic concentration, mixture requirement, consensus on nomenclatures, and various types of ultrasound-guidedtechniques would be a subject of future research. For example, a recent cadaver study demonstrated that cervical ESPB applied with 20 mL dye from C6–7 level passes from C5 to C7 in all cadavers to the brachial plexusand also spreads to the dorsal rami [36]. In our opinion this is a promising direction for development of new IPB techniques for the treatment of head, neck, back and shoulder pain.

Clinical Pearls

- Erector spinae plane block is an easy to perform and safe procedure. It can be utilized in patients with rib fractures, postoperative pain, myofascial pain syndrome, back pain, radiculopathy, postherpetic neuralgia, some other acute, and chronic painful conditions.
- The utilization of corticosteroids for IPBs is controversial because of their common side effects [37]. Some reports indicated that they might lead to tissue calcifications.

Table 2 Samples of published cases in other interfascial plane blocks for head, neck and back pain

Authors	indication	Block and level	Volume and content of LA	Tricks and follow-up
Taketa et al. [28]	Lower cervical and Interscapular myofascial pain, 15 patients	Serrates posterior muscle plane block-second-third rib	15 mL of 0.25% ropivacaine per side	Between serrates posterior muscle and rhomboid major muscle. Reduced rate of NRS before and after the procedure was 80% on average
Ahiskalioglu et al. [32]	Low back pain (no discopatia)-one patient	Modified TLIP block (L3)	20 mL of 0.25% bupivacaine, methylprednisolone 40 mg, bilaterally	Between the longissimus and iliocostalis muscle planes in a medial to lateral direction with in-plane technique. After the TLIP block, the VAS score of the patient has not increased over 20 for 4 weeks
Ueshima et al.	Lumbar back pain due to spondylosis--two patients	TLIP block (L2)	20-mL bolus injection of 0.25% levobupivacaine, bilaterally	Between the multifidus and longissimus muscles. Twice a week for 2 months pain could be managed by oral analgesic/no complaint pain

Arrow: Needle direction and target for the injection

References

1. Rafi AN. Abdominal field block: a new approach via the lumbar triangle. Anaesthesia. 2001;56(10):1024–6.
2. Hebbard P, Fujiwara Y, Shibata Y, Royse C. Ultrasound-guided transversus abdominis plane (TAP) block. Anaesth Intensive Care. 2007;35(4):616–7.
3. Stecco C, Macchi V, Porzionato A, Duparc F, De Caro R. The fascia: the forgotten structure. Ital J Anat Embryol. 2011;116(3):127–38.
4. Piraccini E, Maitan S. Ultrasound guided rhomboid plane hydrodissection for fascial adhesion. J Clin Anesth. 2019;59:13.
5. Domingo T, Blasi J, Casals M, Mayoral V, Ortiz-Sagristá JC, Miguel-Pérez M. Is interfascial block with ultrasound-guided puncture useful in treatment of myofascial pain of the trapezius muscle? Clin J Pain. 2011;27(4):297–303.
6. Tulgar S, Selvi O, Senturk O, Serifsoy TE, Thomas DT. Ultrasound-guided erector spinae plane block: indications, complications, and effects on acute and chronic pain based on a single-center experience. Cureus. 2019;11(1):e3815. https://www.cureus.com/articles/16824-ultrasound-guided-erector-spinae-plane-block-indications-complications-and-effects-on-acute-and-chronic-pain-based-on-a-single-center-experience
7. Tulgar S, Ahiskalioglu A, De Cassai A, Gurkan Y. Efficacy of bilateral erector spinae plane block in the management of pain: current insights. J Pain Res. 2019;12:2597–613. https://doi.org/10.2147/jpr.s182128.

8. Elsharkawy H, Maniker R, Bolash R, Kalasbail P, Drake RL, Elkassabany N. Rhomboid intercostal and subserratus plane block: a cadaveric and clinical evaluation. Reg Anesth Pain Med. 2018;43(7):745–51.
9. Elsharkawy H, Pawa A, Mariano ER. Interfascial plane blocks: back to basics. Reg Anesth Pain Med. 2018;43(4):341–6. https://doi.org/10.1097/AAP.0000000000000750.
10. Xu JL, Tseng V. Proposal to standardize the nomenclature for paraspinal interfascial plane blocks. Reg Anesth Pain Med. 2019. https://doi.org/10.1136/rapm-2019-100696.
11. Tulgar S, Selvi O, Senturk O, Ermis MN, Cubuk R, Ozer Z. Clinical experiences of ultrasound-guided lumbar erector spinae plane block for hip joint and proximal femur surgeries. J Clin Anesth. 2018;47:5–6.
12. Forero M, Rajarathinam M, Adhikary SD, Chin KJ. Erector spinae plane block for the management of chronic shoulder pain: a case report. Can J Anaesth. 2018;65(3):288–93.
13. Darling CE, Pun SY, Caruso TJ, Tsui BCH. Successful directional thoracic erector spinae plane block after failed lumbar plexus block in hip joint and proximal femur surgery. J Clin Anesth. 2018;49:1–2.
14. Tulgar S, Thomas DT, Suslu H. Ultrasound guided erector spinae plane block relieves lower cervical and interscapular myofascial pain, a new indication. J Clin Anesth. 2018;53:74.
15. Piraccini E, Corso RM, Maitan S. Ultrasound guided erector spinae plane block for myofascial pain syndrome. J Clin Anesth. 2019;57:121. https://doi.org/10.1016/j.jclinane.2019.04.016.
16. Ueshima H, Otake H. Successful cases of bilateral erector spinae plane block for treatment of tension headache. J Clin Anesth. 2019;54:153.
17. Takahashi H, Suzuki T. Erector spinae plane block for low back pain in failed back surgery syndrome: a case report. JA Clin Rep. 2018;4(1):60.
18. Tulgar S, Senturk O, Thomas DT, Deveci U, Ozer Z. A new technique for sensory blockage of posterior branches of sacral nerves: ultrasound guided sacral erector spinae plane block. J Clin Anesth. 2019;57:129–30.
19. Piraccini E, Antioco M, Maitan S. Ultrasound guided sacral erector spinae plane block: a useful tool for radicular pain treatment. J Clin Anesth. 2019;59:11–2.
20. Tulgar S, Selvi O, Thomas DT, Ozer Z. ESRA19-0505 new indication for novel block: sacral erector spinae plane block for inferior cluneal/sacral nerve entrapment syndrome. Reg Anesth Pain Med. 2019;44(Suppl 1):A230.
21. Celik M, Tulgar S, Ahiskalioglu A, Alper F. Is high volume lumbar erector spinae plane block an alternative to transforaminal epidural injection? Evaluation with MRI. Reg Anesth Pain Med. 2019. https://doi.org/10.1136/rapm-2019-100514.
22. Schwartz RH, Urits I, Viswanath O, Kaye AD, Eskander J. Extended pain relief utilizing lumbar erector spinae plane block in a patient with discogenic low back pain. Pain Physician. 2019;22(5):E519–21.
23. Sullivan TR, Kanda P, Gagne S, Costache I. Harlequin syndrome associated with erector spinae plane block. Anesthesiology. 2019;131(3):665.
24. Tulgar S, Selvi O, Thomas DT, Manukyan M, Özer Z. Rhomboid intercostal block in a modified radical mastectomy and axillary curettage patient; a new indication for novel interfascial block. J Clin Anesth. 2019;54:158–9.
25. Elsharkawy H, Saifullah T, Kolli S, Drake R. Rhomboid intercostal block. Anaesthesia. 2016;71:856–7.
26. Piraccini E, De Lorenzo E, Maitan S. Rhomboid intercostal block for myofascial pain syndrome in a patient with amyotrophic lateral sclerosis. Minerva Anestesiol. 2019;85(12):1367–9. https://doi.org/10.23736/S0375-9393.19.13791-1.
27. Vilensky JA, Baltes M, Weikel L, Fortin JD, Fourie LJ. Serratus posterior muscles: anatomy, clinical relevance, and function. Clin Anat. 2001;14(4):237–41.
28. Taketa Y, Irisawa Y, Fujitani T. Ultrasound guided serrates posterior superior muscle block relieves interscapular myofascial pain. J Clin Anesth. 2018;44:10–1.
29. Hand WR, Taylor JM, Harvey NR, Epperson TI, Gunselman RJ, Bolin ED, Whiteley J. Thoracolumbar interfascial plane (TLIP) block: a pilot study in volunteers. Can J Anaesth. 2015;62(11):1196–200.

30. Ahiskalioglu A, Yayik AM, Alici HA. Ultrasound-guided lateral thoracolumbar interfascial plane (TLIP) block: description of new modified technique. J Clin Anesth. 2017;40:62.
31. Ahiskalioglu A, Alici HA, Selvitopi K, Yayik AM. Ultrasonography-guided modified thoracolumbar interfascial plane block: a new approach. Can J Anaesth. 2017;64(7):775–6.
32. Ahiskalioglu A, Yayik AM, Celik EC, Aydin ME, Uzun G. Ultrasound guided modified thoracolumbar interfascial plane block for low back pain management. J Clin Anesth. 2019;54:138–9.
33. Kuniya H, Aota Y, Kawai T, Kaneko K-I, Konno T, Saito T. Prospective study of superior cluneal nerve disorder as a potential cause of low back pain and leg symptoms. J Orthop Surg Res. 2014;9:139.
34. Nielsen TD, Moriggl B, Barckman J, Jensen JM, Kolsen-Petersen JA, Søballe K, Børglum J, Bendtsen TF. Randomized trial of ultrasound-guided superior cluneal nerve block. Reg Anesth Pain Med. 2019;44(8):772–80.
35. Cornish P. Ultrasound-guided superior cluneal nerves block: raising the bar. Reg Anesth Pain Med. 2019. https://doi.org/10.1136/rapm-2019-100619.
36. Elsharkawy H, Ince I, Hamadnalla H, Drake RL, Tsui BCH. Cervical erector spinae plane block: a cadaver study. Reg Anesth Pain Med. 2020;45(7):552–6. https://doi.org/10.1136/rapm-2019-101154.
37. Buntragulpoontawee M, Chang KV, Vitoonpong T, Pornjaksawan S, Kitisak K, Saokaew S, Kanchanasurakit S. The effectiveness and safety of commonly used injectates for ultrasound-guided hydrodissection treatment of peripheral nerve entrapment syndromes: a systematic review. Front Pharmacol. 2021;11:621150. https://doi.org/10.3389/fphar.2020.621150.

Further Reading

Atalay YO. A comparison of the ultrasound-guided modified-thoracolumbar interfascial plane block and wound infiltration for postoperative pain management in lumbar spinal surgery patients. Agri. 2020;32(3):140–6; English. https://doi.org/10.14744/agri.2019.97759.

Mavarez AC, Ahmed AA. Transabdominal plane block. In: StatPearls [Internet]. Treasure Island, FL: StatPearls Publishing; 2022.

Superior Cluneal Nerve Block

Josianna Henson, Justin Merkow,
and Narayana Varhabhatla

Essential Concepts

- Superior cluneal nerve pain accounts for up to 14% of low back pain. It should be considered in the differential for patients who have not responded to other interventions for low back pain.
- The SCN may become entrapped where it crosses the thoracolumbar fascia in the osteofibrous tunnel at the level of the iliac crest.
- SCN injection can be done at the bedside with landmark-based or ultrasound-guided techniques. An accurate injection may provide significant long-term relief in some patients.
- Patients with superior cluneal nerve entrapment whose pain is not relieved with pharmacologic management and injections may benefit from surgical release of the nerve.

1 Overview

Low back pain affects 70–85% of adults at some point in life, and no causative pathology is found in 50% of cases [1]. The superior cluneal nerves (SCN) originate from T12-L4 and provide sensation to the lumbar area and buttock. They traverse over the iliac crest, where they split into two to six branches that can be described as medial, middle and lateral branches [2]. SCN pathology accounts for as much as 14% of low back pain and can mimic SI joint pain, facet arthropathy, and lumbar radiculopathy [3]. Physical exam findings include a Tinel-sign over the posterior iliac crest 5–7 cm lateral to the midline that recreates the patient's pain [4]. Maigne

J. Henson · J. Merkow · N. Varhabhatla (✉)
Department of Anesthesiology, University of Colorado School of Medicine,
Aurora, CO, USA
e-mail: josianna.henson@cuanschutz.edu; narayana.varhabhatla@cuanschutz.edu

D. Souza et al. (eds.), *Bedside Pain Management Interventions*,
https://doi.org/10.1007/978-3-031-11188-4_36

syndrome, which is confirmed with a T12/L1 facet injection, is referred pain to the iliac crest via the cluneal nerves [5]. However, the most accurate way to block the nerves and obtain a diagnosis is with blockade of these nerves. This can be done with a landmark-based technique or ultrasound guidance when performed at the bedside.

2 Indications and Contraindications

Superior cluneal nerve pain was first described by Strong and Davila in 1957 as a potential cause of low back pain [6]. It generally presents as unilateral low back pain that can be exacerbated by lumbar movement but can also present as "pseudo-sciatica" in 47-84% of patients with radiation to the legs [2, 7]. Risk factors include bone graft harvesting from the posterior iliac crest, lumbar fusion, and repetitive flexion and extension as with golf or tennis [8].

Physical examination should include palpation of painful areas, with specific attention to the response to palpation over the posterior iliac crest. A myofascial trigger point over the iliac crest may also indicate superior cluneal nerve pathology [9] (Table 1). Imaging with magnetic resonance imaging or computerized tomography is not helpful for diagnosis, because the superior cluneal nerves are very thin (mean nerve size is 1.1 mm) and difficult to visualize using these modalities [3, 10]. Contraindications to the procedure include patient refusal, active infection or evidence of sepsis/bacteremia, or allergy to any of the planned injectates.

Table 1 Proposed diagnostic criteria of superior cluneal neuropathy [2]

1. Low back pain involving the iliac crest and buttocks
2. Symptoms aggravated by lumbar movement or posture
3. Trigger point over the posterior iliac crest corresponding to the nerve compression zone
4. Patients report numbness and radiating pain in the SCN area (Tinel sign) when the trigger point is compressed.
5. Symptom relief by SCN block at the trigger point

3 Clinical Anatomy

The SCN is the cutaneous branch of the dorsal rami of T12-L4 (Fig. 1). From there, it traverses inferolaterally through the psoas major and paraspinal muscles and crosses the iliac crest. It pierces the quadratus lumborum fascia at the lateral border of the erector spinae, and remains between the quadratus lumborum and the thoracolumbar fascia. There are at least 2 branches of the cluneal nerve and as many as 5 [3]. The lateral superior cluneal nerve is the largest of the branches, which range in

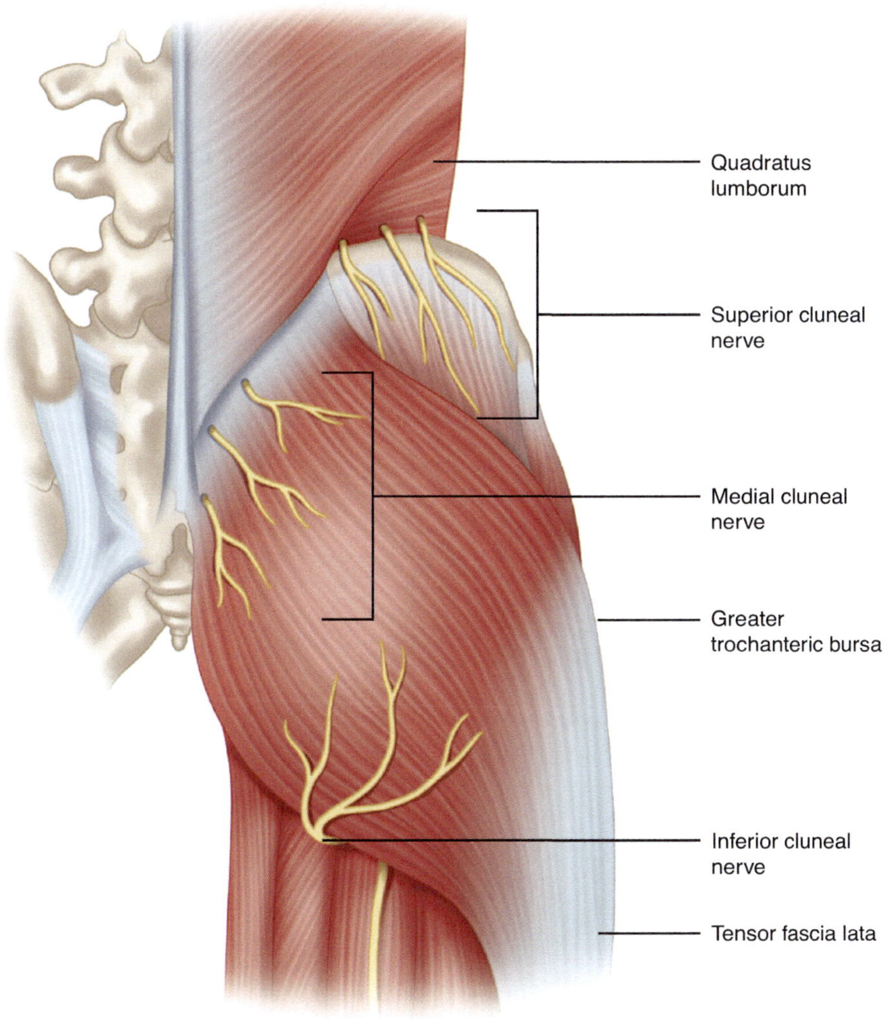

Fig. 1 Location of the superior cluneal nerves relative to the iliac crest. Image courtesy Springer

size from 0.8 to 2.1 mm [3]. In an anatomical study done by Kuniya et al., 56% of cadavers had at least 1 branch of the SCN passing through an osteofibrous tunnel at the level of the iliac crest, 39% of which were medial branches [11]. However, Tubbs did not note any osteofibrous tunnels or obvious compression sites in the area between the iliac crest and the thoracolumbar fascia [3]. This remains a controversial point. There are no known significant vascular structures in this region.

4 Equipment and Supplies

The procedure can be done with a landmark approach or with sonographic guidance when performed at the bedside [12, 13]. A 27 g or 30 g needle is used for anesthetizing the skin with lidocaine (Table 2). We prefer to use a 22 g spinal needle or an 80 mm echogenic needle with a 5 mL syringe for the injectate. The anesthetic solution usually consists of lidocaine or bupivacaine, or a combination of the two, with or without a corticosteroid. The patient can be in the lateral or prone position.

Table 2 Required supplies for superior cluneal nerve block

Syringe	5 mL
Needle	27 or 30 g needle for local anesthesia 22 g spinal needle or 80 mm echogenic needle
Anesthetic	0.25–0.5% bupivacaine 1% lidocaine
Corticosteroid	Triamcinolone 20–40 mg, Methylprednisolone 20–40 mg

5 Superior Cluneal Nerve Block, Landmark Technique

The blocks can be done using a landmark-based technique. The iliac crest is palpated 5-7 cm from the midline [12]. The point of maximal pain is palpated. The skin is anesthetized with 1% lidocaine and a 27 g 1.5-in. needle is inserted perpendicular to the skin until the iliac crest is contact. The needle is withdrawn slightly, negative aspiration is confirmed, and 1–2 mL of a local plus steroid mixture is injected at each of the medial, middle, and lateral branches.

6 Superior Cluneal Nerve Block, Ultrasound Technique

The superior cluneal nerve block can also be done using an ultrasound-guided technique [13–15]. The target is between the lateral border of the erector spinae muscle and the posterior thoracolumbar fascia at the level of the iliac crest. The block is done with a linear transducer in a transverse orientation (Fig. 2). First, the erector spinae muscle is identified, and the lateral border is traced to the level of the iliac crest. When this junction is visualized under ultrasound at the level of the iliac crest, a block needle is inserted in-plane medially to laterally. The needle is advanced until it is deep to the posterior thoracolumbar fascia and medial to the point of fusion between the anterior and posterior thoracolumbar fascia. Upon injection, visualization of separation between the posterior thoracolumbar fascia and the erector spinae should occur.

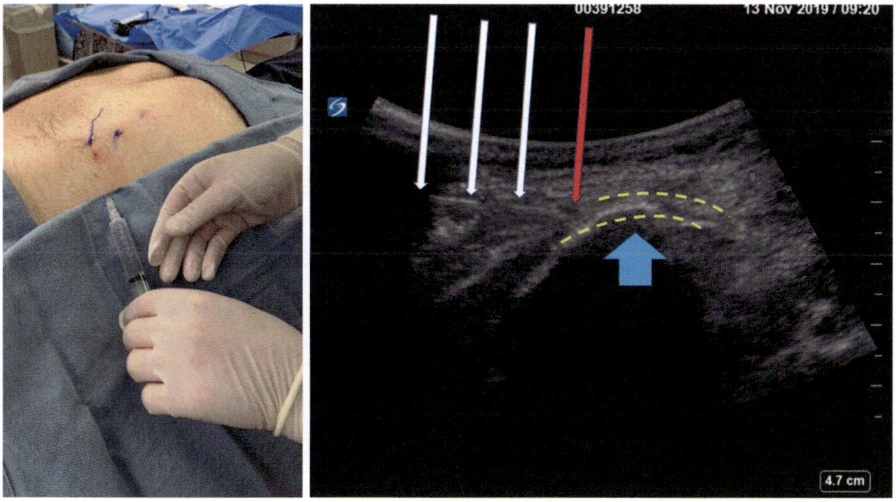

Fig. 2 Superior cluneal nerve block. The needle trajectory presented on the left side, designated with a blue marker. White arrows on the ultrasonogram points towards the needle. The red arrow points to the tip of the needle and the injectate. The iliac crest marked with blue arrow. The spread of the injectate marked with yellow doted lines extends within the same fascial plane as cluneal nerves. (Image: courtesy of Dmitri Souza, MD, PhD)

7 Potential Complications and Adverse Effects

The procedure is generally well tolerated by patients. Injection site pain and muscle spasms are the most likely adverse effects. Rare adverse events include nerve damage, dizziness, lightheadedness, systemic absorption/toxicity [14, 15]. Other important complications and relevant considerations are presented in Table 3.

Table 3 Additional potential complications and adverse effects

• Pressure should be applied to prevent hematoma production in patients with bleeding disorders or on anticoagulation
• Patients must be made aware of the potential for slightly unpleasant cosmetic disfigurement with local hair loss, hyperpigmentation, or cutaneous atrophy due to the corticosteroids utilized in the treatment. Local myotoxicity has been reported with bupivacaine
• Risks should be weighed against potential benefits when utilizing cluneal nerve blocks during pregnancy
• Anaphylaxis can occur with lidocaine or bupivacaine anesthetic, and blocks should not be performed if there has been a prior allergic reaction to the anesthetic
• Patients receiving frequent injections or perhaps using corticosteroids, either orally or as a result of other interventional procedures, are at risk for developing Cushing syndrome or adrenal insufficiency [16]. Clinicians must be diligent in questioning patients specifically about the potential recent use of steroids as this medication history is often not reported by the patient

Clinical and Technical Pearls

- The point of maximal tenderness over the iliac crest should be palpated before beginning the procedure. This allows confirmation with a sonotinel sign.
- The local anesthetic should be seen to spread between the thoracolumbar fascia and the erector spinae.
- The procedure can be done in-plane or out-of-plane, but in our experience, it is often easier to do this in-plane.
- Patients should be informed with the possibility of developing lipodystrophy with the use of steroids or punctate scars, especially with repeated blocks.
- Meticulous attention should be paid to an immunocompromised patient to prevent the development of infections. Although it is rare, early detection is imperative to prevent deleterious fatal consequences.

References

1. Becker A, et al. Low back pain in primary care: Costs of care and prediction of future health care utilization. Spine (Phila PA). 2010;35:1714–20.
2. Isu T, Kim K, Morimoto D, Iwamoto N. Superior and middle cluneal nerve entrapment as a cause of low back pain. Neurospine. 2018;15:25–32.
3. Tubbs RS, et al. Anatomy and landmarks for the superior and middle cluneal nerves: application to posterior iliac crest harvest and entrapment syndromes. J Neurosurg Spine. 2010;13(3):356–9.
4. Lu J, Ebraheim NA, Huntoon M, Heck BE, Yeasting RA. Anatomic considerations of superior cluneal nerve at posterior iliac crest region. Clin Orthop. 1998;347:224–8.
5. Maigne JY, Lazareth JP, Surville HG, Maigne R. The lateral cutaneous branches of the dorsal rami of the thoraco-lumbar junction. Surg Radiol Anat. 1989;11:289–93.
6. Strong EK, Davila JC. The cluneal nerve syndrome; a distinct type of low back pain. Ind Med Surg. 1957;26:417.
7. Konno T, Aota Y, Kuniya H, Saito T, Qu N, Hayashi S, Kawata S, Itoh M. Anatomical etiology of "pseudo-sciatica" from superior cluneal nerve entrapment: a laboratory investigation. J Pain Res. 2017;10:2539.
8. Aly TA, et al. Medial superior cluneal nerve entrapment neuropathy in teenagers: a report of two cases. Tohoku J Exp Med. 2002;197(4):229–31.
9. Kuniya H, Aota Y, Kawai T, Kaneko K, Konno T, Saito T. Prospective study of superior cluneal nerve disorder as a potential cause of low back pain and leg symptoms. J Orthop Surg. 2014;9:139.
10. Kim K, et al. Low back pain due to middle cluneal nerve entrapment neuropathy. Eur Spine J. 2018;27(3):309–13.
11. Kuniya H, et al. Anatomical study of superior cluneal nerve entrapment. J Neurosurg Spine. 2013;19(1):76–80.
12. Trescot AM. Cryoanalgesia in interventional pain management. Pain Physician. 2003;6:345–60.
13. Chang KV, et al. Ultrasonographic technique for imaging and injecting the superior cluneal nerve. Am J Phys Med Rehabil. 2017;96(6):e117–8.

14. Nielsen TD, Moriggl B, Barckman J, Jensen JM, Kolsen-Petersen JA, Søballe K, Borglum J, Bendtsen TF. Randomized trial of ultrasound-guided superior cluneal nerve block. Reg Anesth Pain Med. 2019:rapm-2018-100174.
15. Jeng CL, Torrillo TM, Rosenblatt MA. Complications of peripheral nerve blocks. Br J Anaesth. 2010;105:i97–i107.
16. Jacobs S, Pullan PT, Potter JM, Shenfield GM. Adrenal suppression following extradural steroids. Anaesthesia. 1983;38:953–6.

Further Reading

Fujihara F, Isu T, Kim K, Sakamoto K, Matsumoto J, Miki K, Ito M, Isobe M, Inoue T. Clinical features of middle cluneal nerve entrapment neuropathy. Acta Neurochir. 2021;163(3):817–22. https://doi.org/10.1007/s00701-020-04676-0. Epub 2021 Jan 6

Middle Cluneal Nerve Injections

Jay Karri, Tuan Tang, and Alaa Abd-Elsayed

Essential Concepts

- Pathology of the middle cluneal nerves (MCN) may be implicated in persons with chronic low back pain that radiates across the medial gluteal surface.
- MCN pathology has been associated with bone harvests from the iliac crest via the posterior approach.
- MCN blocks offer both diagnostic and therapeutic benefit in persons with chronic low back pain and can be performed at the bedside.
- Pain relief with MCN blocks can be rapid given immediate effects of local anesthetics and therapeutic benefit may persist across days to weeks, and possibly longer, especially if chemoneurolysis is performed.
- In cases where MCN blocks provide meaningful but only temporary relief, neurolysis may be pursued to provide patients with a longer duration of analgesic benefit.

1 Overview

Pathology of the middle cluneal nerves (MCN) is an often overlooked phenomenon in persons presenting with chronic low back pain [1–3]. Affected patients endorse low back pain with particular radiation of symptoms across the medial aspect of the gluteal region. Given the higher prevalence of other axial low back pain and

J. Karri (✉)
Baylor College of Medicine, Houston, TX, USA

T. Tang
University of Texas HSC at Houston, Houston, TX, USA

A. Abd-Elsayed
Department of Anesthesiology, Medical Examining Board, Wisconsin, Chronic Pain Physician, University of Wisconsin-Madison, Madison, WI, USA

D. Souza et al. (eds.), *Bedside Pain Management Interventions*,
https://doi.org/10.1007/978-3-031-11188-4_37

sacroiliac joint disorders in persons with similar symptoms, the diagnosis of MCN pathology is sometimes delayed and/or overlooked.

Despite the precise mechanism of MCN pathology, MCN injection procedures can be employed with good benefit [1, 4, 5]. These procedures are readily performed at the bedside using anatomical landmarks or ultrasound guidance. They can carry diagnostic and often therapeutic benefit with variable reported success rates. In certain cases where MCN entrapment or chronic neuropathy are implicated, more advanced procedures such as peripheral nerve stimulation and surgical decompression may be necessary for analgesic benefit.

2 Indications and Contraindications

MCN neuralgia can be secondary to a host of etiologies and thus, efforts towards diagnosing the precise underlying pathophysiology can help direct goal directed management with good benefits [1–3]. Despite the precise underlying mechanisms, MCN pathology produces lower back pain with radiation across the medial gluteal aspect. Given that the MCN are purely sensory, there are no associated motor deficits with MCN compromise. While no true diagnostic criteria for MCN neuralgia exist, the spectrum of diagnostic considerations is delineated in Table 1.

The most common complication of posterior iliac crest bone harvest procedures is cluneal nerve damage, which can produce sensory impairments and/or chronic pain [1–3]. While the superior cluneal nerves (SCN) are most implicated with this procedure, the MCN is still vulnerable depending on patient habitus, anatomical nerve trajectory, and laterality of instrumentation.

Entrapment neuropathy is thought to be far more likely with the SCN relative to the MCN. However, MCN entrapment was reported by Aota in 2016 and was thought to be likely in other unreported cases given the susceptibility for MCN compression along the posterior sacral ligaments [1].

Maigne syndrome refers to the referral of pain from lower thoracic-high lumbar facet arthropathy to the iliac crest via cluneal nerves [1–3, 6]. While Maigne syndrome has conventionally implicated the SCN, MCN neuralgia might be secondary to referral pain from lumbosacral facet arthopathy.

Table 1 Diagnosis of Chronic Pain secondary to Middle Cluneal Nerve pathology

(A) Low back pain with usually unilateral referral to the medial gluteal aspect
(B) Focal tenderness to palpation along the long posterior sacroiliac ligament below the posterior superior iliac spine
(C) Moderate-significant analgesic response with local anesthetic nerve block.
(D) Above symptoms not otherwise implicated by other diagnoses including lumbosacral or sacroiliac pathology

Table 2 Injections for the management of Middle Cluneal Nerve pathology

Procedure	Indications	Analgesic Duration	Techniques
Anesthetic block	Diagnostic Therapeutic	Days to weeks	Landmark technique and/or ultrasound-guided
Chemoneurolysis	Therapeutic only	Often months	
Prolotherapy	Therapeutic only	Variable	

Lastly, idiopathic MCN neuralgia is also a very likely phenomenon. Given the only recent recognition and interest in chronic pain from cluneal neuropathies, robust literature and epidemiological data are lacking.

In persons where MCN pathology may be implicated, local anesthetic nerve blocks can be useful for both diagnostic and therapeutic benefit. Nerve blocks, as delineated in Table 2, can also involve the use of neurolysis or prolotherapy [4, 7]. Chemoneurolysis, usually with aqueous phenol, can produce longer term analgesic benefit, sometimes up to 6 months of more. However, it is usually performed only after a diagnosis of MCN neuralgia is well established with an anesthetic nerve block.

When assessing patients for the candidacy of MCN injections, standard practice patterns and contraindications for peripheral nerve blocks are similarly applicable [8]. Namely, judicious strategies are necessary to mitigate the risks of infection, bleeding complications, inadvertent damage to peripheral structures, and drug toxicity. Practitioners should exercise necessary precautions and discretion when assessing clinically vulnerable patients, including but not limited to those who are underaged, pregnant, and immunocompromised.

3 Clinical Anatomy

The MCN is a pure sensory nerve that is derived from the dorsal rami of the S1 to S3 foramina [1–3, 9]. Upon exiting the sacral foramina, the MCN travels inferolaterally under the posterior superior iliac spine (PSIS) and across the long posterior sacroiliac ligament (LPSL). The MCN overlies the gluteus maximus muscle and provides cutaneous innervation to the medial aspect of the buttock (Fig. 1).

Of note, cadaveric studies from multiple groups found varying nerve routes in relation to the LPSL. While Tubbs et al. found the MCN to be superficial to the LPSL, others found the MCN to course underneath or even through LPSL [2, 10–12]. There exists only one report of MCN entrapment in the literature, but underdiagnosis and/or underreporting of MCN entrapment may be possible [1].

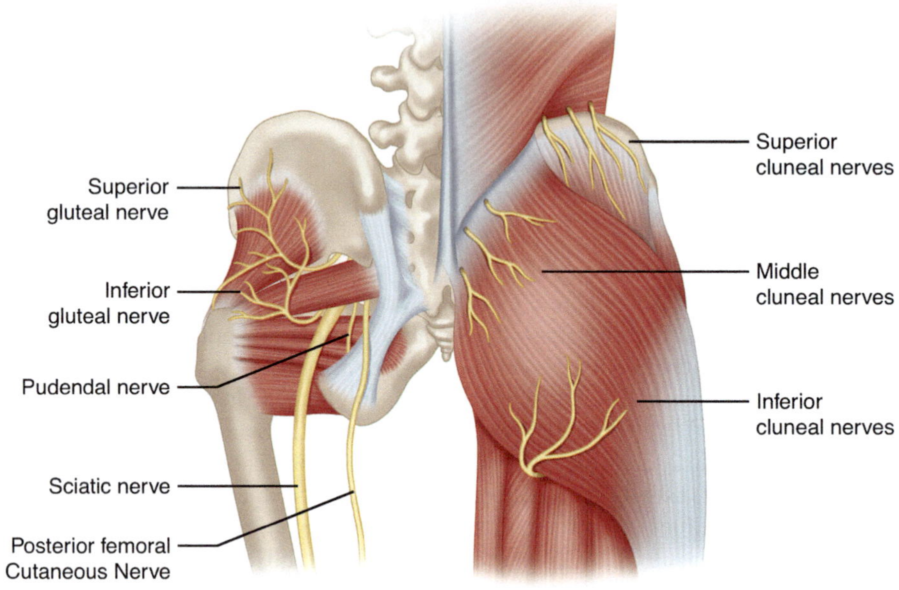

Fig. 1 Medial cluneal nerve anatomy

4 Equipment and Supplies

MCN blocks are easily performed at the bedside. While experienced practitioners may only utilize anatomical landmarks to perform the injection, ultrasound guidance may be utilized to directly visualize the nerve. Given the absence of major arteries, nerves, or other vital structures in immediate proximity to the MCN, ultrasound guidance is not a necessity. However, direct MCN visualization may not only optimize targeted injectate delivery, but also increase the safety profile associated with this procedure.

Typically, a small syringe with a 22–25 gauge, 1.5 in. needle is utilized to inject 2–5 mL of the injectate (Table 3). Anesthetic solutions usually consist of lidocaine or bupivacaine, or less commonly, a lidocaine-bupivacaine combination. They may be mixed with a corticosteroid solution, especially if the injection is being administered for therapeutic benefit.

While limited evidence for corticosteroid addition for treating MCN neuralgia exists, there exist data suggesting that corticosteroid can have several chronic detrimental effects [13]. The incorporation of corticosteroids should be practitioner and patient dependent. Corticosteroid dose should be judiciously considered, especially in patients with diabetes mellitus with poor glycemic control or steroid sensitivity.

Table 3 Supplies utilized for Middle Cluneal Nerve injections

Syringe	3 or 5 mL
Needle	22 or 25 gauge 1½ in. needle
Anesthetic	Bupivacaine 0.25–0.5% Lidocaine 1-2% Lidocaine/bupivacaine combination: 1:1–1:3 ratio
Corticosteroid	Triamcinolone 5–40 mg (t1/2 life: 18–36 h) Betamethasone 18 mg (t1/2 life: 36–54 h) Dexamethasone 4 mg (t1/2 life: 36–54 h) Methylprednisolone 80–125 mg (t1/2 life: 18–36 h)
Phenol	Aqueous phenol solution, 5–8%
Prolotherapy	Dextrose in sterile water, 12.5–25%

5 Anatomical Landmark Technique

The procedure is optimally performed with the patient in a prone position. The ipsilateral low back and gluteal surface are exposed with the contralateral side appropriately draped for patient comfort and privacy. The posterior iliac crest is identified and followed medially until the PSIS is located. The 1-5 cm below the PSIS is carefully palpated to identify tender points that reproduce the patient's painful symptoms [1–3, 5, 9]. The skin is marked approximately 1 cm medial to the identified tender points and standard aseptic technique is utilized to prepare the skin.

A 22 or 25 gauge, 1½ in. needle is introduced at the marked targets and advanced infero-laterally at a shallow angle until immediately below the subcutaneous tissue. Following negative aspiration, the injectate can be administered in a fanlike distribution. A gauze dressing should be used to hold pressure over the injection site once the needle is withdrawn.

6 Ultrasound Technique

Given the small diameters of MCNs, concordance of ultrasound imaging to the aforementioned anatomical landmarks is essential. Start with the ultrasound probe in a vertical position immediately below the PSIS. Attempt to localize the MCNs in short axis by moving rotating the superior aspect of the probe laterally towards the iliac crest. The needle and probe positioning are presented at the Fig. 2.

Once identified, the injection may be performed in ether short axis or long axis to the ultrasound probe. A 3–5 mL syringe with a 25–30 gauge, 1½ in. needle is advanced, with a shallow angle, below the thoracolumbar fascia, above the gluteus maximus, and towards the MCN. The injectate is administered overlying the identified MCN. The ultrasonogram of the injection presented at the Fig. 3.

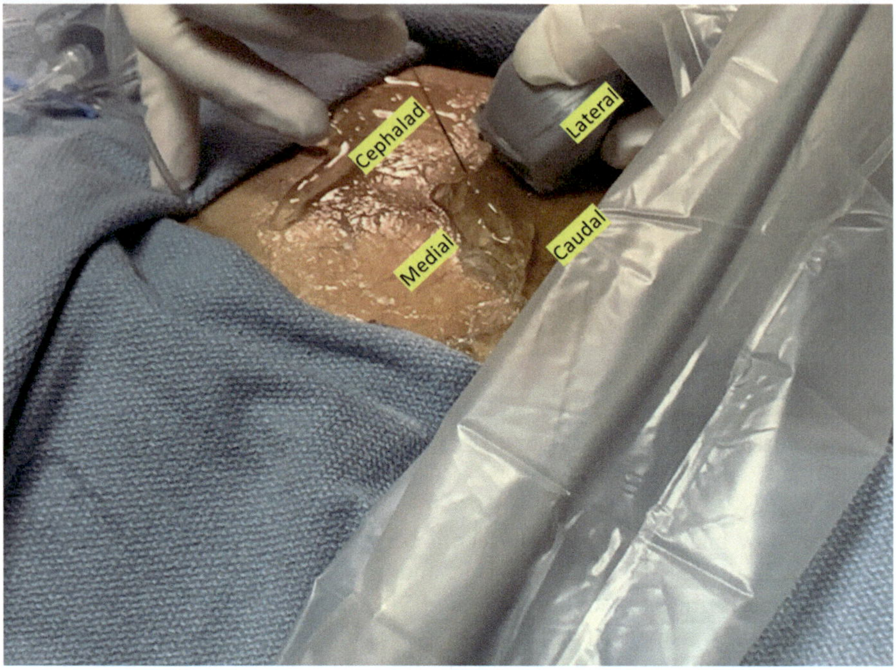

Fig. 2 The probe and the needle positioning for the medial cluneal nerve injection. (Image—courtesy of Dmitri Souza, MD, PhD)

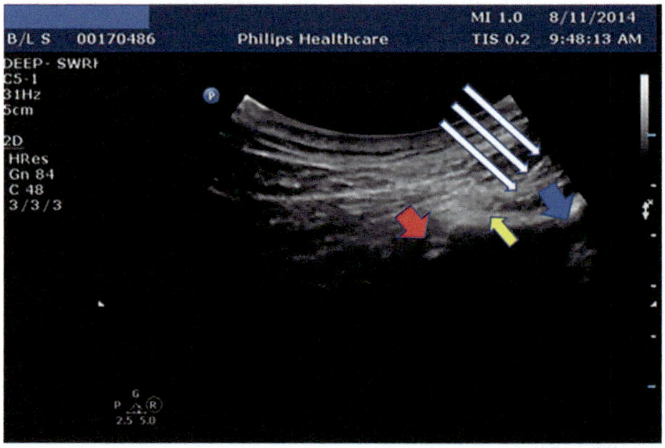

Fig. 3 Ultrasonogram of the medial cluneal nerve injection. White arrows: represents needle shaft. Red arrow points towards sacroiliac joint. Yellow arrow indicates the location over the medial cluneal nerve in close proximity to the S2 foramen (blue arrow). (Image—courtesy of Dmitri Souza, MD, PhD)

7 Potential Complications and Adverse Effects

Given the absence of major arteries, nerves, or other vital structures in immediate proximity to the MCN, this procedure is often well tolerated. However, standard precautions are instrumental in maintaining the favorable safety profile associated with this procedure. Namely, precautionary measures to prevent the risks of

Table 4 Notable potential Complications and Adverse Effects

Standard sterile technique and precautions are necessary to minimize the risk of infection. Additionally, immunocompromised patients warrant specific consideration and possible monitoring
Bleeding risk is mostly limited to hematoma formation, which may be mitigated with careful consideration of physiology or iatrogenic anticoagulation. Additionally, pressure should be maintained over the injection site if oozing or prolonged bleeding occurs
Local anesthetics carry notable risk for anaphylaxis and systemic drug toxicity. Anesthetics should not be utilized if the patient reports previous allergic reactions specific to the anesthetic. If signs or symptoms of systemic absorption of the anesthetic develop, further anesthetic use should be immediately aborted to prevent lethal neuro- and/or cardiotoxicity
Corticosteroids can cause local chondrotoxicity, myotoxcity, or lipodystrophy, cutaneous scarring, or even ligamentous compromise. These adverse effects are thought to be secondary to repeat injections and with high steroid dosages
Corticosteroid use should be judiciously considered in persons with high and/or chronic steroid exposure via intravenous or oral steroid formulations or repeat joint injections with corticosteroid injectates. These patients may be at risk for developed adrenal insufficiency

infection, bleeding complications, inadvertent damage to peripheral structures, and drug toxicity are vital (Table 4).

Infection risk can be decreased by utilizing sterile procedural technique, avoiding needle placement through cutaneous infection sites, and careful monitoring and/or judicious candidacy considerations in immunocompromised patients including those with diabetes mellitus.

Bleeding complications are largely limited to hematoma formation given the absence of major arterial supply overlying the MCN anatomical course. Nonetheless, the use of ultrasound guidance and doppler imaging may help prevent vascular injury. The risk of bleeding can also be minimized using societal guidelines from the American Society of Regional Anesthesia and Pain Medicine (ASRA), which provides recommendations for pre-procedural cessation of anti-platelet and anticoagulant medications [14]. However, the temporary discontinuation of these medications should occur in concert with their prescribing providers and be considered only if deemed reasonable and appropriate.

Depending on patient habitus and practitioner expertise, ultrasound guidance may be utilized to decrease risk of needle trauma to nearby structures. Additionally, appropriate patient positioning can help optimize ease of injection.

Lastly, drug toxicity can result secondary to anaphylaxis, local, or systemic adverse effects [8]. Anaphylaxis, usually secondary to local anesthetics like lidocaine or bupivacaine, may be prevented by surveying patients for prior allergic or adverse reactions to injectates being administered. Localized adverse effects with nerve blocks are often secondary to corticosteroid medications, which have been associated with local chondrotoxicity, muscle damage, and even ligamentous compromise [13]. Myotoxicity has also been associated with bupivacaine use [15]. Phenol use has been associated with risk of local dysesthesias [7]. Systemic adverse effects can occur with systemic absorption of injectate medications, especially if large volumes and/or high doses are utilized. The most threatening adverse effects are secondary to anesthetic toxicity and initially manifest via symptoms of dizziness, lightheadness, blurred vision, slurred speech, metallic taste, perioral numbness, and/or tinnitus [15]. If the patient reports these symptoms, further anesthetic use should be immediately aborted to prevent lethal neuro- and/or cardiotoxicity.

Clinical and Technical Pearls

- MCN pathology may be implicated in persons with chronic low back pain that radiates across the medial gluteal surface.
- Nerve blocks to the MCN are fairly safe and are readily performed at the bedside using anatomical landmarks or ultrasound guidance.
- Chemoneurolysis or prolotherapy injections can also be considered in patients with a confirmed diagnosis of neuralgia or neuropathy from the MCN.
- Appropriate patient selection and safety considerations can help optimize the safety profile associated with MCN injections.

References

1. Aota Y. Entrapment of middle cluneal nerves as an unknown cause of low back pain. World J Orthop. 2016;7(3):167.
2. Tubbs RS, Levin MR, Loukas M, Potts EA, Cohen-Gadol AA. Anatomy and landmarks for the superior and middle cluneal nerves: application to posterior iliac crest harvest and entrapment syndromes. J Neurosurg Spine. 2010;13(3):356–9.
3. Isu T, Kim K, Morimoto D, Iwamoto N. Superior and middle cluneal nerve entrapment as a cause of low back pain. Neurospine. 2018;15(1):25.
4. Inklebarger J, Galanis N. The Management of Cluneal Nerve Referred Pain with Prolotherapy. J Prolother. 2018;10:982–91.
5. Nielsen TD, Moriggl B, Barckman J, et al. Randomized trial of ultrasound-guided superior cluneal nerve block. Reg Anesth Pain Med. 2019:rapm–2018.
6. Maigne J-Y, Maigne R. Trigger point of the posterior iliac crest: painful iliolumbar ligament insertion or cutaneous dorsal ramus pain? An anatomic study. Arch Phys Med Rehabil. 1991;72(10):734–7.
7. Ramamurthy S, Walsh NE, Schoenfeld LS, Hoffman J. Evaluation of neurolytic blocks using phenol and cryogenic block in the management of chronic pain. J Pain Symptom Manag. 1989;4(2):72–5.
8. Jeng CL, Torrillo TM, Rosenblatt MA. Complications of peripheral nerve blocks. Br J Anaesth. 2010;105(suppl_1):i97–i107.
9. Konno T, Aota Y, Saito T, et al. Anatomical study of middle cluneal nerve entrapment. J Pain Res. 2017;10:1431.
10. Grob KR, Neuhuber WL, Kissling RO. Innervation of the sacroiliac joint of the human. Z Rheumatol. 1995;54(2):117–22.
11. McGrath MC, Zhang M. Lateral branches of dorsal sacral nerve plexus and the long posterior sacroiliac ligament. Surg Radiol Anat. 2005;27(4):327–30.
12. Horwitz MT. The anatomy of (a) the lumbosacral nerve plexus—its relation to variations of vertebral segmentation, and (b), the posterior sacral nerve plexus. Anat Rec. 1939;74(1):91–107.

13. Brinks A, Koes BW, Volkers AC, Verhaar JA, Bierma-Zeinstra SM. Adverse effects of extra-articular corticosteroid injections: a systematic review. BMC Musculoskelet Disord. 2010;11(1):206.
14. Narouze S, Benzon HT, Provenzano D, et al. Interventional spine and pain procedures in patients on antiplatelet and anticoagulant medications: guidelines from the American Society of regional anesthesia and Pain medicine, the European Society of regional anaesthesia and pain therapy, the American Academy of pain medicine, the International neuromodulation Society, the North American neuromodulation Society, and the world Institute of pain. Reg Anesth Pain Med. 2018;43(3):225–62.
15. Batinac T, Sotošek Tokmadžić V, Peharda V, Brajac I. Adverse reactions and alleged allergy to local anesthetics: analysis of 331 patients. J Dermatol. 2013;40(7):522–7.

Further Reading

Fujihara F, Isu T, Kim K, Sakamoto K, Matsumoto J, Miki K, Ito M, Isobe M, Inoue T. Clinical features of middle cluneal nerve entrapment neuropathy. Acta Neurochir. 2021;163(3):817–22. https://doi.org/10.1007/s00701-020-04676-0. Epub 2021 Jan 6

Sacroiliac Joint Intraarticular and Periarticular injections

Mohamed Attia and Mowafak Abdelghani

Essential Concepts

- Sacro-iliac (SI) joint is an important source of chronic axial low back pain; with frequency of its occurrence increasing with age. Pain originating from the SIJ can be intra-articular or extra-articular [1].
- The intra-articular causes include infection, arthritis, spondyloarthropathies, and malignancies while enthesopathy, fractures, ligamentous injuries, and myofascial pain constitute the extra-articular causes of SI joint pain [1].
- The International Association for the Study of Pain (IASP) has developed criteria for diagnosing sacroiliac joint pain. Sacroiliac joint pain is defined as pain localized to the region of the SI joint, reproducible by stress and provocation tests, and reliably relieved by selective infiltration of the SI joint with a local anaesthetic [2].

M. Attia (✉) · M. Abdelghani
Manchester University NHS Foundation Trust, Manchester, UK
e-mail: Mohamed.attia@mft.nhs.uk; Mowafak.abdelghani@mft.nhs.uk

D. Souza et al. (eds.), *Bedside Pain Management Interventions*,
https://doi.org/10.1007/978-3-031-11188-4_38

- Even though definitive criteria for the degree of pain improvement to confirm a diagnosis of sacroiliac joint syndrome is insufficient, greater than 50–75% reduction in post injection pain has been suggested as a useful threshold. Since intra-articular steroid injections may effectively reduce the pain associated with sacroiliac joint syndrome (SIJS), low-grade synovial inflammation has been proposed as a potential cause [3].
- The effectiveness of periarticular sacroiliac joint injection has been compared with that of intraarticular injection in several studies. Although periarticular and intra-articular injections may result in similar pain relief, intraarticular injections have been the main stay of treatment used to verify a diagnosis of sacroiliac joint syndrome and to guide more advanced therapies, such as radiofrequency ablation [4].

1 Overview

Sacroiliac joint pain is usually underdiagnosed with 20% of patients with low back pain generated from the sacroiliac joint. Patients with SIJS often present with pain near the posterior superior iliac spine. Both the articular and extraarticular elements of the SIJ have been described as causes of sacroiliac joint pain.

However, pain patterns associated with SIJS can overlap with multiple contributions to its origin, with pain originating from the lower lumbar disk especially the L5 level and that of the adjacent facet joints. As a result, SIJS is mostly underdiagnosed.

2 Indications and Contraindications

The diagnosis of SI joint pain proves challenging due to the lack of definitive medical history, physical exam, or imaging findings. Most pain physicians use a positive response to SI joint injections to make a diagnosis.

Arthritis and infection are two examples of intraarticular causes of SI joint pain. Extra-articular sources are more common and include enthesopathy, fractures, ligamentous injury, and myofascial pain.

In addition to etiologic sources, there are several factors that can subject the individual to gradually developing SI joint pain. Those entail increasing the stress borne by the SI joints include true and apparent leg length discrepancy, gait abnormalities, prolonged vigorous exercise, scoliosis, and spinal fusion to the sacrum [5] (Tables 1 and 2).

Table 1 Diagnostic criteria of Sacroiliac joint syndrome [6]

A. **History:** Pain from the SI joint is generally localized in the gluteal region (94%). Referred pain may also be perceived in the lower lumbar region (72%), groin (14%), upper lumbar region (6%), or abdomen (2%)
B. **Examination:** 1. **Compression test:** The patient lies on their non-painful side, the patient's hips are flexed 45° with the knees flexed 90°. While standing behind the patient both hands are placed on the iliac crest and then pressure is exerted downward and medially which elicits pain in SIJS 2. **Distraction test (gapping test)** Patient lies supine and the examiner places their hands on the painful ipsilateral anterior superior iliac spine (ASIS). The examiner then applies pressure in a posterior-lateral direction which elicits pain on the ipsilateral side in SIJS 3. **Patrick's sign (FABER) (Flexion Abduction External Rotation test):** The patient is positioned supine with the examiner standing next to the painful side. The leg of the affected side is flexed at the hip and knee, with the foot positioned over the opposite knee. Downward pressure is then applied to the knee of the affected side. Pain is elicited upon applying pressure
C. **Diagnostic Block:** The IASP criteria mandate that pain should disappear after intra- articular SI joint infiltration with local anesthetic in order to confirm the diagnosis, before the injection of steroids or radiofrequency treatment

Table 2 Intraarticular and Periarticular Sacroiliac joint injection for the management of Sacroilitis

Procedure	Indications	Techniques	Contraindications
Intraarticular Sacroiliac joint block	Diagnosis and treatment of Sacroiliac joint pain	Landmark technique Ultrasound-guided	Absolute: • Patient refusal • Systemic or local infection • Local malignancy Relative: • Coagulopathy or current/recent use of blood thinning agents • Diabetes Mellitus, Type II, with history of poor glycemic control
Periarticular Sacroiliac joint block and Lateral branch block	Treatment of Sacroiliac joint pain and diagnostic block for Radiofrequency ablation	Landmark technique Ultrasound-guided	Absolute: • Patient refusal • Systemic or local infection • Local malignancy Relative: • Coagulopathy or current/recent use of blood thinning agents • Diabetes Mellitus, Type II, with history of poor glycemic control

3 Clinical Anatomy

The SI joint (Fig. 1) is most often characterized as a large, auricular-shaped, diarthrodial synovial joint. In reality, the synovial characteristics are limited only to the distal third and anterior third of the joint [6].

The posterior part is a syndesmosis consisting of the sacroiliac ligament, the gluteus medius and minimus muscles, and the piriformis muscle. The SI joint cannot function independently because all of these muscles are shared with the hip

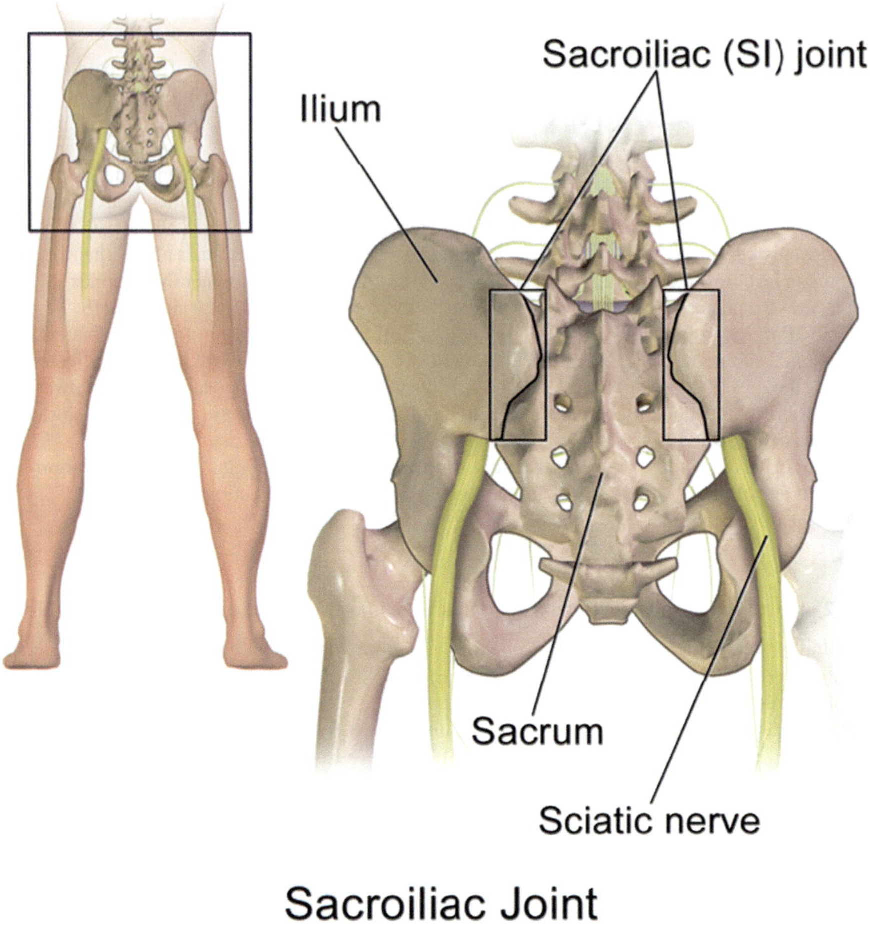

Fig. 1 Anatomy and relations of Sacroiliac joint [10]

joint. That is why the ligamentous structures and the muscles they support have a great influence on the stability of the SI joint [6].

Hence, the choice of inferior approach (targeting the inferior 1/3 of the joint) as a point of needle entry has always been the mainstay of treatment, with recent studies evaluating the efficacy of the superior approach (targeting the superior 2/3 of the joint) to needle placement with weak evidence of apparent effectiveness of such technique.

A combined ventral and dorsal innervation of the SIJ was described in earlier anatomic studies, however, recent studies demonstrate a predominant dorsal innervation of the sacroiliac joint extending from the L5 dorsal ramus to the S4 dorsal ramus. The lateral branches of these rami divide into multiple branches and form the posterior sacral network, which supply the sacroiliac joint with sensory input [7, 8].

The first, second, and third transverse sacral tubercles of the lateral sacral crest were found to be consistent bony landmarks that could be used to demarcate the superior and inferior borders of the posterior sacral network [9].

4 Equipment and Supplies (Table 3)

Table 3 Required supplies for Sacroiliac intra-articular, peri-articular joint injection

Syringe	20 mL Local Anaesthetic or 10 ml Injectate Mixture
Needle	22 or 25 gauge spinal needle 10–12 mm
Anaesthetic	1% Lidocaine 20 mL syringe 0.25–0.5% bupivacaine 10 mL syringe
Corticosteroid	Methylprednisolone 40–80 mg (t1/2 life: 18–36 h) Dexamethasone 6.6 mg (t1/2 life: 36–54 h)
Ultrasound	Linear Probe

5 [Intraarticular and Periarticular Sacroiliac Joint Local Anaesthetic and Steroid Injection] Landmark Techniques

Patient is positioned in the prone position with pillow underneath his pelvis and legs internally rotated for easier access to the SIJ.

Needle entry point is located at a thumb's width inferior to the posterior superior iliac spine (PSIS) and 3.5 cm lateral from the midline (approximately at the level of the second sacral spinous process), as shown on Fig. 2. A 22 G spinal needle is utilized and angled obliquely and slightly towards cranial direction and advanced.

The needle is advanced until it either contacts bone or an increase in resistance is reached, suggesting penetration into a ligament or muscle. Penetration of the SI joint is characterized by a change in resistance (gripping sensation).

The anesthetic-steroid mixture of Bupivacaine 0.25% and methylprednisolone 40 mg or Dexamethasone 6.6 mg are injected intraarticularly into the SIJ after negative aspiration for blood. The capacity of SI joint has been reported to be 2–5 mL after this the injectate becomes periarticular.

The aim of periarticular injections is to spread the local anesthetic and steroid over the S1–3 lateral branches and the posterior ligaments. With recent anatomic studies showing an intimate relationship between the posterior sacroiliac ligaments and the S1–3 lateral branch nerves, the changes in tension on the ligaments may be the cause of pain generated by these branches (Figs. 3 and 4) [11–13].

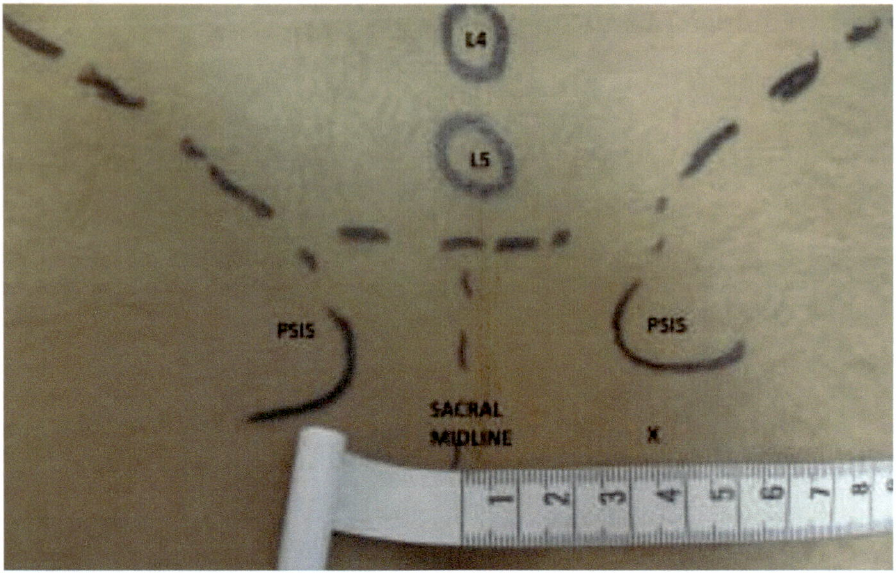

Fig. 2 Landmark-guided sacroiliac joint injection, the needle entry point is marked x (PSIS-Posterior Superior Iliac Spine, L4, L5 indicate spinous process of respective vertebra). Reprinted from (open access) [11]

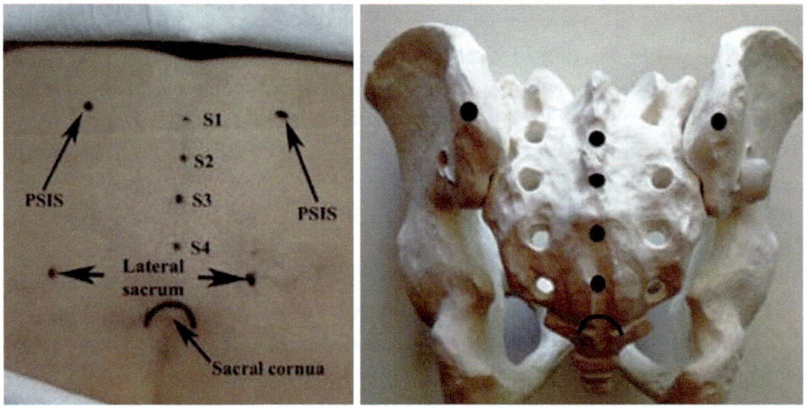

Fig. 3 Skin landmarks for SIJ injection. The posterior superior iliac spines (PSIS) are palpated and marked. Sacral spinous processes (S1–S4), Sacral cornu are marked with sacral edges marked as point of entry. Reprinted from (open access) [12]

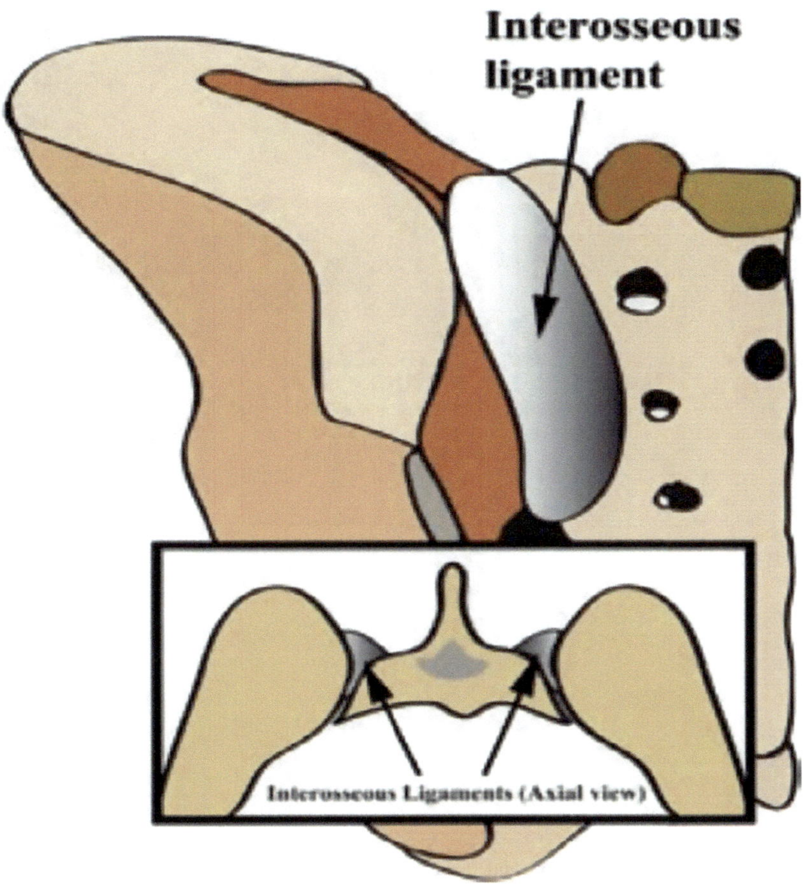

Fig. 4 Anatomical illustration of dorsal sacroiliac ligaments with deeper interosseous component. Reprinted from (open access) [12]

6 Ultrasound Guided Intraarticular Sacroiliac Joint Injection Technique

Patient is lying prone with pillow under pelvis. Anatomical landmarks identified being the posterior superior iliac spine, sacral spinous processes, and sacral cornu (Fig. 5).

The transducer (Linear probe 4–12 Hz) is placed in the transverse plane in the midline over the sacrum. After identifying the sacral spinous process, the probe was moved up until L5-S1 space was located. Then the probe is moved laterally till the PSIS is located. Once the PSIS is visualized the probe is moved caudally to reach the cleft between the iliac bone and sacrum which represent the sacroiliac joint space. Then the probe is rotated to an oblique position such that the posterior sacroiliac ligament is visualized indicating needle entry point (Fig. 6) [13–15].

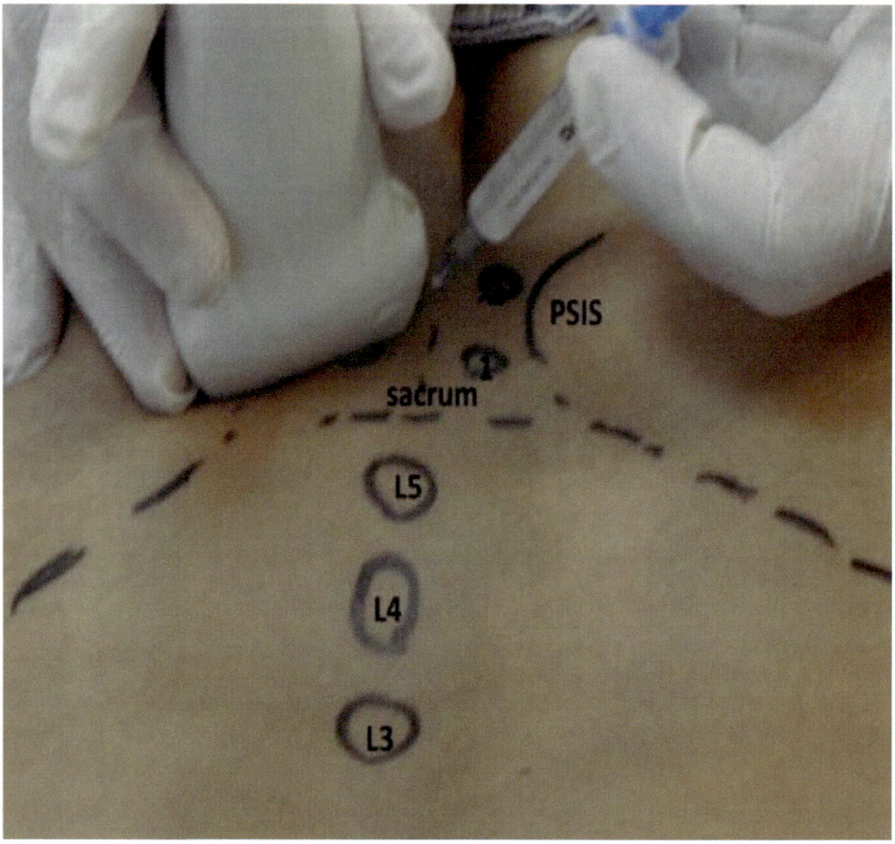

Fig. 5 Ultrasound probe position and posterior superior iliac spine, Sacral spinous processes marked. Reprinted from (open access) [11]

The skin is anaesthetized with 1% lidocaine, then a 22-gauge spinal needle is advanced starting medially and moving laterally, using in-plane technique while needle tip is visualized at all times.

Advancing the needle through the posterior ligament encounters resistance. Further pushing of the needle should result in an abrupt decrease in resistance that is often described as a "pop" which indicates needle entry into the joint; needle advancement may result in a feeling of the needle being gripped in the joint which indicates proper placement. Once the needle tip is positioned precisely in the joint space, 2–5 mL of local anesthetic and steroid mixture of Bupivacaine 0.25% with Methylprednisolone 40 mg is injected. (Fig. 7) [13].

The efficacy of ultrasound versus fluoroscopy guided sacroiliac joint injections is comparable however, ultrasound facilitates the identification and avoidance of the critical vessels around or within the sacroiliac joint (SIJ) [14–16].

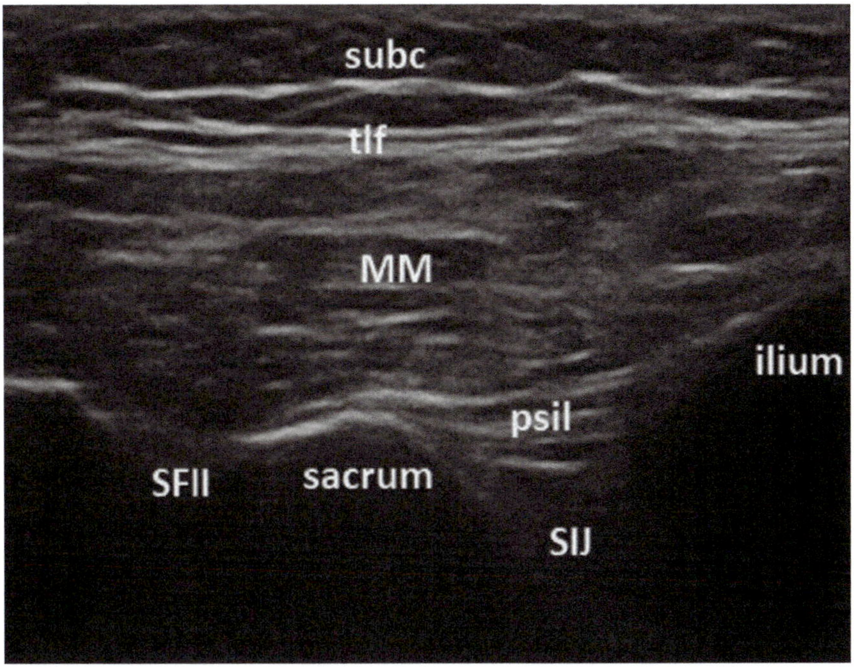

Fig. 6 Ultrasound image of the sacroiliac joint with the transducer in position as in Fig. 5. (SIJ Sacroiliac joint; SFII Second Sacral Foramne; tlf thoracolumbar facias; psil posterior sacroiliac ligament; MM multifidus muscle; psil-posterior superior iliac spine). Reprinted from (open access) [11]

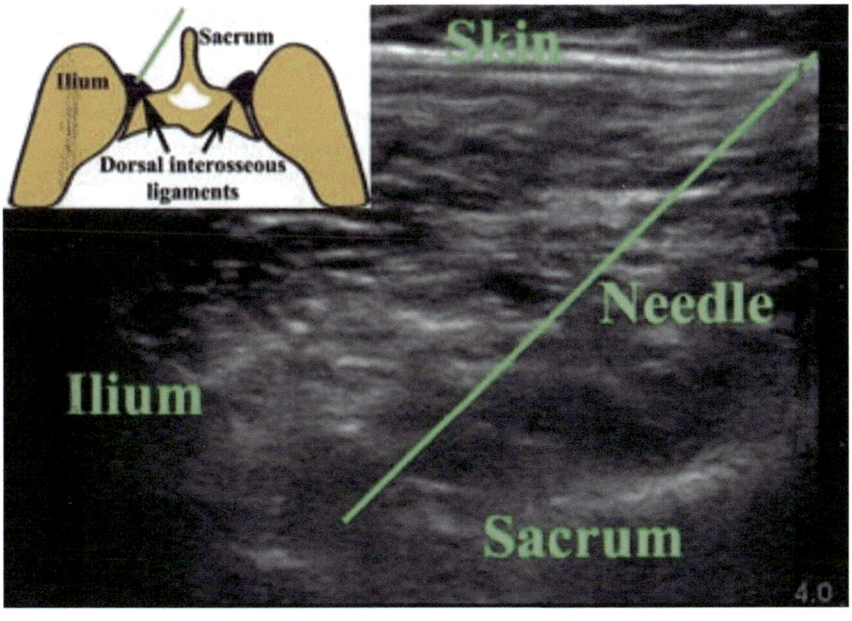

Fig. 7 Ultrasound landmarks identified. The ilium and sacrum are identified as echogenic structures with ilium being cephalad and lateral and the sacrum being central and curved. The cleft between the two is the location of the SIJ. Reprinted from (open access) [12]

7 Potential Complications and Adverse Effects

When guided by ultrasound, SIJ intra-articular or peri-articular injections are generally thought to be safe procedures. Recent review has documented an 11.5% incidence of minor adverse events; most commonly vasovagal reactions [17] (Table 4).

Clinical and Technical Pearls

- Sacroiliac joint presents usually with gluteal stabbing pain with difficulty sitting down for prolonged period of time.
- Patient should be informed of the possible side effects of steroids including weight gain, Increased Blood pressure, Increased blood sugar levels, skin thinning, increased risk of infection and immunosuppression, retinal hemorrhages.
- Extra caution must be taken in patients on anticoagulation. Patients should be observed for at least 15 min after the injection.
- During the procedure it is imperative to get a clear image of the lower 1/3 of the sacroiliac joint this can be achieved by tilting of the ultrasound probe.
- Increased resistance during injection indicates intraarticular injection and slight retraction of the needle may facilitate injection.

Table 4 Summary of potential Complications and Adverse Effects [17]

• Vasovagal reaction
• Cutaneous atrophy due to the corticosteroids utilized in the treatment. Local myotoxicity has been reported with bupivacaine
• The SIJ is drained by the lower volume external vertebral venous plexus, previous studies have documented a low incidence of vascular spread
• Anaphylaxis
• Bruising, Hematoma formation in patients with coagulopathy and bleeding tendency
• Needle placement complications, such as complete penetration of the joint and contact with the sciatic nerve and injury have been reported

References

1. DePalma MJ, Ketchum JM, Saullo T. What is the source of chronic low back pain and does age play a role? Pain Med. 2011;12(2):224–33.
2. Merskey H, Bogduk N. International Association for the Study of Pain. Task Force on Taxonomy. In: Classification of chronic pain: descriptions of chronic pain syndromes and definitions of pain terms. Seattle: IASP Press; 1994.
3. Yoshihara H. Sacroiliac joint pain after lumbar/lumbosacral fusion: current knowledge. Eur Spine J. 2012;21(9):1788–96.
4. Rashbaum RF, Ohnmeiss DD, Lindley EM, Kitchel SH, Patel VV. Sacroiliac joint pain and its treatment. J Spinal Disorders Tech. 2016;29(2):42–8.
5. Zlomislic V, Lee YP, Schwartz A, Garfin S. Management of sacroiliac joint dysfunction. Contemp Spine Surg. 2012;3(3):1–7.
6. Laslett M. Clinical diagnosis of sacroiliac joint pain. Tech Orthop. 2019;34(2):76–8.
7. Yin W, Willard F, Carreiro J, Dreyfuss P. Sensory stimulation-guided sacroiliac joint radiofrequency neurotomy: technique based on neuroanatomy of the dorsal sacral plexus. Spine. 2003;28(20):2419–25.
8. Cusi M, Van der Wall H, Saunders J, Wong L, Pearson M, Fogelman I. Sacroiliac Steroid Injections Do Not Predict Ablation Relief—Not a Surprise. Pain Med. 2013;14(1):163–4.
9. Lim S, Gilligan C. Sacroiliac joint radiofrequency. In: Deer's treatment of pain. Champions: Springer; 2019. p. 433–45.
10. Blausen.com staff Medical gallery of Blausen Medical 2014. WikiJ Med. 1(2) https://doi.org/10.15347/wjm/2014.010. ISSN 2002-4436. is licensed with CC BY 3.0
11. Todorov P, Batalov A. A comparative study between ultrasound guided and landmarks guided intraarticular sacroiliac injections in spondyloarthritis patients. Arch Clin Exp Orthop. 2020;4:1–8.
12. Saunders J, Cusi M, Hackett L, Van der Wall H. An exploration of ultrasound-guided therapeutic injection of the dorsal interosseous ligaments of the sacroiliac joint for mechanical dysfunction of the joint. JSM Pain Manag. 2016;1(1):1003.
13. Kothari K, Sahu DK. Ultrasonography versus fluoroscopy in modern pain management. Indian J Pain. 2016;30(2):71.
14. Cohen SP, Chen Y, Neufeld NJ. Sacroiliac joint pain: a comprehensive review of epidemiology, diagnosis and treatment. Expert Rev Neurother. 2013;13(1):99–116.
15. Chang WH, Lew HL, Chen CP. Ultrasound-guided sacroiliac joint injection technique. Am J Phys Med Rehabil. 2013;92(3):278–9.
16. Plastaras CT, Joshi AB, Garvan C, Chimes GP, Smeal W, Rittenberg J, Lento P, Stanos S, Fitzgerald C. Adverse events associated with fluoroscopically guided sacroiliac joint injections. PM R. 2012;4(7):473–8.
17. Cheng J, Abdi S. Complications of joint, tendon, and muscle injections. Tech Reg Anesth Pain Manag. 2007;11(3):141–7.

Further Reading

Falowski S, Sayed D, Pope J, Patterson D, Fishman M, Gupta M, Mehta P. A Review and Algorithm in the Diagnosis and Treatment of Sacroiliac Joint Pain. J Pain Res. 2020;13:3337–48. https://doi.org/10.2147/JPR.S279390.

Interventions for Coccygeal Pain

Nirav M. Patel and Harsh Sachdeva

Essential Concepts

- Coccydynia is pain in the coccyx region.
- Coccydynia pain can be acute or chronic.
- It impairs the ability of patients to sit. Coccydynia is usually worse with prolonged sitting, standing up from sitting position, and leaning back while sitting. It may get worse with sexual intercourse or defecation in some patients. It is frequently debilitating for patients.
- Management of coccydynia involves a multidisciplinary approach, including injections that can be used at the bedside.
- Bedside interventions for coccydynia can be performed using landmarks or ultrasonography. They typically provide rapid short-term relief, but the effect commonly lasts for months.

1 Coccygeal Nerve Injection

Tailbone pain is referred as coccydynia or coccygodynia [1] Patients with coccydynia usually present with focal pain over the coccyx. Coccydynia is usually worse with prolonged sitting, standing up from sitting position, and leaning back while sitting. It may get worse with sexual intercourse or defecation in some patients [2–4]. Etiologies of tailbone pain include trauma, childbirth, immobility, poor posture, underweight or overweight, cancer, ankylosing spondylitis and lumbar spinal stenosis [1, 3, 5, 6]. Coccydynia is more prominent in females most likely due to trauma during childbirth and because the coccyx in females is located more posteriorly than in males making it more prone to trauma [2, 4, 5]. Interventional treatment of coccydynia is a conventional part of the interdisciplinary management of tailbone pain [7, 8].

N. M. Patel · H. Sachdeva (✉)
University of Cincinnati, Cincinnati, OH, USA
e-mail: sachdehh@ucmail.uc.edu

D. Souza et al. (eds.), *Bedside Pain Management Interventions*,
https://doi.org/10.1007/978-3-031-11188-4_39

2 Indications and Contraindications

The most common indication for coccygeal nerve injection is tailbone pain secondary to trauma, childbirth, immobility, poor posture, being underweight or overweight, hypertrophy of the muscles of the pelvis area, cancer, lumbar spinal stenosis, ankylosing spondylitis, and a variety of other inflammatory arthropathies. Additionally sacrococcygeal ligament overuse or inflammation and other acute or chronic conditions may cause coccygeal pain.

Typical contraindications include local infection at the planned injection site, severe systemic infection, allergy or intolerance to injectate or its components, including local anesthetics and corticosteroids. Another absolute contraindication is patient's refusal. Coagulopathy, including iatrogenic, and platelet dysfunction, including iatrogenic, are not considered to be contraindications for this injection.

3 Clinical Anatomy

The coccyx is located at the end of the sacrum and is the lowest portion of vertebral spine [1, 4]. The coccyx with its two ischial tuberosities makes a tripod that bears weight while person sits. It also serves as an insertion site for multiple muscles, ligaments, and tendons. The coccyx usually has three to five vertebral segments attached by fibrocartilaginous joints [4]. It superiorly attaches to the sacrum. At the inferior portion of the sacrum, there are vestigial remnants of inferior articular processes known as sacral cornua (Fig. 1).

The sacral hiatus is U-shaped space between two sacral cornua created by lower portion of S4 and entire S5 vertebrae and the space (Fig. 1) [9]. The sacral hiatus is covered posteriorly by the sacrococcygeal ligament and penetration of this ligament provides direct excess in epidural space [4, 5, 9].

Treatment for coccygeal pain may involve multiple treatment options including ganglion impar injections, sacrococcygeal injections, and caudal epidural injections. These procedures could be diagnostic and therapeutic in nature and can provide relief from days to weeks, to months.

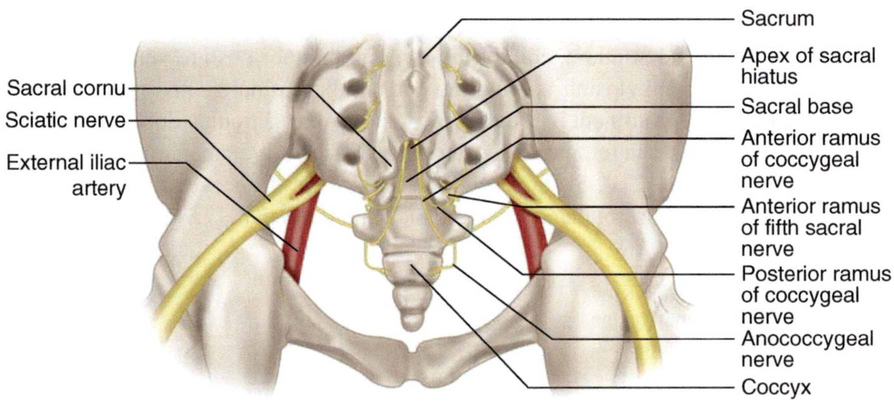

Fig. 1 Posterior view of sacrum and coccyx, as labeled

Table 1 Equipment and supplies for the sacrococcygeal ligament injection and coccygeal nerve injection

Syringe	3–5 mL syringes
Needle	22–25 g needle 1.5–3.5 inch v
Anesthetic	0.25–0.5% bupivacaine 1–2% lidocaine
Corticosteroid	Triamcinolone 40–80 mg (t1/2 life: 18–36 h) or other corticosteroids

4 Equipment and Supplies

Sacrococcygeal ligament injection or coccygeal nerve blocks can be performed at the bedside either using a landmark technique or ultrasound guidance. An antiseptic solution, typically 4% chlorhexidine, 22–25 Gauge 1.5–3.5-in. needle, 5–10 mL syringe for injectate, mask, and sterile gloves should be typically prepared for this procedure. Local anesthetic with or without corticosteroids is typically prepared for this injection as well. Normal saline or local anesthetic can be utilized for ultrasound guidance during hydrolocalization. An ultrasound unit with either a curvilinear or linear transducer will be typically needed. (Table 1).

5 Description of the Procedure

Landmark Technique

The patient is placed in the prone position. The patient's legs and heels can be abducted to avoid tightening of gluteal muscles. A wide skin area over the sacral hiatus is prepared with the 4% chlorhexidine or another conventional antiseptic solution The sacral hiatus, located between the two sacral cornua, is palpated with a finger. After identification of sacral hiatus, the skin over the sacral hiatus is anesthetized using 1% lidocaine. A lidocaine syringe is then attached to a 22–25 Gauge, 1.5–3.5 in. needle, and the needle is inserted through the anesthetized area at a 90-degree angle into the sacrococcygeal ligament. As the needle passes through the sacrococcygeal ligament, a pop can be potentially felt, and advancement should be stopped. After negative aspiration, a local anesthetic or normal saline is injected with or without corticosteroid. The total volume of the injectate is 5 to 10 mL. While landmark-based coccygeal nerve block was commonly used in the past [10], we do not recommend it because of the inability to directly visualize needle advancement and injectate spread that may lead to complications.

Ultrasound-Guided Injection

The patient is placed in the prone position. The patient's legs and heels can be abducted to avoid tightening of gluteal muscles. A wide skin area over the sacral hiatus. is prepared with 4% chlorhexidine or another conventional antiseptic solution. The sacral hiatus located, between two sacral cornua, is palpated with a finger before placing the ultrasound transducer. A transducer is placed in the short axis first over the sacrum (Fig. 2) [9].

The transducer is then moved caudally until the sacral cornua, which looks like two peaks or reversed U-shaped structures, are visualized (Fig. 3).

Between these two reversed U-shaped structures are two hyperechoic bands like structures [9]. The superior band-like structure is the sacrococcygeal ligament and the inferior hyperechoic structure is the base of the sacrum. The space between these two structures contains both anterior and posterior rami of the coccygeal nerves. The space between the sacrococcygeal ligament and the sacral base is the target for the placement of the tip of the needle and the injectate. An area of skin just inferior to the transducer is localized using 1–2% lidocaine. A 22–25 Gauge 1.5–3.5-in. needle is introduced through the anesthetized area using out of plane technique at 90 degrees until it pierces through the sacrococcygeal ligament and enters the caudal canal, the space between sacral base and the sacrococcygeal ligament (Figs. 2 and 3). As the needle passes through the sacrococcygeal ligament, a pop will likely be felt. Since the needle advanced towards the target in an out-of-plane fashion, its visualization may be limited. Needle advancement can be visualized with ultrasound using hydrolocalization with normal saline or local anesthetic. We do not recommend using corticosteroid solution for hydrolocalization. Filling the space between sacral base and sacrococcygeal ligament with local anesthetic solution with or without corticosteroid, and visualization of the injectate spread would complete this procedure [9]. The volume of injectate can be significantly less with ultrasound-guided technique compared to landmark-based technique because of the precise placement of the injectate. The total volume of injectate with ultrasound-guided technique is usually 3 to 5 mL.

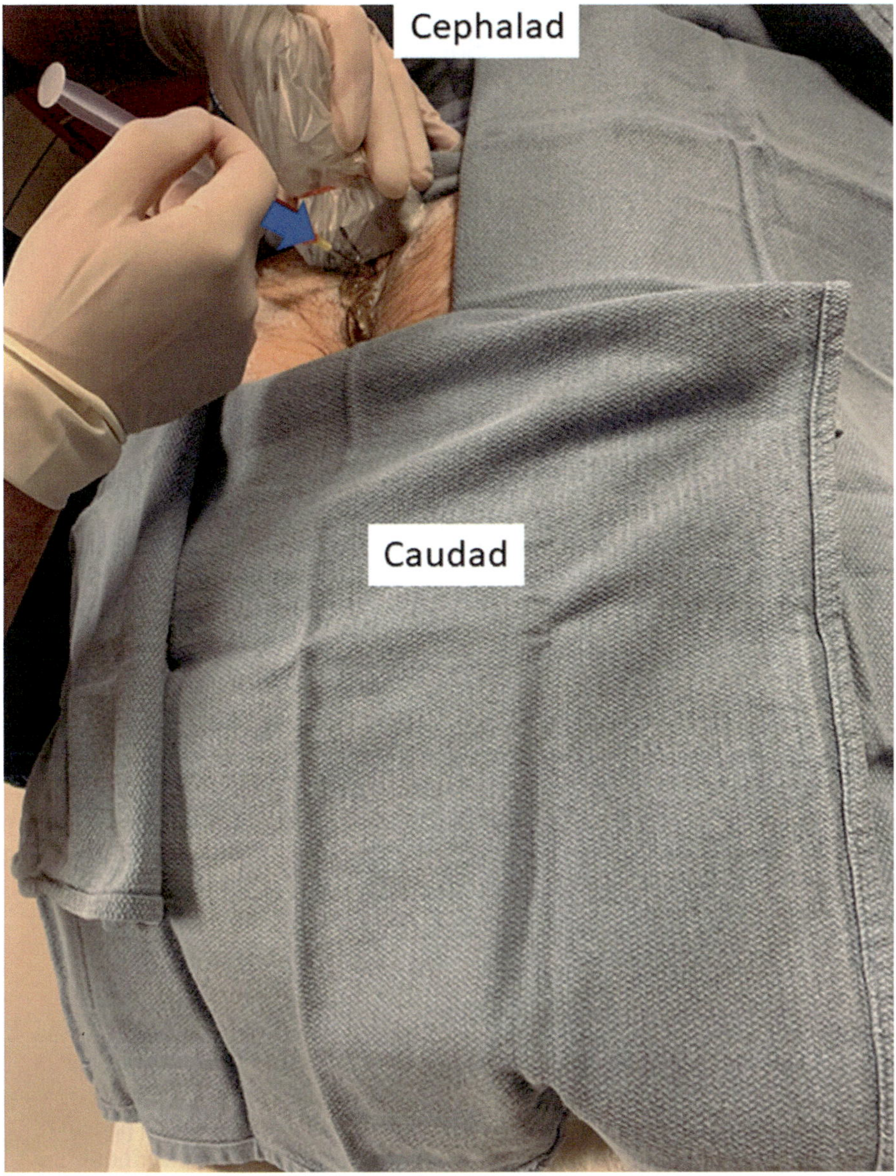

Fig. 2 Patient positioning and ultrasound transducer orientation. The sacral hiatus located, between two sacral cornua, is palpated with a finger before placing the ultrasound transducer. A transducer is placed in the short axis first over the sacrum. The blue arrow indicates the needle trajectory. The curvilinear transducer was used in this patient because of the patient's obesity. (Image–courtesy of Dmitri Souza, MD, PhD)

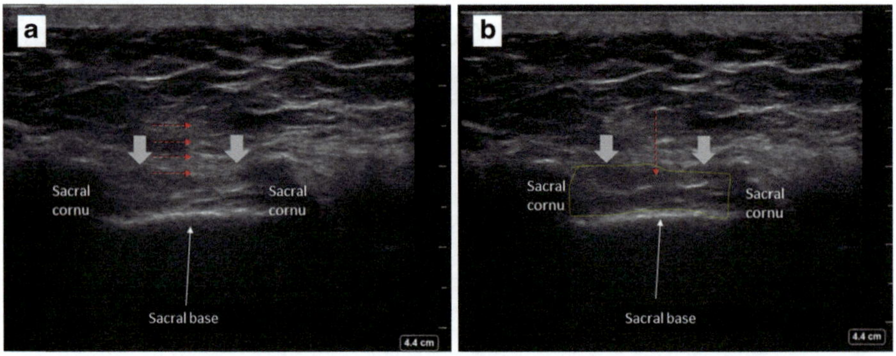

Fig. 3 Transverse ultrasound view of sacral hiatus. (**a**) before the procedure. (**b**) after the injection. Gray arrows point towards the sacrococcygeal ligament. Red dashed arrow points to the needle shaft on image **a**. The needle visualization is limited with the out-of-plane technique utilized for this procedure. The yellow line indicates the spread of the injectate on the same patient on image **b**. The injectate spread is visible under the sacrococcygeal ligament spreading towards the above arterial and posterior rami of the coccygeal nerve that are located just medial to the sacral cornua. The needle visualization (red dashed arrow on image **b**) is limited with the out-of-plane technique utilized for this procedure, however, the hydrolocalization and injectate spread indicate the correct placement of the needle just below the sacrococcygeal ligament, with the injectate likely reaching both anterior and posterior rami of the coccygeal nerves on both sides (yellow line). (Image–courtesy of Dmitri Souza, MD, PhD)

6 Potential Complications

Bleeding is an uncommon, but possible complication of coccygeal nerve blocks. To avoid hematoma formation pressure should be applied in patients with bleeding disorders or on anticoagulation [2, 4, 11]. Other potential complications are presented in Table 2.

Clinical Pearls

1. Coccygeal nerve blocks are relatively easy to perform and can be done at the bedside. We recommend using ultrasonography for this injection.
2. Meticulous attention should be paid to an immunocompromised patient to prevent infection. Although the infections are rare, early detection of the complication is imperative to prevent untoward consequences.

Table 2 Potential complications

If the needle is inadvertently advanced too far anteriorly because the sacrococcygeal ligament penetration ("pop") was not detected during landmark technique injection, it may trigger a bowel perforation. It is expected that in some patients the sacrococcygeal ligament will be seen, or not fused is an anatomical variant
Anaphylaxis can happen as a reaction to a local anesthetic if the history of the patient's allergies was not verified
Pregnancy is not an absolute contraindication to the coccygeal nerve blocks, but a detailed discussion about the risks and benefits of this procedure should be offered to the patient
There are significant concerns with repeated corticosteroid use, especially in the elderly and patients with diabetes mellitus. Repeated injections would patients at risk of developing osteopenia or osteoporosis, weight gain, Cushing syndrome, adrenal insufficiency, worsening of blood sugar control, and others. Clinicians must be diligent in questioning patients specifically about the potential recent use of steroids as this medication history is often not reported by the patient

References

1. Foye PM. Coccydynia: Tailbone pain. Phys Med Rehabil Clin N Am. 2017;28(3):539–49.
2. Foye PM, Varghese CA, Singh R. Looking below the Sacrococcygeal Joint in patients with Coccydynia (Coccyx Pain). Indian J Orthop. 2020;54(1):104.
3. Terlemez R. Coccydynia in a patient with ankylosing spondylitis: enthesitis or structural disorder? Am J Phys Med Rehabil. 2019;98(8):E101.
4. Patel R, Appannagari A, Whang PG. Coccydynia. Curr Rev Musculoskelet Med. 2008;1(3–4):223–6.
5. Skalski MR, Matcuk GR, Patel DB, Tomasian A, White EA, Gross JS. Imaging coccygeal trauma and coccydynia. Radiographics. 2020;40(4):1090–106.
6. Garg B, Ahuja K. Coccydynia-A comprehensive review on etiology, radiological features and management options. Journal of Clinical Orthopaedics and Trauma. 2021;12(1):123–9.
7. White WD, Avery M, Jonely H, Mansfield JT, Sayal PK, Desai MJ. The interdisciplinary management of coccydynia: A narrative review. PM R. 2021;Aug 1. https://doi.org/10.1002/pmrj.12683.
8. Andersen G, Milosevic S, Jensen MM, Andersen M, Simony A, Rasmussen MM, et al. Coccydynia—the efficacy of available treatment options: a systematic review. Global Spine J. 2021.
9. Lirette LS, Chaiban G, Tolba R, Eissa H. Coccydynia: An overview of the anatomy, etiology, and treatment of coccyx pain. Ochsner J. 2014;14(1):84–7.
10. Wray CC, Easom S, Hoskinson J. Coccydynia aetiology and treatment from leicester royal infirmary. J Bone Joint Surg Br. 1991;73(2):335–8.
11. Finsen V. Corticosteroid injection for coccygodynia. Tidsskr Nor Laegeforen. 2001;121(24):2832–3.

Further Reading

Patijn J, Janssen M, Hayek S, Mekhail N, Van Zundert J, van Kleef M. 14. Coccygodynia. Pain Pract. 2010;10(6):554–9. https://doi.org/10.1111/j.1533-2500.2010.00404.x. Epub 2010 Sep 6

Piriformis Muscle Injection

Hemkumar Pushparaj and Anuj Bhatia

Essential Concepts

- Piriformis syndrome (PS) is a cause of deep gluteal pain syndrome and radiculopathy in the lower limb of non-spinal origin.
- Relief from piriformis spasm and contraction may resolve both neuropathic and myofascial symptoms.
- Piriformis injection can be performed accurately and safely with ultrasound guidance.
- Therapeutic injectate choices include local anesthetics, steroids or botulinum toxin.

1 Overview

Low back or gluteal pain with radiculopathy is one of the most common presenting complaints encountered in pain clinics. Although this pain originates from the spine in the majority of patients, extra-spinal etiology needs to be considered when spinal etiologies have been ruled out. Piriformis syndrome (PS) is a common non-spinal

H. Pushparaj
Department of Anesthesia, Faculty of Medicine, University of Toronto, Toronto, ON, Canada

Department of Anesthesia and Pain Medicine, Toronto Western Hospital, Toronto, ON, Canada

A. Bhatia (✉)
Department of Anesthesia, Faculty of Medicine, University of Toronto, Toronto, ON, Canada

Department of Anesthesia and Pain Medicine, Toronto Western Hospital, Toronto, ON, Canada

Institute of Health Policy Management and Evaluation, University of Toronto, Toronto, ON, Canada
e-mail: Anuj.Bhatia@uhn.ca

D. Souza et al. (eds.), *Bedside Pain Management Interventions*,
https://doi.org/10.1007/978-3-031-11188-4_40

cause of lumbar radiculopathy that accounts for about 5–6% of cases [1]. It is more commonly seen in middle-aged female population [1].

2 Piriformis Syndrome

Piriformis syndrome (PS) – compression of the sciatic nerve by the piriformis muscle – usually presents as localized myofascial pain in the gluteal region with features of compression neuropathy in the lower limb [1]. Patients with piriformis syndrome often present with hip pain, buttock pain, dyspareunia (in female patients), and sciatica [2]. Intense and excessive contraction of the piriformis leads to pain in the gluteal region that is often worsened by sitting or by rising from a seated position while irritation of the sciatic nerve that is in close proximity to the muscle causes neuropathic symptoms radiating down the leg [3]. Pathologies responsible for this syndrome include variations of the course of the sciatic nerve or the anatomy of the piriformis muscle with part of or the entire nerve traversing through the muscle, piriformis muscle trauma, hypertrophy, and spasm. However, a systematic review reported no significant difference in the incidence of piriformis syndrome between patients with traditional anatomy compared to those with anatomical variations [4].

This syndrome was first described by Robinson with the following features: (i) history of gluteal trauma, (ii) buttock or sacroiliac pain, which may radiate down the leg, (iii) gluteal muscle wasting, (iv) a palpable sausage-shaped muscle (v) a positive Lasegue sign, (vi) worsening pain with bending or lifting (vi) tenderness at the greater sciatic notch, (vii) improvement with conservative therapy [5]. A 12-point clinical scoring system has been proposed to have a sensitivity and specificity of 96.4% and 100% respectively with a positive predictive value of 100% and a negative predictive value of 86.9% [6]. Specific diagnostic tests that can be used to diagnose PS are listed in Table 1. Most of these rely on reproduction of PS-associated pain with passive internal rotation of the hip. Differential diagnoses include

Table 1 Manoeuvres to diagnose piriformis syndrome [1, 5, 7]

Sign	Description
Freiberg's sign	Pain on passive forced internal rotation of the hip in the supine position
Pace's sign	Pain and weakness on resisted abduction and external rotation of the thigh in a sitting position
FAIR test	Pain on the affected side on voluntary flexion, adduction, and internal rotation
Beatty's maneuver	Active test that involves elevation of the flexed leg on the painful side while the patient lies on the asymptomatic side
Hughes test	External isometric rotation of the affected lower extremity following maximal internal rotation

radiculopathy, lumbar spinal stenosis, sacroiliac (SI) joint–mediated pain, hip joint–mediated pain, facet joint–mediated pain, greater trochanteric pain syndrome, and pain intrinsic to the buttock musculature (deep gluteal pain syndrome) including superior or inferior gemelli, and obturator internus muscles [5].

There is no gold standard investigation to diagnose PS. Computed tomography, magnetic resonance (MR) imaging, MR neurography, and ultrasound can be used to image the piriformis muscle and the sciatic nerve but there are no specific diagnostic features for PS on imaging. These imaging modalities can be used to exclude other causes of lumbar radiculopathy [5].

3 Indications and Contraindications

Treatment for PS is initiated with conservative strategies. Physical exercises (stretching exercises and isometric relaxation techniques) supplemented by oral pharmacological options such as non-steroidal anti-inflammatory drugs, muscle relaxants, and anti-neuropathic agents are often recommended [5]. Injection into the piriformis muscle with local anesthetics (LA), steroids or botulinum toxin A (BTA) are performed when the conservative treatment options fail. Surgical options may also be offered as a last resort which involves decompression of the sciatic nerve and piriformis muscle tenotomy [5].

Contraindications include infection at the injection site and patient refusal.

4 Clinical Anatomy

The piriformis is a biarticular muscle bridging the sacroiliac joint and the hip joint. It originates from the anterior surface of the second, third, and fourth sacral vertebrae, sacrotuberous ligament and the capsule of the sacroiliac joint. It courses across the greater sciatic foramen and inserts onto the medial aspect of the greater trochanter of femur [7]. The action of this muscle relies on the position of the hip. It is predominantly a lateral rotator when the hip is extended but it acts as an abductor when the hip is flexed. Nerve supply to the piriformis is from the posterior divisions of the fifth lumbar and first and second sacral ventral rami. The piriformis divides the deep gluteal space into superior and inferior parts. The superior gluteal neurovascular bundle traverses superior to the piriformis whereas the inferior gluteal vessels and nerve, sciatic nerve and pudendal nerve passes inferior to it (Fig. 1) [7]. In PS, the muscle can be palpated 1 to 2 cm inferior to the middle third of the line joining the posterior superior iliac spine (PSIS) and greater trochanter of the femur [7].

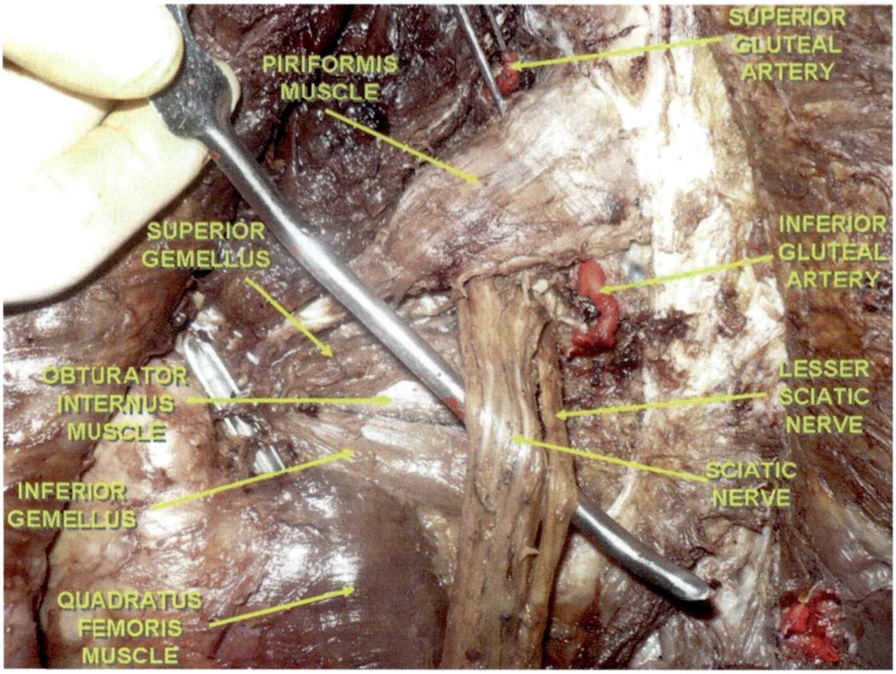

Fig. 1 Anatomy of structures passing through the greater sciatic foramen. The sciatic nerve exits usually beneath the piriformis. The neurovascular bundle above and below the piriformis are named superior and inferior gluteal vessels and nerves respectively. Left is lateral and right is medial in the figure

Table 2 Equipment required for injection into the piriformis muscle

Syringe	1–3 cm^3
Needle	22 or 25-gauge hyperechoic needle (length: 80–120 mm)
Local anesthetic	0.25–0.5% bupivacaine 1–2% lidocaine
Corticosteroid	Methylprednisolone or triamcinolone 40–80 mg
Botulinum Toxin A	50–100 IU diluted in 1–3 cm^3 of normal saline

5 Equipment and Supplies

Piriformis muscle injections can be performed accurately with ultrasound guidance [8, 9]. A 22 or 25-gauge, 80 mm echogenic needle is used for the procedure after infiltrating the skin with local anesthesia (LA). Length of the needle (8 or 12 cm) may vary based on the patient's body habitus (Table 2). Therapeutic medication in a volume of 1–3 cm^3 is injected into the belly of the muscle. There is a lack of evidence to support the use of steroids over LA [10]. Botulinum toxin A (BTA) is often administered and the onset of analgesia from this agent may take a few days but the benefit usually lasts for three to six months [11].

6 Piriformis Injection – Ultrasound-Guided Technique

The patient is positioned prone for this procedure. The gluteal area is prepped and draped on the side to be blocked, from the ipsilateral iliac crest to the inferior gluteal fold and medially up to the midline while taking care not to allow seepage of solution into the perineum as it may be irritating to mucosa. A low frequency curvilinear transducer (2–5 MHz) is used for the procedure. The probe is initially placed just lateral to the posterior superior iliac spine with its long-axis parallel to the course of the piriformis muscle, i.e. a line drawn from the lateral sacral border to the greater trochanter. Iliac crest is visualized as a straight hyper echoic line beneath the gluteal muscles (Fig. 2). The probe is then moved caudally and the straight hyperechoic ilium disappears. This is the cephalad end of greater sciatic notch (GSN). The piriformis muscle is visualized traversing the GSN from deep sacrum and travelling across to insert into the greater trochanter of femur, deep to the gluteus maximus (Fig. 3). To aid in identification of piriformis, the patient can be asked to flex the knee to 90° and to rotate the hip joint externally and internally. This slides the piriformis into and out of GSN while the gluteus maximus remains static. Position of the sciatic nerve is also noted in relation to piriformis to denote any anatomical variation.

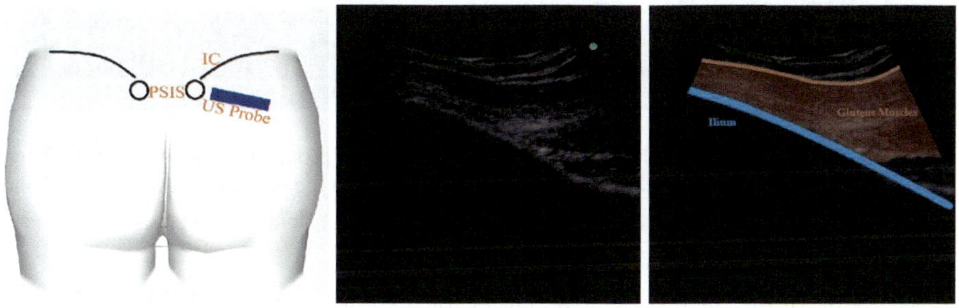

Fig. 2 Ultrasound scan at the level of the ilium, just inferior to the iliac crest. Left is medial and right is lateral in the scans

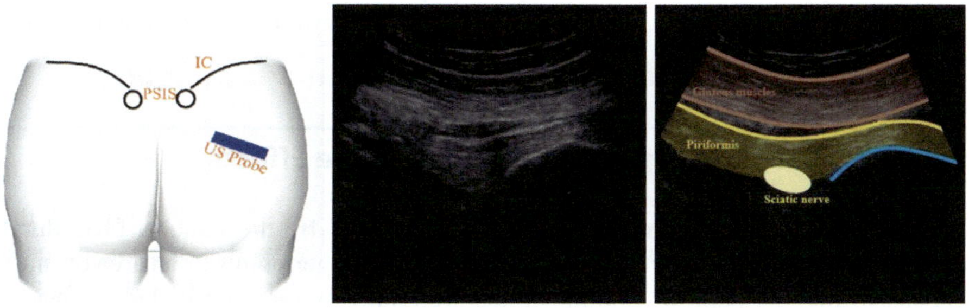

Fig. 3 Ultrasound scan at the level of the ischium. Left is medial and right is lateral in the scans

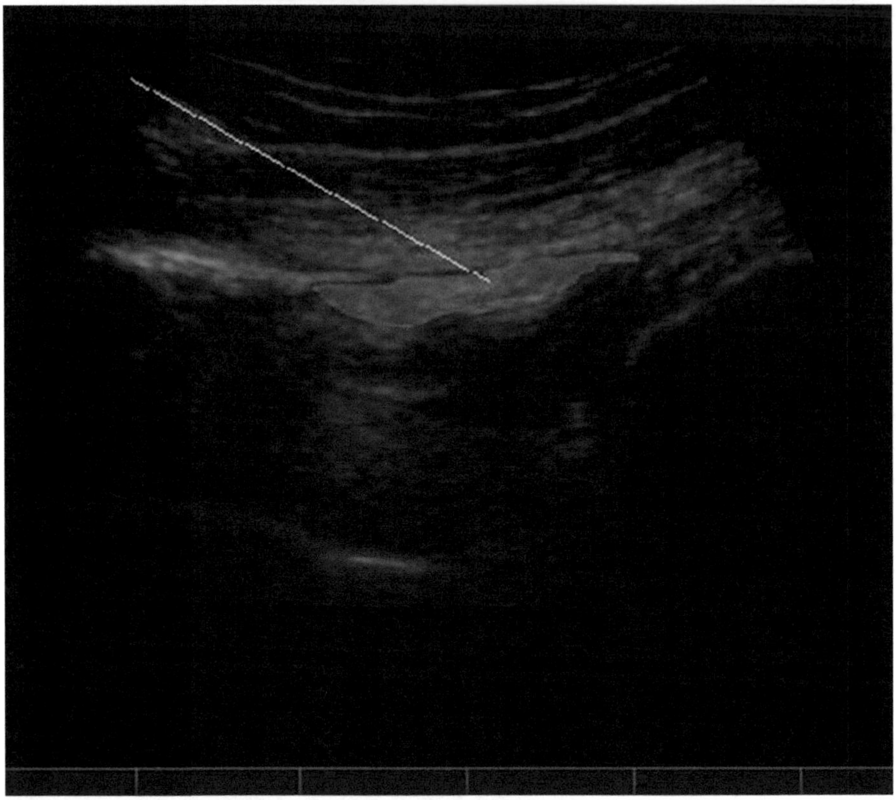

Fig. 4 Needle trajectory from the medial side of the ultrasound probe (left side of the scan) showing the target for needle tip placement and spread of injectate in the piriformis. Left is medial and right is lateral in the scans

The belly of the piriformis is the target for injection. The needle insertion point may be chosen either medial or lateral to the probe. The authors prefer needle entry around 2 cm away from the medial edge of probe in a near-vertical direction. A needle is advanced to reach the belly of the muscle. After injecting 0.2 cm^3 of saline to confirm appropriate position of the needle tip, therapeutic medication is administered (Fig. 4). Care is taken to ensure there is no spread of the medication inferiorly towards the sciatic nerve.

7 Potential Complications and Adverse Effects

Piriformis muscle injection is usually well tolerated by the patient. Procedural adverse effects include discomfort as injection into trigger points or an area of muscle spasm may be painful. Complications are relatively rare and include transient worsening of pain, infection, injection around or into the sciatic nerve, and allergic reaction to the injected medications (Table 3).

Table 3 Potential complications and adverse effects of injection into the piriformis muscle

Sciatic nerve block due to the spread of LA leading to possible transient foot drop or injury from needle trauma and or intraneural injection
Injury to the vasculature in the vicinity of the muscle (superior or inferior gluteal muscles) leading to the formation of a hematoma
Steroid injection into the muscle can cause muscle weakness, osteopenia, transient hypertension and hyperglycemia, and other systemic adverse effects

Clinical and Technical Pearls

- The needle should be inserted through the skin approximately 2 cm medial to the medial edge of the transducer.
- "Toeing in" of the ultrasound transducer towards the needle could help to visualize the needle better.
- Visualization of the ischial spine, seen as a flat hyperechoic structure, indicates that the scan is caudal to the piriformis.
- Bilateral piriformis injection is avoided to prevent possible bilateral sciatic nerve block.
- Pain relief has been shown to last for up to 6 months with injection of botulinum toxin A.

References

1. Jankovic D, Peng P, van Zundert A. Brief review: Piriformis syndrome: etiology, diagnosis, and management. Can J Anesth. 2013;60(10):1003–12.
2. Halpin RJ, Ganju A. Piriformis syndrome. Neurosurgery. 2009;65(suppl_4):A197–202.
3. Hopayian K, Danielyan A. Four symptoms define the piriformis syndrome: an updated systematic review of its clinical features. Eur J Orthop Surg Traumatol. 2018;28(2):155–64.
4. Bartret AL, Beaulieu CF, Lutz AM. Is it painful to be different? Sciatic nerve anatomical variants on MRI and their relationship to piriformis syndrome. Eur Radiol. 2018;28(11):4681–6.
5. Probst D, Stout A, Hunt D. Piriformis syndrome: A narrative review of the anatomy, diagnosis, and treatment. PM R. 2019;11(1):S54–63.
6. Cass SP. Piriformis syndrome: A cause of nondiscogenic sciatica. Curr Sports Med Rep. 2015;14(1):41–4.
7. Michel F, Decavel P, Toussirot E, et al. The piriformis muscle syndrome: An exploration of anatomical context, pathophysiological hypotheses and diagnostic criteria. Ann Phys Rehabil Med. 2013;56(4):300–11.
8. Finnoff JT, Hurdle MFB, Smith J. Accuracy of ultrasound-guided versus fluoroscopically guided contrast-controlled piriformis injections: A cadaveric study. J Ultrasound Med. 2008;27(8):1157–63.
9. Fowler IM, Tucker AA, Weimerskirch BP, Moran TJ, Mendez RJ. A randomized comparison of the efficacy of 2 techniques for piriformis muscle injection: Ultrasound-guided versus nerve stimulator with fluoroscopic guidance. Reg Anesth Pain Med. 2014;39(2):126–32.
10. Misirlioglu TO, Akgun K, Palamar D, Erden MG, Erbilir T. Piriformis syndrome: Comparison of the effectiveness of local anesthetic and corticosteroid injections: A double-blinded, randomized controlled study. Pain Physician. 2015;18:163–71.
11. Rodríguez-Piñero M, Vidal Vargas V, Jiménez Sarmiento AS. Long-term efficacy of ultrasound-guided injection of incobotulinumtoxinA in piriformis syndrome. Pain Med. 2018;19(2):408–11.

Further Reading

Fishman LM, Anderson C, Rosner B. BOTOX and physical therapy in the treatment of piriformis syndrome. Am J Phys Med Rehabil. 2002;81:936–42.

Part V

Bedside Procedures for Thoracic, Abdominal and Pelvic Pain

Intercostal Nerve Blocks

Wenyu Pan, Sarah C. Corral, and Dalia H. Elmofty

Essential Concepts

- Intercostal nerve blocks are an effective method to provide postoperative analgesia after thoracic and upper abdominal surgery.
- Two major techniques are used to perform intercostal nerve blocks: the ultrasound-guided technique and the landmark technique also known as the "blind approach."
- Compared to thoracic epidural anesthesia, intercostal nerve blocks may reduce duration of hospital stay and pulmonary complications following major thoracic surgery [1, 2].
- Potential complications of intercostal nerve blocks are pneumothorax, arterial puncture, hemothorax, and local anesthetic toxicity; performing successful intercostal nerve blocks requires technical expertise.

1 Overview

Intercostal nerve blocks are an effective method in providing analgesia in a variety of acute and chronic pain conditions, including after thoracic and abdominal surgery. The major parts of the skin and muscles of the chest and abdominal wall are innervated by the intercostal nerves. In several settings, intercostal nerve blocks are shown to be effective. For major thoracic surgery, intercostal nerve blocks with liposomal bupivacaine may lessen duration of hospital stays and reduce pulmonary complications compared to thoracic epidural anesthesia [1, 2]. Ultrasound-guided intercostal nerve blocks have been shown to be as effective in pain relief for thoracic

W. Pan · S. C. Corral · D. H. Elmofty (✉)
Department of Anesthesia and Critical Care, University of Chicago, Chicago, IL, USA
e-mail: wenyu.pan@uchospitals.edu; sarah.corral@uchospitals.edu; delmofty@dacc.uchicago.edu

D. Souza et al. (eds.), *Bedside Pain Management Interventions*,
https://doi.org/10.1007/978-3-031-11188-4_41

Table 1 Intercostal nerve blocks for the management of thoracic and upper abdominal surgeries

Procedure	Indications	Techniques
Intercostal nerve block	• Major thoracic surgery: thoracotomy and thoracostomy • Mastectomy • Chest wall trauma • Chest wall tumors • Upper abdominal/flank surgery: gastrostomy, cholecystectomy, and percutaneous nephrolithotomy • Herpes zoster pain • Diagnostic nerve block	• Landmark technique • Ultrasound-guided technique

herpes zoster as fluoroscopy-guided epidural nerve blocks [3]. The accessibility of ultrasound makes intercostal nerve blocks an attractive choice. Ultrasound-guided intercostal nerve blocks at the 11th and 12th intercostal spaces have been shown to provide effective analgesia for percutaneous nephrolithotomy [4].

2 Indications and Contraindications

Intercostal nerve blocks can provide postoperative pain relief after major thoracic surgery, upper abdominal, and flank surgery [1, 2, 4, 5]. They can also provide analgesia for shingles and postherpetic neuralgia [3], chest wall trauma [6], tumors, and as diagnostic nerve blocks to determine if an intercostal nerve is responsible for chest wall pain (Table 1).

Contraindications of intercostal nerve blocks are coagulopathy (relative contraindication) and localized infection at needle entry site.

3 Clinical Anatomy

The intercostal nerves carry both motor and sensory fibers. They originate from the ventral rami of thoracic nerves T1 to T11, while thoracic spinal nerve 12 gives rise to the subcostal nerve. The nerves travel parallel to the ribs in the subcostal groves after piercing the posterior intercostal membrane distal to the intervertebral foramen. They run between the parietal pleura and intercostalis intimus and culminate in two branches: the lateral cutaneous branch near the midaxillary line and the anterior cutaneous branch near the midline. There are many anatomic variations of these nerves, for example, the lateral cutaneous branch innervates the skin and musculature of the lateral torso, reaching the skin at the lateral edge of the rectus abdominis anteriorly and the latissimus dorsi posteriorly. The anterior cutaneous branches of T2 through T6 innervate the skin of the anterior thorax, while the anterior cutaneous branches of T7 through T12 innervate the skin of the anterior abdominal wall and the rectus muscle [7].

Table 2 Required supplies for intercostal nerve blocks

Syringe	3 or 5 mL
Needle	Single shot: 20- or 22-gauge, 2 in. Catheter placement: 18- or 20-gauge Tuohy needle
Anesthetic	0.25–0.5% bupivacaine 1–2% lidocaine with epinephrine 1:200,000 0.2–0.5% ropivacaine
Sterilizing and Resuscitation	Chlorapep, Intralipid

4 Equipment and Supplies

Intercostal nerve blocks are easily performed at the bedside. A 5 cm^3 syringe with a 20- or 22-gauge, 2 in. needle is utilized to inject 3 or 5 mL of the anesthetic solution at each level during a single-shot, multi-injection intercostal nerve block. An 18- or 20-gauge Tuohy needle can be utilized to place a local anesthetic catheter if desired. The local anesthetic solution usually consists of 0.25–0.5% bupivacaine, 0.2–0.5% ropivacaine, or 1–2% lidocaine with or without epinephrine. Resuscitation equipment such as intralipid should be readily available to treat local anesthetic systemic toxicity. Blood levels of local anesthetics after intercostal nerve blocks are higher than for most regional anesthetic procedures (Table 2).

5 Intercostal Nerve Blocks, Landmark Technique

For the landmark technique, the patient is placed in a prone, sitting, or lateral position with the block side up. The patient's arms are positioned forward or hanging down allowing the scapula to retract laterally. This positioning is especially important when performing nerve blocks above the level of the fifth rib. Using aseptic technique, the inferior edge of the rib to be blocked is palpated and marked 6–8 cm laterally from the midline at the lateral border of the paraspinous muscles, which correlates to the angle of the rib. A small amount of 1–2% Lidocaine is injected at the site of needle entry. The skin is then drawn cephalad by about 1 cm and a 20 or 22 gauge needle is introduced at a 20 degree angle cephalad with the bevel facing up. After about 1 cm, the needle should make contact with the rib. The skin is allowed to slide back over the rib and the needle is advanced a few millimeters while scraping the bottom of the rib to enter the subcostal groove (Fig. 1) [7]. A "give" or "pop" may be felt while advancing the needle. Prior to injection, aspirate and then inject 3–5 mL of anesthetic fluid. This can be repeated on multiple levels and should be done one level cephalad and one level caudal to the intercostal nerve being targeted for adequate coverage.

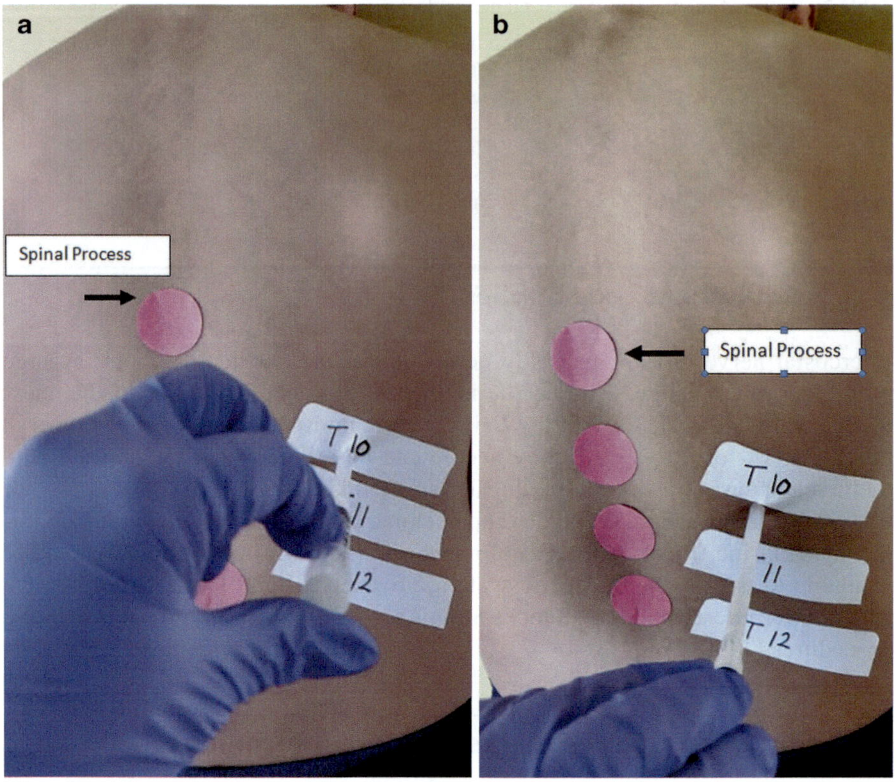

Fig. 1 Landmark Technique for intercostal nerve blocks (**a**) Needle contacting 10th rib (**b**) Needle scraping the bottom of the 10th rib into the subcostal grove

6 Ultrasound Technique

For the ultrasound-guided technique, the same patient positioning can be used as in the Landmark technique. Using a high-resolution linear probe, the ultrasound probe is placed 4–5 cm lateral to the spinal process in a sagittal plane with a slightly oblique tilt. The intercostal neurovascular bundle is expected to lie between the internal intercostal muscle and the innermost intercostal muscle (Fig. 2). Needle entry occurs at the upper margin of the rib, one level caudal to the intercostal nerve being targeted at the angle of the rib as described above. Using the same 20-degree entry angle, insert the needle in an in-plane approach (Fig. 3) as this approach has an advantage of visualizing the needle shaft more clearly compared to an out-of-plane approach (Fig. 4). As the needle advances, it is important to hydrodissect repeatedly to confirm needle tip positioning. Continue to advance under direct visualization until the needle tip reaches the level of the internal intercostal muscle (Fig. 5) [8]. Color Doppler may help visualize the intercostal vessels in the inferior intercostal grove (Fig. 6). First aspirate and then inject 3–5 mL of anesthetic fluid

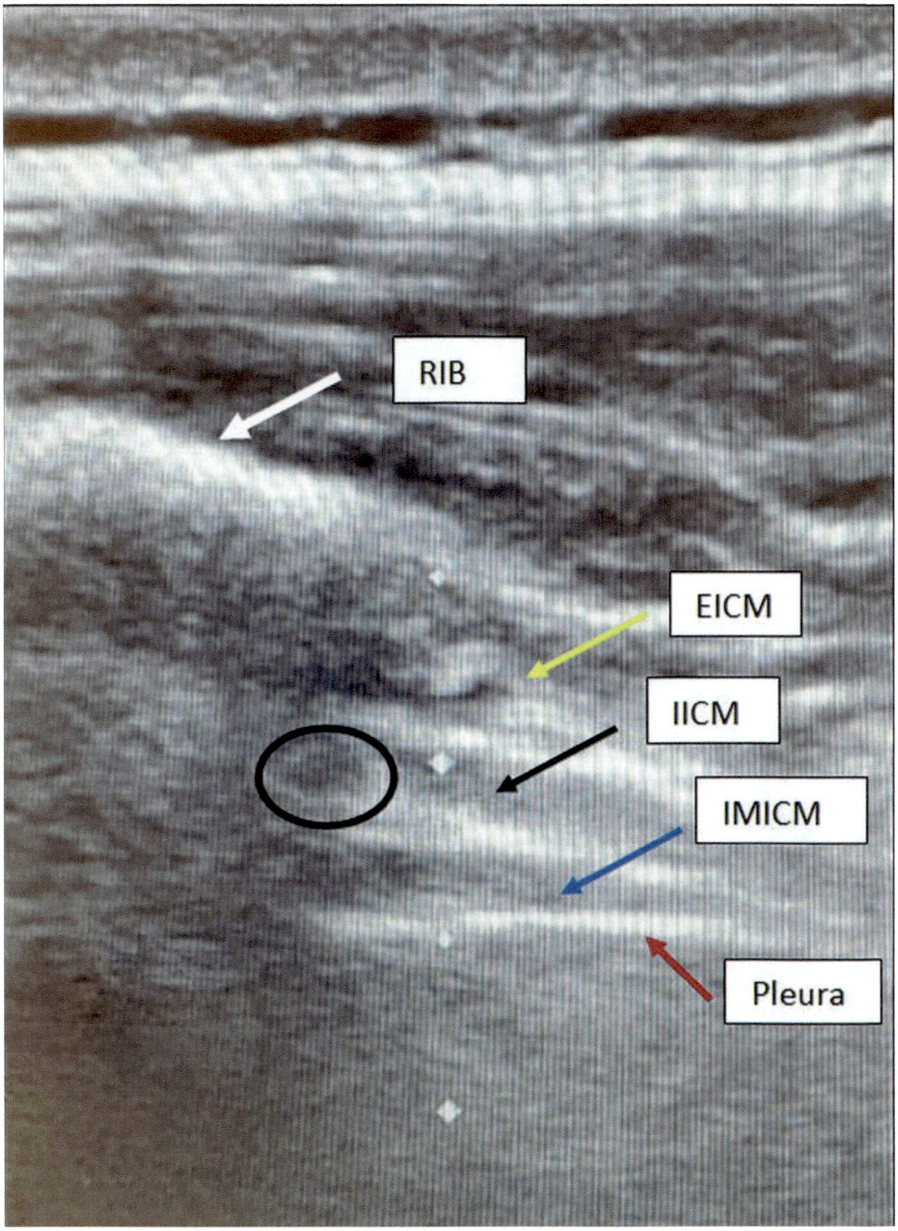

Fig. 2 Sonoanatomy of the intercostal space. White arrow demonstrates the rib, yellow arrow demonstrates the external intercostal muscle (EICM), black arrow demonstrates the internal intercostal muscle (IICM), blue arrow demonstrates the innermost intercostal muscle (IMICM), red arrow demonstrates the parietal pleura, and black circle demonstrates neurovascular bundle

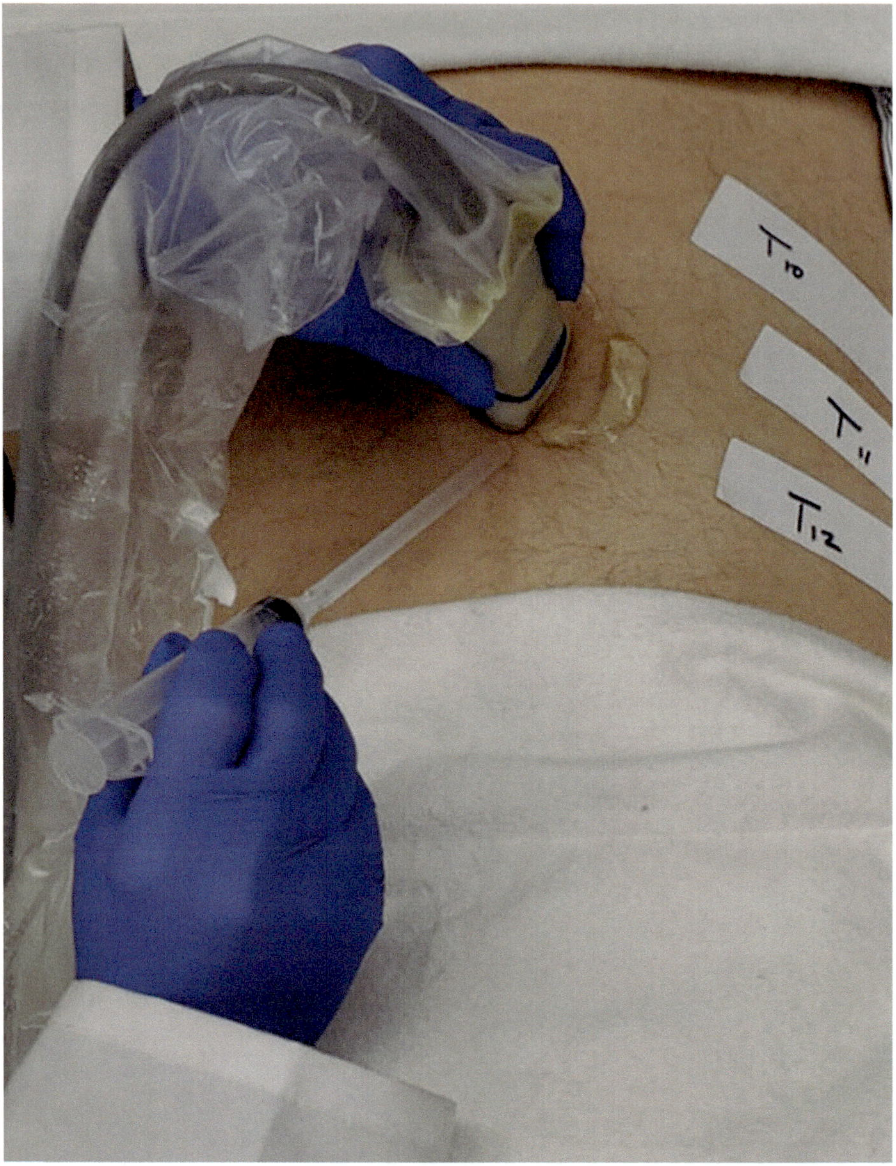

Fig. 3 Ultrasound-guided In-plane Approach. Patient is placed in the prone position with ultrasound probe placed in a sagittal and slightly oblique tilt

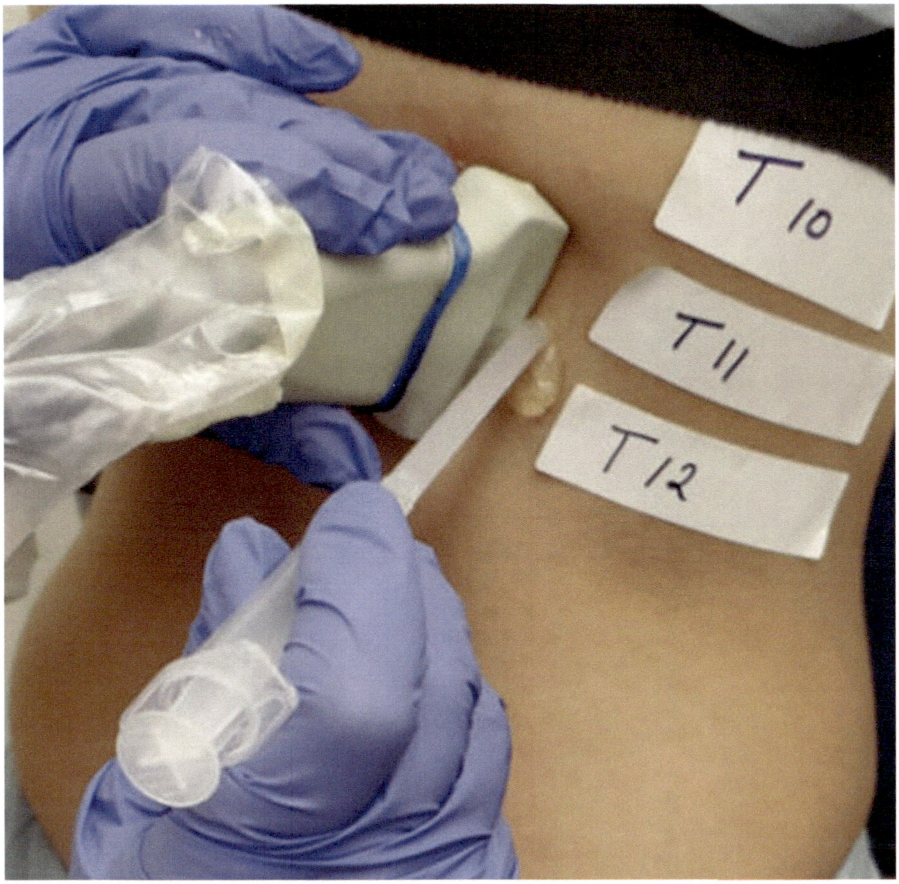

Fig. 4 Ultrasound-guided Out-of Plane Approach

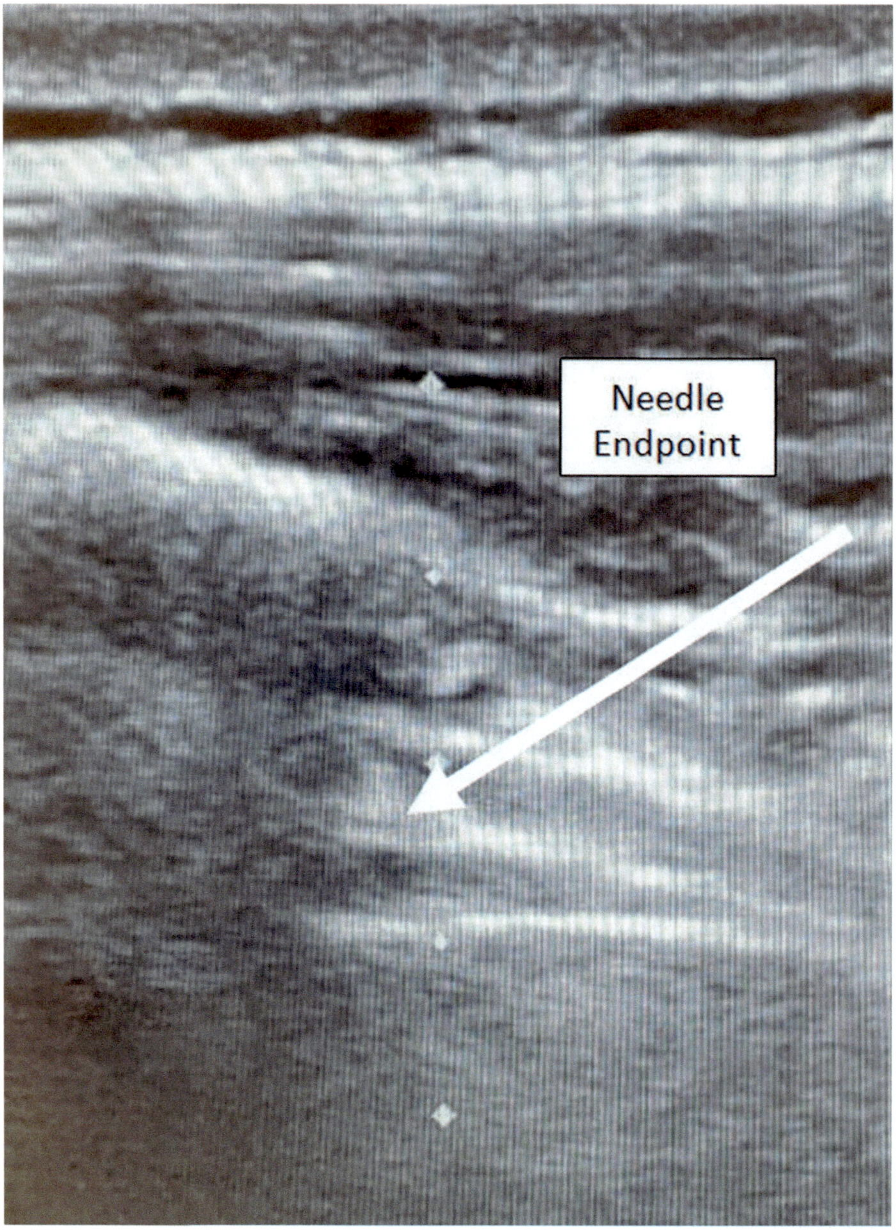

Fig. 5 Needle Endpoint. Needle is advanced until the needle tip reaches the level of the internal intercostal muscle

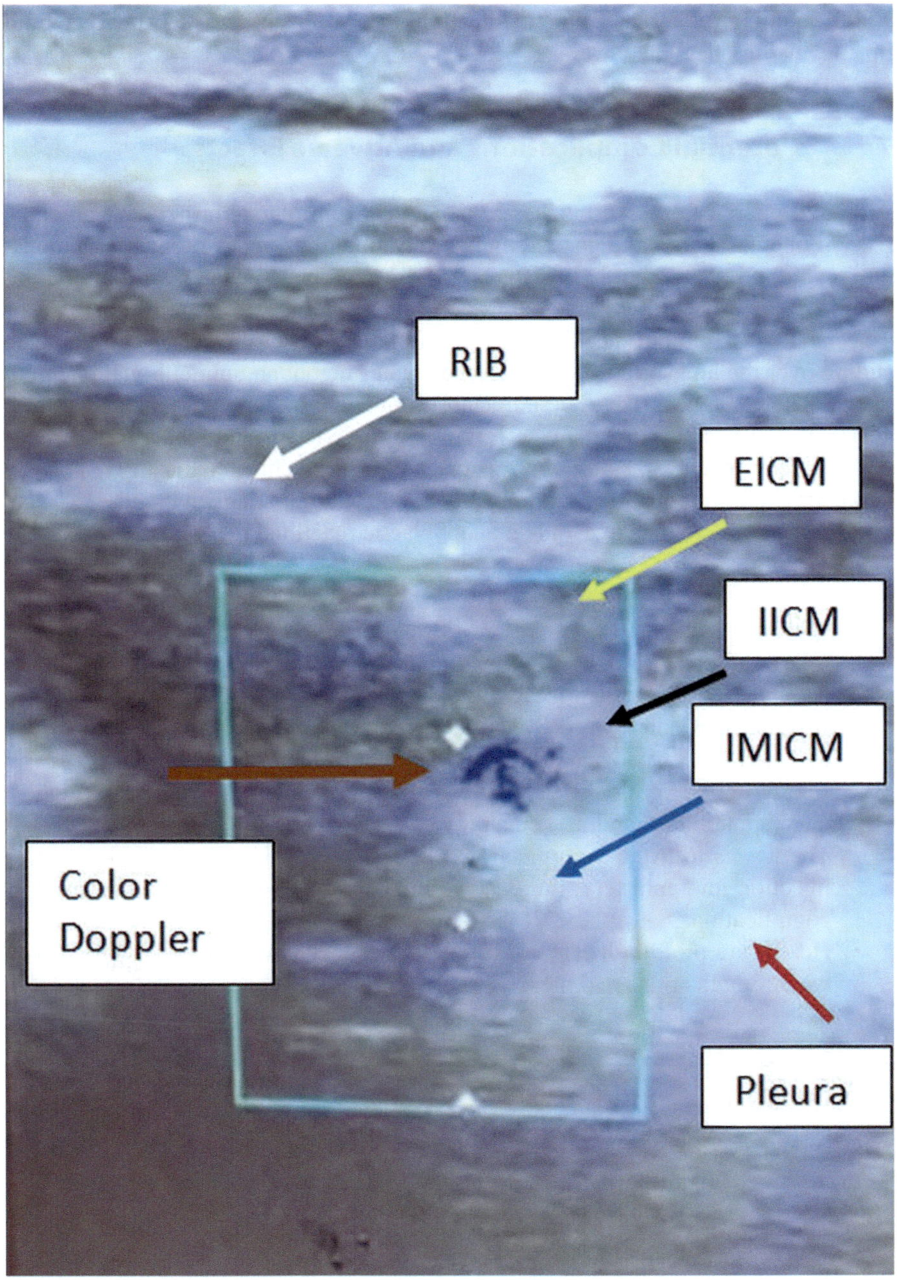

Fig. 6 Color Doppler demonstrating intercostal vessels in the inferior intercostal grove

while watching for spread of the medication. Repeat this process as above on multiple levels for adequate coverage.

7 Potential Complications and Adverse Effects

Although intercostal nerve blocks are generally well tolerated, there are potential risks of pneumothorax and, in extremely rarely situations, inadvertent arterial puncture resulting in hemothorax [9, 10]. These risks can be lessened by utilizing ultrasound to guide needle and catheter placement. Patients with emphysema can be especially susceptible to needle puncture of the pleura. Visualization of the pleura sliding over the lungs after block placement can rule out an unintentional pneumothorax. There can be a risk of systemic absorption and toxicity with the use of local anesthetics, especially in patients receiving multiple levels and bilateral injections. Patients may report dizziness, confusion, slurred speech, metallic taste, perioral numbness, and tinnitus [11]. Caution should be used in patients with allergic reactions to local anesthetics to avoid an anaphylactic reaction [12].

Clinical and Technical Pearls

- Intercostal nerve blocks provide a reliable unilateral dermatomal band for the vertebral level performed.
- If more than one level or bilateral coverage is required, multiple blocks may be necessary to achieve analgesia.
- Intercostal nerve blocks are relatively simple to perform with a thorough understanding of landmark anatomy and sonoanatomy.
- The key is to avoid complications such as pneumothorax or inadvertent injection into an artery; ultrasound guidance may decrease the chance of complications.
- Healthcare professionals performing these blocks must know how to deal with complications and have resuscitation materials nearby.

References

1. Khalil KG, Boutrous ML, Irani AD, Miller CC 3rd, Pawelek TR, Estrera AL, et al. Operative intercostal nerve blocks with long-acting bupivacaine liposome for pain control after thoracotomy. Ann Thorac Surg. 2015;100(6):2013–8.
2. Rice DC, Cata JP, Mena GE, Rodriguez-Restrepo A, Correa AM, Mehran RJ. Posterior intercostal nerve block with liposomal bupivacaine: an alternative to thoracic epidural analgesia. Ann Thorac Surg. 2015;99(6):1953–60.
3. Lee HJ, Park HS, Moon HI, Yoon SY. Effect of ultrasound-guided intercostal nerve block versus fluoroscopy-guided epidural nerve block in patients with thoracic herpes zoster: a comparative study. J Ultrasound Med. 2019;38(3):725–31.

4. Ozkan D, Akkaya T, Karakoyunlu N, Arik E, Ergil J, Koc Z, et al. Effect of ultrasound-guided intercostal nerve block on postoperative pain after percutaneous nephrolithotomy: prospective randomized controlled study. Anaesthesia. 2013;62(12):988–94.
5. Nunn JF, Slavin G. Posterior intercostal nerve block for pain relief after cholecystectomy. Anatomical basis and efficacy. Br J Anaesth. 1980;52(3):253–60.
6. Ho AM, Karmakar MK, Critchley LA. Acute pain management of patients with multiple fractured ribs: a focus on regional techniques. Curr Opin Crit Care. 2011;17(4):323–7.
7. Brown DL. Intercostal Nerve Blocks. In: Brown DL, editor. Atlas of Regional Anesthesia. 3rd ed. Philadelphia: Elsevier Inc; 2006. p. 239–43.
8. Peng PWH, Narouze S. Ultrasound-guided interventional procedures in pain medicine: a review of anatomy, sonoanatomy, and procedures. Reg Anesth Pain Med. 2009;34:458–74.
9. Shanti CM, Carlin AM, Tyburski JG. Incidence of pneumothorax from intercostal nerve block for analgesia in rib fractures. J Trauma. 2001;51(3):536–9.
10. Dangoisse M, Collins S, Glynn CJ. Haemothorax after attempted intercostal catheterization. Anaesthesia. 1994;49(11):961–3.
11. Dickerson DM, Apfelbaum JL. Local anesthetic systemic toxicity. Aesthet Surg J. 2014;34(7):1111–9.
12. Al-Dosary K, Al-Qahtani A, Alangari A. Anaphylaxis to lidocaine with tolerance to articaine in a 12 year old girl. Saudi Pharm J. 2014;22(3):280–2.

Further Reading

Detterbeck FC. Efficacy of methods of intercostal nerve blockade for pain relief after thoracotomy. Ann Thorac Surg. 2005;80(4):1550–9.

Bedside Injections for Costochondral Pain

Ankit Maheshwari and Daniel Gotlib

Essential Concepts

- Costochondral pain is generally self-limited, with symptoms lasting weeks, months, or rarely longer.
- Tietze syndrome involves a single tender and swollen costochondral joint.
- Uncertain diagnosis should have further clinic workup for more life threatening pathologies.
- Local analgesic and steroid injections therapies may be beneficial to patients with more prolonged or severe symptoms.
- Costochondral joint injection may be an effective therapeutic tool in treating a variety of costochondral pain. Parasternal Blocks are an effective therapeutic tool in treating costochondral pain due to sternal fractures and pain from post-surgical anterior chest procedures.
- Costochondral pain can be managed with broader coverage blocks including Pectoralis nerve block (PEC1, PEC2), Serratus Anterior Plane (SAP), Erector Spinae Plane (ESP), Paravertebral, and Thoracic Epidural.

1 Overview

Costochondral pain, also known as costosternal syndrome, parasternal chondrodynia, or costochondritis, involves nociceptive signals originating from the costosternal joints, or the associated sternum or ribs. Although the actual etiology is relatively unknown [1], patients usually report a history of chest trauma, or a musculoskeletal

A. Maheshwari (✉)
Texas Pain Intervention Clinic, McKinney, TX, USA

D. Gotlib
Department of Anesthesiology & Perioperative Medicine, University Hospitals Case Western Reserve, Cleveland, OH, USA
e-mail: Daniel.gotlib@uhhospitals.org

D. Souza et al. (eds.), *Bedside Pain Management Interventions*,
https://doi.org/10.1007/978-3-031-11188-4_42

injury including exertional exercise, heavy lifting, coughing, or sneezing. Pain is most commonly unilaterally located across multiple costosternal joints between second to fifth ribs [1]. Pain is exacerbated by repetitive activities, tenderness to palpation, deep breathing, or coughing. Pain may be severe enough to cause changes in respiratory effort, and may exacerbate dyspnea especially in patients with underlying pulmonary pathology. This condition is relatively self-limited, with symptoms lasting weeks, months, or rarely years [2]. Although costochondral pain is a common complaint and diagnosis, a thorough history and physical must be obtained to differentiate other etiologies or life-threatening disease processes for chest pain [2].

Swelling associated with costochondral joint pain can occur in Tietze syndrome. Compared to costochondritis, Tietze syndrome is rare, and affects a single costochondral joint most commonly at the second or third costosternal joint [3]. Possible etiologies include infection, rheumatologic, or neoplastic processes. Infectious etiologies are associated with stab wounds, post-surgery, or IV drug use [4, 5]. Neoplasm etiologies include primary or metastatic neoplasm to the costochondral joint and closely associated anatomy [6]. If suspected, additional workup may be required to determine and treat the primary pathology.

Initial treatment options include manual therapies such as physical therapy [7], osteopathic manipulation, chiropractic manipulation, or acupuncture. Medical treatment involves analgesics, and nonsteroidal anti-inflammatories to help temporize pain. For more recurrent or severe symptoms, local analgesic and steroid injection therapies are beneficial [8].

2 Costochondral Joint Injection

Indications and Contraindications

Costochondral joint injection can be used in the treatment of refractory costochondral pain. Absolute contraindications include local infection, local tumor, local anesthetic allergy, lack of technical expertise, and patient refusal. Coagulopathy is a relative contraindication. Complications include pain, bleeding, infection, pneumothorax, and local anesthetic toxicity. Uncertain diagnosis should have further clinic workup for more life-threatening pathologies.

Clinical Anatomy

The first seven ribs are called true ribs since they attach directly to the sternum by cartilage. Ribs 2–7 contain a synovial joint since they contain a fibrous joint capsule connecting the rib to the sternum. Rib 1 joint is a synchondrosis since the hyaline cartilage is connected directly to the manubrium. Ribs 8–10 are called false ribs, and attach to the cartilage portion of the rib above each corresponding rib, forming a synovial interchondral articulation. Ribs 11–12 are floating ribs, and do not attach at the anterior ends. These joints allow for rib articulation with respiration and truncal movements.

The synovial joints of ribs 2–7 are most affected by costochondritis and Tietze syndrome. Subcutaneous tissue and pectoralis major muscle lie superficial to these joints. The intercostal muscles lie between the ribs and joints, and house the intercostal vessels and intercostal nerves. The pleura and lung lie deep to these joints (Fig. 1).

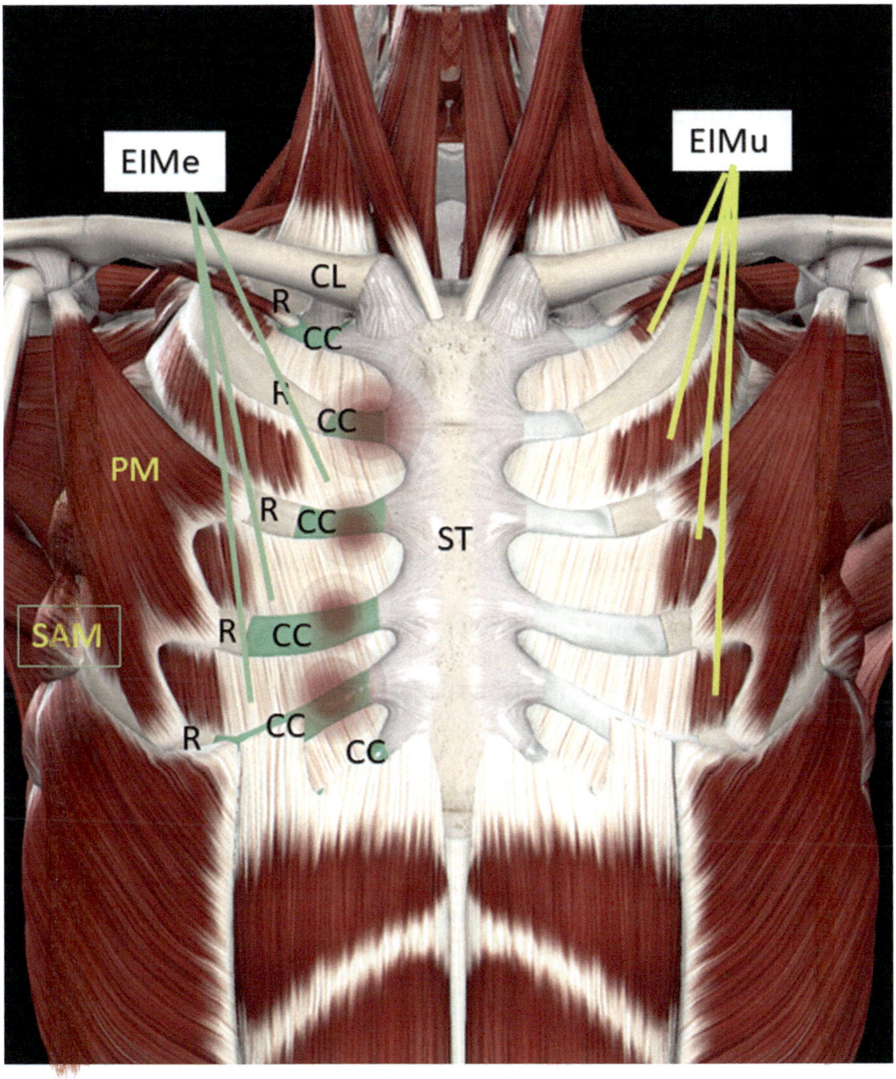

Fig. 1 Anatomy of the costochondral junctions, schematic. *CL* clavicle, *R* rib, *ST* sternum, *CC* cosochondral cartilage, *EIMe* external intercostal membrane, *EIMu* external intercostal muscle, *PM* pectoralis minor muscle, *SAM* serratus anterior muscle, Costochondral cartilage marked in yellow, Red spheres represent common sites of costochondral pain

Table 1 Required supplies for costochondral injection

Syringe	3–10 mL
Needle	22–27 gauge 1–1.5 in.
Single Injection	1–3 mL
Local Anesthetic	0.25–0.75% bupivacaine 0.5–2% lidocaine
Corticosteroid	10 mg triamcinolone parasite, with maximal dose of 40 mg/inj. or alternative corticosteroid

Equipment and Supplies

Costochondral injections for costochondral pain can readily be performed at the bedside. Skin prep will be necessary for appropriate skin sterilization with chlorhexidine 4% (or betadine in those allergic to it). A 3 to 10 mL syringe with local anesthetic (lidocaine 0.5 to 2% of bupivacaine 0.25 to 0.75%, or other), with or without corticosteroids, attached to a 22–27 gauge 1–1.5 in. needle will be needed to attain cutaneous anesthesia and advancement to the target tissue using anatomical landmark technique.

A linear high-frequency ultrasound probe with sterile probe cover is utilized for identifying target muscles, critical structures, and needle guidance. Adjustments in needle size and ultrasound probe of choice may be required depending on the patient's body habitus (Table 1).

Costochondral Injection—Landmark Technique

The patient is positioned in supine position. Palpate the costochondral joints to determine maximal local tenderness for needle insertion. Prep the chest in a standard aseptic fashion, and use sterile technique throughout the procedure. Insert the needle at the maximal tender point to the costochondral cartilage, then withdrawn 1 mm. Obtain negative blood aspiration, and inject local anesthetic into the area. Repeat for multiple costochondral joints as indicated. Superficial tissue infiltration of the costochondral joint is sufficient to provide appropriate analgesia [9]. Advancement of the needle into the costochondral joint is not recommended using this technique.

Ultrasound is an excellent bedside imaging modality which can make this injection more precise and safer. Fluoroscopic guidance can be very effective for localizing the joints but is hard to obtain at the bedside and for this reason is not covered in detail in this chapter.

Costochondral Injection Ultrasound Technique

The patient is positioned in supine position. Prep the chest in a standard aseptic fashion, and use sterile technique throughout the procedure. Place the probe parallel to the ribs approximately 4–5 cm lateral to sternum. The desired rib, costochondral junction, and pleura should be clearly identified. In parasagittal orientation, the costochondral joint will appear oval, and in the transverse orientation, the

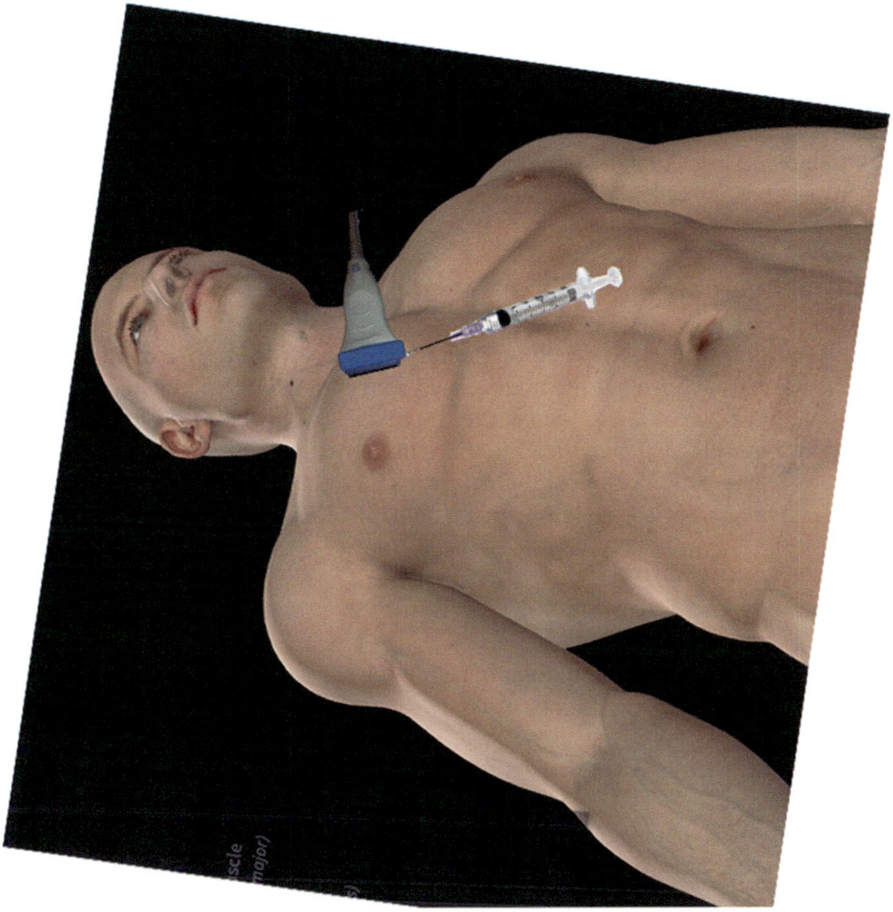

Fig. 2 Bedside injections for costochondral pain. Ultrasound probe and needle orientation, schematic

costochondral joint will show as ribbon-shaped. The costochondral joint can appear homogenously hypoechoic, however hyperechoic echos in the joint with posterior acoustic shadowing have been associated with Tietze's Syndrome [10]. Advance the needle in plane from lateral to medial until needle passes through the cartilage. Ensure tip of the needle is visualize at all times to avoid deeper penetration. Obtain negative blood aspiration, and inject local anesthetic into the targeted area (Fig. 2).

3 Parasternal Block

Indications and Contraindications

Parasternal Block can be used in the treatment of anterior chest and sternal pain supplied by the anterior cutaneous branch of the intercostal nerve:

- Sternal fracture [11]
- Post-surgical anterior chest (sternotomy) [12]

Absolute contraindications include local infection, local tumor, local anesthetic allergy, lack of technical expertise, and patient refusal. Coagulopathy is a relative contraindication. Complications include pneumothorax, pericardium puncture, local anesthetic toxicity, and hematoma.

Clinical Anatomy

The Anterior Cutaneous Branch of Intercostal Nerve (ACB) pierces through the intercostal muscles around the midline and split into lateral and medial branches. These supply innervation to the anterior thorax. The ACB lies deep to the internal intercostal muscle, and superficial to the transversus thoracis muscle. The internal thoracic vein and artery run parallel along the sternum, and also lie between these muscles. For appropriate analgesic effect, bilateral blocks should be performed [13].

Equipment and Supplies

The same as for costochondral joint injection. Please see Table 1.

Parasternal Block Ultrasound Technique

Place the probe in parasagittal plane alone the midclavicular line and scan medially toward the sternum. Continue to scan medially until the transverse thoracic muscle comes into frame. The desired ribs, pleura, and innermost intercostal muscle, and transverse thoracic muscle should be clearly identified. The target area is between the innermost intercostal muscle and transverse thoracic muscle. Advance the needle in plane from caudad to cephalad. Obtain negative blood aspiration, and inject local anesthetic into the targeted area. Pleural displacement should be visualized [13] (Fig. 3).

Potential Complications and Adverse Effects

Any interventional treatment has inherent risks of bleeding and infectious complications. The risks of catastrophic bleeding or infection is extremely low with these injections.

Costochondral injection, especially with landmark-based/blind technique, is associated with pleural injury and pneumothorax risk. Performing this injection at multiple levels further accentuates this risk. While performing this injection, special care must be taken to avoid this complication, and imaging should be utilized whenever possible.

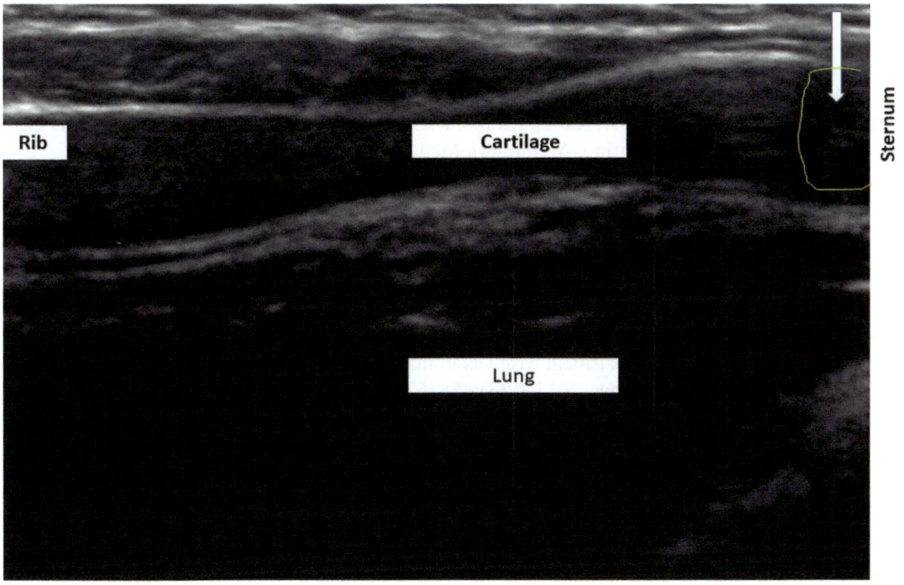

Fig. 3 Parasternal injections. Ultrasonogram, as labeled. The figure demonstrates an ultrasound image of costal cartilage at the junction with the sternum—the parasternal inflammation/painful side labeled with a yellow line. The white arrow points to the injection target. The injection should be performed while visualizing the depth of the pleura and lung to avoid injury to these structures

Clinical and Technical Pearls

- Adequate analgesia can be achieved with local anesthesia into the costochondral joint, or local anesthesia infiltration superficial to the joint.
- Costochondritis is common, and affects multiple unilateral sternocostal joints most commonly second-fifth joints. Tietze syndrome is rare, affects a single sternocostal joint most commonly second-third joint, and associated with swelling.
- Costochondral blocks have risk for pneumothorax. Parasternal blocks have risk for pneumothorax and pericardial puncture.
- Costochondral pain can be managed with broader fascial plane blocks and neuraxial blocks. These include Pectoralis nerve block (PEC1, PEC2), Serratus Anterior Plane (SAP), Erector Spinae Plane (ESP), Paravertebral, and Thoracic Epidural. The advantages and limitations of these blocks are discussed in other chapters.
- For paraspinal block, pleural displacement should be visualized to ensure appropriate local anesthetic placement.

References

1. Proulx AM, Zryd TW. Costochondritis: diagnosis and treatment. Am Fam Physician. 2009;80(6):617–20.
2. Disla E, Rhim HR, Reddy A, Karten I, Taranta A. Costochondritis. A prospective analysis in an emergency department setting. Arch Intern Med. 1994;154(21):2466–9.
3. Proulx AM, Zryd TW. Wright State University Boonshoft School of Medicine, Dayton, Ohio. Am Fam Physician. 2009;80(6):617–20.
4. Zapatero J, López Longo J, Monteagudo I, Carreño L. Costal chondritis in heroin addicts: a comparative study with postsurgical chondritis. Br J Dis Chest. 1988;82(4):341–6.
5. Heckenkamp J, Helling HJ, Rehm KE. Post-traumatic costochondritis caused by Candida albicans. Aetiology, diagnosis and treatment. Scand Cardiovasc J. 1995;31(3):165–7.
6. Meyer CA, White CS. Cartilaginous disorders of the chest. Radiographics. 1998;18(5):1109–23.
7. Zaruba RA, Wilson E. Impairment based examination and treatment of costochondritis: A case series. Int J Sports Phys Ther. 2017;12(3):458–67.
8. Freeston J, Karim Z, Lindsay K, Gough A. Can early diagnosis and management of costochondritis reduce acute chest pain admissions? J Rheumatol. 2004;31(11):2269–71.
9. DeLisa JA, Gans BM, Walsh NE. Physical medicine and rehabilitation: principles and practice, vol. 1. Philadelphia: Lippincott Williams & Wilkins; 2005. p. 345–6.
10. Cho JY, Park D. Ultrasound-guided corticosteroid injection in a patient with tietze syndrome combined with costochondral joint swelling. Am J Phys Med Rehabil. 2019;98(7):71–3. From the Department of Rehabilitation Medicine, Daegu Fatima Hospital, Daegu, South Korea
11. Thomas KP, Sainudeen S, Jose S, Nadhari MY, Macaire PB. Ultrasound guided parasternal block allows optimal pain relief and ventilation improvement after a sternal fracture. Pain Ther. 2016;5(1):115–22.
12. Doğan Bakı E, Kavrut Ozturk N, Ayoğlu RU, Emmiler M, Karslı B, Uzel H. Effects of parasternal block on acute and chronic pain in patients undergoing coronary artery surgery. Semin Cardiothorac Vasc Anesth. 2016;20(3):205–12.
13. Mott T, Jones G, Roman K. Costochondritis: rapid evidence review. Am Fam Physician. 2021;104(1):73–8. PMID: 34264599

Further Reading

Expert Panel on Thoracic Imaging, Stowell JT, Walker CM, Chung JH, Bang TJ, Carter BW, Christensen JD, Donnelly EF, Hanna TN, Hobbs SB, Johnson BD, Kandathil A, Lo BM, Madan R, Majercik S, Moore WH, Kanne JP. ACR appropriateness Criteria® nontraumatic chest wall pain. J Am Coll Radiol. 2021;18(11S):S394–405. https://doi.org/10.1016/j.jacr.2021.08.004.

Transversus Abdominis Plane Blocks

Jeffrey S. Grzybowski and Kristopher M. Schroeder

Essential Concepts

- Transversus abdominis plane blocks (TAP blocks) target the ventral rami of the T7-L1 thoracolumbar nerves to the abdominal wall muscular layers: the external oblique, internal oblique, and the transversus abdominis muscles in addition to their fascial sheaths, overlying skin, and underlying parietal peritoneum.
- Both blind and ultrasound guided techniques to a classic TAP block have been described providing post-operative analgesia for incisions typically below the level of the umbilicus.
- An ultrasound-guided subcostal TAP block technique has been described which can allow for improved cephalad distribution of analgesia.
- TAP blocks can be used as a diagnostic and/or therapeutic tool in the chronic pain population to identify a somatosensory origin of abdominal pain as well as to achieve pain relief while minimizing side effects of chronic opioid use.
- TAP blocks are large volume tissue plane blocks, which are very safe when performed appropriately.

1 Overview

The landmark-based abdominal field block, now more commonly known as a transversus abdominis plane (TAP) block was first described by Rafi in 2001 [1]. In his description, the "lumbar triangle of Petit" (see Fig. 1) is the critical landmark through which a large volume (20 mL) of local anesthetic is deposited following

J. S. Grzybowski (✉) · K. M. Schroeder
Department of Anesthesiology, University of Wisconsin School of Medicine and Public Health, Madison, WI, USA
e-mail: JGrzybowski@wisc.edu; Kmschro1@wisc.edu

D. Souza et al. (eds.), *Bedside Pain Management Interventions*,
https://doi.org/10.1007/978-3-031-11188-4_43

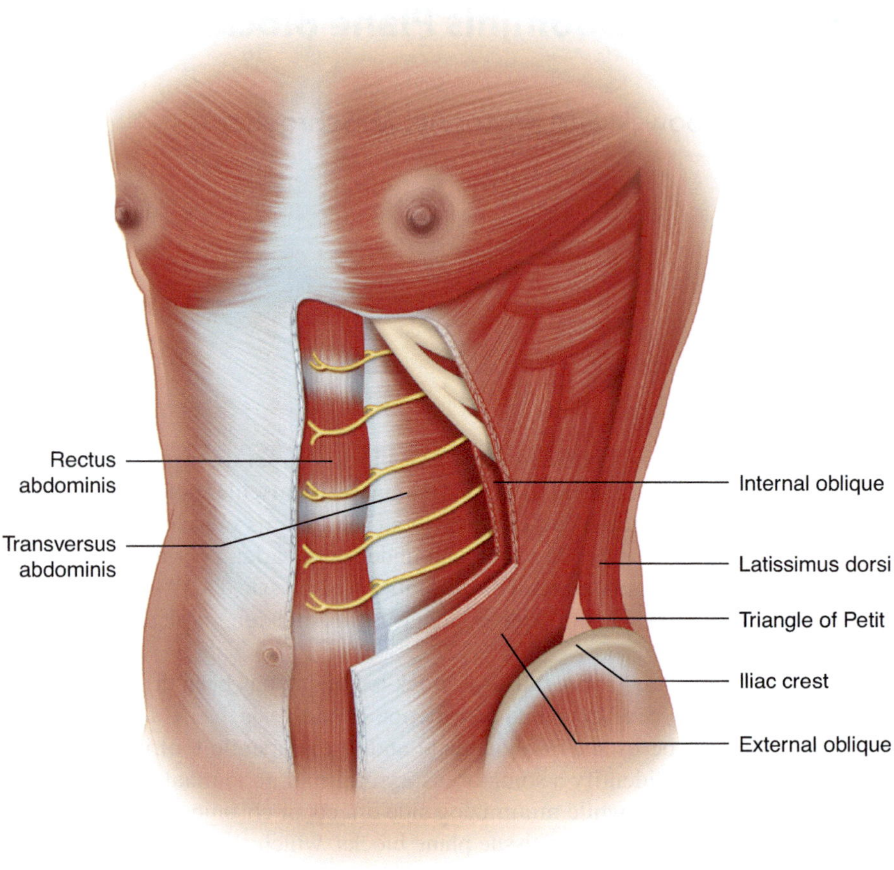

Fig. 1 Anatomy of the transversus abdominis plane

tactile identification of the plane between the internal oblique and transversus abdominis muscles. Improvements in anatomical understanding and ultrasound imaging technology have facilitated contemporary interest in utilizing ultrasound guidance for this block. Following a period of initial rampant enthusiasm, the classic TAP block now seems most suited to provide significant perioperative analgesia for patients undergoing lower abdominal surgeries [2]. Both single-shot and continuous catheter techniques have been used successfully to provide intermediate and sustained analgesia. TAP blocks also have diagnostic utility and may be utilized to delineate somatic pain originating from the abdominal muscular wall from visceral pain transmitted via sympathetic innervation. The classic TAP block provides analgesia below the level of the umbilicus. However, both recent cadaveric and volunteer studies have called into question the perceived maximal cephalad spread as well as overall dermatomal distribution of analgesia [3, 4]. One study cites potential limitations in midline abdominal analgesic coverage of TAP blocks that may be better managed with either rectus sheath or quadratus lumborum blocks [4].

2 Indications and Contraindications

Exact dermatomal analgesic coverage provided by a classic TAP block is variable. Bilateral blocks have been used for midline and transverse incision, whereas, unilateral blockade may be sufficient for a lateralized incision. Classical TAP has been reported to provide adequate analgesia following caesarian section, hysterectomy, hernia repair, kidney transplant, colostomy closure, and multiple other lower abdominal surgeries [2].

Fischer et al. provided a review of potential indications for TAP block in the setting of chronic abdominal pain [5]. A positive response to a diagnostic TAP confirms somatosensory origin, can contribute to therapeutic planning, and can also prevent the treating clinician from pursuing a course targeting visceral pain, potentially including celiac plexus or splanchnic nerve blocks, both with higher risk profiles. Tables 1, 2, 3 discuss chronic post-surgical pain and application of the TAP block.

See Table 4 below for a listing of both absolute and relative contraindications to administration of a TAP block.

Table 1 Criteria Defining Chronic Post-Surgical Pain [6]

1. The pain should have developed after a surgical procedure
2. The pain should be of at least 2 months duration
3. Other causes for the pain should be excluded, for example, continuing malignancy (after oncologic surgery) or chronic infection
4. The possibility that the pain is continuing from a pre-existing problem should be explored and exclusion attempted

Table 2 Prevalence of persistent post-surgical pain and pre-procedure pain for various abdominal surgeries [7]

Surgical procedure	Prevalence of chronic pain	Prevalence of preoperative pain
Cesarean section	6%	Common, intermittent, acute labor pain
Cholecystectomy	23%	Common, variable, from acute cholecystitis to chronic vague abdominal pain
Colectomy	28%	Uncommon
Hernia repair, inguinal	12%	Common, incident pain with peritoneal stretch

Table 3 Reported Outcomes from and Indications for TAP blocks in Patients with Chronic Abdominal Pain

Etiology of pain	Number of patients	Injectate and Technique	Single shot or catheter	Duration of pain relief
Pain secondary to chronic pancreatitis [8]	54	40 mg depot Methylprednisolone and 10 mL of 0.25% levobupivacaine injected bilaterally via ultrasound-guided Subcostal TAP block	Single Shot	In patients with myofascial pain there was clinically significant pain relief at three months (95%, 20/21) and durable pain relief lasting six months (62%, 13/21). With visceral pain, the block provided transient benefit for two-three weeks in 6/17 patients
Chronic abdominal wall pain following surgery [9]	5	Unstated in one, between 40 and 80 mg triamcinolone acetate with between 0.375% and 1% ropivacaine for the others	Variable	Variable follow up and levels of pain resolution. Best case resulted in complete resolution of pain for 266 days following the single shot procedure
Chronic Abdominal Pain [10]	30	Unilateral blocks: 8 mL bupivacaine 0.25% with 80 mg triamcinolone Bilateral blocks: 9 mL bupivacaine 0.25% with 40 mg triamcinolone on each side (some performed at the subcostal level to treat high abdominal pain conditions)	Single Shot	Pain improved in 79.5% of the performed blocks. Percentage of pain improvement was 54.7% ± 36.4% for an average of 84 ± 108 days
Persistent post-surgical pain following laparoscopic cholecystectomy [11]	1	Ultrasound-guided TAP with 15 mL 0.5% ropivacaine followed by infusion of ropivacaine 0.2% at 8 mL/h with a patient controlled bolus of 12 mL with a 60-min lockout interval	Single shot with catheter after	Marked improvement of pain level and functional status for 9 months from day of catheter insertion
Refractory cancer pain due to metastasis to abdominal wall [12]	1	Ultrasound-guided subcostal TAP. Performed with 10 mL 1% lidocaine and 10 mL 0.75% levobupivacaine for diagnostic block injected on each side. Performed with 20 mL of 6% aqueous phenol to each side for therapy	Single shot	70% reduction in dynamic pain, 100% reduction in static pain maintained for 2 months

Table 4 Contraindications to TAP block [13]

Absolute	Relative
Patient refusal	Hemorrhagic diathesis
Local infection	Anticoagulation treatment
Allergy to local anesthetic	Abdominal wall hernias (particularly a lumbar hernia through the "Triangle of Petit" in the classic TAP approach)

3 Clinical Anatomy

The three lateral abdominal wall muscular layers: the external oblique, the internal oblique, and the transversus abdominis and their associated fascial sheaths (as well as the parietal peritoneum) are innervated by the ipsilateral ventral rami of T7 to L1 [2] (Fig. 2).

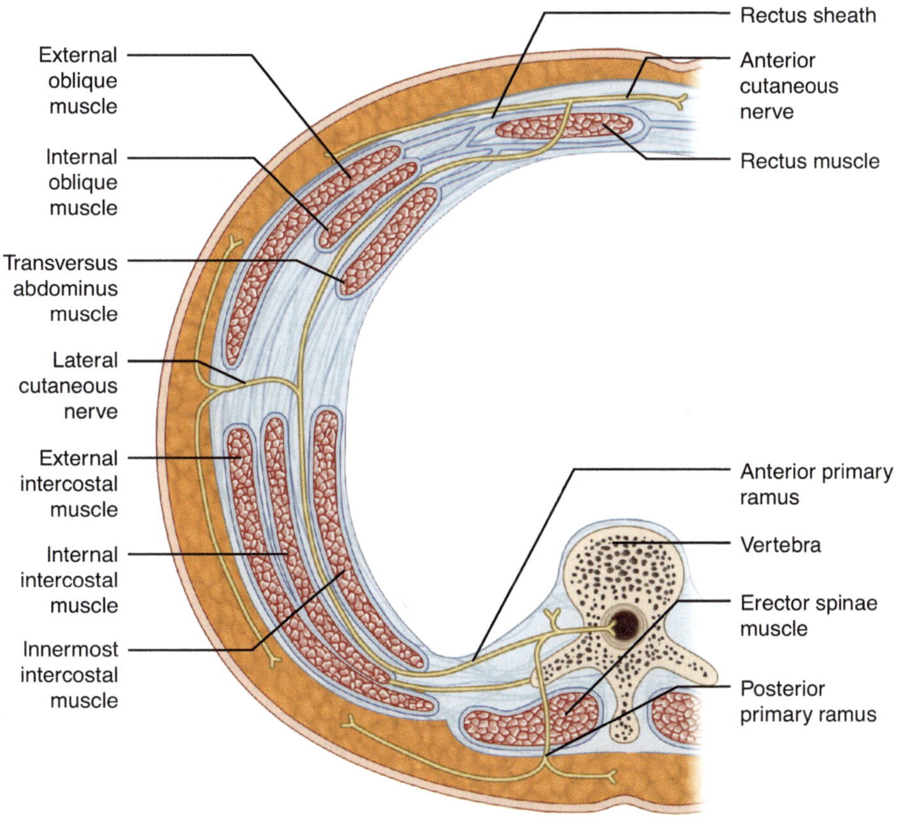

Fig. 2 Innervation of the abdominal wall. The mixed motor-sensory nerve travels anteriorly between the internal oblique and transversus abdominis muscles. They branch in the midaxillary line

The external oblique aponeurosis and the anterior lamella of the internal oblique aponeurosis join and pass anteriorly to the rectus abdominis muscle forming the anterior rectus sheath. The aponeuroses from the posterior lamella of the internal oblique muscle and the transversus abdominis muscle pass posteriorly to the rectus muscle forming the posterior layer of the sheath. At this point, the ventral rami of the lower thoracic nerves are located between the posterior rectus sheath and the rectus muscle. They run antero-medially within the sheath traverse the rectus, and emerge from the muscle anteriorly to form the anterior cutaneous branches. Within the TAP, the lower thoracic spinal nerves give origin to the lateral cutaneous branches posterior to the midaxillary line.

4 Equipment and Supplies

A needle for injection of the local anesthetic solution of at least 50 mm in length is required to identify two losses of resistance if the landmark based (blind) technique is chosen. A blunt needle will reduce the risk of iatrogenic injury to abdominal viscera or other structures. As the TAP block is a fascial plane block, large volumes of local anesthetic solution (15–30 mL/side) are generally required to provide the desired analgesic benefit. Additional equipment needed will vary depending upon the technique chosen. If an ultrasound-guided TAP block is planned, a high-frequency linear ultrasound probe is appropriate for use on thin adults and children. A low-frequency curvilinear probe may be helpful in large or obese adults. See Table 5 below for additional supplies/equipment.

Table 5 Equipment and Supplies Needed for Performing a TAP block

Sterile gloves
Procedure mask
Skin marker
50 mm-22 gauge insulated injection needle, 100 mm-21 gauge insulated injection needle, or other comparable sterile needle for injection of local anesthetic
Desired local anesthetic medication, between 10 mL and 30 mL for most adults depending on medication concentration, patient weight, and unilateral or bilateral planned block
Sterile skin prep
Sedation medication, if desired/requested in an awake patient
Sterile extension tubing for local anesthetic injection
(If planning on catheter placement)18 gauge Touhy needle with sterile catheter and appropriate sterile tubing, securing devices, etc. often packaged together for neuraxial/peripheral nerve catheter insertion
(If performing US-guided block)- sterile US conducting gel
(If performing US-guided block)- US probe: a high-frequency (10–13 MHz) linear transducer is often best or a low frequency (2–5 MHz) transducer for larger patients
(If performing US-guided block)- Ultrasound machine
(If performing US-guided block)- Sterile US probe cover

5 Landmark Technique

With the patient in a supine position, the operator stands on the targeted side and palpates the iliac crest. The triangle of Petit is identified as a finger is moved posteriorly from the anterior crest and a gap is felt in the musculature of the lateral abdominal wall just posterior to the mid-axillary line. After sterile prep and draping, a blunt 50–100 mm needle (21–24 gauge) is inserted perpendicular to the skin approximately 1 to 2 cm above the iliac crest, toward the apex of the triangle (Fig. 3). Two distinct pops (loss of resistance) are felt. The first pop is appreciated as the internal oblique muscle is traversed and a second as the transversus abdominis fascial plane is entered. After negative aspiration to exclude vascular puncture, 15–20 mL of local anesthetic is injected [13, 14].

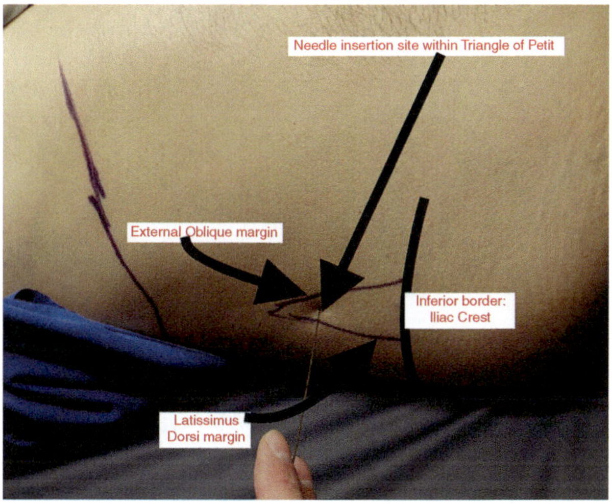

Fig. 3 Landmarks for the transversus abdominis plane block

6 Ultrasound Technique

With the patient in a supine position, the operator stands on the side to be blocked with the ultrasound machine on the opposite side. The patient is prepped and draped in sterile fashion and a sterile ultrasound transducer is used. The lateral abdominal wall is scanned using a high frequency linear transducer oriented transversely over the lateral abdominal wall between the iliac crest and the costal margin (Fig. 4). At this level, the abdominal wall exhibits three muscle layers with their surrounding connective tissue sheaths (Fig. 5). A blunt needle connected to flushed extension tubing is introduced anterior to the transducer and visualized in-plane along its entire path. The target is visualization of hydrodissection in the space bounded by the hyperechoic fascial sheath of the internal oblique and transversus abdominis layers (deep) such that the internal oblique lifts off the transversus abdominis. After appropriate hydrodissection, local anesthetic is injected in the plane [2, 13].

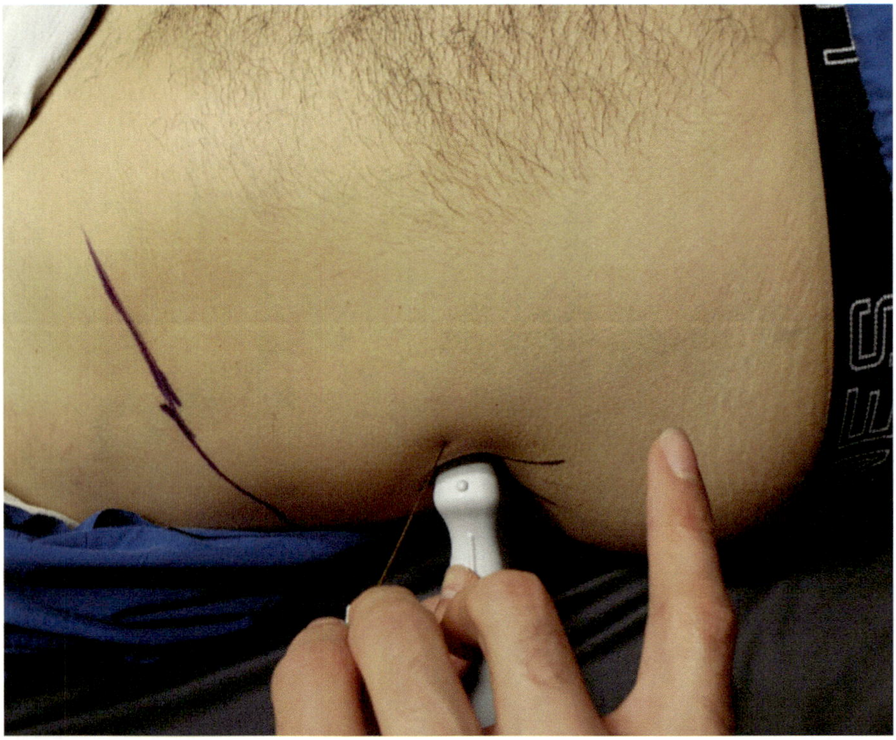

Fig. 4 Ultrasound transducer positioning

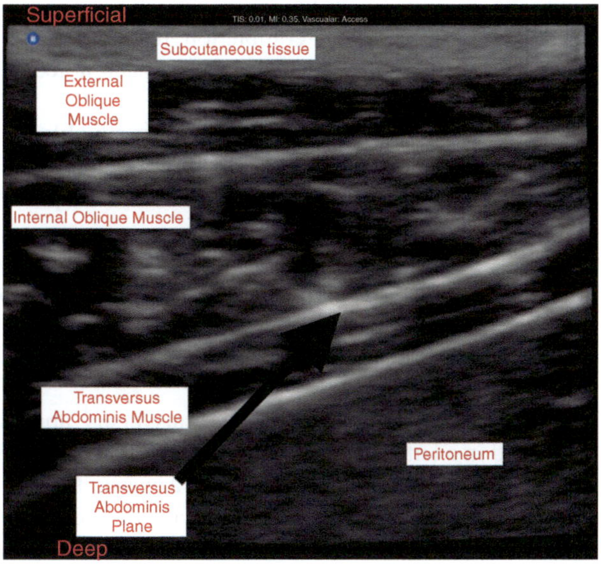

Fig. 5 Ultrasonogram of the transversus abdominis plane. The black arrow indicates the target structure, a fascial plane between transversus abdominis muscle and internal oblique muscle

7 Complications and Adverse Effects

As TAP blocks rely on administration of relatively large volumes of local anesthetic, there is the potential for systemic toxicity. Little is known, however, as to the pharmacokinetics of local anesthetic agents injected into the TAP [13]. Care should be taken not to exceed safe maximal weight-based dosing of local anesthetic. Abdominal organ injury is a risk which is greatly reduced by careful attention to technique and ultrasound guidance. There has been a case reported of inadvertent injury in a patient with undiagnosed hepatomegaly. Localized swelling is possible after injection. A transient femoral nerve block is possible and is associated with local anesthetic tracking between the transversus abdominis muscle and the transversalis fascia.

Clinical and Technical Pearls

- Although a classic anterior needle approach is described above, placement of the needle as far posteriorly as possible (by the mid-axillary line or behind) has the theoretical advantage of blocking the lateral cutaneous branches before they exit the TAP [2].
- An intramuscular needle location is identified by swelling of the internal oblique as opposed to separation from the transversus abdominis on ultrasound [2].
- The internal oblique is usually identified as the largest of the three lateral abdominal wall muscles while the transversus abdominis appears as the most hypoechoic muscle.

- A “flank bulge” sign has been described to indicate a successful TAP block. Within 10 min of block completion, flank bulging believed to indicate relaxation of lateral abdominal musculature has been noted along with diminution of cold sensation in thin patients [15].
- An out-of-plane technique may be more suitable in obese patients when the needle path is not easily seen. In addition, lateral positioning may facilitate plane identification and block performance in obese patients.

8 Subcostal Transversus Abdominis Plane Block

Overview

The ultrasound guided subcostal transversus abdominis plane block was first described in a letter to the editor by Hebbard [16] in which he found superior cephalad analgesic coverage, compared with a classic TAP block, via a subcostal approach. Improved cephalad coverage along with the possibility to place a subcostal TAP catheter made the block a viable alternative to epidural analgesia for supra-umbilical surgeries. He described deposition of local anesthetic between the transversus abdominis and the rectus abdominis muscles or between the rectus and the posterior rectus sheath depending upon the anatomy visualized on ultrasound with the transducer placed parallel and immediately beneath the subcostal margin. Since its introduction, the subcostal TAP block has shown great utility in both the acute perioperative period for upper abdominal surgeries as well as in the chronic abdominal pain population.

Indications and Contraindications

Similar to a classical TAP block (Tables 1, 2, 3 above), subcostal TAP single shot blocks and catheters have a variety of applications in acute perioperative analgesia. With improved mean block height per Hebbard [16], subcostal TAPs have been shown anecdotally to have efficacy for patients undergoing either open or laparoscopic cholecystectomy [17, 18]. After four hours, patients receiving a subcostal TAP for laparoscopic cholecystectomy had significantly lower pain scores than patients receiving a posterior TAP block [18].

Described chronic pain applications include use of a subcostal TAP injection with phenol performed after diagnostic block for intractable cancer pain due to metastatic involvement of the abdominal wall [12]. Additional applications for subcostal TAP blocks are described for both heterogeneous causes of chronic abdominal pain as well as that specifically due to chronic pancreatitis [8, 10].

See Table 4 for contraindications, similar to those for classical TAP block.

Clinical Anatomy

There are four paired muscles of the anterolateral abdominal wall: the anterior rectus abdominis muscles and, from deep to superficial, the three lateral muscles: transversus abdominis, internal oblique, and external oblique muscles. (Figs. 1 and 2) Medially the three muscle layers form tendinous aponeuroses. Under ultrasound, once the rectus abdominis is identified near mid-line, moving the probe laterally the transversus abdominis muscle will appear beneath the rectus abdominis muscle [19]. In this technique, the local anesthetic is to be deposited between the transversus abdominis and the rectus abdominis muscles. Dermatomal coverage up to T6–T8, depending on the authors, is possible as local anesthetic hydrodissects the TAP on a line connecting the xiphoid to the anterior iliac crest [5].

Equipment and Supplies

As the subcostal TAP block is a fascial plane block, a large volume of local anesthetic is typically required. Appropriately sized blunt injection needles will be needed depending on whether a single shot block or a catheter placement is planned. An ultrasound machine with a linear, high frequency transducer is required for this technique. Additional necessary equipment is the same as with a classic TAP block, see Table 5.

Ultrasound Technique

The ultrasound probe is placed over the anterior abdominal wall immediately inferior and parallel to the costal margin. (Fig. 6) The rectus abdominis muscle is identified medially, and the probe then moved laterally until the transversus abdominis muscles are identified. Using the in-plane approach, the needle is inserted from the posterolateral position and advanced anteromedially until its tip is in the fascial plane between the rectus abdominis and transverse abdominis muscles [19] (Fig. 7). There, 15–20 mL of local anesthetic solution is injected and visualized on ultrasound.

Complications and Adverse Effects

Similar to the classic TAP block, a large volume of local anesthetic is typically injected in this fascial plan block. Thus, the potential for systemic toxicity exists and care should be taken not to exceed safe maximal weight-based dosing of local anesthetic. Localized swelling as well as allergic reactions to the local anesthetic itself are possible. Careful attention to ultrasound and needle technique must be taken to avoid inadvertent injury to abdominal viscera or the pleural cavity in this approach.

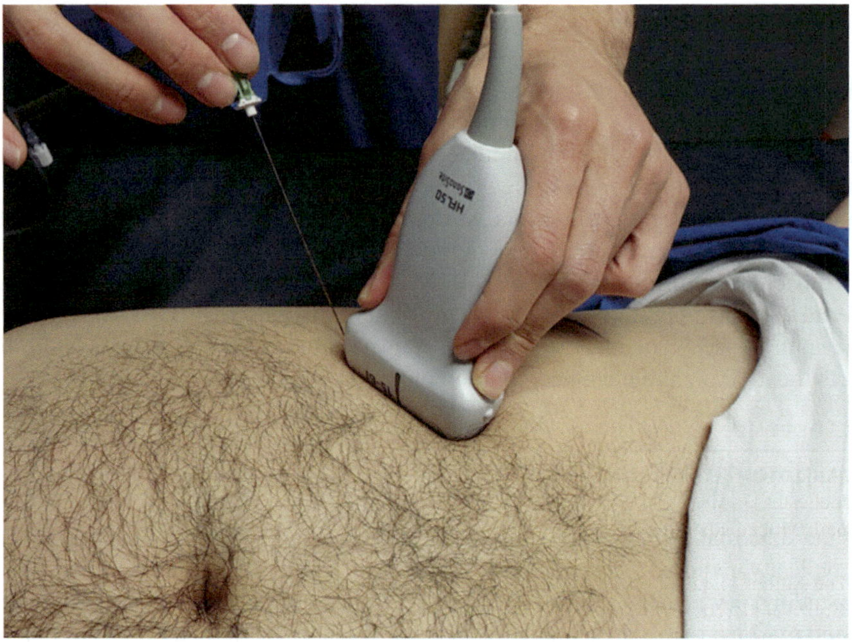

Fig. 6 Ultrasound transducer positioning for the subcostal transversus abdominis plane block

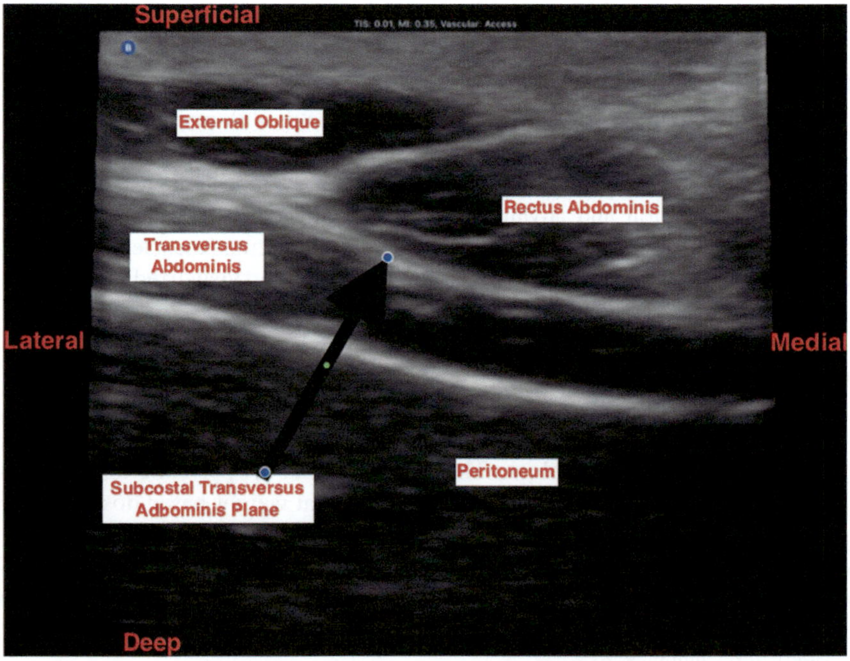

Fig. 7 Ultrasonogram of the subcostal transversus abdominis plane. The black arrow indicates the target structure, a fascial plane between transversus abdominis muscle and rectus abdominis muscle

Clinical and Technical Pearls

- When performing a right-sided block, care should be taken not to injure the liver, especially in patients with hepatomegaly or with very thin abdominal wall tissue.
- Subcostal TAP blocks with adjuvant steroid (triamcinolone) have been used to treat chronic pain resistant to other treatment modalities [10].
- Alternatively, a rectus sheath block can be performed with a needle insertion point medial to the transducer, near the xiphoid process with local anesthetic injected between the rectus muscle and the posterior rectus sheath if the transversus abdominis is not visible in this supero-medial location and midline analgesia is desired.

References

1. Rafi AN. Abdominal field block: a new approach via the lumbar triangle. Anaesthesia. 2001;56:1024–6.
2. Mounir-Soliman L. Chapter 40, Transversus Abdominis Plane Block (Classic Approach). In: Brown's Atlas of Regional Anesthesia. 5th ed. Amsterdam: Elsevier; 2017. p. 249–50.
3. Carney J, Finnerty O, Rauf J, Bergin D, Laffey JG, Mc Donnell JG. Studies on the spread of local anaesthetic solution in transversus abdominis plane blocks. Anaesthesia. 2011;66:1023–30.
4. Stoving K, Rothe C, Rosenstock CV, Aasvang EK, Lundstrom LH, Lange KHW. Cutaneous sensory block area, muscle-relaxing effect, and block duration of the transversus abdominis plane block. Reg Anesth Pain Med. 2015;40(4):355–62.
5. Fischer M, Guirguis M, Abd-Elsayed A. Review of transversus abdominis plane blocks and their application to chronic adbominal pain. ASRA Pain Medicine News. Aug 7, 2019. https://www.asra.com/news-publications/asra-newsletter/newsletteritem/asra-news/2019/08/07/review-of-transversus-abdominis-plane-blocks-and-their-application-to-chronic-abdominal-pain. Accessed 8/2/22.
6. Macrae WA. Chronic post-surgical pain: 10 years on. Br J Anaesth. 2008;101(1):77–86.
7. Perkins FM, Franklin JS. Chapter 19 Prediction and prevention of persistent post-surgical pain. In: Practical Management of Pain. 5th ed. Maryland Heights: Mosby; 2014. p. 298–303.
8. Niraj G, Kamel Y. Ultrasound-guided subcostal TAP block with depot steroids in the management of chronic abdominal pain secondary to chronic pancreatitis: a three-year prospective audit in 54 patients. Pain Med. 2019:1–7.
9. Baciarello M, Migliavacca G, Marchesini M, Valente A, Allegri M, Fanelli G. Transversus abdominis plane block for the diagnosis and treatment of chronic abdominal wall pain following surgery: a case series. Pain Pract. 2018;18(1):109–17.
10. Abd-Elsayed A, Malyuk D. Efficacy of transversus abdominis plane steroid injection for treating chronic abdominal pain. Pain Pract. 2018;18(1):48–52.
11. Guirguis M, Abd-Elsayed AA, Girgis G, Mounir SL. Ultrasound-guided transversus abdominis plan catheter for chronic abdominal pain. Pain Pract. 2013;13(3):235–8.
12. Restrepo-Garces CE, Asenjo JF, Gomez CM, Jaramillo S, Acosta N, Ramirez LJ, Lopera LM, Vargas JF. Subcostal transversus abdominis plane phenol injection for abdominal wall cancer pain. Pain Pract. 2014;14(3):278–82.
13. McDonnell J, O'Donnell B. Chapter 34, Transversus abdominis plane block. In: Peripheral nerve blocks and peri-operative pain relief. 2nd ed. Amsterdam: Elsevier; 2011. p. 234–8.
14. Narchi P, Singelyn F, Paqueron X, Nicholls B. Chapter 55, Truncal Blocks. In: Practical management of pain. 5th ed. Maryland Heights: Mosby; 2014. p. 745–54.
15. Grady MV, Cummings KC. The "Flank Bulge" Sign of a Successful Transversus Abdominis Plane Block. Reg Anesth Pain Med. 2008;33:387.

16. Hebbard P. Subcostal transversus abdominis plane block under ultrasound guidance. Anesth Analg. 2008;106(2):674–5.
17. Laffey JG, McDonnell JG. In response to: subcostal transversus abdominis plane block under ultrasound guidance. Anesth Analg. 2008;106(2):675.
18. Bhatia N, Arora S, Wig J, Kaur G. Comparison of posterior and subcostal approaches to ultrasound-guided transverse abdominis plane block for postoperative analgesia in laparoscopic cholecystectomy. J Clin Anesth. 2014;26:294–9.
19. Farag E. Chapter 41, Subcostal transversus abdominis plane block. In: Brown's Atlas of regional anesthesia. 5th ed. Amsterdam: Elsevier; 2017. p. 251–3.

Further Reading

Mounir-Soliman L. Chapter 40, Transversus abdominis plane block (Classic Approach). In: Brown's Atlas of Regional Anesthesia. 5th ed. Amsterdam: Elsevier; 2017. p. 249–50.

Perkins FM, Franklin JS. Chapter 19 Prediction and prevention of persistent post-surgical pain. In: Practical management of pain. 5th ed. Maryland Heights: Mosby; 2014. p. 298–303.

McDonnell J, O'Donnell B. Chapter 34, Transversus abdominis plane block. In: Peripheral nerve blocks and peri-operative pain relief. 2nd ed. Amsterdam: Elsevier; 2011. p. 234–8.

Abdominis Rectus Sheath Block

Jonathan M. Hagedorn and Ryan S. D'Souza

Essential Concept

- The rectus abdominis muscle (RAM) is the principal medial abdominal muscle.
- The paired vertical RAM are separated by the midline linea alba.
- The muscle is entirely enclosed by the rectus sheath cephalad to the umbilicus, but the posterior wall of the rectus sheath is absent caudal to the umbilicus leaving epimysium and transversalis as the posterior border.
- The mechanism of action is the result of blockade of nociceptive afferent fibers from T9 to T11 that enter by piercing the posterior RAM and supply cutaneous sensation to the midline anterior abdominal wall and umbilical area.
- The rectus sheath block (RSB) can be performed by either landmark or ultrasound technique, and are used for pain control following midline abdominal surgeries from umbilical hernias to laparotomy.

J. M. Hagedorn (✉) · R. S. D'Souza
Department of Anesthesiology and Perioperative Medicine, Division of Pain Medicine, Mayo Clinic, Rochester, MN, USA
e-mail: Hagedorn.jonathan@mayo.edu

D. Souza et al. (eds.), *Bedside Pain Management Interventions*,
https://doi.org/10.1007/978-3-031-11188-4_44

1 Overview

The rectus sheath block (RSB) was first described in 1899 to provide abdominal wall relaxation before an operation [1]. It has been described by both landmark and ultrasound-guidance, and is performed by placing injectate between the RAM and the posterior border of the rectus sheath. It is primarily used for post-operative pain control following midline abdominal surgery, including laparotomy, umbilical, and periumbilical operations (Table 1) [2, 3]. Studies have reported both significantly decreased intraoperative and postoperative opioid requirements, as well as reduced postoperative pain scores in patients undergoing abdominal surgery who received RSB [4–6]. Occasionally, in select high-risk patients with poor cardiovascular and physiological reserves, cases have been reported with successful use of bilateral RSBs as the sole primary anesthetic in simple periumbilical surgery [7].

2 Indications and Contraindications (Table 1)

Table 1 Rectus sheath blocks for the management of midline abdominal pain [2, 3, 8]

Procedure	Indications	Techniques	Contraindications
Rectus sheath block	Treatment of midline perioperative pain, including midline laparotomy and periumbilical surgeries	1. Landmark technique 2. Ultrasound-guided	Absolute: 1. Patient or guardian refusal 2. Systemic or local infection 3. Allergy to injectate medications

3 Clinical Anatomy

The anterolateral abdominal wall is innervated by the anterior rami of spinal nerves T7–T12 [1, 3]. These spinal nerves become the intercostal, subcostal, and iliohypogastric/ilioinguinal nerves. These nerves will exit their initial course and run between the internal oblique and the transversus abdominis muscles. Eventually, the T7–T12 nerves puncture the rectus sheath and RAM before ending as anterior cutaneous nerves [8] (Fig. 1).

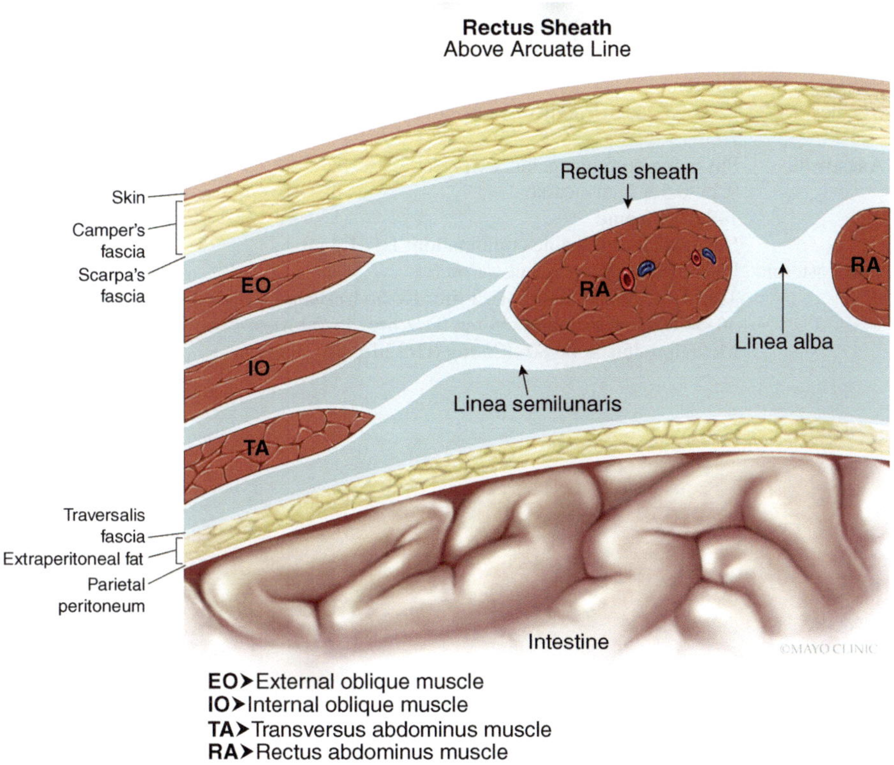

Fig. 1 Cross-sectional orientation of the abdominal wall musculature with other surrounding structures

4 Equipment and Supplies

Rectus sheath blocks can be performed at the bedside or intraoperatively. The physician will need a two to five-inch needle (depending on body habitus of the patient), extension tubing (optional), a 20 milliliter (mL) syringe, and 20 mL of injectate (10 mL per side). Anesthetic solution usually consists of the local anesthetic lidocaine or bupivacaine, or a combination of the two, with or without a corticosteroid. For longer lasting pain relief, a catheter can be threaded into this area during the block procedure to allow additional future boluses to be provided as needed (Table 2).

Table 2 Required supplies for rectus sheath block

Syringe	20 mL
Needle	22 or 25 gauge Tuohy or short-beveled needle 2–5″
Anesthetic	Physician preference, but we prefer: 0.25–0.5% bupivacaine 1–2% lidocaine Lidocaine/bupivacaine combination: 1:1–1:3 ratio
Corticosteroid	Physician preference, but we prefer: Triamcinolone 5–40 mg (t1/2 life: 18–36 h) Betamethasone 18 mg (t1/2 life: 36–54 h) Dexamethasone 4 mg (t1/2 life: 36–54 h) Methylprednisolone 80–125 mg (t1/2 life: 18–36 h)

5 Rectus Sheath Block, Landmark Technique

In a supine patient, a location cephalad to the umbilicus and approximately two to three centimeters from the midline is chosen (Fig. 2). A five-centimeter needle is directed through the skin at a right angle. An initial tactile pop indicates penetration

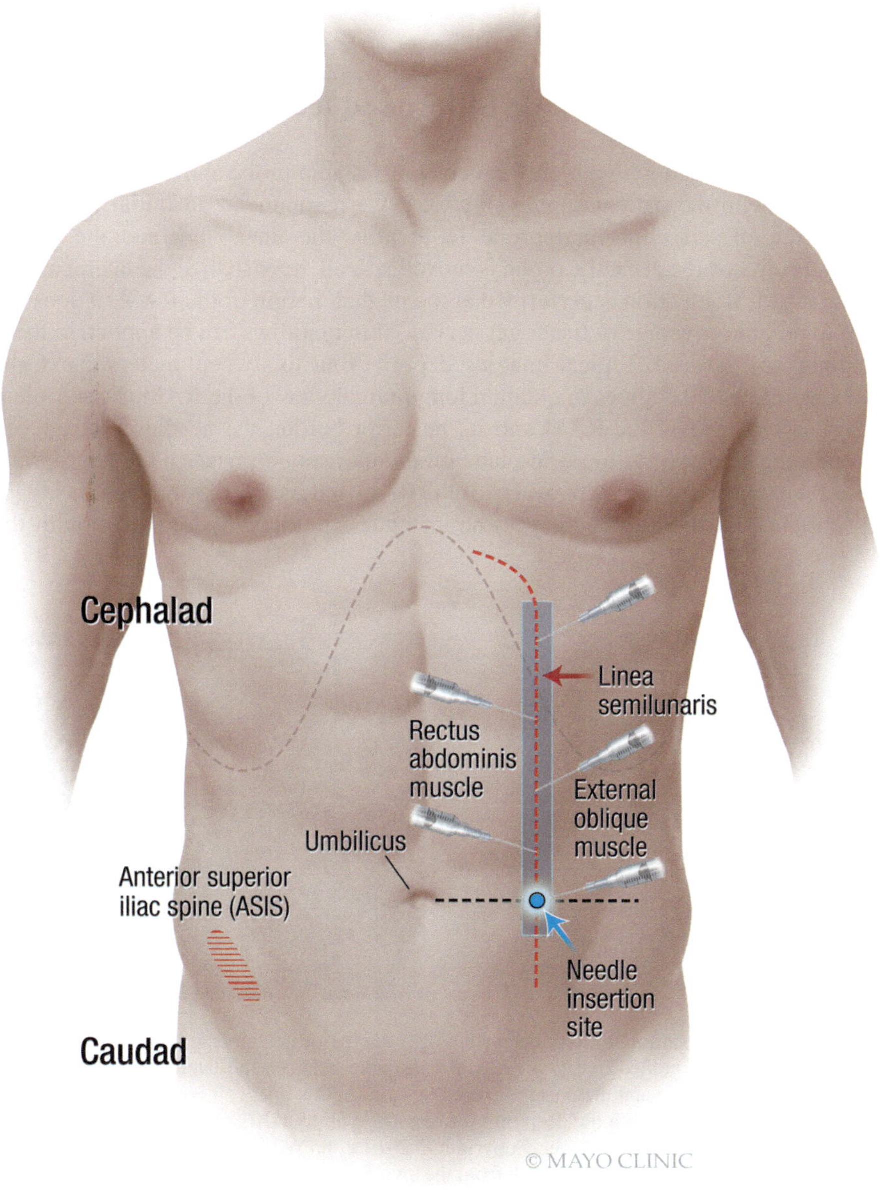

Fig. 2 Relevant surface anatomy for performance of the landmark technique injection

of the anterior rectus sheath. The needle is advanced through the RAM until further resistance is met. This indicates the needle location is at the posterior rectus sheath [1, 8]. Ten mL of solution should be injected here. The procedure should be repeated on the contralateral side. The blind technique should be avoided caudal to the umbilicus given the absence of the posterior rectus sheath [1]. Recently, a neurostimulator guided approach to RSB was described as a feasible approach that results in optimal local anesthetic spread and blockade in about 75% of patients without the use of ultrasound [9].

6 Rectus Sheath Block, Ultrasound Technique

The RAM is imaged with a high-frequency ultrasound probe above the level of the umbilicus with the patient supine (Fig. 3a). We recommend an initial transverse orientation of the ultrasound probe to identify the linea alba and the paired RAM. From this location, the probe is moved laterally to visualize the lateral aspect of the RAM. If injection is performed at the medial margin of the RAM, it does not lead to reliable coverage of the target nerves. Skin markings can be applied to these landmarks, if desired. Typical imaging depth is four to six centimeters. Next, the probe is rotated 90 degrees to obtain a longitudinal view of the RAM. Once a clear image is obtained of the RAM and its posterior border, the needle is introduced through the skin and followed in-plane on the ultrasound image to the appropriate position between the posterior aspect of the RAM and the posterior rectus sheath [1, 8] (Fig. 3b). Lastly, introduction of the injectate will allow hydrodissection of the

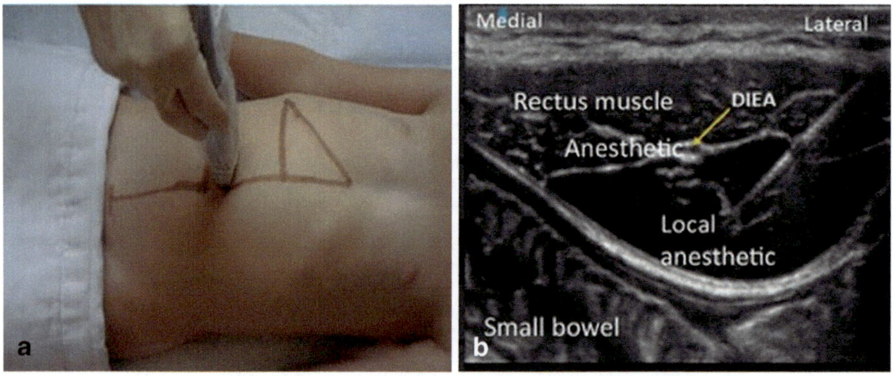

Fig. 3 (**a**) Probe orientation for Rectus sheath blocks to provide analgesia at the level of the umbilicus; (**b**) Ultrasound-guided injection of local anesthetic between the lateral border of the left rectus abdominis muscle and the posterior rectus sheath. In this image, it is noted that the nerves run craniocaudally along with the deep inferior epigastric artery (DIEA). (Reprinted from Visoiu et al. with permission of the publisher. Copyright © 2019, John Wiley and Sons Inc. Authorization for this adaptation has been obtained both from the owner of the copyright in the original work and from the owner of copyright in the translation or adaptation)

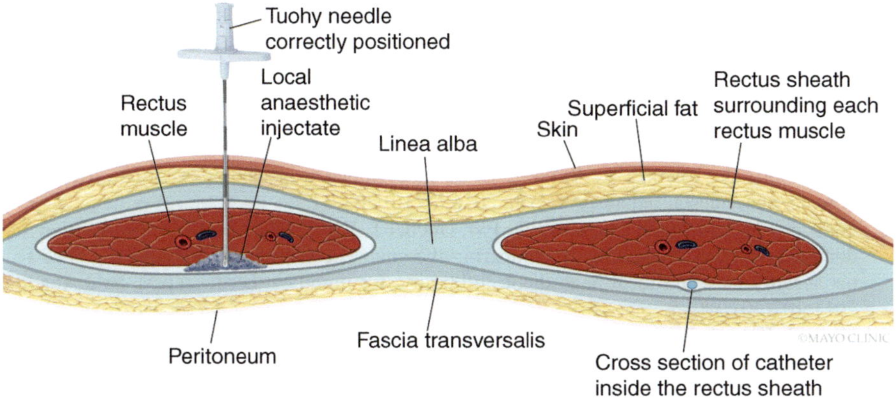

Fig. 4 Cross-sectional depiction of the block needle in appropriate position with initial placement of the injectate

muscle away from the rectus sheath (Fig. 4). This should be performed bilaterally. An initial 10 mL bolus is applied to each side after calculating the maximum dosages and selecting an appropriate local anesthetic concentration to avoid toxicity. If desired, a catheter can be threaded five to six inches into this space so that intermittent additional boluses can be given.

7 Potential Complications and Adverse Effects

In addition to the expected risks from any procedure (i.e. infection, bleeding, pain, damage to surrounding structures, local anesthetic toxicity, etc.), RSBs carry the risk of inadvertent needle entry into the peritoneal cavity with potential puncture of an organ within this space or injection into the superior and/or inferior epigastric vessels [1, 2, 8]. These risks are quite rare, particularly with ultrasound guidance.

Clinical and Technical Pearls

- Given the proximity of the needle tip to the peritoneal cavity, we strongly recommend ultrasound guidance throughout the procedure.
- Rectus sheath blocks should be used following midline abdominal surgeries. Lateral incisions will not be covered with this technique.
- Special attention will be required to provide this injection safely in the patient with a past history of prior abdominal surgeries.
- We do not recommend performing this technique below a level one-third of the distance from the umbilicus to the pubic symphysis due to anatomical loss of the posterior rectus sheath and increased risk of inadvertent entry into the peritoneal cavity.

References

1. Yarwood J, Berrill A. Nerve blocks of the anterior abdominal wall. Continuing education in anaesthesia critical care and pain. 2010;10(6):182–6.
2. Webster K. Ultrasound guided rectus sheath block – analgesia for abdominal surgery. Update in Anaesthesia. 2010;26(1):12–7.
3. Chakraborty A, Khemka R, Datta T. Ultrasound-guided truncal blocks: A new frontier in regional anaesthesia. Indian J Anaesth. 2016;60(10):703–11.
4. Gurnaney HG, Maxwell LG, Kraemer FW, Goebel T, Nance ML, Ganesh A. Prospective randomized observer-blinded study comparing the analgesic efficacy of ultrasound-guided rectus sheath block and local anaesthetic infiltration for umbilical hernia repair. Br J Anaesth. 2011;107(50):790–5.
5. Hong S, Kim H, Park J. Analgesic effectiveness of rectus sheath block during open gastrectomy: A prospective double-blinded randomized controlled clinical trial. Medicine (Baltimore). 2019;98(15):e15159.
6. Kartalov A, et al. The Effect of rectus sheath block as a supplement of general anesthesia on postoperative analgesia in adult patient undergoing umbilical hernia repair. Pril (Makedon Akad Nauk Umet Odd Med Nauki). 2017;38(3):135–42.
7. Quek KH, Phua DS. Bilateral rectus sheath blocks as the single anaesthetic technique for an open infraumbilical hernia repair. Singap Med J. 2014;55(3):e39–41.
8. Chin KJ, McDonnell JG, Carvalho B, Sharkey A, Pawa A, Gadsden J. Essentials of our current understanding: abdominal wall blocks. Reg Anesth Pain Med. 2017;42(2):133–83.
9. Albokrinov AA, Perova-Sharonova VM, Fesenko UA. A new neurostimulator guided technique of rectus sheath block: study of feasibility and local anesthetic spread in children. Anaesthesiol Intensive Ther. 2019;51(2):83–7.

Further Reading

Chapter 57—Rectus Sheath Block. Atlas of Ultrasound-Guided Regional Anesthesia (Third Edition). 2019; 249–258.

Ilioinguinal and Iliohypogastric Nerve Block

Dominika Lipowska James and Maryam Jowza

Essential Concepts

- Iloinguinal and iliohypogastric neuralgias can occur as a consequence of trauma or iatrogenic injury such as surgery.
- Blockade of these nerves can be helpful with symptom control.
- Nerve blocks can be performed using landmark technique or ultrasound guidance.
- The nerves can be blocked with an injection targeting the neurovascular bundle layer located between internal oblique and transversus abdominis muscle.

1 Overview

The ilioinguinal (II) and iliohypogastric (IH) nerves are frequently blocked to provide pain relief for the lower abdominal wall pain. Blockade of these nerves can be helpful in setting of acute pain, for example as the analgesic for an inguinal hernia repair or for chronic pain related to neuralgias [1]. Blockade can be performed at the bedside and can be done either utilizing landmark technique or with ultrasound. The ilioinguinal (II) and iliohypogastric (IH) blocks are also suitable in management of acute perioperative pain in both the adult and pediatric population [2, 3].

D. L. James (✉) · M. Jowza
University of North Carolina at Chapel Hill, Chapel Hill, NC, USA
e-mail: Dominika_James@med.unc.edu; Maryam_Jowza@med.unc.edu

D. Souza et al. (eds.), *Bedside Pain Management Interventions*,
https://doi.org/10.1007/978-3-031-11188-4_45

2 Indications and Contraindications

Ilioinguinal and iliohypogastric nerve blocks are indicated for treatment of pain secondary to ilioinguinal and iliohypogastric neuralgias. Neuralgias of iliohypogastric (IL) and ilioinguinal (II) nerves are often a result of accidental mechanical trauma, or iatrogenic injury following surgical intervention. Mechanical trauma to the lower abdomen such as blunt trauma from motor vehicle collision or stretch injury with pregnancy, may result in neural injury and/or nerve impingement. Iatrogenic neuropathy is prone to occur as a result of low abdominal surgeries such as appendectomy, hysterectomy, orchiectomy, abdominoplasty, inguinal hernia repair, and cesarean section. In most cases, neuralgias occur secondary to intraoperative nerve injury either as a result of transection or traumatic trochar placement [4]. Neuralgias with delayed onset of symptoms are often secondary to nerve entrapment due to postsurgical scar tissue formation or surgical mesh implantation [5]. Some patients may experience II/IH neuralgia as a result of tissue adherence secondary to endometriosis [6].

Diagnosis of the ilioinguinal neuralgia requires a careful history and physical examination (Table 1). Patients will often report pain involving lower abdomen and upper thigh, as well as pain referring to anterior genital region. Patients may also report diminished sensation or increase in sensitivity in the region [7]. On examination, there is tenderness on palpation medial and inferior to the anterior superior iliac spine and impaired sensation along the sensory distribution of the II/IH nerves. Complete neurologic examination is mandatory to exclude genitofemoral neuralgia, lumbosacral radiculopathy, plexopathy, or other neuropathic conditions. Genitofemoral nerve neuralgia is often difficult to discern from ilioinguinal/iliohypogastric neuralgia as the cutaneous innervation of those nerves shows significant overlap [8]. II/IH blocks may be used as diagnostic tools to rule out other causes of low abdominal neuropathic pain.

Some studies suggest that visual evaluation of the II/IH nerves using ultrasonography and/or MR neurography, as well as functional evaluation with electromyography may aid in identification of injured nerves [9–11].

Contraindications to ilioinguinal and iliohypogastric nerve blocks include patient refusal or inability to cooperate, allergy to medications used (local anesthetics and/or steroids) or infection at the site of injection. One should consider peripheral nerve

Table 1 Diagnostic Features of Ilioinguinal/Iliohypogastric Neuralgia

History	Symptoms	Physical
Trauma Surgery Pregnancy	Burning, lancinating lower abdominal/upper thigh pain Sensory disturbance (hypoesthesia, hyperalgesia, hyperesthesia) lower abdomen/upper thigh Pain referring to groin/genitalia	Tenderness to palpation medial to ASIS Pain with hip extension Sensory impairment in distribution of II/IH nerve supply Pain at site where nerve exits inguinal canal

Table 2 Interventional Treatment Options

Procedure	Indications	Techniques	Contraindications
IL/IH nerve block	Diagnosis and treatment of IH/IL neuralgia	Landmark technique Nerve stimulator Ultrasound-guided	Absolute: Patient refusal Local infection Allergy to local anesthetic Inability to cooperate Relative: Coagulopathy
Pulsed RF Cryoablation	Treatment of IH/IL neuralgia	Ultrasound-guided	Same
Peripheral Nerve Stimulation	Treatment of chronic refectory neuralgia	Ultrasound	Same

Table 3 Sensory and motor innervation of low abdominal nerves

Nerve/root	Cutaneous innervation	Motor innervation
Ilioinguinal (T12/L1) Iliohypogastric (T12/L1) Genitofemoral (L1/L2)	Anterior branch: Lower abdomen Area superior to pubis Lateral branch Lateral gluteal region Medial thigh Female—pubis and labia majora Male—base of penis and anterior scrotum Superior aspect of thigh Female—labia Male—scrotum	Internal oblique muscle Internal oblique muscle Cremaster

blocks with caution in patients with preexisting neural deficits, history of bleeding disorder or on anticoagulation therapy (Tables 2 and 3).

3 Clinical Anatomy

The II nerve and the IH nerve arise as a trunk from the anterior ramus of the T12 and L1 nerves. The trunk divides into the II/IH nerves at the lateral edge of the psoas muscle anterior to the quadratus lumborum, with the II nerve running parallel but inferior to the IH nerve (Fig. 1). They then course in the inferior and anterior direction to pierce the transversus abdominis and internal oblique muscle superior to the anterior superior iliac spine. The II/IH nerve bundle traverses superiorly to the ilio-inguinal ligament to finally enter the inguinal canal ultimately exiting at the level of the superficial inguinal ring.

The ilioinguinal nerve functions as a sensory nerve to the superior medial thigh with the IH nerve providing innervation primarily to the region superior to pubis. In women, II and IH nerves also provide sensation to the anterior one third of the labia

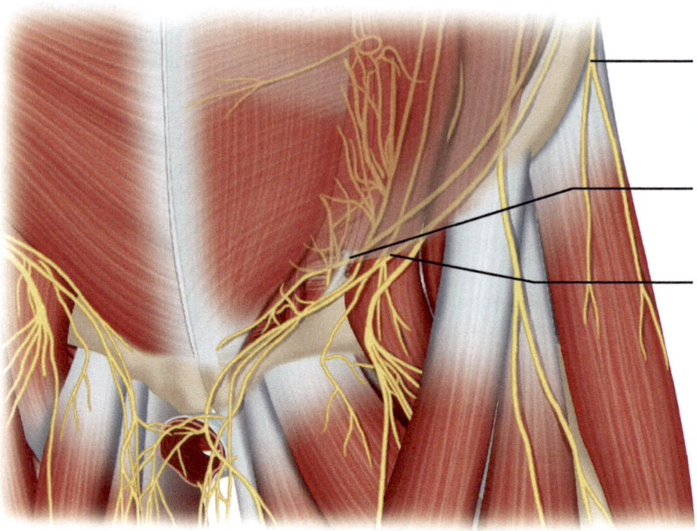

Fig. 1 Anatomy of ilioinguinal and iliohypogastric nerves (LIHN- lateral cutaneous branch of iliohypogastric nerve, AIHN - anterior branch of iliohypogastric nerve, IIN- ilioinguinal nerve)

and the root of clitoris. In men, the nerves supply the anterior one third of the scrotum and base of the penis. The cutaneous distribution of these nerves often overlaps and may be difficult to distinguish from involvement of various branches of the genitofemoral nerve [8].

4 Equipment and Supplies (Table 4)

Table 4 Ilioinguinal/Iliohypogastric block supplies

Syringe	3 mL and 10 mL
Needle	27 g ½ to 1½ for skin local 22 g echogenic needle (author preference)
Anesthetic	1–2% lidocaine (skin local) (1–2 mL) 0.5% Bupivacaine (6 mL)
Corticosteroid	Triamcinolone 40 mg or Methylprednisolone 80 mg

5 Ilioinguinal and Iliohypogastric Nerve Blocks, Landmark Technique

Landmark based approaches to II and IH nerve blocks vary tremendously throughout the literature. One of the most commonly cited techniques, identifies point of needle entry for the II/IH block as localized 2 cm medial and 2 cm superior from the

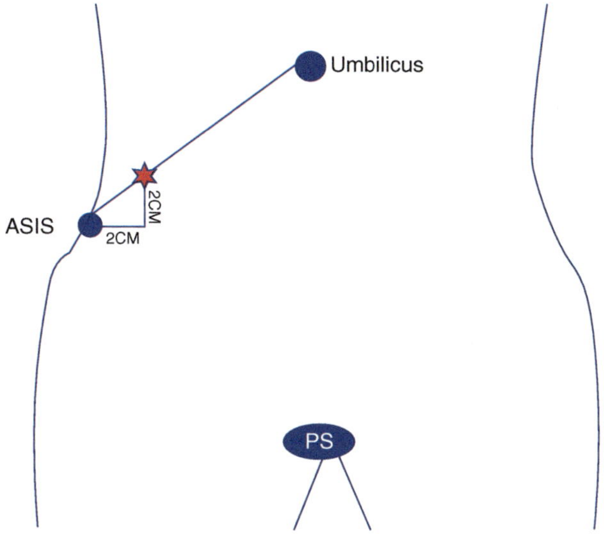

Fig. 2 Anatomic landmarks for IL/IH block

anterior superior iliac spine (ASIS), along the diagonal line between the ASIS and the umbilicus (Fig. 2). A needle is advanced perpendicular to the skin until two pops are felt. The first "pop" is penetration of the external oblique aponeurosis. At this juncture about 5 mL of injectate is deposited. The needle is then advanced until a second "pop" is felt. This marks penetration of the aponeurosis of the internal oblique muscle. At this juncture, the needle tip is presumed to be in the plane between the external oblique muscle and transversus abdominus muscle. A further 5 mL of injectate is deposited. Some publications advise needle insertion to be 1 inch medial and 1 inch inferior from ASIS towards the pubic symphysis for the IH nerve block, and 2 in. medial and 2 in. inferior for the II nerve block [6, 12].

Caution should be taken while performing this technique as the anatomy of the abdominal muscular layers may be altered in patients with prior history of low abdominal surgery.

6 Ultrasound Technique

Due to anatomical variability, success with the landmark-based technique is estimated to be between 55 and 90% with a common reason for failure being deposition of local anesthetic in the incorrect muscle layer [12]. Ultrasound helps to improve the success rate.

In the ultrasound guided technique, the key to effective block is clear visualization of the muscle layers. With the patient in the supine position, the ASIS is identified. A high frequency linear probe (6–13 MHz) is placed parallel to the inguinal ligament with the lateral border of the probe over the iliac crest. In this position, the bony drop out of the iliac crest can be identified and the iliac crest itself will be seen as a hyperechoic structure. Alternatively, the transducer can be pointed towards the umbilicus (Fig. 3).

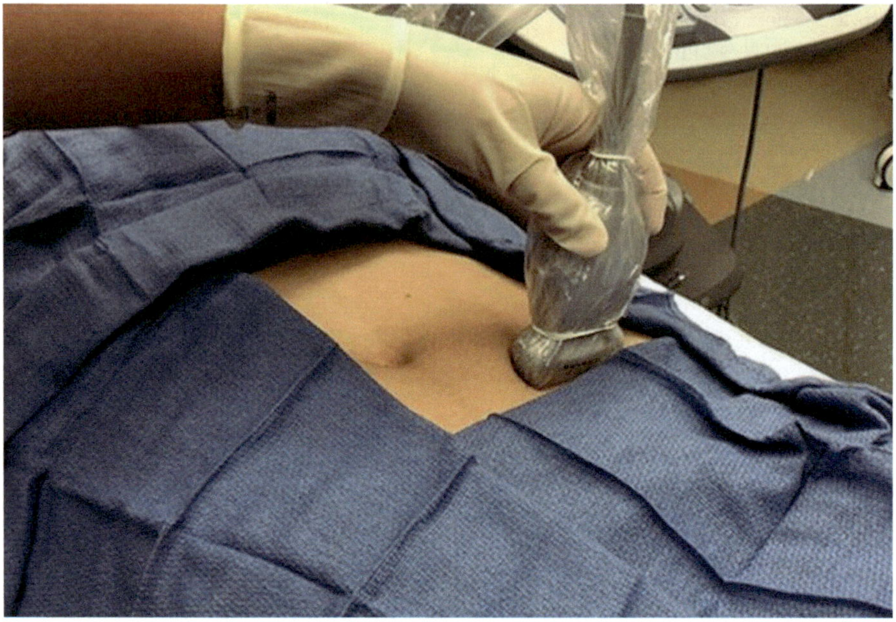

Fig. 3 Positioning for ultrasound guided block

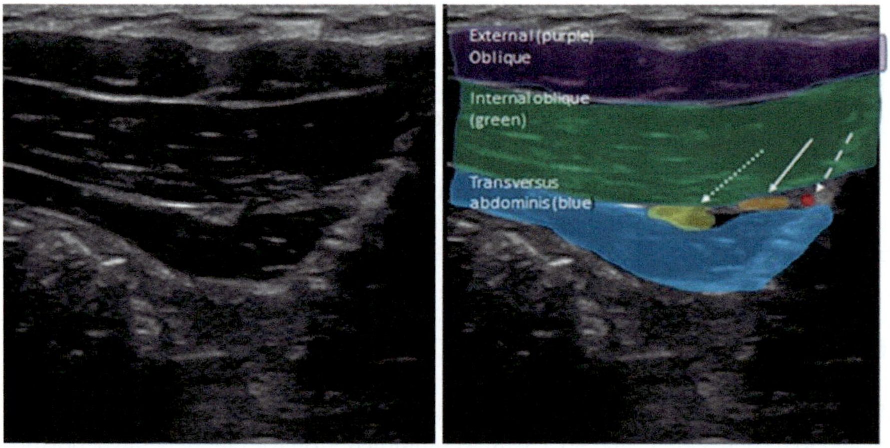

Fig. 4 Ultrasound anatomy of abdominal wall and II/IH neurovascular bundle (internal oblique muscle (purple), internal oblique muscle (green), transversus abdominis muscle (blue), iliohypogastric nerve (yellow/dotted arrow), ilioinguinal nerve (orange/solid arrow), circumflex ilioinguinal artery (red/interrupted arrow)

The layers of the abdominal wall, from superficial to deep are: skin, external oblique muscle, internal oblique muscle, transverse abdominis muscle, and peritoneum (Fig. 4). The peritoneum is easily identified by its peristaltic movements. The probe may need to be tilted in the cephalad or caudad direction for improved visualization. The II and IH nerves may be visualized as oval structures in the facial plane between the internal oblique and transverse abdominis muscles. It is not uncommon that visualization of the neurovascular bundle housing the II and the IH nerves may be challenging.

Direct visualization of the nerve is not necessary for effective block placement, whereas successful identification of the facial layers is essential. The deep circumflex iliac artery courses in close proximity lateral to II/IH nerves and may be detected by employing color doppler [13, 14].

After identification of the facial layers, the needle can be advanced from the lateral to medial direction if using an in-plane technique until the needle tip lies in the plane between the internal oblique and transversus abdominis muscles. Caution must be taken to avoid needle placement beyond the transversus abdominis muscle to avoid breach of the peritoneum, as this may result in inadvertent bowel injury. Continuous visualization of the needle tip during the needle advancement is of outmost importance [15]. Upon confirming a proper needle placement, a solution of 6–10 mL of injectate deposited under real time ultrasound should show lateral to medial spread with separation of transversus abdominis and external oblique muscles. An out of plane technique may also be used.

The technique described above can be used for pulsed radiofrequency treatment or cryoablation of the nerves. These techniques are thought to potentially provide longer duration of pain relief as compared to steroid injections [16]. Discussion on merits of peripheral nerve block vs ablation or stimulation is beyond the scope of this chapter, however, these techniques have also been described in treatment of II/IH neuralgias (Fig. 5) [17].

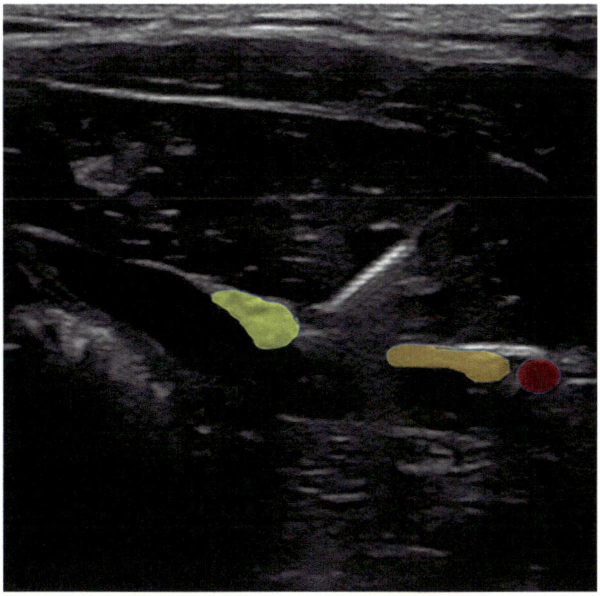

Fig. 5 Ultrasound image of II/IH block with evidence of hypoechoic needle aiming at iliohypogastric nerve (yellow) with the ilioinguinal nerve lateral (orange) and circumflex ilioinguinal artery in (red)

7 Potential Complications and Adverse Effects

Complications related to II and IH nerve block are rare. The most common complication is worsening of pain post injection. The most serious complication includes inadvertent entry to the peritoneal cavity with possible bowel perforation [18] due to advancement of the needle past the transversus abdominis muscle. Direct needle visualization during ultrasound guidance can help minimize this risk.

As with any other injection the risk of bleeding resulting in hematoma or infection at the injection site, allergic reaction to injected medications as well as lack of post-procedural pain relief may occur [19].

Local anesthetic toxicity is also a rare complication as the dose of local anesthetic typically used for this block is generally too low to reach toxic levels [20]. Occasional spread of local anesthetic to involve femoral nerve has also been described [21].

Clinical and Technical Pearls

- II and IH neuralgias commonly occur as a result of iatrogenic injury during surgery or abdominal trauma.
- Blockade of II and IH nerves can be both diagnostic and therapeutic for pain involving the lower abdomen with radiation to the scrotum or labia and inner thigh.
- II and IH blocks can be performed based on anatomical landmarks or with assistance of ultrasonography.
- Care must be taken to avoid needle advancement past the two superficial muscle layers (external and internal oblique muscles), as advancement of the needle pass the third layer (transversus abdominis) will result in peritoneal perforation
- Complications of this procedure are rare.

References

1. Baerentzen F, Maschmann C, Jensen K, et al. Ultrasound-guided nerve block for inguinal hernia repair: a randomized, controlled, double-blind study. Reg Anesth Pain Med. 2012;37:502–7.
2. Benzon HT, Rathmell JP, Wu CL, et al. Practical management of pain. 5th ed. Philadelphia: Elsevier Mosby; 2014. p. 683–800.
3. Tarun B, et al. Ultrasound-guided trunk and core blocks in infants and children. J Anesth. 2013;27:109–23.
4. Cardosi RJ, Cox CS, Hoffman MS. Postoperative neuropathies after major pelvic surgery. Obstet Gynecol. 2002;100(2):240–4.
5. Demirer S, Kepenecki I, Evirgen O, et al. The effect of polypropylene mesh on ilioinguinal nerve in open mesh repair of groin hernia. J Surg Res. 2006;131920:175–81.
6. Nagpal A, Moody EL. Interventional Management for Pelvic Pain. Phys Med Rehabil Clin N Am. 2017;28(3):621–46.

7. Prendergast SA, Weiss JM. Screening for musculoskeletal causes of pelvic pain. Clin Obstet Gynecol. 2003;46(4):773–82.
8. Elchins N, Hunt J. Neurogenic Pelvic Pain. Phys Med Rehabil Clin N Am. 2017;28:551–69.
9. Chhabra A, Rozen S, Scott K. Three-dimentional MR neurography of the lumbosacral plexus. Semin Musculoskelet Radiol. 2015;19(2):149159.
10. Feng P, et al. Role of MR Neurography in Groin and Genital Pain: Ilioinguinal, Iliohypogastric, and Genitofemoral Neuralgia. Am J Roentgenol. 2019;212(3):632–43.
11. Cho H, et al. Diagnosis of ilioinguinal nerve injury based on electromyography and ultrasonography: a case report. Ann Rehabil Med. 2017;41(4):705–8.
12. Trainor D, Moeschler S, Pingree M, et al. Landmark-based versus ultrasound-guided ilioinguinal/iliohypogastric nerve blocks in the treatment of chronic postherniorrhaphy groin pain: a retrospective study. J Pain Res. 2015;8:767–70.
13. Gofeld M, Christakis M. Sonographically guided ilioinguinal nerve block. J Ultrasound Med. 2006;25:1571–5.
14. Eichenberger U, Greher M, Kirchmair L, et al. Ultrasound-guided blocks of the ilioinguinal and iliohypogastric nerve: accuracy of a selective new technique confirmed by anatomical dissection. Br J Anaesth. 2006;97(2):238–43.
15. Peng PW, Tumber PS. Ultrasound guided interventional procedures for patients with chronic pelvic pain – a description of techniques and review of literature. Pain Physician. 2008;11(2):215–24.
16. Kastler A, Aubry S, Piccand V, et al. Radiofrequency neurolysis versus local nerve infiltration in 42 patients with refractory chronic inguinal neuralgia. Pain Physician. 2012;15(3):327–44.
17. Banh DPT, et al. Permanent implantation of peripheral nerve stimulator for combat injury-related ilioinguinal neuralgia. Pain Physician. 2013;16(6):E789–91.
18. Martin J, Sossai MD. Colonic puncture during ilioinguinal nerve block in a child. Anesth Analg. 1999;88(5):1051–2.
19. Vaisman J. Pelvic hematoma after an ilioinguinal nerve block for orchialgia. Anesth Analg. 2001;92(4):1048–9.
20. Jeng CL, Torrillo TM, Rosenblatt MA. Complications of peripheral nerve blocks. Br J Anaesth. 2010;105:97–107.
21. Rosario DJ, Jacob S, Luntley J, Skinner PP, Raftery AT. Mechanism of femoral nerve palsy complicating percutaneous ilioinguinal field block. Br J Anaesth. 1997;78(3):314–6.

Further Reading

Khaled M, Elsakka KM, Basit H, Allam A, Khaled M. Ilioinguinal Neuralgia. StatPearls.com. Last updated 07/2019. Bookshelf ID: NBK538256. PMID: 30855844.

Genitofemoral Nerve Block

Melanie G. Wood, Kanishka Rajput, and Robert M. Chow

Essential Concepts

- The GFN block is a useful diagnostic and treatment tool for acute or chronic groin/pelvic pain.
- GFN blocks are commonly used in the perioperative period for inguinal hernia surgeries, but have been used for other groin surgeries as well.
- GFN blocks cover visceral pain that transversus abdominis plane (TAP) blocks do not
- GFN blocks can be easily and safely performed at the bedside.

1 Indications and Contraindications

The GFN block is a useful diagnostic and treatment tool for pelvic or groin pain that may occur as a complication of groin surgeries or abdominal surgeries that result in possible damage to nerves due to trocar or retractor placement or entrapment with the scar tissue formation. In addition, the genitofemoral nerve block can be used for analgesia in the perioperative setting for inguinal hernia repairs as well as other surgeries. Its value is found in blocking the visceral pain that ilio-inguinal and ilio-hypogastric blocks cannot cover [1]. As such, it has been utilized in conjunction with ilio-inguinal and ilio-hypogastric blocks for other groin surgeries including femoral endarterectomies, endovascular aneurysm repair (EVAR), and extracorporeal membrane oxygenation (ECMO) cannulation [2–4]. GFN blocks and GFN ablations have also been used for both chronic inguinal and scrotal pain [5–7]. Contraindications include infection at the planned procedure site or severe systemic infection, patient refusal, allergy or intolerance to injectate or its components.

M. G. Wood · K. Rajput · R. M. Chow (✉)
Department of Anesthesiology, Yale University School of Medicine, New Haven, CT, USA
e-mail: melanie.wood@yale.edu; kanishka.rajput@yale.edu; robert.chow@yale.edu

D. Souza et al. (eds.), *Bedside Pain Management Interventions*,
https://doi.org/10.1007/978-3-031-11188-4_46

Coagulopathy, including iatrogenic, and platelet dysfunction, including iatrogenic, and not typically contraindications for this procedure. However, an assessment of the risks and benefits of the procedure, and a detailed discussion with the patient are mandatory.

2 Clinical Anatomy

The genitofemoral nerve arises from L1-L2 segments of the lumbar plexus. The nerve then passes inferiorly, piercing the psoas muscle and then splitting into two divisions.

The genital branch carries mostly sensory fibers along with the motor component of the cremaster reflex. It courses through the deep inguinal ring and through the inguinal canal, where it innervates the anterior scrotum in males and the mons pubis and labia majora in females.

The femoral branch passes deep to the inguinal ligament within the muscular section of the femoral canal. It provides sensory innervation to the upper, medial, and anterior thigh as well as the sensory component of the cremaster reflex (Fig. 1).

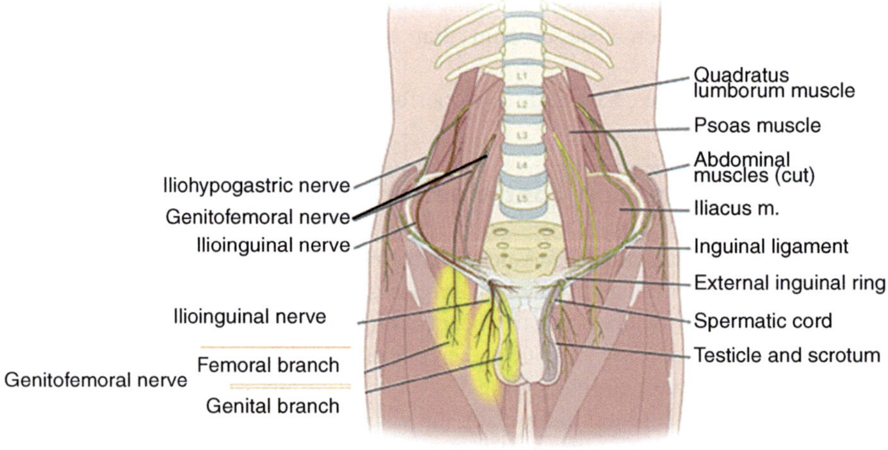

Fig. 1 Genitofemoral nerve anatomy, as labeled

3 Equipment and Supplies

Genitofemoral nerve blocks can be performed at the bedside. A sterile interventional procedure tray with 4% chlorhexidine or another antiseptic solution are typically used. A 5-10 mL syringe with 22–25 Gauge 1.5–2.5-in. needle are typically used. The anesthetic solution usually consists of 5–10 mL of a medium to long-acting local anesthetic (LA) is used. The block that specifically targets the genital branch can utilize 5 mL of LA injected inside and/or around the spermatic cord. Corticosteroids can be utilized for chronic pain, if no contraindications, and no concerns about potential side effects (Table 1).

Table 1 Equipment and supplies for genitofemoral nerve block

Needle	22 g or 25 g
Syringe	5 mL × 2 or 10 mL
Anesthetic	**For genital branch:** 5–10 mL of 0.25% bupivacaine or 0.2% ropivacaine around the spermatic cord/round ligament **For femoral branch:** 5–10 mL of 0.25% bupivacaine or 0.2% ropivacaine **Combined:** 10 mL of 0.25% bupivacaine or 0.2% ropivacaine

4 Genitofemoral Nerve Block, Landmark Technique

The genitofemoral nerve block usually refers to block of the genital branch of the nerve. The patient is placed in the supine position, then a 22 g or 25 g needle is introduced 1 cm superior and lateral to the pubic tubercle with a field block aimed towards the inguinal canal. This blind landmark technique can put structures such as the spermatic cord and peritoneum at risk for accidental injury and is not commonly used [8].

5 Genitofemoral Nerve Block, Ultrasound Technique

Genital Branch

The patient is placed in supine position. A linear probe is placed inferior to the inguinal canal in the transverse orientation to locate the femoral artery. The probe is then rotated to the longitudinal orientation and moved cephalad until the artery is seen diving deep toward the inguinal ligament. The probe is then rotated to the oblique position, and the spermatic cord, an oval or circular shape with 1–2 arteries, will then be identifiable (Fig. 2).

In women, the round ligament will be seen. A 21 g or 22 g echogenic needle is introduced in plane. Total of 5–10 mL of local anesthetic is injected adjacent to the spermatic cord. In women, the local anesthetic is administered around the round ligament. [8–10]

Femoral Branch

In order to block the femoral branch of the GFN, a linear ultrasound probe is placed parallel and superior to the inguinal ligament to visualize the external iliac artery (EIA) (Fig. 3).

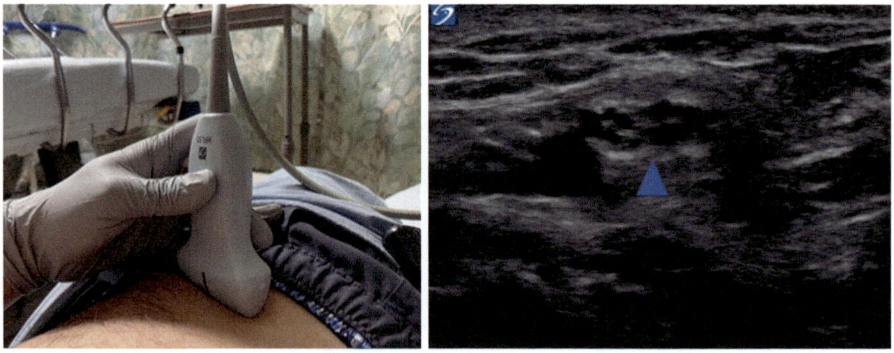

Fig. 2 Genitofemoral Nerve Block (Genital Branch) in male. Probe and needle orientation, on the left. Ultrasonogram, on the right. Blue Arrowhead—Spermatic Cord

The nerve is typically not seen but is found in the same fascial layer as the EIA. A 21 g or 22 g echogenic needle is inserted until it is directly lateral to the EIA. Then 5–10 mL of local anesthetic is deposited in the peri-arterial region [3].

A second approach has been described, which also uses a 21 g or 22 g echogenic needle and 10 mL of LA deposited lateral to the femoral artery and caudal to the inguinal ligament between the fascia lata and the fascia iliaca [4].

Combined Genitofemoral Block

A novel approach for the GFN block has been described by Yoshida et al., which is performed in conjunction with a quadratus lumborum (QL) block. This technique uses the “shamrock view”, which can be obtained just superior to the iliac crest in the axial plane. It is formed by the “stem” or transverse process of L4, and the “leaves” or the QL, psoas major and erector spinae muscles (Fig. 4).

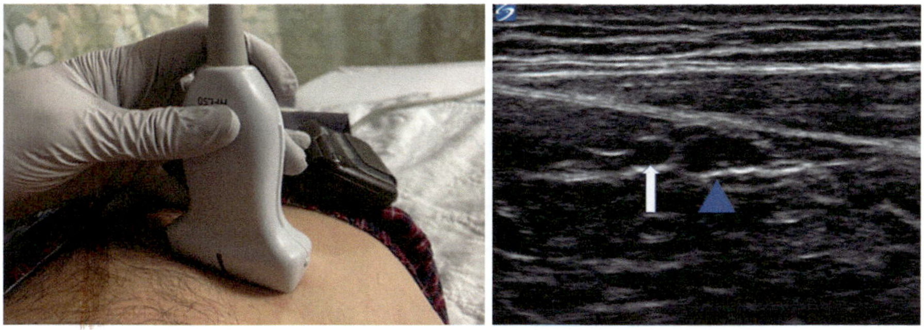

Fig. 3 Genitofemoral Nerve Block (Femoral Branch). Probe and needle orientation, on the left. Ultrasonogram, on the right. White Arrow—External Iliac Artery. Blue Arrowhead—External Iliac Vein

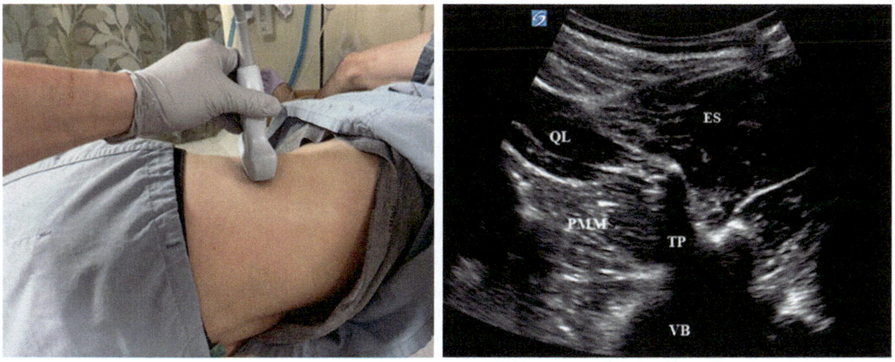

Fig. 4 Combined Genitofemoral Nerve Block. Probe and needle orientation, on the left. Ultrasonogram, on the right. Shamrock View: Q—Quadratus Lumborum Muscle, E—Erector Spinae Muscle, PMM—Psoas Major Muscle, T—Transverse Process, VB—Vertebral Body

After the quadratus lumborum block is completed, the needle is advanced through the fascia of the psoas major muscle (PMM) and 10 mL of local anesthetic is deposited in the sub-fascial layer of the PMM. In the original pilot study, 9 out of 11 patients had blocks of both branches with this approach [11]. Of note, cadaveric studies have shown that local anesthetic spread to the GFN after a standard quadratus lumborum block occurs in 20% of cases [12].

6 Potential Complications and Adverse Effects

This procedure is considered to be extremely safe. Few complications of the genitofemoral nerve block have been described, but several are theoretically possible. With injection into the spermatic cord, there is danger of damage to the internal spermatic cord structures or of a spermatic cord hematoma. There is also concern for unintentional blockage of the femoral nerve. If the landmark technique is utilized, there is also the possibility of puncture of the peritoneum.

Clinical and Technical Pearls

- The GFN can be performed at the bedside for management of acute or chronic groin and scrotal pain.
- The GFN block significantly reduces the amount of intraoperative opioid required for inguinal hernia repair surgeries.
- Although useful for perioperative analgesia, Stav et al. demonstrated that the GFN block is most effective when performed in conjunction with a TAP block [13]. Thus, the GFN block can be used with other peripheral nerve blocks to obtain surgical anesthesia or perioperative analgesia for groin surgeries.

References

1. Huang Z, Xia W, Peng X, Ke J, Wang W. Evaluation of ultrasound-guided genitofemoral nerve block combined with ilioinguinal/iliohypogastric nerve block during inguinal hernia repair in the elderly. Curr Med Sci. 2019;39:794–9. https://doi.org/10.1007/s11596-019-2107-2.
2. Ohgoshi Y, Takeda M, Miura M, Kori S, Matsukawa M. Combination of femoral and genitofemoral nerve blocks is effective for endovascular aneurysm repair. J Clin Anesth. 2017;37:97–8. https://doi.org/10.1016/j.jclinane.2016.12.024. Epub 2017 Jan 5
3. Romano V, Burke C, Hou J, Xu JL. The analgesic efficacy of transversus abdominis plane block combined with femoral branch of genitofemoral nerve block for femoral endarterectomy. Anesth Essays Res. 2019;13(1):191–2. https://doi.org/10.4103/aer.AER_46_19.
4. Brisard L, Belaidi M, Bizouarn P. Ultrasound-guided transversus abdominis plane/genitofemoral blocks for a patient receiving extracorporeal life support. AA Case Rep. 2014;2(12):155–6. https://doi.org/10.1213/XAA.0000000000000030.
5. Lee KS, Sin JM, Patil PP, et al. Ultrasound-guided microwave ablation for the management of inguinal neuralgia: a preliminary study with 1-year follow-up. J Vasc Interv Radiol. 2019;30(2):242–8. https://doi.org/10.1016/j.jvir.2018.10.031.

6. Terkawi AS, Romdhane K. Ultrasound-guided pulsed radiofrequency ablation of the genital branch of the genitofemoral nerve for treatment of intractable orchalgia. Saudi J Anaesth. 2014;8(2):294–8. https://doi.org/10.4103/1658-354X.130755.
7. Shanthanna H. Successful treatment of genitofemoral neuralgia using ultrasound guided injection: a case report and short review of literature. Case Rep Anesthesiol. 2014;2014:371703. https://doi.org/10.1155/2014/371703.
8. Peng PW, Tumber PS. Ultrasound-guided interventional procedures for patients with chronic pelvic pain—a description of techniques and review of literature. Pain Physician. 2008;11:215–24.
9. Frassanito L, Zanfini BA, Pitoni S, et al. Ultrasoundguided genitofemoral nerve block for inguinal hernia repair in the male adult: a randomized controlled pilot study. Minerva Anestesiol. 2018;84(2):189–95.
10. Singh SK, Vadera HB. Ultrasound guided hernia blocks. Anaesth Pain Intensive Care. 2015;19(3):366–71.
11. Yoshida T, Nakamoto T, Kamibayashi T. ESRA19-0050 A subfascial local anesthetic injection to the psoas major muscle combined with the anterior approach for quadratus lumborum block: technical description and retrospective evaluation. Reg Anesthesia Pain Med. 2019;44:A231.
12. Das Adhikary S, El-Boghdadly K, Nasralah Z, Sarwani N, Nixon AM, Chin KJ. A radiologic and anatomic assessment of injectate spread following transmuscular quadratus lumborum block in cadavers. Anaesthesia. 2017;72(1):73–79. https://doi.org/10.1111/anae.13647. Epub 2016 Oct 12.
13. Stav A, Reytman L, Stav MY, et al. Transversus abdominis plane versus ilioinguinal and iliohypogastric nerve blocks for analgesia following open inguinal herniorrhaphy. Rambam Maimonides Med J. 2016;7(3):e0021. Published 2016 Jul 28. https://doi.org/10.5041/RMMJ.10248.

Further Reading

Standing, Susan. *Gray's Anatomy.* 41st ed. Philadelphia: Elsevier Limited; 2016. Chapter 62, Posterior abdominal wall and retroperitoneum; p. 1083–97.

Pudendal Nerve Block

Adi Cosic and Ankit Maheshwari

Essential Concepts

- Pudendal nerve blocks were previously used for pain relief in the perineal area for the parturient during labor but have since fallen out of favor due to adverse complications such as fetal acidosis.
- Goals for bedside use of ultrasound for pudendal nerve block are accurate identification of the pudendal nerve at Alcock canal prior to nerve termination.
- A combination of local anesthetic and steroid use, decided by the practitioner, will quickly provide pain relief with minimal effect on the sacral plexus with the use of ultrasound.
- The mechanism of action includes blockade of nociceptive fibers innervating the perineal area via the three endings of the pudendal nerve, which include the anal and rectal, perineal, and clitoral or penile nerves.

1 Overview

The pudendal nerve, a nerve arising from the sacral plexus, has been previously studied as a potential target for treatment of intractable pain in the perineal and genital area. Given its distribution, it is a desired target for perioperative pain control in patients undergoing colorectal, perineal, and urological procedures. In addition, it is used in the diagnosis of pain syndromes such as pudendal nerve entrapment [1, 2]. It is frequently the target of chronic pain syndromes involving the superficial genital and perineal regions. As recently as 2013, advancements in ultrasound technology

A. Cosic
University Hospitals, Cleveland, OH, USA
e-mail: adi.cosic@uhhospitals.org

A. Maheshwari (✉)
Texas Pain Intervention Clinic, McKinney, TX, USA
e-mail: dr.m@texaspainclinic.com

D. Souza et al. (eds.), *Bedside Pain Management Interventions*,
https://doi.org/10.1007/978-3-031-11188-4_47

have made this an accessible option in bedside scenarios for the treatment of perineal and superficial genital perioperative pain, as well as chronic and intractable pain syndromes.

2 Indications and Contraindications

Pudendal nerve blocks (PNB) can be utilized for diagnosis and treatment of pudendal nerve entrapment syndrome with unilateral or bilateral nociceptive pain, as well as providing perioperative pain relief for various surgeries. It can also be used in pregnant patients in the second stage of labor.

It is contraindicated in patients with infection at the planned injection site, severe systemic infection, allergy or intolerance to injectate or its components, and patient refusal.

Other concerns to generalized deep nerve blocks include low platelet counts, ongoing anticoagulation, incompatible body habitus, amongst others. However, anticoagulation, including iatrogenic and platelet dysfunction, is not an absolute contraindication. It requires shared decision making with the patient and other providers (Table 1).

3 Clinical Anatomy

The pudendal nerve, a paired nerve, arises from the ventral rami of the S2-4 spinal nerves. Both left and right nerves form from three roots that, soon after exiting the sacral plexus, become cords that further merge into the pudendal nerve on the inferior border of the piriformis and superior portion of the coccygeus muscle and sacrospinous ligament. Following its formation and initial descent it leaves the pelvis briefly via the greater sciatic foramen, accompanied by the internal pudendal artery and vein. It then crosses posteriorly to the sacrospinous ligament, close to its insertion point, and reenters the pelvis through the lesser sciatic foramen. Here it changes course to an anterosuperior route through Alcock's canal (also known as the pudendal canal, formed from the fascia of the obturator internus muscle) where

Table 1 Indications and contraindications for pudendal nerve

Indications	Contraindications or concerns
Pain in distribution of pudendal nerve (pudendal nerve entrapment)	Patient refusal
Urological procedure involving external genitalia, including lower vagina	Systemic or local infection
Colorectal procedures involving anus	Platelet counts less than 50,000 required shared decision making
Gynecological procedures involving lower 1/5 of vagina	INR > 1.5 or currently on anticoagulation, required shared decision making
Chronic pain syndromes in distribution of pudendal nerve	

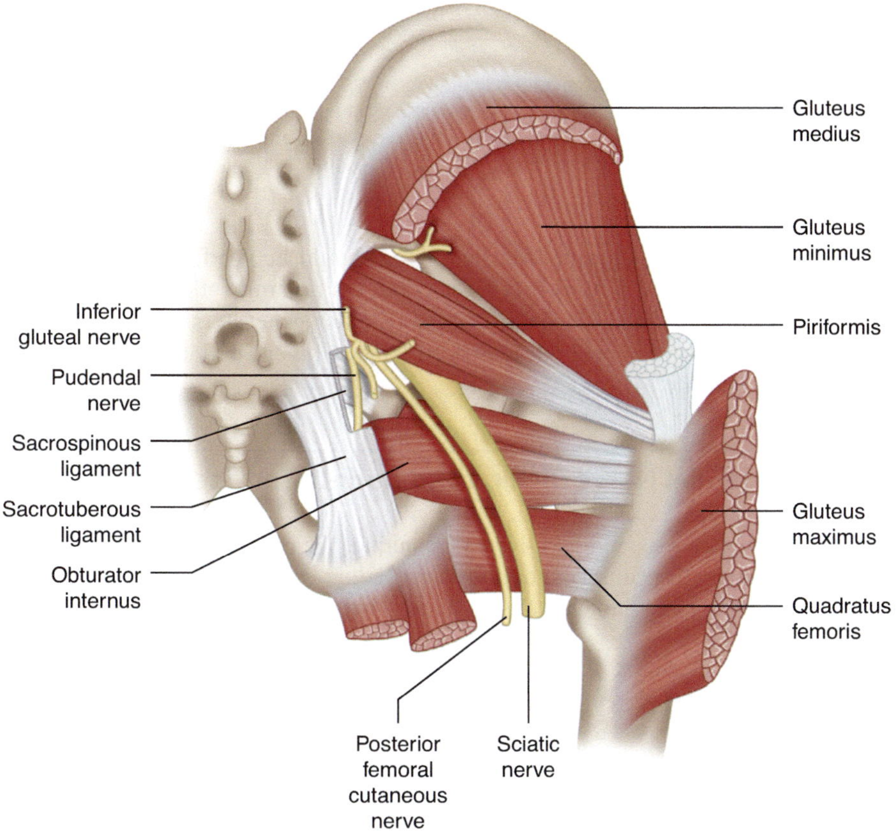

Fig. 1 Pudendal nerve anatomy, as labeled

it continues forward through the floor of the pelvic musculature. Branches in this portion include the inferior rectal nerve, the perineal nerve, and the continuation as the dorsal nerve of the penis or clitoris. It carries sensation from the external genitalia, including the lower 1/5 of the vagina, the perineal area, and the skin around anus. Of note, the pudendal nerve does not supply the anterior portion of the perineal area or the upper vagina and cervix. Motor supply granted by this nerve includes portions of the pelvic musculature, the male and female external urethral sphincter, and the external anal sphincter [3] (Fig. 1).

4 Equipment and Supplies

Pudendal nerve blocks can be performed at the bedside with the use a of a 10 mL syringe and 2 in 22 gauge needle if using the anterior approach, and a short bevel 4 in needle if using the posterior technique. Injectable solutions consist of local anesthetic (lidocaine, bupivacaine, ropivacaine) with the option of adding a

Table 2 Equipment and supplies

Syringe	5–10 mL
Needle	2 in 22 gauge (anterior technique) 5 in 22 gauge short bevel (posterior technique)
Anesthetic	Combination of local anesthetic and/or steroid chosen by the practitioner

corticosteroid and epinephrine. Sterile gloves should be used, as well as sterile draping. An ultrasound with a curvilinear probe is recommended, given its deep field of imaging. (Table 2). Radiofrequency (RF) generators and needles are needed if RF ablation is desired. However, RF equipment may be challenging to obtain at the bedside [4].

5 Pudendal Nerve Block, Landmark-Based Technique

Some practitioners use landmark-based technique. We recommend using imaging-guided technique. The ultrasound-guided procedure provides real-time procedure visualization, and can be effectively used at the bedside.

6 Pudendal Nerve Block, Ultrasound-Guided Technique

Two ultrasound-guided techniques are available for pudendal nerve block: the anterior perineal approach and the posterior transgluteal approach. Anterior perineal blocks are performed with the patient in lithotomy position with appropriate monitoring and sterile field protocol. Given the superficial depth of the pudendal nerve at this region, transducers with high or intermediate frequency transducers should be used. The junction of the genitals and rectum should be targeted with the transducer at an angle of 45 degrees, and the anatomy of the pudendal neurovascular bundle identified along the medial side of the ischial tuberosity. Doppler imaging should be used to identify the pudendal artery and the hyperechoic three-millimeter nerve surrounding it, corresponding to the branching of the pudendal nerve [2]. After proper local anesthesia, a 2-in. 22 gauge needle, with a provider chosen combination of local anesthetic and/or steroid, is used to inject between a 3 and 5 mL volume.

The posterior approach is performed in the prone or lateral decubitus position with the affected side facing upwards (Fig. 2).

Following proper patient positioning, sedation, and aseptic technique, a curvilinear transducer is introduced to the skin and pudendal nerve structures identified between 5 to 6 cm beneath the skin. An oblique angle at the junction of the sacrum and ileum along the proximal gluteal surface, following the curved track of the nerve, should be employed. Identify the posterosuperior iliac spine, the greater sciatic foramen, the iliac spine, the sacral plexus, the piriformis muscle, and the superior gluteal artery. The sacrospinous ligament, the sacrotuberous ligament, and laterally the sciatic nerve and inferior gluteal artery can be finally visualized (Fig. 3).

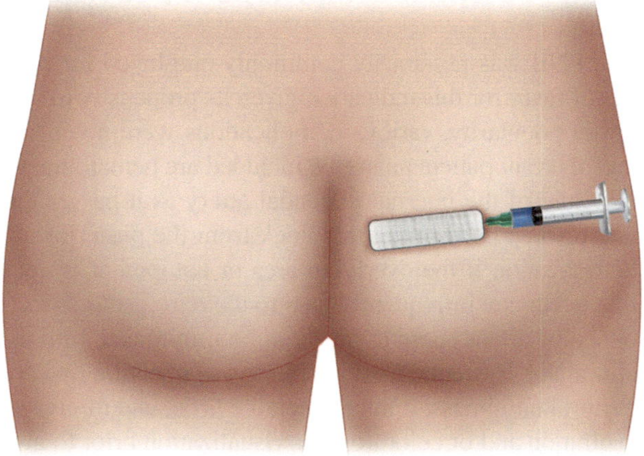

Fig. 2 Pudendal nerve block, posterior approach. Ultrasonographic probe and needle/syringe positioning

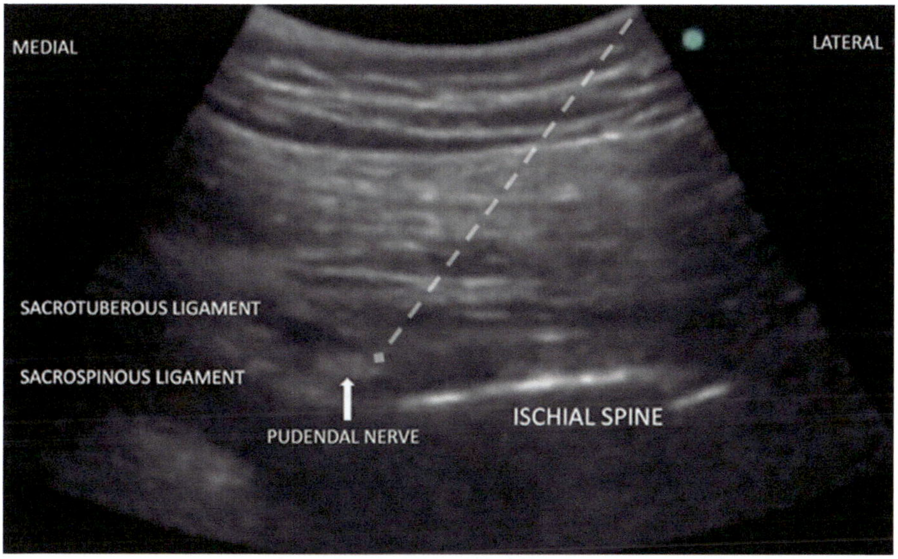

Fig. 3 Ultrasonogram of the pudendal nerve block, as labeled. Ultrasound showies the sacrotuberous and sacrospinous ligaments in relation to the ischial spine. Needle is advanced until it penetrates the sacrotuberous ligament and the injection performed with local anesthetic spread between the two ligaments. The needle trajectory marked with dhsed line

In this position, at the medial half of the image, the internal pudendal artery and pudendal nerve can be identified. Given its small size (averaging 3.5 mm), the pudendal nerve is challenging to identify consistently, most often being found medial to the pudendal vessels. Once identified, a 5in 22 gauge needle is advanced in-plane or out-of-plane. After insertion and positioning, neurostimulation can be used to confirm positioning [2].

7 Potential Complications and Adverse Effects

The PNB was previously commonly employed for the parturient but has since faded out of favor for this indication given its propensity to induce fetal acidosis. Through its initial popularity, various complications were noted from use of incorrect technique and aberrant patient anatomy. Included are hematoma, which most likely occurs due to puncture of the internal pudendal artery as it passes through Alcock's canal with the nerve when performing the block from the posterior position. Infection could be a re complication if the overlying area or equipment is not properly sterilized. Infections that occur can infrequently pass to the retro psoas space, forming an abscess. The incidence of direct nerve trauma can be minimized with the use of ultrasound and nerve stimulator. Systemic toxicity, by way of injection into arterial vessels, can identified by perioral numbness, tinnitus, metallic taste, and rarely seizures. These are prevented by aspiration and or color doppler visualization prior to injection of local anesthetic.

Clinical and Technical Pearls

- Pudendal nerve blocks have a wide utility in gynecological, urological, and colorectal surgeries, along with chronic pain syndromes involving the nerve.
- Proper positioning of patient and transducer is key to successful identification of the pudendal nerve in the posterior block.
- Utilize standard of care for regional blocks, including aseptic technique, appropriate sedation, and employ caution with patients on anticoagulants.
- Use of nerve stimulator to confirm positioning of needle is advised.

References

1. Rojas-Gómez MF, Blanco R, Roa VT, González AMG. Regional anesthesia guided by ultrasound in the pudendal nerve territory. Colomb J Anesthesiol. 2017;45(3):200–9.
2. Bendtsen TF, et al. Ultrasound-Guided Pudendal Nerve Block at the Entrance of the Pudendal (Alcock) Canal. Reg Anesth Pain Med. 2016;41(2):140–5.
3. "The Pudendal Nerve." TeachMeAnatomy. https://teachmeanatomy.info/pelvis/other/pudendal-nerve/. Acessed March 15 2022.
4. Fang H, et al. Clinical effect and safety of pulsed radiofrequency treatment for pudendal neuralgia: a prospective, randomized controlled clinical trial. J Pain Res. 2018;11(16):2367–74.

Further Reading

Ghanavatian S, Derian A. Pudendal nerve block. In: StatPearls. Treasure Island (FL): StatPearls Publishing; 2021.

Takashima Y, Handler SJ, Zeno A, Alvarez P, Miyazaki B, Del Canto I, Khamis C, Yazdany T, Le TH. The anatomical distribution of the pudendal nerve block injection: a cadaveric study. Female Pelvic Med Reconstr Surg. 2021;27(2):e306–8.

Part VI

Bedside Procedures for Upper Extremity Pain

Shoulder Joint Injections

Sahna Reddy, Alexander Hynes, and Maxim Eckmann

Essential Concepts The anatomy of the shoulder joint involves 3 main articulations and 2 gliding planes.

- Osteoarthritis and impingement syndrome are the most common indications for shoulder injections.
- Injections for the shoulder can result in pain relief for months at a time and can delay or serve as a bridge to surgery in some patients.
- The most employed method is glenohumeral intraarticular corticosteroid injection, however, multiple injectates are available and actively used.
- Ultrasound has been shown to have superior results for most of the injection approaches to the joints and bursae.
- Ultrasound techniques are simple and easily performed at the bedside.

1 Overview

Shoulder pain is the third most common musculoskeletal complaint with a lifetime prevalence as high as 66.7% and a peak incidence from 45 to 64 years of age [1–3]. Pain involving the shoulder, especially if chronic, can lead to significant morbidity and interruption in work and activities of daily living.

The shoulder is one of the most intricate and complex joints in the human body. It is composed of three articulations (the glenohumeral joint (GHJ), acromioclavicular joint (ACJ), and sternoclavicular joint (SCJ)) and two gliding planes (subacromial/subdeltoid and scapulothoracic). These articulations along with the many muscles, tendons and ligaments that cross or span the shoulder allow for the greatest mobility of any joint in the human body [4]. This also allows for many pathological

S. Reddy · A. Hynes · M. Eckmann (✉)
Department of Anesthesiology and Pain Medicine, University of Texas Health San Antonio, San Antonio, TX, USA
e-mail: ReddySP@uthscsa.edu; HynesA@uthscsa.edu; eckmann@uthscsa.edu

D. Souza et al. (eds.), *Bedside Pain Management Interventions*,
https://doi.org/10.1007/978-3-031-11188-4_48

processes to involve the shoulder. Since the GHJ (commonly referred to as the shoulder joint), ACJ, and subacromial/subdeltoid bursa (SASDB) are the most common areas of pathology and generators of pain in the shoulder, they will be the focus of this chapter. Common indications (Table 1) for injections in the shoulder joint, absolute and relative contraindications (Table 2, 3), and the major bedside techniques of injection and the injectates used will also be discussed.

2 Indications and Contraindications (Tables 1, 2 and 3)

Table 1 Indications for injections around the shoulder for various pathologies

Indications
Glenohumeral Joint
Primary osteoarthritis
Rheumatoid/inflammatory arthritis
Post-traumatic arthritis
Adhesive capsulitis ("frozen shoulder")
Acromioclavicular Joint
Primary osteoarthritis
Post-traumatic arthritis
Osteolysis
Subacromial/Subdeltoid Bursa
Shoulder impingement syndrome
Subacromial bursitis
Rotator cuff tear
Rotator cuff tendinopathy

Table 2 Absolute contraindications for performing interventional procedures around the shoulder joint

Absolute Contraindications
Malignancy
Infection or breakdown of skin at the site of injection
Infection or destruction of the joint
Joint fracture
Bleeding diathesis
Known history of contraindication to individual injectates (adverse reaction to local anesthetic, severely compromised immune status, etc.)

Table 3 Relative contraindications for performing interventional procedures around the shoulder joint

Relative Contraindications
Anticoagulation therapy dependent
Joint instability
Infection near site of injection
Prosthetic joint
Recent corticosteroid injection (within the past 3 months)
Known history of relative contraindication to individual injectates (poorly controlled diabetes, poorly controlled hypertension, hypersensitivity to avian products such as proteins, feather, and egg products that can sometimes be found in viscosupplementation products, etc.)

3 Clinical Anatomy

Relevant clinical anatomy will be discussed in each subsection.

4 Equipment and Supplies

All procedures discussed below can be performed at the patients beside in the office or hospital room setting. They should be carried out under strict sterile technique in accordance with practice guidelines. Sedation is not commonly utilized for these procedures. However, if used, standard ASA monitors should be applied. Equipment needed to complete these procedures include a stand with a sterile drape, sterile gloves, sterile ultrasound cover, sterile syringe (size depends on injectate used and overall volume), a 1.5-inch 25–27-gauge needle, and an ultrasonography machine with linear probe. Additional equipment that can be helpful in some instances include 2–4-inch connector tubing (used between needle and syringe) and potentially a 3.5-inch 25–27-gauge Quincke needle to account for body habitus as needed.

5 Injectates

Corticosteroids

The most common injectate used in shoulder injections are corticosteroids. According to a Cochrane review on corticosteroids in 2003, intra-articular corticosteroids may be beneficial in the short-term for adhesive capsulitis or rotator-cuff disease [5]. The theoretical mechanism involves inflammatory marker modulation with reduced blood flow to the synovium. Corticosteroids have also been shown to alter local collagen fiber synthesis possibly decreasing the formation of scar tissue. There is limited evidence to support the selection of one corticosteroid over another and selection is generally based on the duration of action. It has been shown that branched esters of corticosteroids were superior to non-ester derivatives due to a longer duration at the site of injection [6]. The most common corticosteroids utilized include: Depo-Medrol (Methylprednisolone acetate) 40–80 mg, Kenalog (Triamcinolone acetonide) 10-40 mg and Decadron (Dexamethasone acetate) 4–8 mg. Generally, 5 mL of total injection volume, including diluents, is utilized. Systematic evidence is lacking when it comes to selecting which corticosteroid is ideal for shoulder injections.

Local Anesthetics

Local anesthetics of the amide class are commonly combined with corticosteroids to facilitate needle placement and provide immediate relief that corticosteroids do not offer. Lidocaine, bupivacaine, and ropivacaine are common local anesthetics used in clinical practice.

Viscosupplementation (Hyaluronic Acid derivatives)

The injection of viscosupplementation is a relatively new treatment for intra-articular injections of the shoulder [7]. Although hyaluronic acid is only approved for knee injections by the FDA, initial clinical trials showed potential efficacy for its use in the shoulder joint [8]. Hyaluronic acid is a physiologic component of native synovial fluid with viscoelastic properties that protect and promote joint mobility and anti-inflammatory properties that aid in decreasing pain [7]. Formulations can be categorized as cross-linked versus non-cross-linked and low-molecular weight versus high-molecular weight. Although there is a theoretical benefit of low molecular weight preparations in their ability to interact with synoviocytes in the joint space, they are less viscous in comparison to high molecular weight preparations [9, 10]. Despite these differences, none of the preparations have been shown to make a clinically significant difference in a small number of studies [10, 11]. Below is a list of common viscosupplementation preparations available [11] (Table 4):

Platelet-Rich Plasma

Many studies have been performed recently on the use of platelet-rich plasma (PRP) but have demonstrated an equivocal to minor benefit for shoulder pain, function and healing [12]. There is a small amount of evidence that supports the use of PRP in the non-operative management of rotator cuff tears, particularly in patients that have contraindication to receiving corticosteroids [13–15]. More studies are required to evaluate the potential clinical benefits of PRP in shoulder pathology.

Table 4 Common viscosupplementation preparations

Product structure	Product name	Origin	Molecular weight (kDa)	Injection interval	Dosing volume	Recommended dosing regimen
Cross-linked	Synvisc	Sodium hyaluronate	6000	1 week	2 mL (16 mg hylan polymers A & B)	3
	Synvisc-One	Sodium hyaluronate	6000	N/A	6 mL (48 mg hylan polymers A & B)	Once
Non-cross-linked	Supartz	Sodium hyaluronate	620–1170	1 week	2.5 mL (25 mg)	3 or 5 depending on indication
	Hyalgan	Sodium hyaluronate	500–730	1 week	2 mL (20 mg)	3 or 5 depending on indication
	Orthovisc	Bacterial fermentation (nonavian)	1000–2900	1 week	2 mL (30 mg)	3 or 4 depending on indication
	Euflexxa	Bacterial fermentation (nonavian)	2400–3600	1 week	2 mL (20 mg)	3

Less Common Agents

Botox

Botulinum Toxin A has recently been used for intra-articular injections into the glenohumeral joint. Intra-articular Botulinum toxin was shown to have reduced pain severity and increased range of motion when compared to placebo and triamcinolone [16, 17]. A retrospective cohort study on the use of Botulinum Toxin A into the SASD suggested that it was equally effective to steroid injection and could be considered in cases where steroids are not tolerated by the patient [18]. More studies on the utilization of Botulinum toxin for the treatment of shoulder pain are required before common use in bedside or office procedures.

Morphine

Supplementing local anesthetic solutions with morphine in intra-articular injection techniques has been shown to be efficacious [19–21]. Patients showed improved visual analog pain scores following intra-articular injections with the addition of 5 mg of morphine to bupivacaine than those patients who received bupivacaine alone [20]. Based on these studies, morphine can be considered as an adjunct to intra-articular formulations used in shoulder injections for postoperative pain control.

Hydrodistention

Although not an injectate, hydrodistention of the glenohumeral joint capsule has been described as an effective technique used to treat frozen shoulder since the 1960s. However, it's use in practice is limited secondary to extreme pain for the patient with the procedure. In one particular study, comparing the efficacy of intra-articular corticosteroid injection versus hydrodistention done under interscalene nerve block, hydrodistention done with 40 mg of triamcinolone, 10 cm^3 of 1% lidocaine, and 30 cm^3 of saline solution, patients had improved range of motion and pain relief at 3 months following the procedure with similar results at 1 year follow up. Hydrodistention may be a useful technique to consider for patients with frozen shoulder [22].

6 The Glenohumeral Joint

Anatomy

The glenohumeral joint, the articulation of the humeral head in the glenoid cavity of the scapula, is commonly referred to as the shoulder joint (Fig. 1). It is a ball-and-socket type of synovial joint and is widened by the glenoid labrum [4]. The joint is stabilized internally by the tendons of the four rotator cuff muscles (supraspinatus, infraspinatus, teres minor, and subscapularis), anteriorly by the glenohumeral ligaments, and superiorly by the coracohumeral ligament. It is further stabilized by the transverse humeral ligament, the coraco-acromial arch, and a fibrous capsule [23]. The lateral pectoral nerve, axillary nerve, suprascapular nerve, and nerve to subscapularis innervate the glenohumeral joint [23–25].

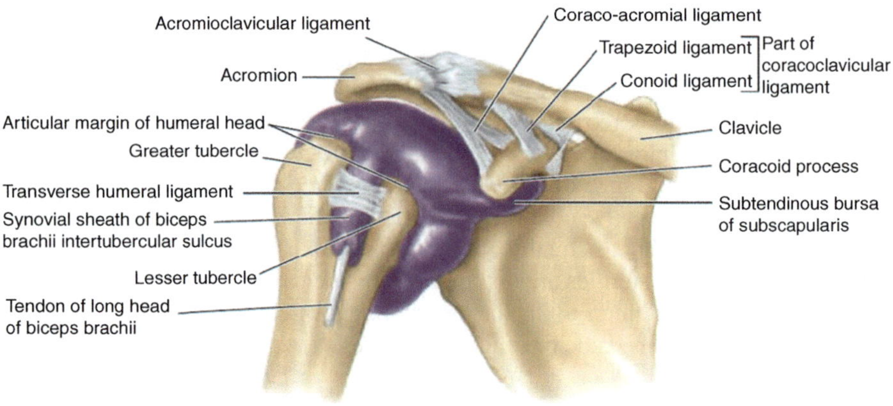

Fig. 1 Articular skeletal anatomy involved in and surrounding the glenohumeral joint. (Image from *Moore, Keith L, Dalley, Arthur and Agur, Anne. Clinically Oriented Anatomy, seventh Edition. Lippincott Williams & Wilkins, 01/21/2013*. Used with permission from Wolvers Kluwer)

Technique & Approach

Injections into and surrounding the glenohumeral joint are commonly employed as part of the non-operative management of shoulder pain. It previously was common to perform these injections in a blind manner using direct palpation and anatomic landmarks. However, there is potentially a high incidence of extra-articular injections. The research on blind needle placement is controversial with accuracy of needle placement between 30 and 85% [26–28]. In a systematic review of ultrasound guidance compared to blind injection, ultrasound demonstrated a significantly greater clinical improvement and greater accuracy [29, 30]. Additionally, fluoroscopy can be employed to verify proper needle placement. Ultrasound is more cost-effective and accessible in comparison to fluoroscopy, and has been increasingly used as it allows for radiation-free, real-time imaging of needle placement. Many studies have demonstrated greater success of ultrasound guidance compared with fluoroscopy on the first attempt [31]. Ultrasound can also be less time consuming [31].

Ultrasound-Guidance

In general regarding any approach, a high-frequency linear probe is used for most patients, however, a convex low-frequency probe can assist with imaging in the obese populations to assess the deeper structures.

Although the anterior approach to the glenohumeral joint is less commonly used, it can be the preferred approach when patients have damage to the posterior joint. Anterior placement theoretically puts therapeutic medication in close proximity to any painful structures such as the biceps or subscapularis muscles, but care should be taken to avoid damage to their tendinous portions. Approach via the anterior shoulder is facilitated with the patient in the seated position and the arm in external rotation at the shoulder and supination. The probe is placed transversely over the anterior joint line inferior to the acromion. The coracoid process (medially) and the head of the humerus on the (laterally) are identified within one image. The needle is passed in-plane, lateral-to-medial, over the humeral head and toward the space bordered by the subscapularis tendon (superior), the head of the humerus (lateral) and the coracoid process (medial) (Fig. 2).

The posterior approach is more commonly utilized due to many advantages: less extravasation, lack of important articular structures, and fewer stabilizing structures [4, 32, 33]. The patient can be positioned in either lateral decubitus or seated positions with easy access to the back. The shoulder is adducted across the anterior body to help facilitate opening of the posterior joint. The ultrasound probe is placed transversely at the lateral edge of the spine of scapula. Identification of the humeral head, posterior glenoid, and posterior labrum will help identify the needle path. The needle is inserted in-plane, lateral-to-medial and traverses the deltoid and infraspinatus. The end point is a hypoechoic triangular-like space medial to the humeral head and lateral to the labrum (Fig. 3).

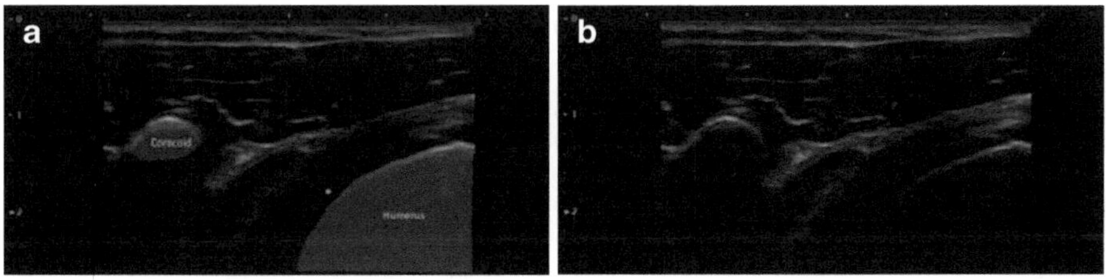

Fig. 2 (**a**) Anterior approach demonstrating osseous and muscular structures appreciated in the ultrasound image on the approach to the glenohumeral joint. (**b**) Standalone ultrasound image of the anterior approach of the glenohumeral joint

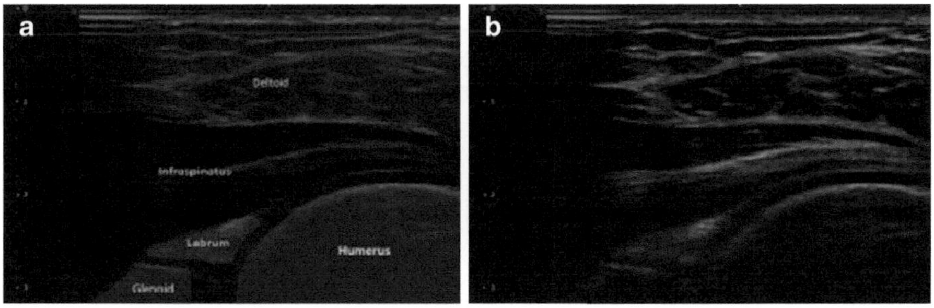

Fig. 3 (**a**) Osseous and muscular structures appreciated in the ultrasound image in the posterior approach to the glenohumeral joint. (**b**) Standalone ultrasound image of the posterior approach to the glenohumeral joint

7 The Acromioclavicular Joint

Anatomy

The acromioclavicular joint is comprised of the lateral articulation of the clavicle, the medial articulation of the acromion, and a central disc. It is a plane type synovial joint that is stabilized horizontally by the acromioclavicular and coraco-acromial ligaments and vertically by the conoid and trapezoid ligaments, which are known together as the coracoclavicular ligaments [34]. The innervation of the joint is comprised of the lateral pectoral nerve, axillary nerve, suprascapular nerve, and the cutaneous lateral supraclavicular nerve [23] (Fig. 4).

Technique & Approach

Similar to glenohumeral joint injections, several studies have shown that the blind technique for AC joint injection is inferior to image-guided techniques [35–39]. One mechanism that has been suggested for the difference in palpation versus image-guided techniques is the relatively small space of the joint and the variation of the anatomy amongst individuals. On average the rates of inaccuracy for successful blind intra-articular ACJ was between 40 and 70% in comparison with a near 100% success rate for both fluoroscopy and ultrasound guided techniques in the studies mentioned above. Additionally, ultrasound has several advantages to fluoroscopy-guided injection in that it offers continuous real-time needle guidance

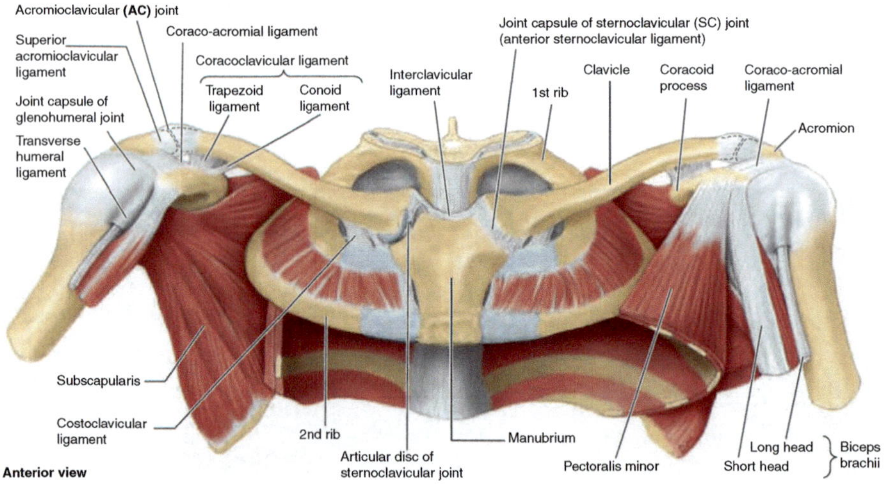

Fig. 4 Anatomy of articulation of the pectoral girdle and upper extremity. Note the acromioclavicular joint and ligaments involved in the stability of the AC joint. (Image from *Moore, Keith L, Dalley, Arthur and Agur, Anne. Clinically Oriented Anatomy, seventh Edition. Lippincott Williams & Wilkins, 01/21/2013*. Used with permission from Wolvers Kluwer)

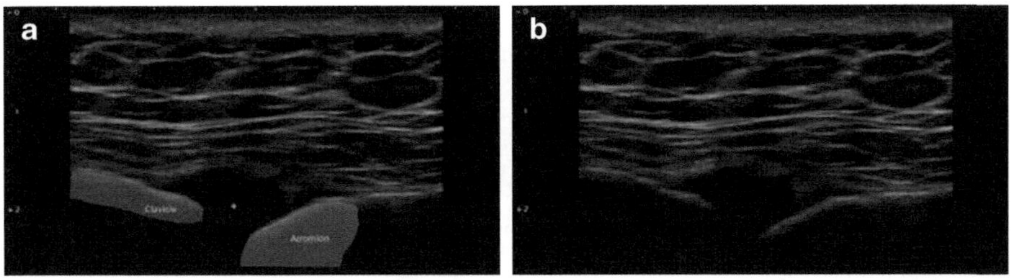

Fig. 5 (**a**) Osseous structures appreciated in the ultrasound image in the approach to the AC joint. (**b**) Standalone ultrasound image of AC joint

and is more practical, cost-effective, and safe for patients in terms of radiation exposure [38].

Intra-articular ACJ injection can be performed via an anterior or lateral approach. Due to the superficial nature of the joint, the anterior approach is preferred over the lateral technique. Yet, in many of the image-guided technique studies, a lateral approach was used due to ease in either placing an ultrasound probe or assessing appropriate needle trajectory under fluoroscopy.

The patient can be either supine or upright with the arm in a neutral anatomical position in order to provide the largest access to the AC joint. A high frequency ultrasound probe is placed in a transverse fashion along the coronal plane with the acromion placed laterally and the clavicle found medially. A small 22G–25G needle is advanced from a superior and anterior approach in an inferior fashion at about 30 degrees until the tip of the needle is visualized between the acromion and clavicle, with care to not infiltrate the underlying subacromial space. Although both out-of-plane and in-plane techniques have been used, the out-of plane technique offers the advantage of approaching the relatively small and superficial joint more easily [11, 40] (Fig. 5).

The needle tip, if placed appropriately, can be confirmed in the AC joint by rotating the ultrasound probe 90 degrees into an in-plane view. In this image, the needle trajectory into the joint can be visualized to confirm appropriate injectate distribution [41].

8 The Subacromial/Subdeltoid Bursa

Anatomy

The SASDB, the largest bursa in the body, is a potential synovial space that separates the deltoid muscle, acromion, and coracoacromial ligament from the supraspinatus tendon. It extends anteriorly covering the bicipital groove, laterally toward the greater tuberosity, and medially to the coracoid process [11]. The bursa serves to reduce friction and wear on the supraspinatus tendon from the humeral head and the acromion during shoulder movement [42]. In a healthy patient, the SASDB is about 1 mm thick and can only be visualized with ultrasound by the hyperechoic peribursal fat lining between the deltoid muscle and supraspinatus tendon [42, 43] (Fig. 6).

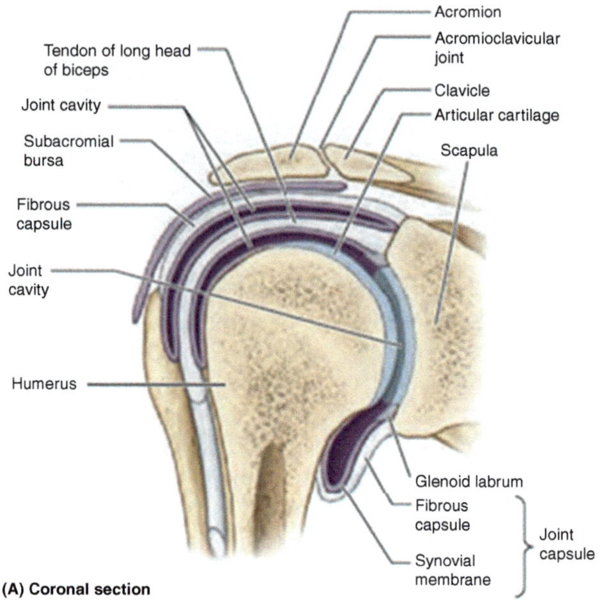

Fig. 6 Coronal section of the shoulder. Note the subacromial (subdeltoid) bursa superior to the glenohumeral joint. (Image from *Moore, Keith L, Dalley, Arthur and Agur, Anne. Clinically Oriented Anatomy, seventh Edition. Lippincott Williams & Wilkins, 01/21/2013*. Used with permission from Wolvers Kluwer)

Technique & Approach

In contrast to GHJ and ACJ injections, the superiority of ultrasound over landmark techniques for SASDB injection in terms of accuracy and efficacy to the patient, is debatable [30]. A Cochrane Review done in 2012 regarding the efficacy of image guided versus landmark techniques found that patients experienced no difference in functional or pain scores between both techniques [44]. In contrast, a more recent systematic review and meta-analysis in 2015 reported that patients do have improved pain and functional scores with ultrasound-guided techniques in comparison to landmark techniques [45]. However, when short and long-term outcomes were compared, a 2018 study discovered that although patients may have short-term improvement in scores with ultrasound, there was no difference in long-term outcomes [46]. Regardless of the patient-relevant efficacy of SASDB injections, in certain cases, such as difficulty with palpation or abnormal anatomy, ultrasound-guided techniques should be considered over landmark techniques [47]. Both landmark and ultrasound-guided techniques will be described here. The use of one over the other should be guided by provider comfort and preference, patient anatomy, history of a previously failed injection, and specific area of pathology within the bursa.

Blind Techniques

Anterior, lateral, and posterior approaches are used in landmark techniques for SASDB injections. For bursitis, the anterior and lateral approaches have some evidence for improved accuracy compared to the posterior approach, with the posterior approach being particularly inaccurate among women [48]. In the treatment of impingement syndrome, all three approaches had similar efficacy [49–51].

In the landmark-based anterior approach, the patient's arm is held in 0 degrees abduction and 20 degrees external rotation. The inferior and anterior edge of the acromion should be palpated with the needle entry point being 1 cm inferior to the clavicle. The needle should be advanced in a posterior, cephalad, and slightly lateral direction until a drop in pressure is felt during needle insertion.

The landmark-based lateral approach is best done with the patient seated and the arm distracted by gravity. After palpation of the mid to lateral aspect of the acromion, the needle is inserted slightly inferior to this point and advanced slightly cephalad until a drop in pressure is felt.

Lastly, the landmark-based posterior approach to SASDB injection is performed with the patient seated and the arm distracted by gravity. The needle should be inserted 1 cm inferior and medial to the palpable posterolateral corner of the acromion. The trajectory of needle insertion should be in an anterior, cephalad, and slightly lateral direction until a drop in pressure is felt, indicating insertion into the SASDB.

It should be noted that in the posterior approach, the distance that the needle must traverse to access the SASDB is significantly greater than the anterior or lateral approach, an average of 5.2 cm versus 2.9 cm respectively [52]. As such, it is recommended to use a needle that is at least 6 cm in length when using the posterior approach.

Ultrasound Techniques

The SASDB is most commonly performed via lateral or anterior approaches [53]. Using ultrasound guidance, no single approach has been shown to have improved accuracy [43].

Irrespective of the approach, the patient is placed in a modified Crass position with the ipsilateral arm extended posteriorly and the palmar surface of the hand on the superior aspect of the iliac wing or buttock [42, 43]. The patient can be in either a lateral decubitus or seated position.

The most common approach under ultrasound guidance is the lateral approach. The ultrasound probe is placed along the long axis of the supraspinatus tendon in the anatomic coronal plane at the proximal end of the humerus. The needle is then advanced in-plane inferior to superior with a cephalad tilt to the bursa found between the deltoid and the supraspinatus muscles [4, 42] (Fig. 7).

In the less commonly used anterior approach, the ultrasound probe is placed in a transverse or axial plane across the short axis of the supraspinatus tendon. The needle is then inserted in the lateral to medial direction into the bursa.

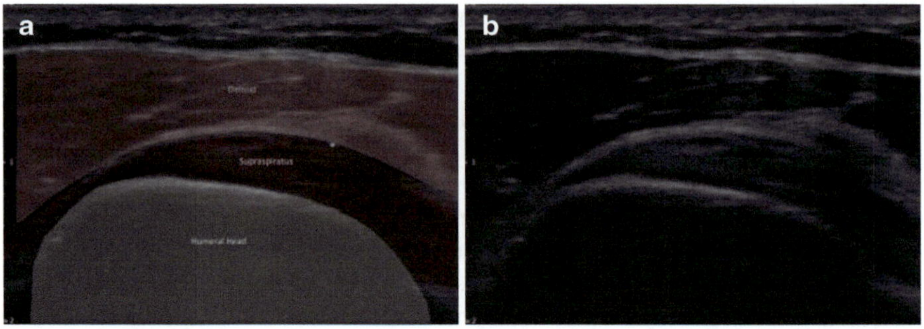

Fig. 7 (**a**) Osseous and muscular structures appreciated in the ultrasound image in the lateral approach to the subacromial/subdeltoid bursa. Note the Bursa is appreciated between the deltoid and supraspinatus muscle. (**b**) Standalone ultrasound image of the lateral approach to the subacromial/subdeltoid bursa

9 Potential Complications and Adverse Effects

Complications include risk of infection, hemarthrosis, and damage to tends, intraarticular structures, and nerves.

10 Conclusion

Bedside shoulder joint injections are useful, cost-effective, and safe treatment modalities in the diagnosis and management of shoulder pain. The increasing accessibility to ultrasound warrants practitioners to be skilled at understanding the various approaches and techniques to shoulder joint injections. Blind and fluoroscopically guided techniques continue to be relevant in trained hands. The vast majority of providers rely on the general use of corticosteroids for their injections, however PRP and viscosupplementation are contemporary options. Continued research is still necessary in order to elucidate best practices in preferred injectate, technique, and patient selection.

Clinical Pearls

- The complexity of the shoulder joint allows for various injections that can be employed depending on the underlying pathology.
- All joints can be accessed with ultrasound guidance which can provide superior results in most cases.
- The posterior approach to the glenohumeral joint is the safest and most utilized.
- The most common injectate used is corticosteroids, however, platelet rich plasma is becoming more commonly used.
- Absolute contraindications to access of the glenohumeral joint include malignancy, bleeding diathesis, fracture, and allergy to the injectate.
- Risk factors include infection, hemarthrosis, damage to tendons, intraarticular structures and nerves.

References

1. Luime JJ, Koes BW, Hendriksen IJ, Burdorf A, Verhagen AP, Miedema HS, et al. Prevalence and incidence of shoulder pain in the general population; a systematic review. Scand J Rheumatol. 2004;33(2):73–81.
2. Urwin M, Symmons D, Allison T, Brammah T, Busby H, Roxby M, et al. Estimating the burden of musculoskeletal disorders in the community: the comparative prevalence of symptoms at different anatomical sites, and the relation to social deprivation. Ann Rheum Dis. 1998;57(11):649–55.
3. Van der Windt DA, Koes BW, de Jong BA, Bouter LM. Shoulder disorders in general practice: incidence, patient characteristics, and management. Ann Rheum Dis. 1995;54(12):959–64.
4. Benzon H, Raja SN, Fishman SM, Liu SS, Cohen SP, Hurley RW. Ultrasound-guided musculoskeletal injections: shoulder, hip, and knee essentials of pain medicine. 4th ed. Philadelphia, PA: Elsevier Health Sciences; 2018. p. 749–62.
5. Buchbinder R, Green S, Youd JM. Corticosteroid injections for shoulder pain. Cochrane Database Syst Rev. 2003;2003(1):Cd004016.
6. Caldwell JR. Intra-articular corticosteroids. Guide to selection and indications for use. Drugs. 1996;52(4):507–14.
7. Tagliafico A, Russo G, Boccalini S, Michaud J, Klauser A, Serafini G, et al. Ultrasound-guided interventional procedures around the shoulder. Radiol Med. 2014;119(5):318–26.
8. Gross C, Dhawan A, Harwood D, Gochanour E, Romeo A. Glenohumeral joint injections: a review. Sports Health. 2013;5(2):153–9.
9. Abate M, Pulcini D, Di Iorio A, Schiavone C. Viscosupplementation with intra-articular hyaluronic acid for treatment of osteoarthritis in the elderly. Curr Pharm Des. 2010;16(6):631–40.
10. Gigante A, Callegari L. The role of intra-articular hyaluronan (Sinovial) in the treatment of osteoarthritis. Rheumatol Int. 2011;31(4):427–44.
11. Benzon HT. Practical management of pain. [electronic resource]. 5th ed. Amsterdam: Elsevier/Saunders; 2014.
12. Schneider A, Burr R, Garbis N, Salazar D. Platelet-rich plasma and the shoulder: clinical indications and outcomes. Curr Rev Musculoskelet Med. 2018;11(4):593–7.
13. Shams A, El-Sayed M, Gamal O, Ewes W. Subacromial injection of autologous platelet-rich plasma versus corticosteroid for the treatment of symptomatic partial rotator cuff tears. Eur J Orthop Surg Traumatol. 2016;26(8):837–42.
14. Zhang JY, Fabricant PD, Ishmael CR, Wang JC, Petrigliano FA, Jones KJ. Utilization of platelet-rich plasma for musculoskeletal injuries: an analysis of current treatment trends in the United States. Orthop J Sports Med. 2016;4(12):2325967116676241.
15. Hussain N, Johal H, Bhandari M. An evidence-based evaluation on the use of platelet rich plasma in orthopedics—a review of the literature. SICOT J. 2017;3:57.
16. Singh JA, Fitzgerald PM. Botulinum toxin for shoulder pain. Cochrane Database Syst Rev. 2010;9:Cd008271.
17. Hashemi S, Khamene S, Nabi BM, M G. Effects of ultrasound-guided intraarticular botox vs. corticosteroids for shoulder osteoarthritis. Anaesth Pain Intensive Care. 2018;22(3):355–60.
18. Wu T, Song HX, Li YZ, Ye Y, Li JH, Hu XY. Clinical effectiveness of ultrasound guided subacromial-subdeltoid bursa injection of botulinum toxin type A in hemiplegic shoulder pain: A retrospective cohort study. Medicine (Baltimore). 2019;98(45):e17933.
19. Joshi GP, McCarroll SM. Intra-articular morphine for the management of frozen shoulder. Anaesthesia. 1992;47(7):627.
20. Seyam S, Elsheshtawy K, Abdelmaboud M. Effects of adding morphine to intra-articular dexamethasone injection on postoperative pain after arthroscopic subacromial decompression shoulder surgery. Al-Azhar Assiut Med J. 2019;17(4):398–403.
21. Tetzlaff JE, Brems J, Dilger J. Intraarticular morphine and bupivacaine reduces postoperative pain after rotator cuff repair. Reg Anesth Pain Med. 2000;25(6):611–4.
22. Buchbinder R, Green S, Forbes A, Hall S, Lawler G. Arthrographic joint distension with saline and steroid improves function and reduces pain in patients with painful stiff shoulder: results of a randomised, double blind, placebo controlled trial. Ann Rheum Dis. 2004;63(3):302–9.

23. Moore K, Dalley AF II, Agur AMR. Clinically Oriented Anatomy. 7th ed. Philadelphia: LWW; 2013.
24. Tran J, Peng PWH, Agur AMR. Anatomical study of the innervation of glenohumeral and acromioclavicular joint capsules: implications for image-guided intervention. Reg Anesth Pain Med. 2019:rapm-2018-100152.
25. Eckmann MS, Bickelhaupt B, Fehl J, Benfield JA, Curley J, Rahimi O, et al. Cadaveric study of the articular branches of the shoulder joint. Reg Anesth Pain Med. 2017;42(5):564–70.
26. Andrews JR. Diagnosis and treatment of chronic painful shoulder: review of nonsurgical interventions. Arthroscopy. 2005;21(3):333–47.
27. Sethi PM, Kingston S, Elattrache N. Accuracy of anterior intra-articular injection of the glenohumeral joint. Arthroscopy. 2005;21(1):77–80.
28. Catalano OA, Manfredi R, Vanzulli A, Tomei E, Napolitano M, Esposito A, et al. MR arthrography of the glenohumeral joint: modified posterior approach without imaging guidance. Radiology. 2007;242(2):550–4.
29. Soh E, Li W, Ong KO, Chen W, Bautista D. Image-guided versus blind corticosteroid injections in adults with shoulder pain: a systematic review. BMC Musculoskelet Disord. 2011;12:137.
30. Aly AR, Rajasekaran S, Ashworth N. Ultrasound-guided shoulder girdle injections are more accurate and more effective than landmark-guided injections: a systematic review and meta-analysis. Br J Sports Med. 2015;49(16):1042–9.
31. Rutten MJ, Collins JM, Maresch BJ, Smeets JH, Janssen CM, Kiemeney LA, et al. Glenohumeral joint injection: a comparative study of ultrasound and fluoroscopically guided techniques before MR arthrography. Eur Radiol. 2009;19(3):722–30.
32. Ogul H, Bayraktutan U, Yildirim OS, Suma S, Ozgokce M, Okur A, et al. Magnetic resonance arthrography of the glenohumeral joint: ultrasonography-guided technique using a posterior approach. Eurasian J Med. 2012;44(2):73–8.
33. Chung CB, Dwek JR, Feng S, Resnick D. MR arthrography of the glenohumeral joint: a tailored approach. AJR Am J Roentgenol. 2001;177(1):217–9.
34. Mazzocca AD, Arciero RA, Bicos J. Evaluation and treatment of acromioclavicular joint injuries. Am J Sports Med. 2007;35(2):316–29.
35. Edelson G, Saffuri H, Obid E, Lipovsky E, Ben-David D. Successful injection of the acromioclavicular joint with use of ultrasound: anatomy, technique, and follow-up. J Shoulder Elb Surg. 2014;23(10):e243–50.
36. Pichler W, Weinberg AM, Grechenig S, Tesch NP, Heidari N, Grechenig W. Intra-articular injection of the acromioclavicular joint. J Bone Joint Surg Br. 2009;91(12):1638–40.
37. Peck E, Lai JK, Pawlina W, Smith J. Accuracy of ultrasound-guided versus palpation-guided acromioclavicular joint injections: a cadaveric study. PM R. 2010;2(9):817–21.
38. Javed S, Sadozai Z, Javed A, Din A, Schmitgen G. Should all acromioclavicular joint injections be performed under image guidance? J Orthop Surg (Hong Kong). 2017;25(3):2309499017731633.
39. Bisbinas I, Belthur M, Said HG, Green M, Learmonth DJ. Accuracy of needle placement in ACJ injections. Knee Surg Sports Traumatol Arthrosc. 2006;14(8):762–5.
40. Waldman SD. Atlas of pain management injection techniques. 4th ed. St. Louis, Missouri: Elsevier; 2017.
41. Furman MB, Goodman B, Berkwits L. Atlas of Image-Guided Spinal Procedures. Amsterdam: Elsevier - Health Sciences Division; 2017.
42. Pourcho AM, Colio SW, Hall MM. Ultrasound-guided interventional procedures about the shoulder: anatomy, indications, and techniques. Phys Med Rehabil Clin N Am. 2016;27(3):555–72.
43. Peng PW, Cheng P. Ultrasound-guided interventional procedures in pain medicine: a review of anatomy, sonoanatomy, and procedures. Part III: shoulder. Reg Anesth Pain Med. 2011;36(6):592–605.
44. Bloom JE, Rischin A, Johnston RV, Buchbinder R. Image-guided versus blind glucocorticoid injection for shoulder pain. Cochrane Database Syst Rev. 2012;8:Cd009147.

45. Wu T, Song HX, Dong Y, Li JH. Ultrasound-guided versus blind subacromial-subdeltoid bursa injection in adults with shoulder pain: A systematic review and meta-analysis. Semin Arthritis Rheum. 2015;45(3):374–8.
46. Fawcett R, Grainger A, Robinson P, Jafari M, Rowbotham E. Ultrasound-guided subacromial-subdeltoid bursa corticosteroid injections: a study of short- and long-term outcomes. Clin Radiol. 2018;73(8):760.e7–e12.
47. Rutten MJ, Maresch BJ, Jager GJ, de Waal Malefijt MC. Injection of the subacromial-subdeltoid bursa: blind or ultrasound-guided? Acta Orthop. 2007;78(2):254–7.
48. Marder RA, Kim SH, Labson JD, Hunter JC. Injection of the subacromial bursa in patients with rotator cuff syndrome: a prospective, randomized study comparing the effectiveness of different routes. J Bone Joint Surg Am. 2012;94(16):1442–7.
49. Ramappa A, Walley KC, Herder LM, Iyer S, Zurakowski D, Hall A, et al. Comparison of anterior and posterior cortico-steroid injections for pain relief and functional improvement in shoulder impingement syndrome. Am J Orthop (Belle Mead NJ). 2017;46(4):E257–e62.
50. Kang MN, Rizio L, Prybicien M, Middlemas DA, Blacksin MF. The accuracy of subacromial corticosteroid injections: a comparison of multiple methods. J Shoulder Elb Surg. 2008;17(1 Suppl):61s–6s.
51. Ogbeivor C. Needle placement approach to subacromial injection in patients with subacromial impingement syndrome: A systematic review. Musculoskeletal Care. 2019;17(1):13–22.
52. Sardelli M, Burks RT. Distances to the subacromial bursa from 3 different injection sites as measured arthroscopically. Arthroscopy. 2008;24(9):992–6.
53. Chang KV, Mezian K, Naňka O, Wu WT, Lin CP, Özçakar L. Ultrasound-guided interventions for painful shoulder: from anatomy to evidence. J Pain Res. 2018;11:2311–22.

Further Reading

Schaefer MP, Fox K. Ultrasound-guided shoulder joint and bursa injections. In: Narouze S, editor. Atlas of ultrasound-guided procedures in interventional pain management. New York, NY: Springer; 2018.
Waldman SD. Atlas of pain management injection techniques, Chap. 26: Intraarticular glenohumeral joint injections. St. Louis, MO: Elsevier Health Sciences; 2017.
Baxi N and Spinner DA. (2014). Chapter 2: Shoulder. In: Spinner DA, Kirschner JS, Herrera JE. Atlas of ultrasound guided musculoskeletal injections. Springer, New York, NY.
Lennard TA. Upper extremity joint injections. In: Lennard, et al., editors. Pain procedures in clinical practice. Philadelphia, PA: Elsevier Health Sciences; 2011.

Periarticular Shoulder Injections

Nirmal G. Aras, Michelle Puszynski, Oscar Coppes, and Dalia H. Elmofty

Essential Concepts

- Subacromial bursa injections offer pain relief and increased functional capacity for shoulder discomfort.
- Biceps tendinitis commonly occurs in conjunction with other rotator cuff pathologies; biceps tendon sheath injections can relieve pain and improve functionality associated with biceps tendinitis.
- Rotator cuff tendon injections can provide significant pain relief for various acute and chronic tendinopathies; targets include the supraspinatus, infraspinatus, and subscapularis tendons.
- Acute tendinopathies can be treated with corticosteroid injections.
- Steroids should be avoided in chronic tendinopathies as they can damage the tenocyte.
- Chronic tendinopathies can be treated with platelet-rich plasma (PRP) and glucose prolotherapy.

1 Periarticular Shoulder Pain

Overview

Periarticular shoulder pain can result from subacromial bursitis, biceps tendonitis, and rotator cuff tendinopathies (supraspinatus, infraspinatus, and subscapularis). Subacromial impingement syndrome (SIS) is a common pathology of shoulder pain

N. G. Aras · M. Puszynski · O. Coppes · D. H. Elmofty (✉)
Department of Anesthesia and Critical Care, University of Chicago, Chicago, IL, USA
e-mail: nirmal.aras@uchospitals.edu; michelle.puszynski@uchospitals.edu; ocoppes@bsd.uchicago.edu; delmofty@dacc.uchicago.edu

D. Souza et al. (eds.), *Bedside Pain Management Interventions*,
https://doi.org/10.1007/978-3-031-11188-4_49

in which the tendinous portion of the rotator cuff becomes entrapped between the coracoacromial ligament, antero-inferior portion of the acromion, and the humeral head [1]. SIS commonly occurs in patients with a history of repetitive use of the shoulder involving overhead movements. It clinically presents as pain during elevation of the arm or while lying on the affected side. This pathology can result in debilitating pain and functional loss of movement in the shoulder joint. Common etiologies of SIS include intrinsic (tendinous) factors such as overuse of the shoulder and degenerative tendon disease as well as extrinsic (extra-tendinous) factors such as acromioclavicular joint degeneration and thickening of the coracoacromial ligament [2].

Inflammation associated with rotator cuff tendinosis or partial tears can be treated with injections at the rotator cuff insertion sites. These are different from subacromial injections, which are inserted in the subacromial bursa (SAB). Inflammation associated with rotator cuff pathology is treated by relieving the subacromial bursitis or by diffusion of the corticosteroid through the undersurface of the bursa and onto the underlying rotator cuff tendons.

The two proximal tendons of the biceps brachii muscle can cause pain within the shoulder joint. The long head of the biceps tendon tends to be the common source. Although biceps tendinitis can present as an isolated condition, in up to 90% of cases it occurs in combination with other shoulder issues such as rotator cuff tears [3]. Biceps tendinitis commonly presents in patients who perform repetitive overhead activities or activities that involve heavy lifting or pulling movements. Presenting symptoms include pain (e.g., a deep, throbbing ache in the anterior shoulder), weakness, and a sense of instability within the shoulder joint.

The various injections in rotator cuff tendons are best classified by chronicity and choice of injectate. Corticosteroid injections have been the mainstay injection therapy for a variety of rotator cuff tendinopathies. A meta-analysis of subacromial corticosteroid injections found no significant reduction in pain for rotator cuff tendinosis compared with placebo at 3 months. However, these injections showed a statistically significant reduction in pain compared to placebo at 4 and 8 weeks [4].

Chronic tendinopathy (degenerative rotator cuff pathologies) can be treated with injections at the tendon sheath. Corticosteroids should be avoided as they can be damaging to tenocytes. Alternatives such as platelet-rich plasma (PRP) and glucose prolotherapy have been shown to be beneficial in treating chronic partial thickness tears and degenerative rotator cuff tendinopathy. PRP is a whole blood byproduct with large concentrations of platelets that endure degranulation, triggering various growth factors with restorative properties, including platelet derived growth factor (PDGF), transforming growth factor B collagen, and vascular endothelial growth factor (VEGF). PRP injections in patients with symptomatic partial rotator cuff tears have demonstrated significant decreases in pain scores at 3 months with improved range of motion [5]. In a comparison study of patients with subacromial impingement syndrome (who had not responded to conservative therapy for >3 months) those receiving PRP or steroid (40 mg methylprednisolone) injections had significantly better pain scores following steroid injection versus PRP at 6 weeks and 6 months. Both groups had comparable improvements in range of motion of their shoulder joints [2]. PRP increases the physiological healing process by stimulating a proliferation of various cell types, such as local stem cells and tenocytes; the latter can aid in the repair of tendons [2].

Glucose prolotherapy consists of injecting a 10% glucose solution into the tendon sheath. The injection leads to lysis of cells which leads to an increase in local growth factors and inflammatory cells. This in turn triggers a cascade of additional wound-healing factors that ultimately yields the deposition of collagen and tendon growth [6]. In a randomized, double-blinded clinical trial conducted on 36 patients with supraspinatus tendinopathy, patients were treated with either glucose prolotherapy injections in the supraspinatus tendon sheath or with corticosteroid injections in the subacromial bursa. Glucose prolotherapy was shown to be statistically equivalent to corticosteroid injections when evaluated for the level of pain during overhead activities at 3- and 6-month follow-ups [6].

Indications and Contraindications of Periarticular Shoulder Injections

Subacromial impingement syndrome is characterized by compression of the rotator cuff against the lateral acromion leading to bursitis and cuff inflammation. This clinically manifests as a significant decrease in horizontal abduction and, if left untreated, can result in frozen shoulder. If the clinical symptoms of subacromial impingement syndrome are present without an underlying acute tendon injury, patients may benefit from subacromial bursa corticosteroid injections. In cases of acute tendon injury, including partial thickness tears of the rotator cuff tendons (supraspinatus, infraspinatus, and subscapularis), injections in the rotator cuff tendon sheath can help relieve pain and inflammation. Calcific tendinopathy, a chronic calcium deposition in the tendon, has historically been treated with corticosteroid injections. However, recent studies demonstrate the benefits of ultrasound guided percutaneous irrigation [7]. Table 1 describes the indications and techniques used for commonly performed periarticular shoulder injections. Landmark and ultrasound -guided techniques have been described [8]. Absolute contraindications to these interventions include bacteremia, cellulitis overlying the injection site, and osteomyelitis adjacent to the injection site. Relative contraindications include chronic infections, allergy to injectate, diabetes, and uncontrolled coagulopathies.

Clinical Anatomy

The anatomy of the shoulder consists of the shoulder joint formed by the humerus as it attaches to the scapula as a ball-and-socket joint. Figure 1a, b demonstrates periarticular injection targets in the anterior and lateral aspect of the shoulder girdle. The rotator cuff is a collection of muscles and tendons that surround the *shoulder*, providing support and allowing a wide range of motion. The subscapularis muscle originates from the subscapular fossa of the scapula and inserts into the lesser tubercle of the humerus; it is innervated by the upper and lower subscapular nerves from

Table 1 Periarticular shoulder injections for acute and chronic shoulder tendinopathies

Procedure	Indication	Techniques
Subacromial bursa injection	• Subacromial-subdeltoid bursitis • Rotator cuff impingement • Rotator cuff tendinosis • Adhesive capsulitis	• Landmark technique • Ultrasound-guided technique
Biceps tendon injection	• Biceps tendinitis • Rotator cuff tendinosis with associated biceps tendinitis	• Landmark technique • Ultrasound-guided technique
Supraspinatus tendon injection	• Subacromial impingement syndrome with underlying supraspinatus tendinopathy • Acute/chronic partial thickness tears • Degenerative supraspinatus tendinopathy • Calcific tendonitis	• Landmark technique • Ultrasound-guided technique
Infraspinatus tendon injection	• Subacromial impingement syndrome with underlying infraspinatus tendinopathy • Acute/chronic partial thickness tears • Degenerative infraspinatus tendinopathy • Calcific tendonitis	• Landmark technique • Ultrasound-guided technique
Subscapularis tendon injection	• Subacromial impingement syndrome with underlying subscapularis tendinopathy • Acute/chronic partial thickness tears • Degenerative infraspinatus tendinopathy • Calcific tendonitis	• Landmark technique • Ultrasound-guided technique

C5, 6, and 7. It medially rotates the arm and stabilizes the shoulder joint. The supraspinatus muscle originates from the supraspinous fossa of the scapula and inserts onto the greater tubercle of the humerus on the anterior aspect. It is innervated by the suprascapular nerve. It initiates abduction of the shoulder and stabilizes the shoulder joint. The infraspinatus muscle originates from the infraspinous fossa of the scapula and inserts into the greater tubercle of the humerus on the posterior aspect. It is innervated by the suprascapular nerve and laterally rotates and adducts the arm at the shoulder joint.

The subacromial bursa (SAB) has three distinct portions: subacromial, subdeltoid, and subcoracoid. Some texts refer to the bursa as the subacromial-subdeltoid (SA-SD) bursa. A limited number of studies have confirmed that the subacromial and subdeltoid bursa are two communicating yet distinct bursa [9, 10].

The SAB is circular-shaped and lies beneath several structures, including the acromion, coracoacromial ligament, deltoid muscle, and subdeltoid fascia (Fig. 1). The superficial roof layer of the bursa is adherent to the subdeltoid fascia and together they attach to the edge of the acromion. The bursal roof encircles the coracoacromial ligament. The bursa expands laterally and attaches to the greater tubercle and medially expands into the supraspinous fossa [11]. The SAB floor is firmly adherent to the supraspinatus tendon. The bursa serves as a gliding mechanism between the rotator cuff and the coracoacromial arch. The innervation of the SAB arises from the brachial plexus and an extensive network of free nerve endings, including both myelinated and unmyelinated fibers. As the upper trunk of the brachial plexus divides, the suprascapular nerve continues to split into various terminal

Fig. 1 Periarticular targets for shoulder injections: (**a**) anterior targets include the biceps tendon and the subscapularis tendon, (**b**) lateral targets include the subacromial bursa, supraspinatus, and infraspinatus tendons

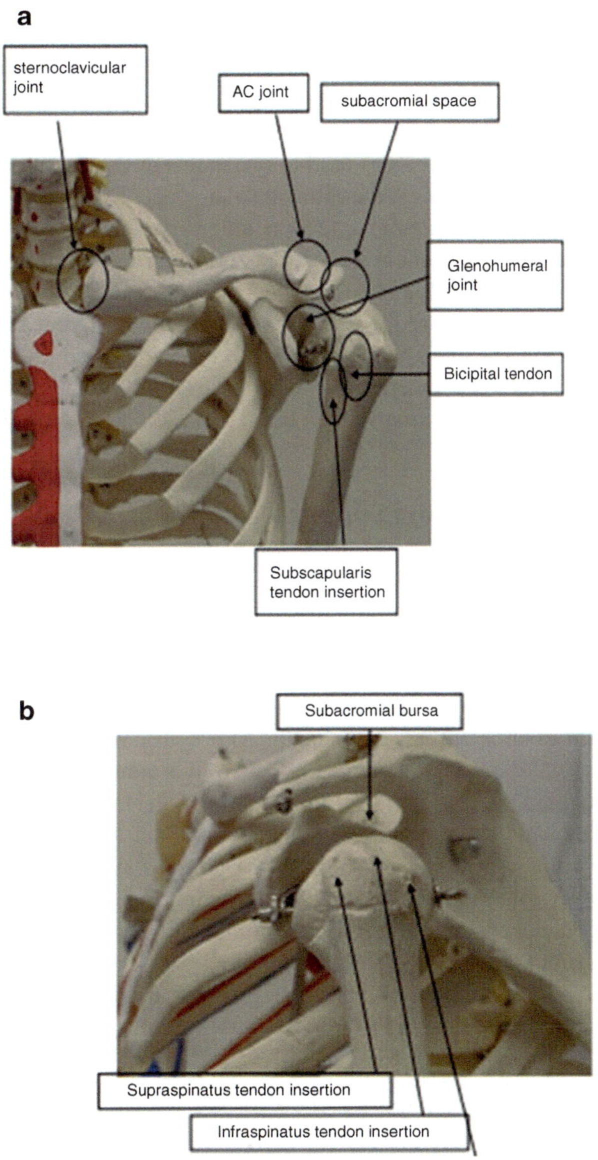

branches that supply the superior portion of SAB. In addition, branches of the lateral pectoral nerve supply both the superior and anterior portions of the SAB. The lateral portion of the SAB is supplied by a small branch of the axillary nerve deriving from the posterior cord of the brachial plexus. It has been suggested that because the SAB has such an extensive sensory nerve supply, the bursa is involved in proprioception, neuromuscular coordination, and nociception of the shoulder. Studies have identified mechanoreceptors within the SAB, including Ruffini endings, Pacinian, and Golgi-Mazzini corpuscles. Proprioception information from these mechanoreceptors "feed into the reflex arc of the suprascapular and axillary nerves, thereby helping protect the shoulder joint from damage resulting from excess movement, compression, or impingement" [11]. The blood supply for the SAB is derived from branches of the thoracoacromial and suprascapular arteries.

The biceps brachii muscle has two proximal tendons: long head and short head. The long-head biceps tendon originates at the supraglenoid tubercle of the scapula and travels through the intracapsular space. Borders of the intracapsular space are as follows: subscapularis tendon anteriorly, supraspinatus tendon posteriorly, coracoacromial ligament superiorly, and superior glenohumeral ligament inferiorly. The long-head tendon then courses along the humeral head into the bicipital groove where it is secured by the transverse humeral ligament and surrounded by the bicep tendon sheath. The short-head tendon of biceps brachii is attached to the coracoid process. The biceps brachii muscle is supplied by the musculocutaneous nerve (C5–6) and vascularly by a branch of the anterior circumflex humeral artery.

Equipment and Supplies

Periarticular shoulder injections are easily performed at the bedside. A list of equipment and supplies are listed in Table 2. Typically, a 5–10 mL syringe with a 25-gauge, 1.5-in. needle is utilized to perform the injection. For corticosteroid injections, 5–7 mL of 1% lidocaine, 0.25–0.5% bupivacaine, or 0.2–0.5% ropivacaine, with the addition of 1–2 mL methylprednisolone (40 mg/mL), is injected at the rotator cuff tendon sheath. Although lidocaine and bupivacaine are commonly used, some studies have shown ropivacaine to be less chondrotoxic than bupivacaine [3, 12, 13]. In addition to classic injections with steroids and/or local anesthetics, multiple regenerative injection therapies exist, including PRP, glucose prolotherapy, and stem cells [3]. Using the syringe and needle as described above, a PRP injection can be done at the same rotator cuff targets. PRP is a preparation of platelet concentrate, cryoprecipitate of fibrinogen, and thrombin that can be obtained from the hospital's transfusion medicine service or prepared using disposable kits. Approximately 2–3 mL of PRP is mixed with 1–2 mL of 10% calcium gluconate solution that is used to activate the PRP solution immediately prior to injection. PRP

Table 2 Required supplies for periarticular shoulder injections

Syringe	5–10 mL
Needle	22–25 gauge, 1.5 in.
Anesthetic	5 or 7 mL of 1% lidocaine 0.25–0.5% bupivacaine 0.2–0.5% ropivacaine
Corticosteroid	1–2 mL betamethasone sodium phosphate and acetate 1–2 mL methylprednisolone, 40 mg/mL
Platelet-rich plasma	2–3 mL of PRP injected at the rotator cuff tear site 1–2 mL of 10% calcium gluconate solution
Glucose prolotherapy	1 mL of 50% glucose (25 g/50 mL solution) 1 mL of 1% lidocaine

is commonly injected at the rotator cuff tendon tear site. Glucose prolotherapy injections require 1 mL of 50% glucose (25 g/50 mL solution) mixed with 1 mL of 1% lidocaine, which creates a 25% glucose prolotherapy solution.

Subacromial Bursitis, Landmark Technique

The patient is placed in a seated position with the arm flexed at the elbow and the hand resting on the thigh. The spine of the scapula is located and is followed laterally as it becomes the acromion process. Once the posterolateral corner of the acromion process is identified, the space approximately 2 cm below this location is the insertion site (Fig. 2). After the location is marked, the needle should be directed

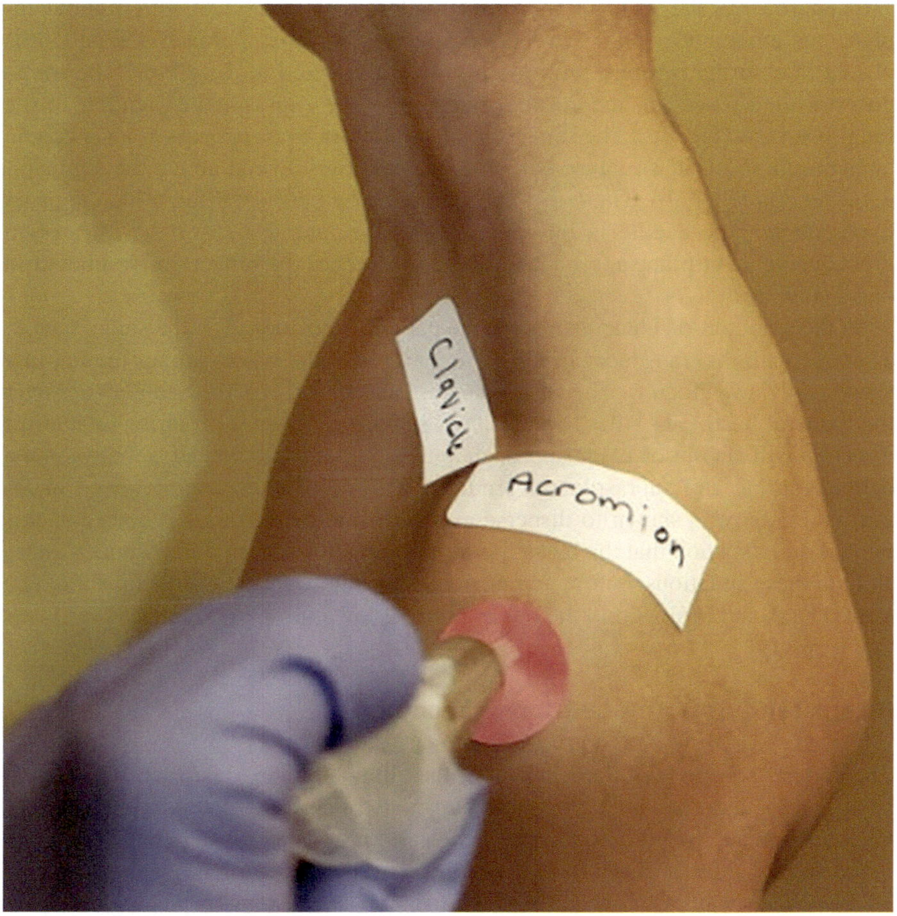

Fig. 2 Landmark technique for subacromial bursa injection: needle is inserted on the lateral aspect of the shoulder approximately 2 cm below the posterolateral corner of the acromion

medially, anteriorly, and slightly superior toward the underside of the midpoint of the acromion and advanced to a depth of approximately 3–4 cm. Aspirate to ensure the needle is not intravascular. The injectate should go in freely; if there is any resistance, withdraw and readjust.

A randomized, double-blind clinical trial assessed the effectiveness of ultrasound-guided versus blind approach subacromial steroid injections to determine improvement in pain and function for subacromial impingement syndrome. Both groups showed decreased pain and increased function 6 weeks after the injection. There was no significant difference in pain or functional scores between the two groups, suggesting high accuracy of blind injections [6, 12].

Subacromial Bursitis, Ultrasound Technique

Two approaches are used in the ultrasound-guided technique: longitudinal in-plane and axial out-of-plane. In the longitudinal in-plane approach, the patient is placed in a sitting position with the arm slightly flexed at the elbow. The transducer is then placed in the coronal plane with the supraspinatus tendon in the long-axis view (Fig. 3a). The subacromial-subdeltoid bursa appears as an anechoic or hypoechoic linear structure below the deltoid muscle and above the supraspinatus tendon (Fig. 3b). The bursa is surrounded by peribursal fat, which appears hyperechoic. The needle is introduced from the lateral side of the ultrasound probe, using an in-plane approach until the tip reaches the subacromial-subdeltoid bursa (Fig. 3c).

In the axial out-of-plane approach, the patient is positioned in the same manner as above with the transducer in the axial plane with the supraspinatus tendon in a short-axis view (Fig. 4a). The supraspinatus muscle and tendon create an arc over the humeral head (Fig. 4b). The needle is introduced from a posterior to anterior direction with an out-of-plane approach until the tip reaches the bursa, between the deltoid muscle and supraspinatus tendon (Fig. 4c). The injectate, viewed under ultrasonography, is shown to disperse evenly within the bursa. If it does not, this may be an indication that the bursa has multi-compartments caused by bursal adhesion. In these situations, before administering the injectate, the needle tip should be moved back and forth within the bursa to break down the adhesions.

Biceps Tendinopathy, Landmark Technique

The patient is seated with arm flexed at the elbow and the hand is in a supinated position. The long-head biceps tendon is palpated inferior to the anterior corner of the acromion and found between the greater and lesser tuberosities of the humerus, in the bicipital groove (Fig. 5). The upper portion of the tendon is enveloped by the tenosynovial sheath. Confirmation of this location can be done by placing fingers in the area and externally and internally rotating the patient's arm; when flexed at 90°, a thick cord will be palpated and, in biceps tendinitis, this area will be exceedingly

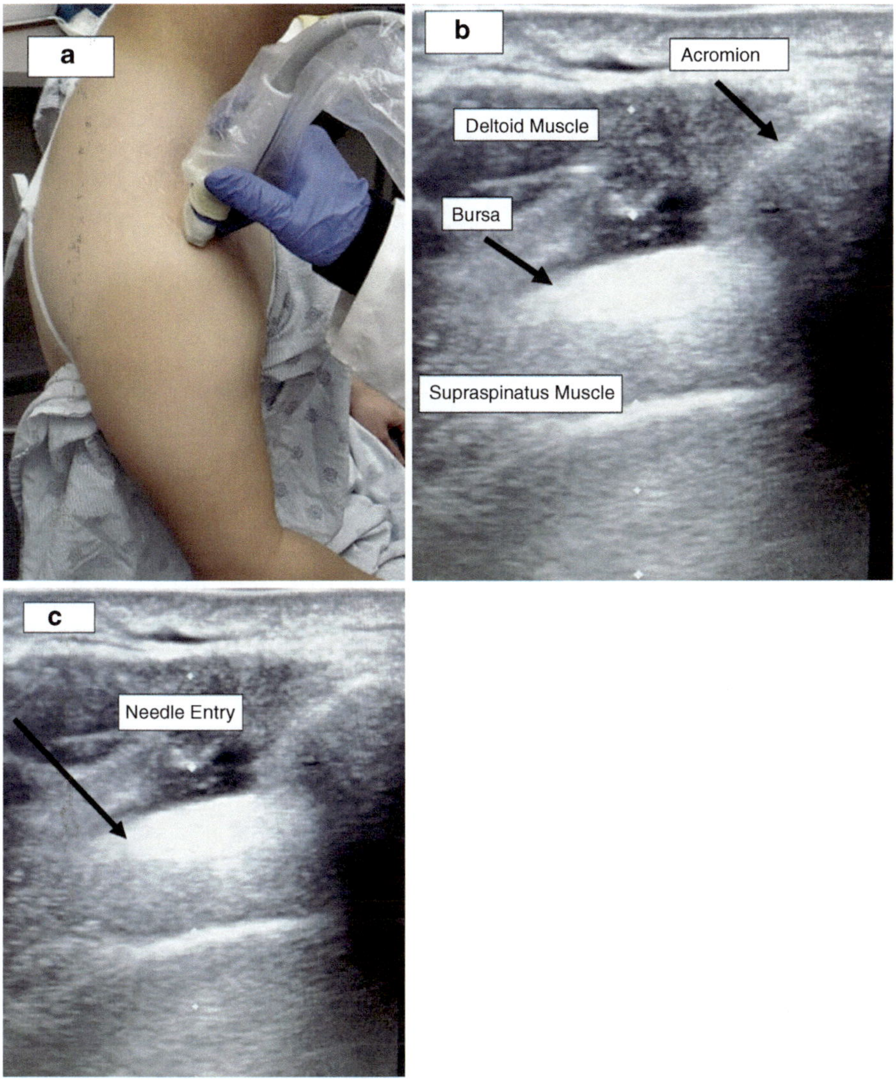

Fig. 3 Longitudinal view of the subacromial/subdeltoid bursa: (**a**) patient is placed in a sitting position with arm flexed at the elbow. The ultrasound probe is placed in long-axis view and the acromion process is visualized cephalad, (**b**) sonoanatomy of the subacromial/subdeltoid bursa, (**c**) needle entry in an in-plane approach with endpoint between deltoid muscle (superior) and supraspinatus (inferior)

tender. Once the area of maximum tenderness is identified, an area slightly distal to this area is marked. When the site is prepped sterile, insert the needle at an angle of 30–45° and advanced from caudal to cranial to a depth of about 3–4 cm (Fig. 5). Aspirate and inject under slight resistance. If there is substantial resistance to the injection, withdraw slightly to avoid intra-tendon injection.

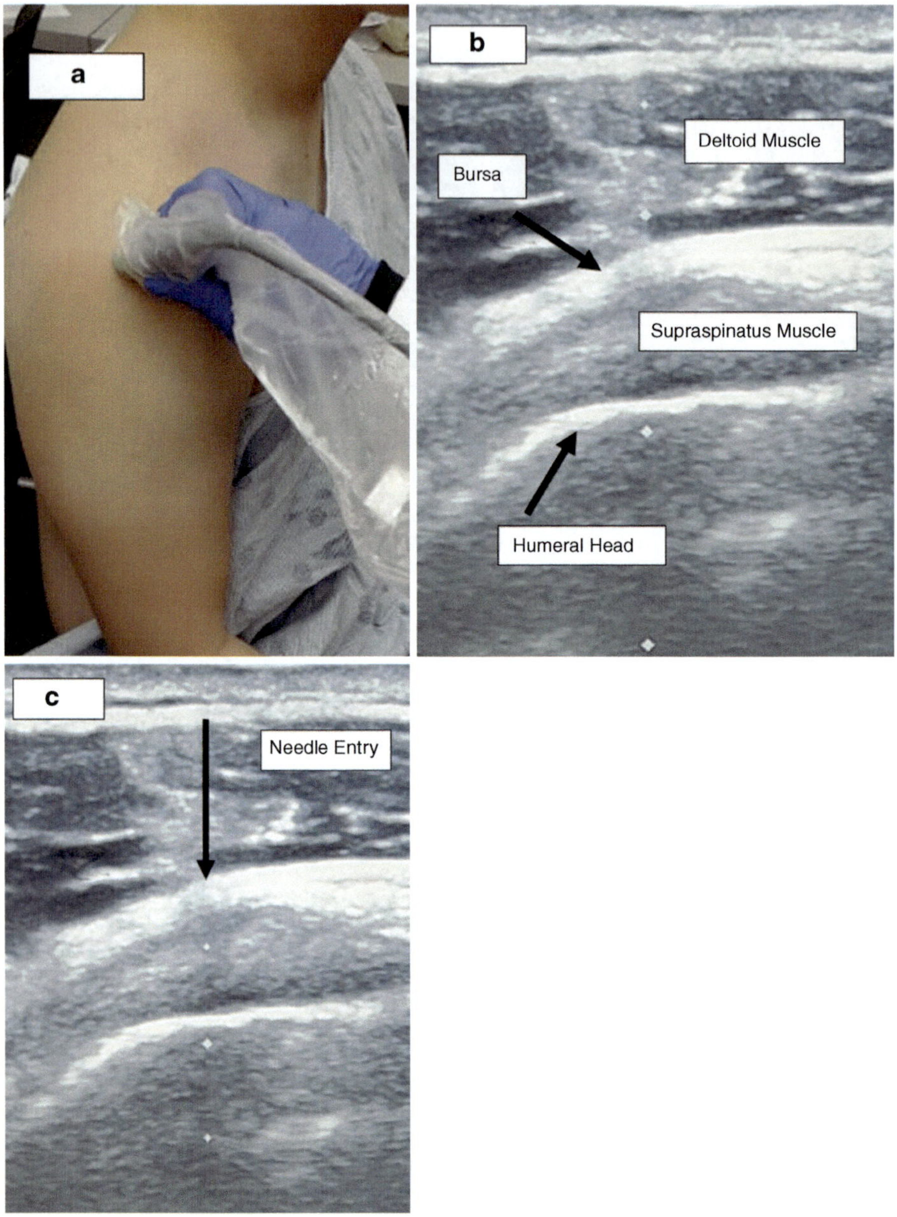

Fig. 4 Axial view of subacromial/subdeltoid bursa: (**a**) patient is placed in a sitting position with arm flexed at the elbow. The ultrasound probe is placed in a short-axis view and the humeral head is visualized inferior, (**b**) sonoanatomy of the subacromial/subdeltoid bursa, (**c**) needle entry in an out-of-plane approach with endpoint between deltoid muscle (superior) and supraspinatus (inferior)

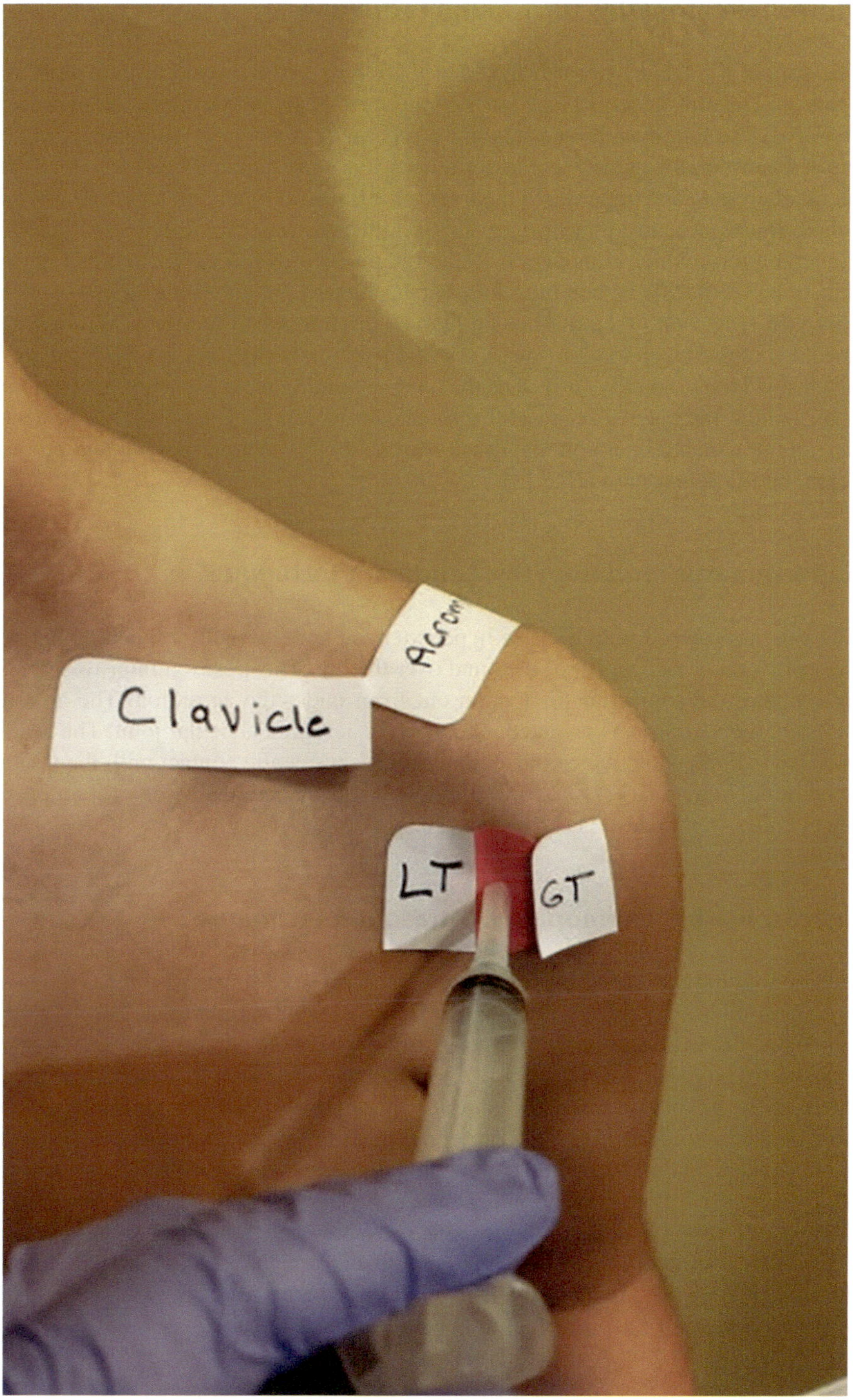

Fig. 5 Landmark technique for long head of biceps tendon injection: *GT* greater tuberosity, *LT* lesser tuberosity

Biceps Tendinopathy, Ultrasound Technique

The patient is seated with arm flexed at the elbow and the hand is in a supinated position. The transducer is placed in the transverse plane below the coracoid process (Fig. 6a). The long-head biceps tendon is seen in the short axis. The tendon will be viewed between the greater and lesser tuberosity of the humeral head, known as the bicipital groove, and underneath the transverse humeral ligament, which is a hyperechoic linear structure that bridges the two tuberosities (Fig. 6b). The circumflex humeral artery, which runs lateral to the bicipital groove, must be avoided during injection. The needle is then introduced at an angle of 30–45° using an out-of-plane approach (Fig. 6c). Once the needle pierces the transverse humeral ligament, the needle is in the bicep tendon sheath and the solution is injected. As the injectate is given slowly, it gradually surrounds the tendon creating what is termed a "doughnut sign," which indicates a successful intra-sheath injection. There is some evidence that an intra-sheath injection may track back to the glenohumeral joint and provide some intra-articular pain relief [3].

Supraspinatus Tendinopathy, Landmark Technique

The patient is seated with the arm hyperextended and internally rotated by placing the ipsilateral dorsal aspect of the hand over the hip. This position improves access by bringing the supraspinatus tendon out from under the acromion. The anterior aspect of the acromion is palpated, lateral to the acromioclavicular joint. The needle is advanced perpendicular to the skin until it makes gentle contact with the periosteum of the humerus (Fig. 7a, b). Withdraw the needle less than 1 cm, aspirate, and inject under slight resistance.

Supraspinatus Tendinopathy, Ultrasound Technique

Ultrasonography of the supraspinatus tendon in both the short and long axis allows for increased accuracy in needle approach toward the desired target. For the short-axis view, the patient is seated with the arm hyperextended and internally rotated by placing the ipsilateral dorsal aspect of the hand over the hip. Placing the transducer in the axial plane over the anterior shoulder affords maximum view of the supraspinatus tendon (Fig. 8a). The corresponding ultrasound image reveals the supraspinatus tendon over the hyperechoic humeral head (Fig. 8b). To ensure complete evaluation of the supraspinatus tendon, sweeping the transducer distally will allow a full view of the supraspinatus as it passes over the facets and terminates. Once the tear or area of tendinopathy is in view, place the needle perpendicular to the skin, and advance in an in-plane approach until the needle tip is seen at the site of the tendon injury; aspirate and inject under slight resistance (Fig. 8c).

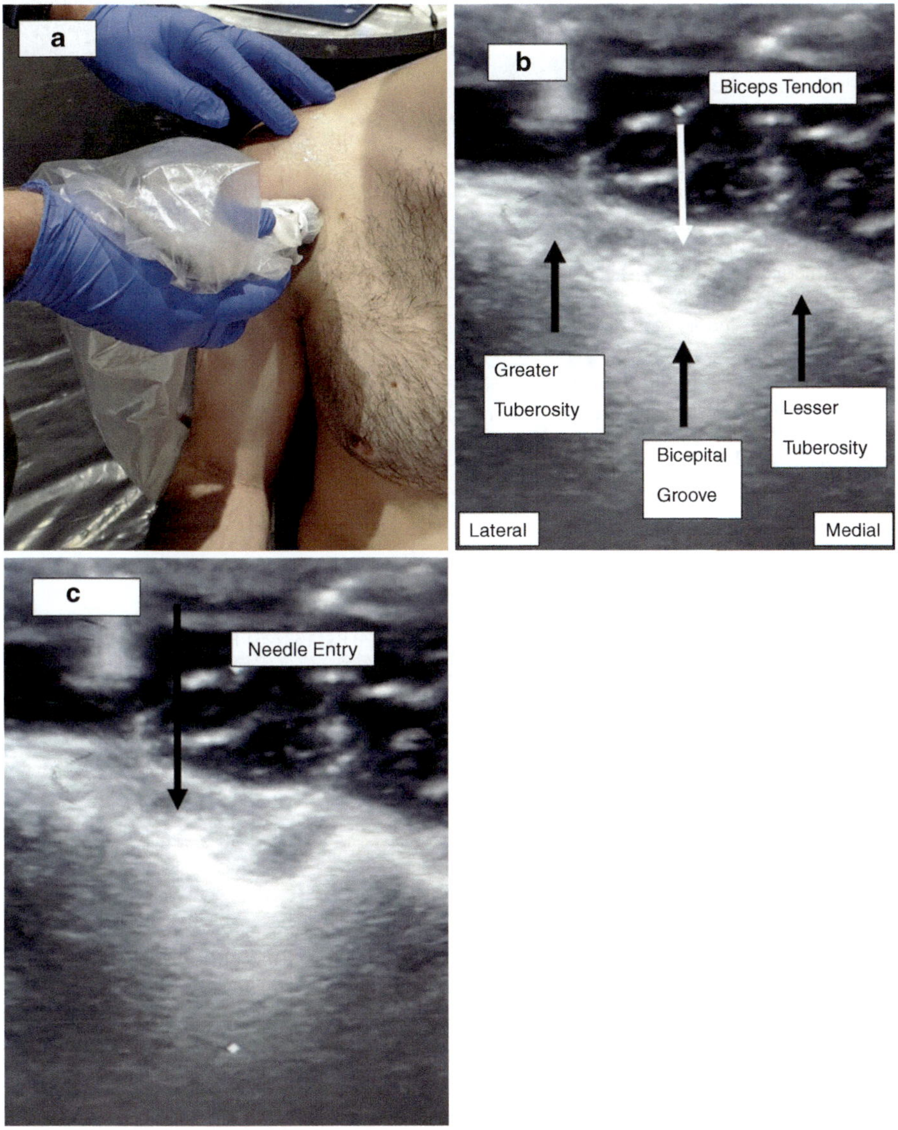

Fig. 6 Axial view long head of biceps tendon: (**a**) patient is placed in sitting position with the elbow flexed and hand supinated. The ultrasound probe is placed in an axial view at the level of the bicipital grove, (**b**) sonoanatomy of the long head of the biceps tendon, (**c**) needle entry in an out-of-plane approach

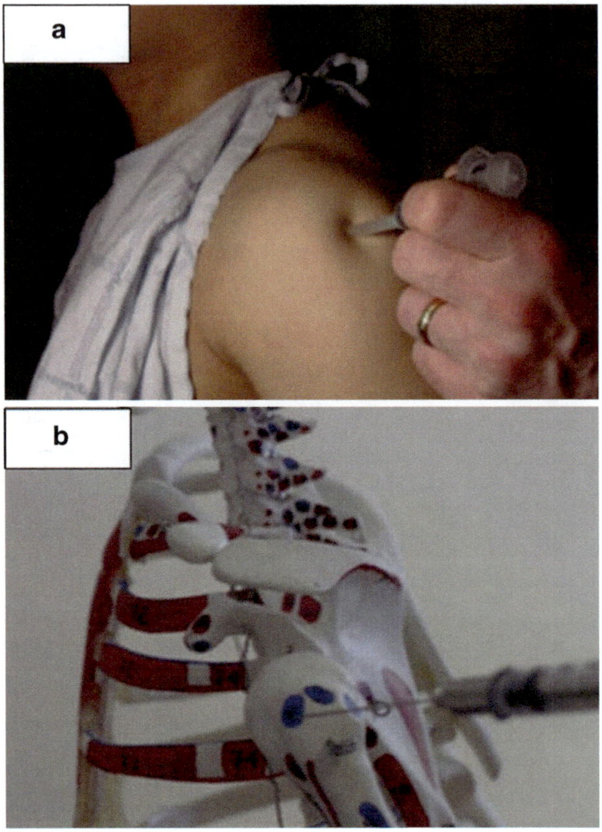

Fig. 7 Landmark technique supraspinatus injection: (**a**) needle entry perpendicular to the skin, (**b**) needle tip contacting anterior aspect of the greater tuberosity of the humerus. Reprinted from Physical Medicine and Rehabilitation Clinics of North America, Volume 15, issue 2, Todd P. Stitik, Patrick M. Foye, Jeffery Fossati, Shoulder injections for osteoarthritis and other disorders, 407–446, 2004, with permission from Elsevier

Infraspinatus Tendinopathy, Landmark Technique

The patient is placed in a seated position. The infraspinatus tendon insertion site is on the posterolateral aspect of the humeral head. Access to the insertion site is best when the patient's arm is relaxed along the side of the body. The needle trajectory is perpendicular to the skin, and advanced until gentle contact is made with the periosteum of the humerus (Fig. 9a, b). Withdraw the needle less than 1 cm, aspirate, and inject under slight resistance.

Infraspinatus Tendinopathy, Ultrasound Technique

Ultrasonography of the infraspinatus tendon is best seen when the patient's hand is in his/her lap with the palm facing upward. Over the posterior humerus, the transducer is placed in an axial plane orientation just below the scapular spine (Fig. 10a). This allows viewing of the infraspinatus tendon in long-axis at its insertion on the posterior aspect of the greater tuberosity. The humeral head is seen with the adjacent

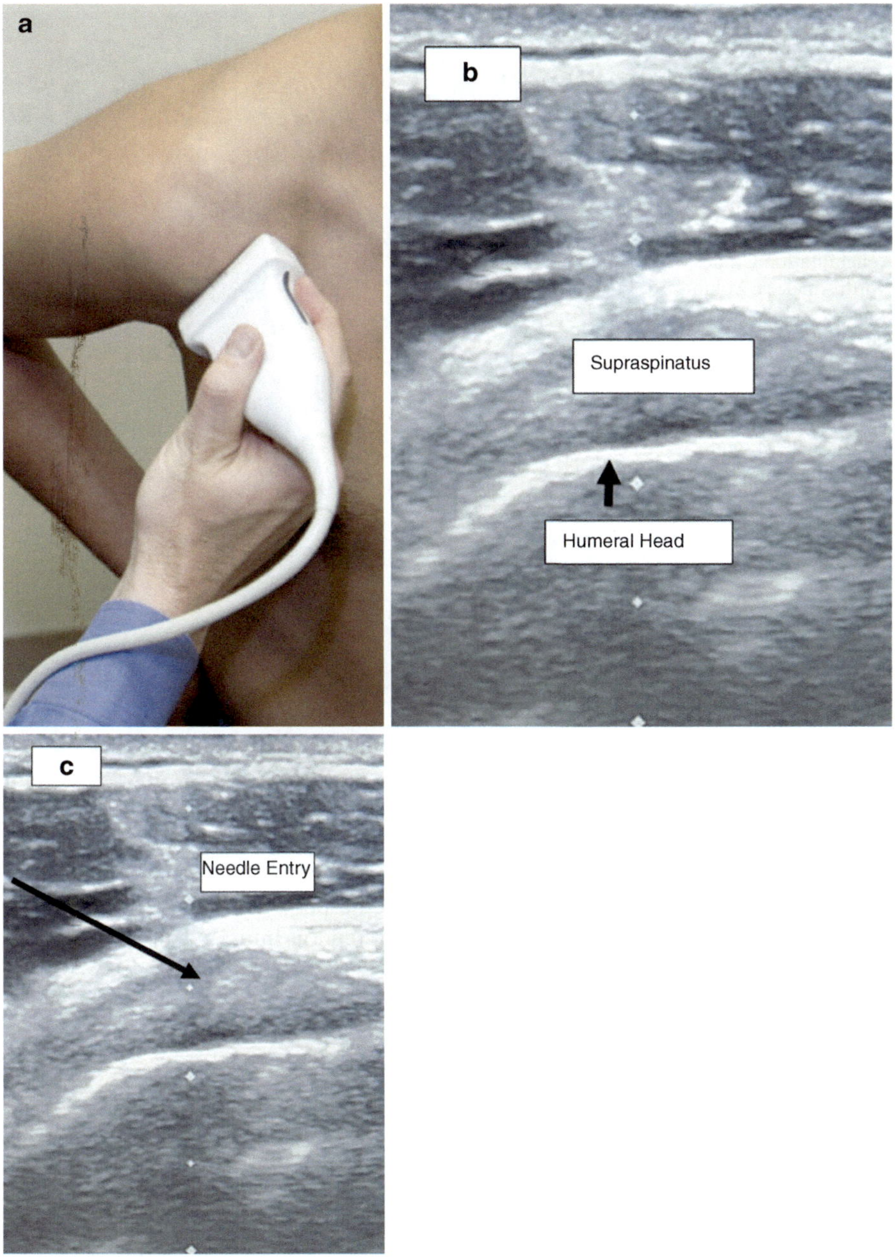

Fig. 8 Supraspinatus short-axis view: (**a**) patient is in a sitting position with the arm hyperextended and internally rotated by placing the ipsilateral dorsal aspect of the hand over the hip, (**b**) sonoanatomy of supraspinatus tendon, (**c**) needle entry using an in-plane approach

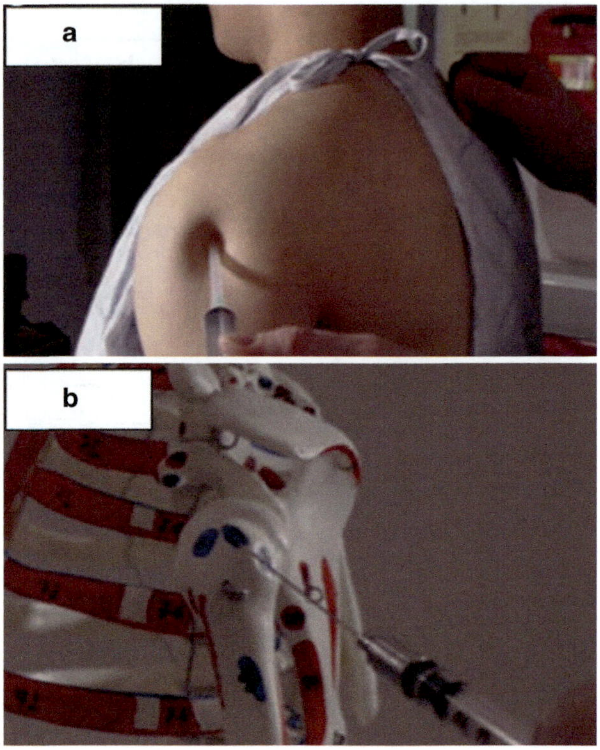

Fig. 9 Infraspinatus tendon landmark technique: (**a**) needle entry perpendicular to the skin, (**b**) needle tip contacting posterior aspect of the greater tuberosity of the humerus. Reprinted from Physical Medicine and Rehabilitation Clinics of North America, Volume 15, issue 2, Todd P. Stitik, Patrick M. Foye, Jeffery Fossati, Shoulder injections for osteoarthritis and other disorders, 407–446, 2004, with permission from Elsevier

infraspinatus tendon and glenoid labrum (Fig. 10b). Rotating the probe 90° allows a view of the infraspinatus tendon in short-axis. Sweeping the transducer along the scapular spine allows full visualization of the infraspinatus tendon. Once the tear or area of tendinopathy is observed, place the needle perpendicular to the skin, and advance until the needle tip is at the site of the tendon injury; aspirate and inject under slight resistance (Fig. 10c).

Subscapularis Tendinopathy, Landmark Technique

The patient is placed in the supine or sitting position with the arm externally rotated to maximize access to the insertion site of the subscapularis tendon on the lesser tuberosity of the humerus. The needle trajectory is perpendicular to the skin, and advanced until it makes gentle contact with the periosteum of the humerus. Withdraw the needle less than 1 cm, aspirate, and inject under slight resistance (Fig. 11a, b).

Subscapularis Tendinopathy, Ultrasound Technique

For ultrasonography of the subscapularis tendon, the patient's hand is placed in his/her lap with the palm facing upward. For the long-axis view, the transducer is in the

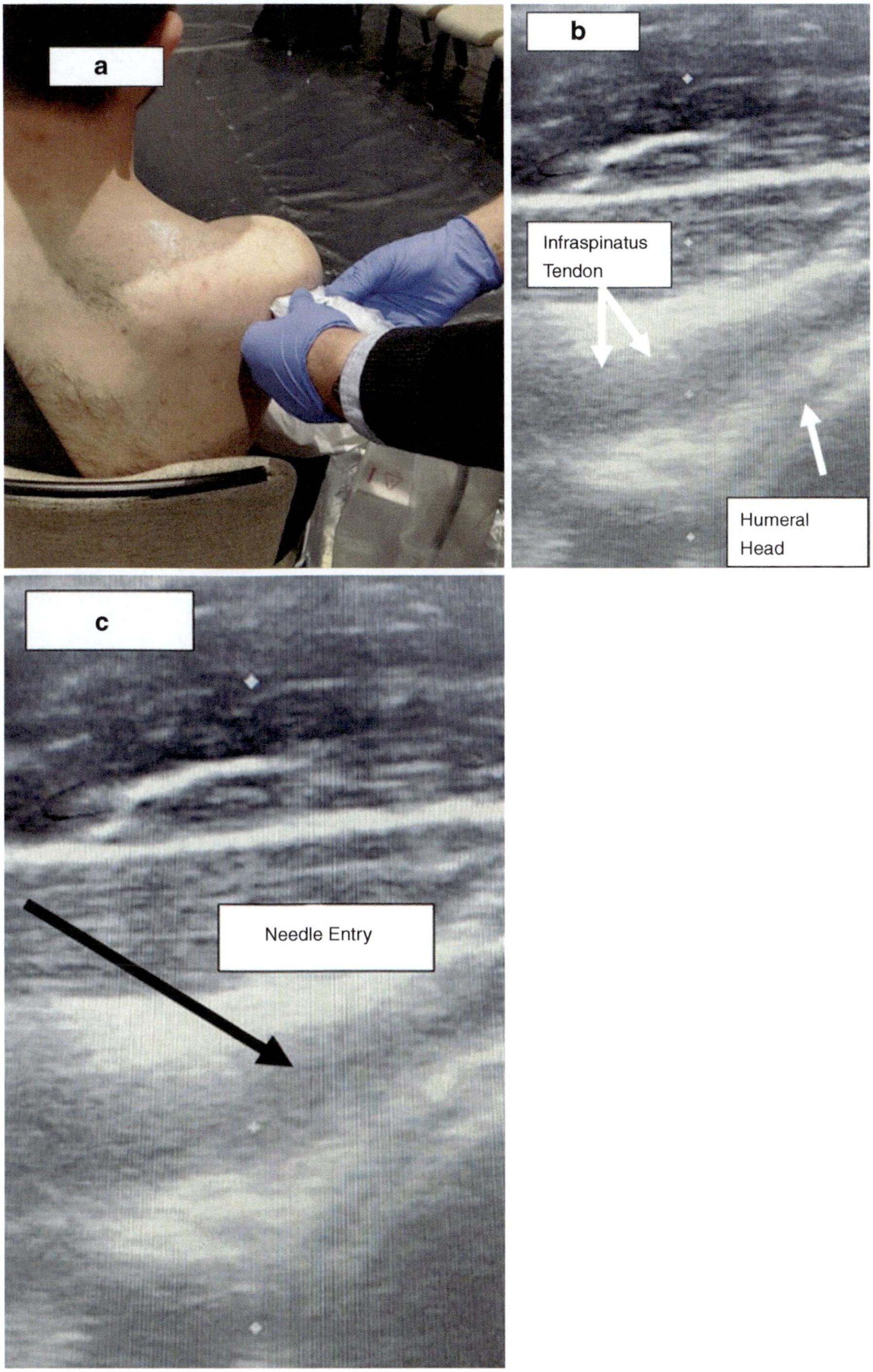

Fig. 10 Infraspinatus tendon long-axis view: (**a**) patient in sitting position with hand in lap and palm facing upward. The transducer is placed over the posterior humerus in an axial plane orientation just below the scapular spine, (**b**) sonoanatomy of the infraspinatus tendon, (**c**) needle entry in an in-plane approach

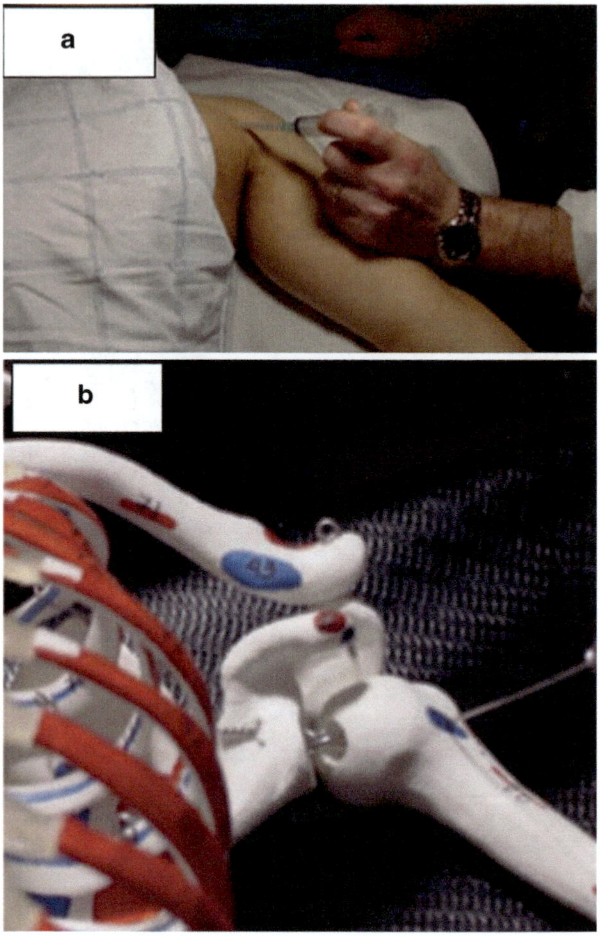

Fig. 11 Subscapularis tendon landmark technique: (**a**) needle entry perpendicular to the skin, (**b**) needle tip contacting lesser tuberosity of the humerus. Reprinted from Physical Medicine and Rehabilitation Clinics of North America, volume 15, issue 2, Todd P. Stitik, Patrick M. Foye, Jeffery Fossati, Shoulder injections for osteoarthritis and other disorders, 407–446, 2004, with permission from Elsevier

axial orientation along the anterior shoulder (Fig. 12a). The transducer is then centered over the lesser tuberosity to provide a long-axis view of the tendon (Fig. 12b). Complete evaluation along the entire tendon requires the patient to externally rotate the shoulder. Rotate the transducer 90° along the anterior shoulder to obtain a short-axis view of the subscapularis tendon. Once the tear or area of tendinopathy is in view, the needle is placed perpendicular to the skin and advanced until the needle tip is seen at the site of the tendon injury; aspirate and inject under slight resistance (Fig. 12c).

Potential Complications and Adverse Effects

Periarticular shoulder injections are well tolerated and complications, while rare, may include joint infection, damage to nearby bone or cartilage, and vascular or nerve damage. The use of corticosteroids in the joint space can cause skin

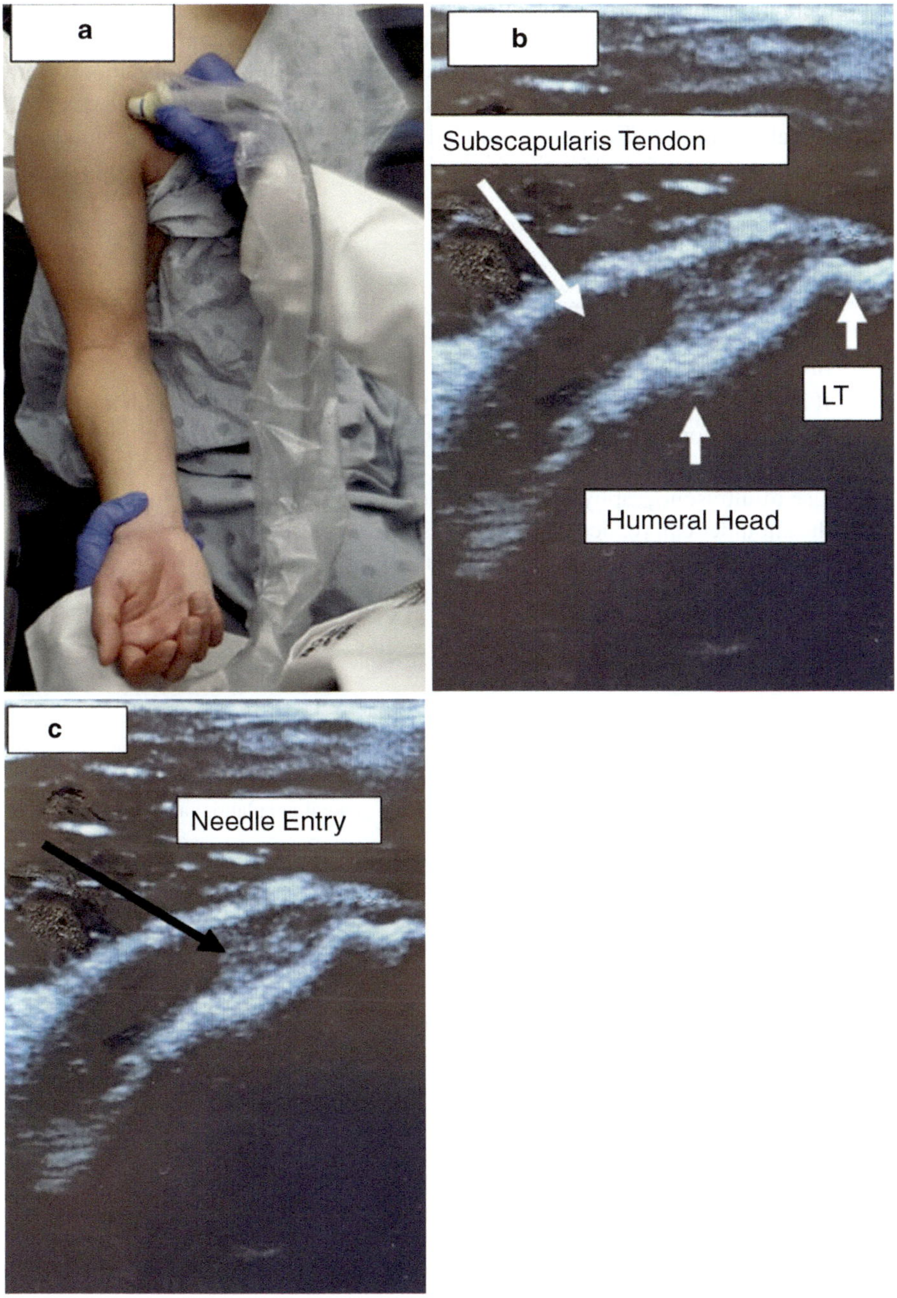

Fig. 12 Subscapularis tendon long-axis view: (**a**) patient in a sitting position with the elbow flexed, palm up, and arm externally rotated to maximize access to the insertion site of the subscapularis tendon, (**b**) sonoanatomy of the subscapular tendon, (**c**) needle entry in-plane approach

depigmentation, fat atrophy, weakening, and rupture of the tendon [2]. Steroids can adversely affect tendons by weakening the tendon fibers, potentially causing or increasing the size of a tear; however, this effect is less relevant in patients with significant pain and reduced functional ability who are not surgical candidates [14]. Systemic absorption of the steroid can lead to facial flushing, increased blood glucose levels, and a weakened immune response.

Clinical and Technical Pearls

- Rotator cuff dysfunction secondary to tendinopathy is a common cause of shoulder pain in adults and is characterized by painful functional limitation of the shoulder.
- It is essential to have an understanding of pertinent anatomy, such as bone surface anatomy and tendon orientation to accurately perform ultrasonography of the shoulder.
- Use of ultrasonography for needle placement for periarticular injections of the shoulder can reduce complications and increase block success rate.
- The choice of injectate (e.g., corticosteroid, PRP, glucose prolotherapy) is dictated by the underlying pathology and chronicity of the injury.

References

1. Luime JJ, Koes BW, Hendriksen IJ, Burdorf A, Verhagen AP, Miedema HS, Verhagen JA. Prevalence and incidence of shoulder pain in the general population; a systematic review. Scans J Rhematol. 2004;33(2):73–81.
2. Say F, Gurler D, Bulbul M. Platelet-rich plasma versus steroid injection for subacromial impingement syndrome. J Orthop Surg. 2016;24(1):62–6.
3. Schickendantz M, King D. Nonoperative management (including ultrasound-guided injections) of proximal biceps disorders. Clin Sports Med. 2016;35:57–73.
4. Lin KM, Wang D, Dines JS. Injection therapies for rotator cuff disease. Orthop Clin N Am. 2018;49:231–9.
5. Sengodan VC, Kurian S, Ramasamy R. Treatment of partial rotator cuff tear with ultrasound-guided platelet-rich plasma. J Clin Imaging Sci. 2017;7:32.
6. Cole BF, Peters KS, Hackett L, Murrell GAC. Ultrasound-guided versus blind subacromial corticosteroid injections for subacromial impingement syndrome: a randomized, double-blind clinical trial. Am J Sports Med. 2016;44(3):702–7.
7. Messina C, Banfi G, Orlandi D, Lacelli F, Serafini G, Mauri G, et al. Ultrasound-guided interventional procedures around the shoulder. Br J Radiol. 2016;89(1057):20150372.
8. Soh E, Li W, Ong KO, Chen W, Bautista D. Image-guided versus blind corticosteroid injections in adults with shoulder pain: a systematic review. BMC Musculoskelet Disord. 2011;12:137.
9. Birnbaum K, Lierse W. Anatomy and function of the bursa subacromialis. Acta Anat (Basel). 1992;145(4):354–63.
10. Duranton LD, Gagey OJ. Anatomy and function for the subdeltoid bursa. Surg Radiol Anat. 2001;23(1):23–5.
11. Kennedy MS, Nicholson HD, Woodley SJ. Clinical anatomy of subacromial and related shoulder bursae: a review of the literature. Clin Anat. 2017;30:213–26.

12. Breu A, Rosenmeier K, Kujat R, Angele P, Zink W. The cytotoxicity of bupivacaine, ropivacaine, and mepivacaine on human chondrocytes and cartilage. Anesth Analg. 2013;117(2):514–22.
13. Piper SL, Kim HT. Comparison of ropivacaine and bupivacaine toxicity in human articular chondrocytes. J Bone Joint Surg Am. 2008;90(5):986–91.
14. Faucet R, Robinson GP, Jafari M, Rowbotham E. Ultrasound-guided subacromial-subdeltoid bursa corticosteroid injections: a study of short- and long-term outcomes. Clin Radiol. 2018;73:780.e7–780.e12.

Further Reading

Stitik TP, Foye PM, Fossati J. Shoulder injections for osteoarthritis and other disorders. Phys Med Rehabil Clin N Am. 2004;15(2):404–46.

Injections for Acromioclavicular Joint Pain

James Sweet, Alexander F. Bautista, and George C. Chang Chien

Essential Concepts

- Acromioclavicular (AC) joint injections are usually performed if pain is persistent after exhausting conservative treatment modalities. Alternatively, this injection also can be offered preemptively, to facilitate physical rehabilitation.
- Acromioclavicular injections have both diagnostic and therapeutic value.
- The injection is superficial, and therefore, caution should be practiced and utilization of proper technique is necessary to minimize side effects of corticosteroids such as skin discoloration and subcutaneous fat atrophy.

1 Acromioclavicular Joint Injection

Overview

Acromioclavicular (AC) joint pain is a common source of shoulder pain, frequently observed in clinical practice. It has been estimated that between 0.5–2.9/1000 people per year present with AC joint pain [1]. The AC joint is very prone to injury from acute trauma to the shoulder following a fall or from sports-related injury. Oftentimes, the pain can become chronic. It is frequently accompanied by

J. Sweet (✉) · A. F. Bautista
Department of Anesthesiology and Perioperative Medicine, University of Louisville, Louisville, KY, USA
e-mail: afbaut01@louisville.edu

G. C. Chang Chien
GCC Institute, Newport Beach, CA, USA

D. Souza et al. (eds.), *Bedside Pain Management Interventions*,
https://doi.org/10.1007/978-3-031-11188-4_50

progressive arthritic changes in the AC joint, and osteolysis of the joint. Diagnosis mainly relies on history and physical examination. Initial treatment often precedes imaging modalities such as X-rays and radiographs. Rest, physical therapy, and analgesics are part of the initial treatment for AC joint pain. However, local corticosteroid injections can be used if previous conservative management fails. Alternatively AC injections can be done to facilitate physical rehabilitation [2].

Indications and Contraindications

Acromioclavicular joint pain is commonly caused by direct injury to the AC joint itself. The injury may be due to direct impact to the joint following a fall from an outstretched arm or as a consequence of repetitive stress on the joint in people who perform overhead lifting activities, e.g., weight lifting. The ongoing microtrauma may lead to acute inflammation followed by chronic changes in the AC joint. Commonly the condition becomes chronic. It may be accompanied by distal clavicular osteolysis [3]. Damage to the AC joint can be associated with damage to the supraspinatus tendon and osteophytes from the arthritic joint can be contributory to subacromial impingement producing further shoulder pain with localization over the AC joint [4].

Indications for AC joint injection include AC joint pain of various etiologies, primary osteoarthritis of AC joint, secondary osteoarthritis of AC joint, including traumatic osteoarthritis, and distal clavicle osteolysis [5]. Contraindications for AC joint injection include infection at the planned injection site, allergy to, or intolerance to injectate, including local anesthetics and corticosteroids, and patient refusal. Relative contraindications include presence of a lesion or mass at the site of the injection, severe joint destruction, bone fracture in proximity to the joint [2]. Coagulopathy or platelet dysfunction including iatrogenic are not considered to be a contraindication to the AC joint injection. However, the clinicians should use the best judgment, and discuss risks and benefits in detail with the patient.

Clinical Anatomy

The acromioclavicular joint is formed by the articulation of the distal end of the clavicle and the acromion. The joint is a diarthrodial joint that is surrounded by a capsule. It is stabilized by different ligaments namely, the superior, inferior, anterior, and posterior ligaments. The AC joint functions as a gliding synovial joint that provides the ability to raise the arm above the head and facilitate arm rotation (Fig. 1).

There are six grades of AC joint separation (Table 1).

Grades 4–6 are typically treated with surgical intervention to correct the deformity (Fig. 2).

Equipment and Supplies

Acromioclavicular joint injection can be performed at the bedside either using a landmark technique or USG. An antiseptic solution, typically 4% chlorhexidine, 25 Gauge 1.5-in. needle, 3–5 ml syringe for injectate, mask, and sterile gloves

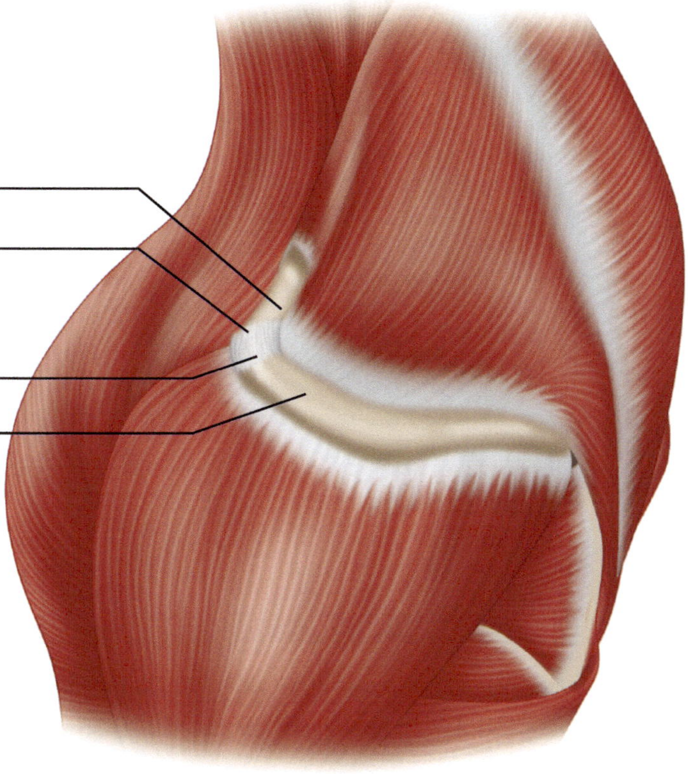

Fig. 1 Acromioclavicular joint anatomy as labeled

Table 1 Acromioclavicular (AC) joint separation

Grade 1	AC joint sprain
Grade 2	AC joint ligaments torn
Grade 3	AC joint 100% dislocated
Grade 4	Collarbone displaced backward
Grade 5	AC joint 100% dislocated, with a markedly greater degree of separation than grade 4.
Grade 6	Collarbone displaced under the coracoid

should be typically available for this procedure. Local anesthetic, typically 1% lidocaine, with or without corticosteroid should be prepared for this injection as well. An ultrasound device with a high-frequency linear transducer will be typically needed (Table 2).

Landmark Technique

AC joint injection can be potentially technically challenging because the joint is very small and narrow. Palpation of the AC joint is achieved by feeling the crevice between the distal end of the clavicle and acromion [2]. After identification of the

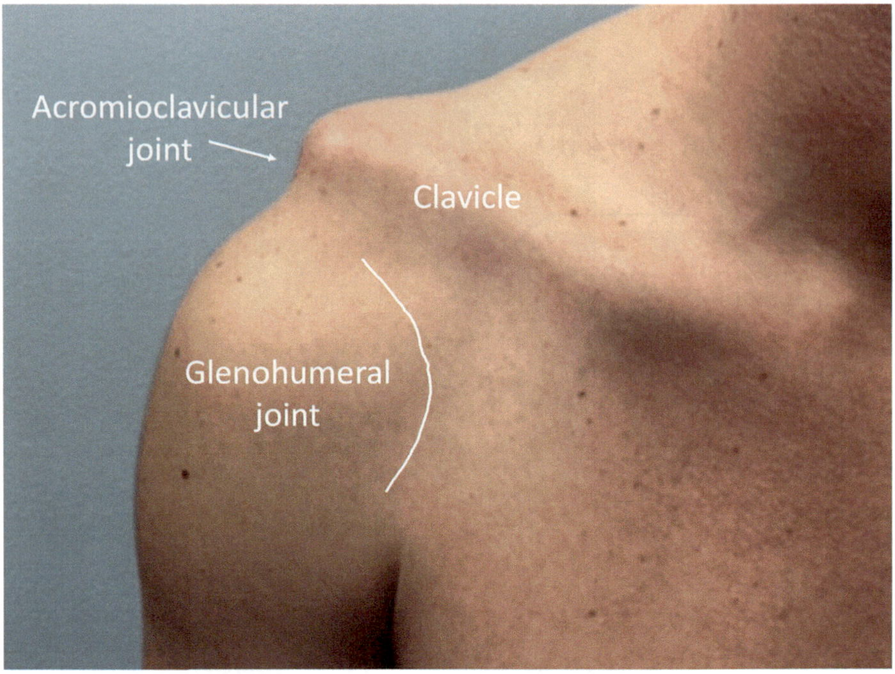

Fig. 2 Acromioclavicular joint separation Grade 3. The distal clavicle has moved superiorly from the acromion

Table 2 Acromioclavicular joint injection. Equipment and supplies

Antiseptic	4% chlorhexidine or 10% povidone-iodine (Betadine)
Ultrasound probe	5–18 MHz linear probe, with sterile cover and sterile gel
Syringe	3–5 ml
Needle	25–30 gauge 0.5–1 in.
Injectate local anesthetics	1–2% Lidocaine
Injectate corticosteroids	Triamcinolone 5–40 mg (*t*1/2 life: 18–36 h) Betamethasone 18 mg (*t*1/2 life: 36–54 h) Dexamethasone 4 mg (*t*1/2 life: 36–54 h) Methylprednisolone 80–125 mg (*t*1/2 life: 18–36 h)

soft spot in the AC joint, local anesthetic injection can be performed to confirm joint localization. The needle is then kept in place and the syringe is exchanged with the steroid solution [6].

Ultrasound Technique

The use of ultrasound guidance can aide the provider in accessing the AC joint. The procedure is performed with the patient seated and the arm resting at their side. The lateral margin of the clavicle is palpated and the gap adjacent to the lateral margin is identified. The ultrasound is then placed in a coronal plan, across the AC joint (Fig. 3).

From this position, the joint capsule is visualized as a hyperechoic fibrillary arc marking the superior joint capsule (Fig. 4).

An out-of-plane approach can proceed from this point from anterior to posterior (Fig. 5).

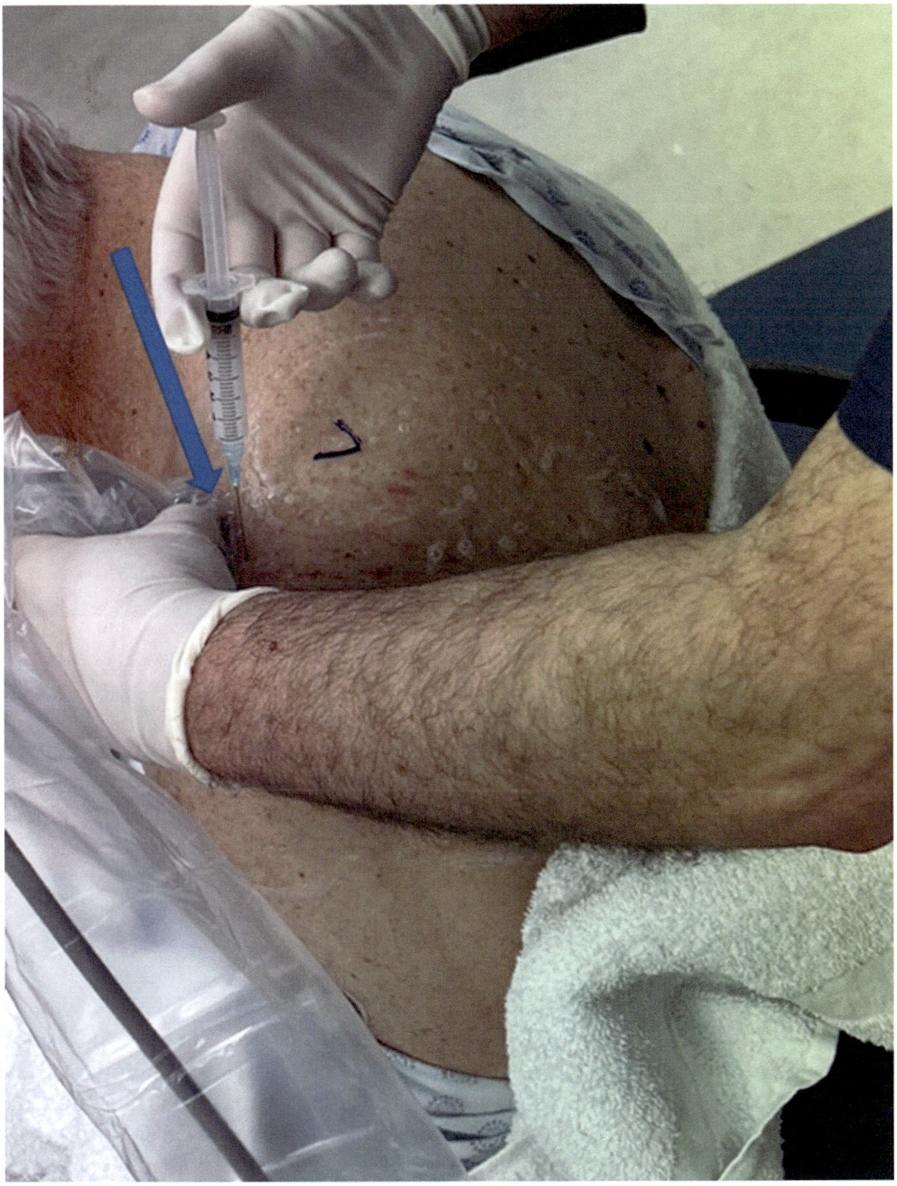

Fig. 3 Ultrasound transducer, needle and syringe positioning. Blue arrow points towards location over the acromioclavicular joint. Image–courtesy of Dmitri Souza, MD, PhD

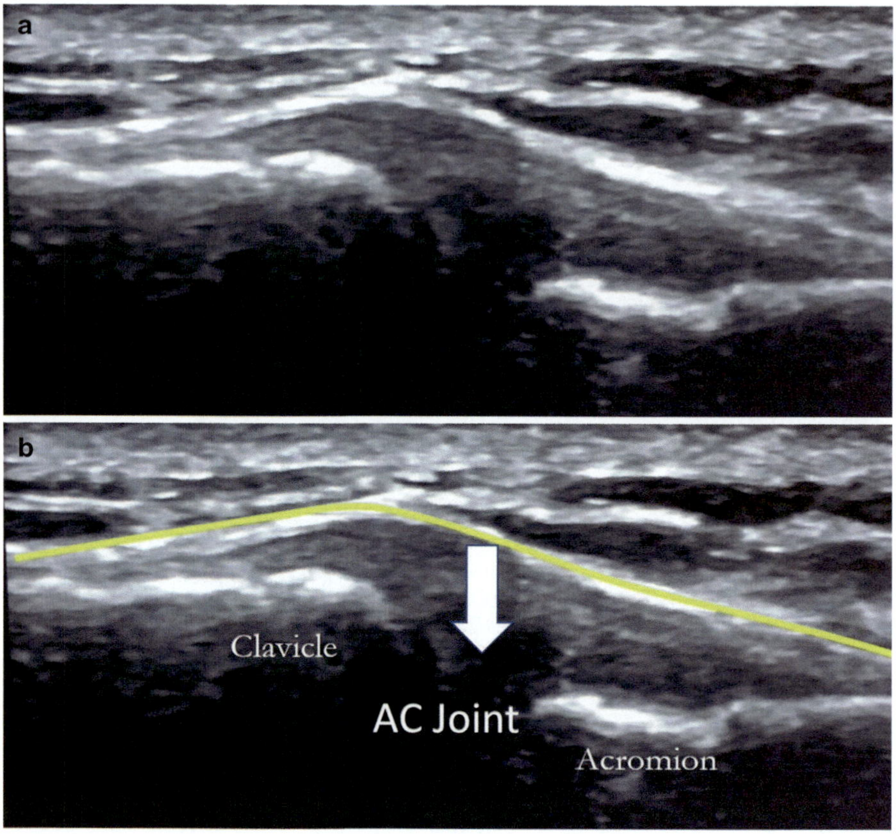

Fig. 4 (**a**) Acromioclavicular joint ultrasound evaluation. (**b**) The clavicle has superior displacement in this image with a distended capsule outlined in yellow and mild joint fluid

Additionally, an in-plane approach can also be utilized from this probe position by accessing the joint in a lateral-medial orientation. Lastly, an alternative in-plane approach can be accomplished with the ultrasound probe oriented in a sagittal plane, and the needle inserted in plane from lateral to medial in to the AC joint capsule [7].

Potential Complications and Adverse Effects

Intraarticular injection of steroid into the AC joint is generally safe with very minimal risk. Aseptic technique should be employed at all times to minimize the risk of infection. Corticosteroids on the other hand carry inherent risks of systemic adverse reaction such as hyperglycemia, post-injection symptom flare, facial flushing, and anaphylaxis. Also, corticosteroids are associated with tendon weakening/rupture, fat atrophy, muscle wasting, skin pigmentation, septic arthritis, potential nerve and blood vessel damage. Avoiding frequent injections and high doses are advised,

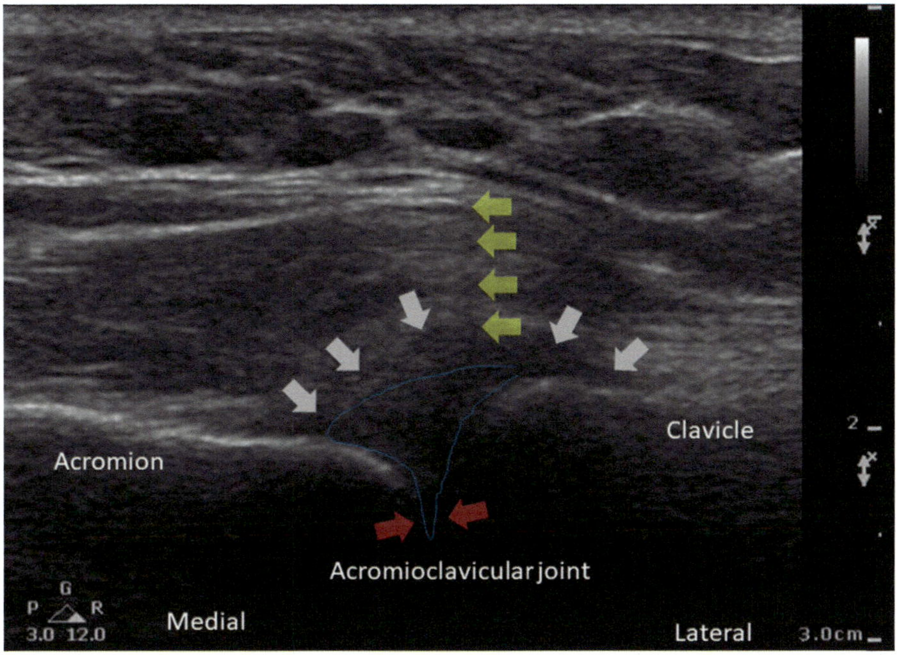

Fig. 5 Acromioclavicular joint injection in a morbidly obese individual. Please note excessive adipose tissue over the acromioclavicular joint. Normally, this joint is easy to palpate. In this case ultrasonography helped to locate the joint because it was not easily palpable. Gray arrows point towards the thickened joint capsule, and hypertrophied synovium. Blue line indicates joint fluid mixed with the injectate. Yellow arrows point towards the out of plane needle placed under the joint capsule. Red arrows indicate acromioclavicular joint. Image–courtesy of Dmitri Souza, MD, PhD

though, there has been paucity of scientific literature to support the specific interval for steroid injections [2].

Clinical and Technical Pearls

- Treatment of AC joint pain involves non-operative treatment that includes activity modification, physical therapy, medication, and joint injection.
- Oftentimes, plain radiographs would indicate arthritic changes in the AC joint but would be clinically insignificant if the joint is non-tender on palpation. However, radiographs may be warranted to exclude fracture, dislocation, or separation of the AC joint.
- AC joint injection can be done utilizing landmark technique or ultrasound guidance at the bedside.
- Although infection risk following steroid injection is rare, it is imperative to be cautious in patients who are on chronic steroid or immunocompromised.

- Anticoagulation need not be stopped for AC joint injection since it has low bleeding risk and the area is compressible and superficial.
- Due to the superficial nature of the injection, care should be taken to decrease the risk of subcutaneous fat atrophy and skin depigmentation.
- Some evidence suggests greater success when using ultrasound as compared to landmark.
- One cadaveric study demonstrated a high peri-articular injection rate when experienced providers used a "blind" technique [8].

References

1. van der Windt DA, Koes BW, de Jong BA, Bouter LM. Shoulder disorders in general practice: incidence, patient characteristics, and management. Ann Rheum Dis. 1995;54(12):959–64.
2. Bell AD, Conaway D. Corticosteroid injections for painful shoulders. Int J Clin Pract. 2005;59(10):1178–86.
3. Beals RK, Sauser DD. Nontraumatic disorders of the clavicle. J Am Acad Orthop Surg. 2006;14(4):205–14.
4. Chaudhury S, Bavan L, Rupani N, et al. Managing acromio-clavicular joint pain: a scoping review. Shoulder Elbow. 2018;10(1):4–14.
5. DeFroda SF, Nacca C, Waryasz GR, Owens BD. Diagnosis and management of distal clavicle osteolysis. Orthopedics. 2017;40(2):119–24.
6. Armstrong A. Evaluation and management of adult shoulder pain: a focus on rotator cuff disorders, acromioclavicular joint arthritis, and glenohumeral arthritis. Med Clin North Am. 2014;98(4):755, xii.
7. Chang KV, Mezian K, Naňka O, Wu WT, Lin CP, Özçakar L. Ultrasound-guided interventions for painful shoulder: from anatomy to evidence. J Pain Res. 2018;11:2311–22.
8. Pichler W, Weinberg AM, Grechenig S, Tesch NP, Heidari N, Grechenig W. Intra-articular injection of the acromioclavicular joint. J Bone Joint Surg. 2009;91(12):1638–40.

Further Reading

Park KD, Kim TK, Lee WY, Ahn JK, Park Y. Palpation versus ultrasound-guided acromioclavicular joint intra-articular injections: a retrospective comparative clinical study. Pain Physician. 2015;18(4):333–41.

Suprascapular Nerve Block

Rahul Rastogi and Justin Wikle

Essential Concepts

- Suprascapular nerve block is an easy to perform, low-risk procedure that is well-tolerated. It can be performed at the bedside.
- It can be useful to treat shoulder pain of various etiologies, including post-operative shoulder pain, osteoarthritis, other degenerative or inflammatory arthropathies of the acromioclavicular or glenohumeral humeral joints, adhesive capsulitis, hemiplegic shoulder pain, cancer, trauma, entrapment neuropathies, and some other conditions.
- Suprascapular nerve block may be performed using landmarks or ultra-sound guidance as a distinct nerve block or in combination with brachial plexus or other peripheral nerve blocks.

R. Rastogi (✉) · J. Wikle
Department of Anesthesia, Division of Pain Medicine, University of Iowa Carver College of Medicine, Iowa City, IA, USA

Department of Anesthesia, University of Iowa Carver College of Medicine, Iowa City, IA, USA
e-mail: rahul-rastogi@uiowa.edu

J. Wikle
Department of Anesthesia, University of Iowa Carver College of Medicine, Iowa City, IA, USA
e-mail: justin-wikle@uiowa.edu

D. Souza et al. (eds.), *Bedside Pain Management Interventions*,
https://doi.org/10.1007/978-3-031-11188-4_51

1 Suprascapular Nerve Block

Overview

Suprascapular nerve block (SSNB) is an easy to perform, well-tolerated and safe procedure for pain relief [1]. It can be utilized for various types of shoulder pain, including postoperative pain, osteoarthritis, other degenerative or inflammatory arthropathies of the acromioclavicular or glenohumeral humeral joints, adhesive capsulitis, hemiplegic shoulder pain, cancer, injury, entrapment neuropathies, and some other conditions presenting with shoulder pain. It can be performed at the bedside [1–3]. The suprascapular nerve block (SSNB) can be performed in addition to the interscalene brachial plexus, supraclavicular, or other peripheral nerve blockades [4, 5]. This is because the commonly performed interscalene brachial plexus block may not completely cover the shoulder, lateral axilla, and posterior upper arm. A combination of SSNB with an axillary nerve block can achieve a near-complete shoulder block [2, 3]. The suprascapular nerve block can be performed using anterior (proximal), distal superior, and distal posterior approaches.

Indications and Contraindications

Suprascapular nerve block can be used as a therapeutic or diagnostic tool [4]. It can provide relief of acute or refractory shoulder pain of various etiologies including degenerative or inflammatory arthropathy of glenohumeral, acromioclavicular joints, or even sternoclavicular joint if performed proximally. It can alleviate pain secondary to trauma, including rotator cuff injury, adhesive capsulitis ("frozen shoulder), and hemiplegic shoulder pain [5, 6]. It can be useful in the treatment of SSN neuritis or SSN entrapment [6, 7]. It can be used perioperatively for patients undergoing shoulder surgery [3]. One recent high-quality meta-analysis established that SSNB can be an effective and safe analgesic technique providing pain control similar to interscalene brachial plexus block with similar utilization of opioid analgesics between these two blocks [4]. It was noted that SSNB resulted in fewer nerve block-related complications during arthroscopic shoulder surgery, especially in patients with severe chronic obstructive pulmonary disease, obstructive sleep apnea, and morbid obesity [4]. Therefore, careful evaluation of risks and benefits of the anterior (proximal) SSNB is critical for patients with respiratory compromise [4, 8]. Suprascapular nerve blocks have diagnostic value in planning for SSN decompression surgery, neurectomy, or even neuromodulation.

Contraindications include infection at the planned injection site, intolerance or allergy to the injectate, including local anesthetic and corticosteroids. Coagulopathy including iatrogenic coagulopathy, or impaired platelet function are typically not considered contraindications for this procedure [4, 7].

Clinical Anatomy

The suprascapular nerve is a mixed sensory and motor nerve originating from ventral rami of C5 and C6 nerve roots leaving the brachial plexus just before the formation of its superior trunk. Sometimes it also receives fibers from the C4 nerve root [1]. It runs posteriorly under the omohyoid muscle towards the trapezius muscle. It is typically accompanied by vessels up to the suprascapular notch. At the suprascapular notch, the superior transverse scapular ligament separates the SSN from the associated vessels [1–3]. The SSN travels under this ligament and over the notch towards the suprascapular fossa. In the suprascapular fossa, the SSN gives rise to the motor branch to the supraspinatus muscle and sensory articular branch to the acromioclavicular joint, posterosuperior glenohumeral joint, rotator cuff elements, and coracohumeral ligaments. The nerve continues and passes between the spinoglenoid ligament and the spinoglenoid notch to enter the infraspinatus fossa. There it gives sensory and motor terminal branches to the infraspinatus muscle and sometimes to the glenohumeral joint [1, 9] (Fig. 1; Table 1).

Equipment and Supplies

Peripheral nerve blocks like the suprascapular nerve can be performed at the bedside either using a landmark technique or USG. An antiseptic solution, typically 4% chlorhexidine, 22–25 Gauge 1.5–3.5-in. needle, 5–10 ml syringe for injectate, mask,

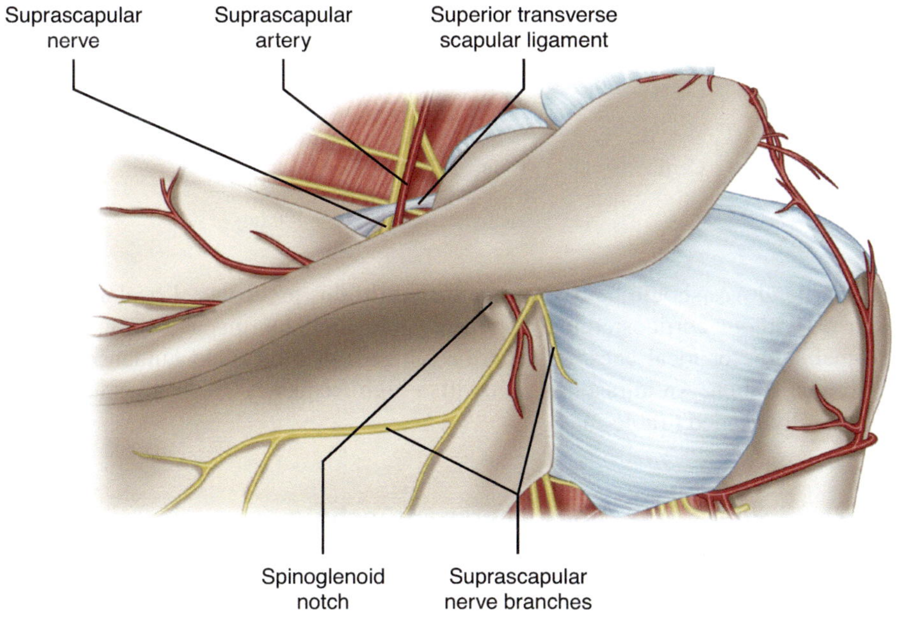

Fig. 1 Anatomy of the suprascapular nerve, as labeled

Table 1 Suprascapular nerve anatomy

Origin	Ventral rami of the C5,6 nerve root.
Formation	The nerve leaves the brachial plexus just before the formation of the superior trunk.
Path	• Runs posteriorly deep to omohyoid muscle and trapezius muscle along the superior border of the scapula • Continues under superior transverse scapular ligament at the suprascapular notch to reach supraspinatus fossa • Passes under spinoglenoid ligament over spinoglenoid notch to give terminal branches in the infraspinatus fossa
Branches	• In supraspinatus fossa—Motor branch to supraspinatus muscles and sensory branch to the acromioclavicular and glenohumeral joints
Relationships	Suprascapular artery and vein pass above the superior transverse scapular ligament, while the suprascapular nerve passes on the that his ligament
Innervation	Motor innervation include supraspinatus and infraspinatus muscles Sensory innervation include acromioclavicular joint, glenohumeral joint, and associated ligaments
Landmarks	Acromion, scapular spine, suprascapular notch
Anatomical variants	Some of the C4 nerve root fibers may contribute to the suprascapular nerve. Suprascapular vein sometimes passes under superior transverse scapular ligament.

Table 2 Suprascapular nerve block. Equipment and supplies

Antiseptic		4% chlorhexidine or 10% povidone-iodine (Betadine)
Ultrasound probe		5–20 MHz linear probe, with sterile cover and sterile gel
Syringes		5–10 ml
Needle		22–25 gauge 1.5–3.5 in.
Injectate for hydrolocalization or hydrodissection		Normal saline or local anesthetic
Injectate	Local anesthetics	0.25–0.5% bupivacaine 0.5% Ropivacaine 1–2% lidocaine
	Corticosteroids	Triamcinolone 5–40 mg Dexamethasone 4 mg Methylprednisolone 80–120 mg

and sterile gloves should be typically prepared for this procedure. Local anesthetic with or without corticosteroids is typically prepared for this injection as well. Normal saline or local anesthetic can be utilized for ultrasound guidance during hydrolocalization. An ultrasound unit with a high-frequency linear transducer will be typically needed (Table 2).

Suprascapular Nerve Block, Landmark Technique

The entry point is identified at the mid–distal scapular spine, just medially from the medial border of the acromion, with the patient in either sitting, prone, or lateral decubitus position using palpation. This technique represents the superior distal approach. Skin is prepped with antiseptic solution, typically 4% chlorhexidine, and anesthetized using 1 ml of 1% Lidocaine. The needle should be advanced caudad from the entry point to reach the supraspinatus fossa floor. A typical volume of the injectate for the landmark technique is large, 10–15 ml. Alternatively, the needle can be introduced below the scapular spine to target spinoglenoid notch for the posterior distal approach.

The anterior (proximal) approach is not recommended with the landmark technique [10–12].

Ultrasound Technique

Ultrasound guidance is preferable for the SSNB as it allows real-time visualization of the needle advancement and observation of the injectate spread. It would likely help to avoid intravascular injection and, with the anterior (proximal) SSNB, may decrease the chance of pneumothorax and incidental phrenic nerve block.

The patient can be in the supine position for the anterior (proximal) approach. The suprascapular nerve can be located under the inferior belly of the omohyoid muscle. Because of the precise localization of the SSN, this approach allows to use of a lower volume of injectate, 3–5 ml, as compared to 10–15 ml with blind injection (Table 3).

Table 3 Suprascapular nerve block. Ultrasound-guided techniques

Position	Siting with holding contralateral shoulder or prone with the arm hanging down (for superior and posterior approaches) or supine with contralateral neck turn (for anterior approach).
USG probe	5–18 MHz linear probe
Superior and posterior (distal) approaches	In-plane: medial to lateral > lateral to medial Also, can be done out of plane
Probe orientation	In-plane or out of plane, over and parallel to the scapular spine over the suprascapular notch and suprascapular fossa for superior distal approach In-plane or out of plane, below and parallel to the scapular spine over the spinoglenoid notch fossa for posterior distal approach
Important structures to visualize with ultrasonography	Suprascapular notch and superior transverse carpal ligament for superior distal approach Spinoglenoid notch for posterior distal approach
Technique and additional tips	Advance needle towards the suprascapular notch using a superior distal approach Advanced needle towards spinoglenoid notch for posterior distal approach Out of plane technique frequently requires hydrolocalization/ hydrodissection Identify suprascapular artery and vein using Doppler
Anterior (proximal) approach	Supine, in-plane, lateral to medial needle passage
Probe orientation	In-plane, parallel to scapula spine and near distal clavicle at supraclavicular fossa.
Important structures to visualize with ultrasonography	Supraclavicular fossa Identify the inferior belly of the omohyoid muscle and brachial plexus
Technique and additional tips	Advance needle lateral to medial through the omohyoid muscle towards inferior to SSN situated under omohyoid muscle and lateral to brachial plexus.
Concerns	Still unable to reliably prevent phrenic nerve block
Injectate volume	3–5 ml

The patient can be located prone or sitting for the distal anterior and distal posterior approaches. The ultrasound transducer should be located parallel to the distal clavicle superiorly, and medially to the acromion. This position of the transducer will allow visualization of the supraclavicular fossa (Figs. 2 and 3). The precise injection allows lower volumes of the injectate, typically 3–5 ml of, to be as clinically effective as higher volumes of local anesthetic used for the blind injections.

The suprascapular nerve block can be performed at the level of spinoglenoid notch. With this approach the transducer is parallel to the distal scapular spine, slowly moved caudad and lateral until the SSN becomes visible under the spinoglenoid ligament (Figs. 4 and 5).

Potential Complications

The suprascapular nerve block is typically well-tolerated, and the complications are rare. The complications may be related to nerve injury, infection, bleeding, allergic reaction, or intolerance to the components of injectate, including local anesthetic and corticosteroids. The patient should be advised that on rare occasions the SSNB

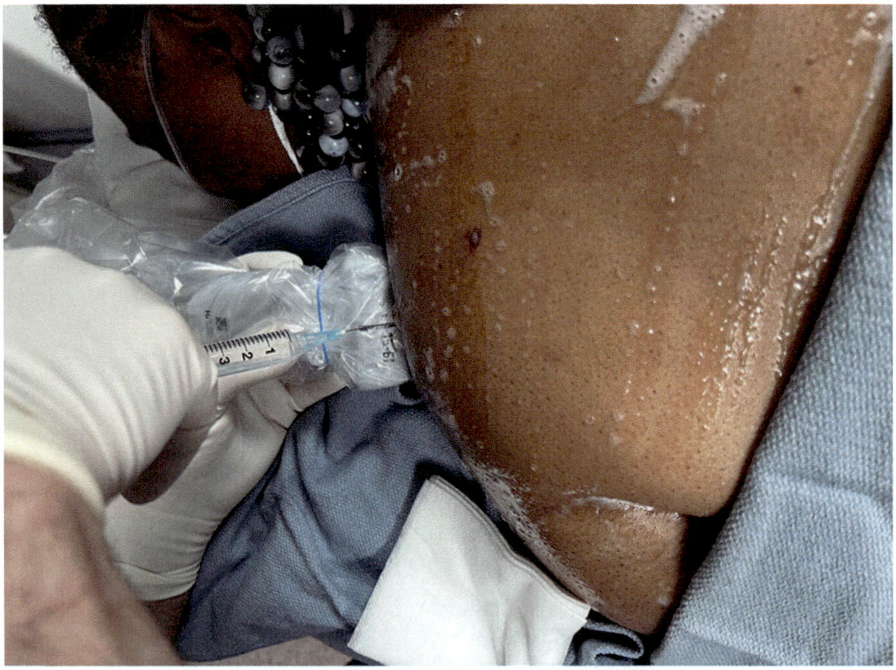

Fig. 2 The superior distal approach for the ultrasound-guided suprascapular nerve block. Ultrasound transducer orientation. Image—courtesy of Dmitri Souza

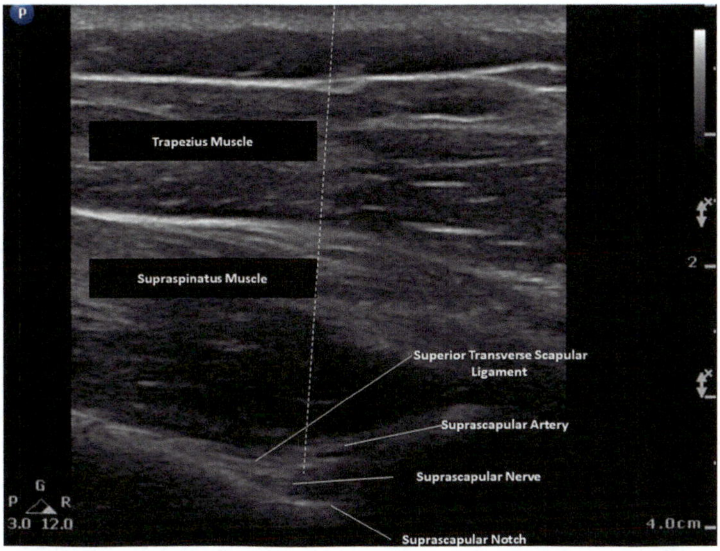

Fig. 3 Ultrasonogram of the suprascapular nerve block, superior distal approach. Dashed line represents out of plane the needle trajectory. Image—courtesy of Dmitri Souza

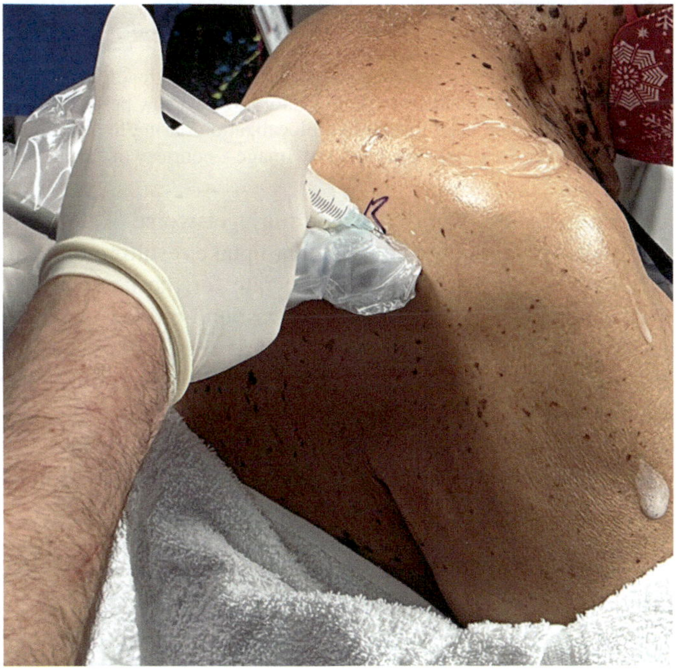

Fig. 4 Ultrasound-guided suprascapular nerve block at the spinoglenoid notch, posterior distal approach. Ultrasound transducer orientation. Image—courtesy of Dmitri Souza

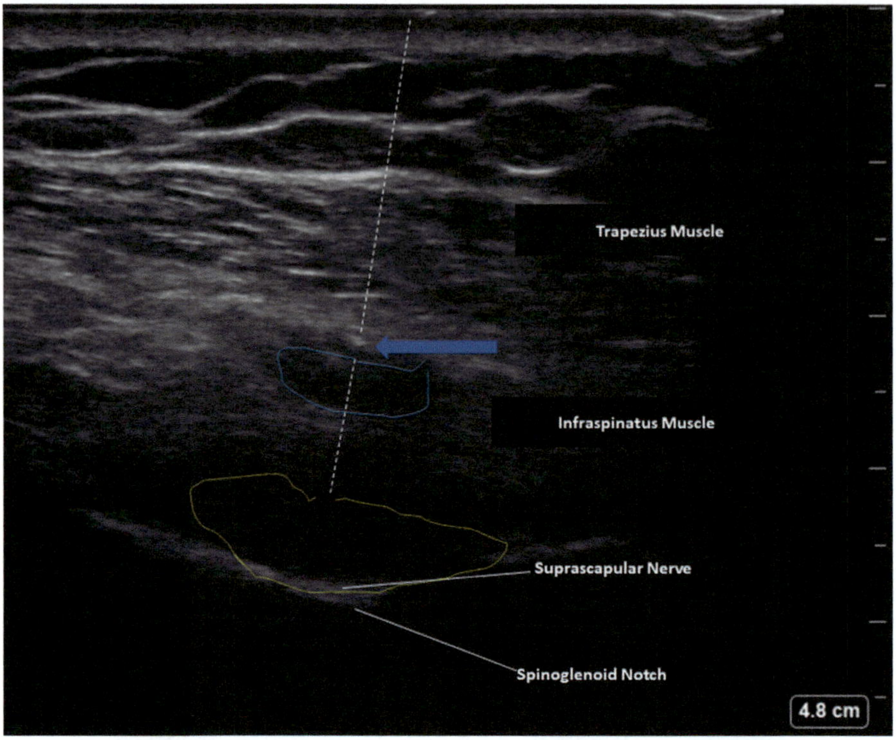

Fig. 5 Ultrasonogram of the suprascapular nerve block at the spinoglenoid notch, posterior distal approach. The dashed line represents the needle trajectory. Blue arrow points to the needle shaft. Blue line delineates the injectate used for the hydrolocalization during the injection. The yellow line delineates injectate over the suprascapular nerve. Image—courtesy of Dmitri Souza

may not work, or, even less likely, the pain may get worse. The landmark-based injection has a higher potential for intravascular uptake resulting in local anesthetic toxicity, partly because of the volume of injectate for the landmark technique is typically significantly higher than with the ultrasound-guided technique [10–12]. The local anesthetic toxicity may be manifested as a metallic taste in the mouth, dizziness, ringing in the ears, perioral numbness, blurred vision, slurred speech, drowsiness, hypotension, and cardiorespiratory arrest.

With the anterior superior approach, especially with the proximal part of the nerve blockade, pneumothorax and phrenic nerve blockade may occur, especially with blind injection [11].

Clinical and Technical Pearls

- Suprascapular nerve and suprascapular artery are two hypoechoic structures that can be easily differentiated with color Doppler.
- Patients should be observed for at least 15 min after the injection.

References

1. Chan CW, Peng PW. Suprascapular nerve block: a narrative review. Reg Anesth Pain Med. 2011;36(4):358–73. https://doi.org/10.1097/AAP.0b013e3182204ec0.
2. Fernandes MR, Barbosa MA, Sousa AL, Ramos GC. Suprascapular nerve block: important procedure in clinical practice. Rev Bras Anestesiol. 2012;62(1):96–104. https://doi.org/10.1016/S0034-7094(12)70108-3.
3. Hewson DW, Oldman M, Bedforth NM. Regional anesthesia for shoulder surgery. BJA Edu. 2019;19:98–104.
4. Sun C, Ji X, Zhang X, Ma Q, Yu P, Cai X, Yang H. Suprascapular nerve block is a clinically attractive alternative to interscalene nerve block during arthroscopic shoulder surgery: a meta-analysis of randomized controlled trials. J Orthop Surg Res. 2021;16(1):376. https://doi.org/10.1186/s13018-021-02515-1.
5. Boonsong P, Jaroenarpornwatana A, Boonhong J. Preliminary study of suprascapular nerve block (SSNB) in hemiplegic shoulder pain. J Med Assoc Thail. 2009;92(12):1669–74.
6. Haque R, Baruah RK, Bari A, Sawah A. Is suprascapular nerve block better than intra-articular corticosteroid injection for the treatment of adhesive capsulitis of the shoulder? A randomized controlled study. Ortop Traumatol Rehabil. 2021;23(3):157–65. https://doi.org/10.5604/01.3001.0014.9152.
7. Harmon D, Hearty C. Ultrasound-guided suprascapular nerve block technique. Pain Physician. 2007;10(6):743–6.
8. Roark GL. Suprascapular nerve block at the spinoglenoid notch. Reg Anesth Pain Med. 2003;28(4):361–2. https://doi.org/10.1016/s1098-7339(03)00181-0.
9. del-Olmo C, de-Diego P, Morillas P, Garcia-Navlet M. Ultrasound-guided pain interventions in shoulder region. Tech Reg Anesth Pain Manag. 2013;17(3):81–95.
10. Laumonerie P, Ferré F, Cances J, Tibbo ME, Roumiguié M, Mansat P, Minville V. Ultrasound-guided proximal suprascapular nerve block: a cadaveric study. Clin Anat. 2018;31(6):824–9.
11. Shanahan EM, Smith MD. The safety of suprascapular nerve block. Reg Anesth Pain Med. 2012;37(1):120–1. https://doi.org/10.1097/AAP.0b013e3182320d59. Author reply 121.
12. Sehmbi H, Johnson M, Dhir S. Ultrasound-guided subomohyoid suprascapular nerve block and phrenic nerve involvement: a cadaveric dye study. Reg Anesth Pain Med. 2019;44(5):561–4. https://doi.org/10.1136/rapm-2018-100075.

Further Reading

Auyong DB, Hanson NA, Joseph RS, Schmidt BE, Slee AE, Yuan SC. Comparison of anterior suprascapular, supraclavicular, and interscalene nerve block approaches for major outpatient arthroscopic shoulder surgery: a randomized, double-blind, noninferiority trial. Anesthesiology. 2018;129(1):47–57. https://doi.org/10.1097/ALN.0000000000002208.

Brachial Plexus Blocks

Joseph M. Hanna and Ramsey N. Saad

Essential Concepts

- Bedside analgesia of the upper limb can be achieved by blocking the brachial plexus at different stages along its course.
- The four most common approaches used are interscalene, supraclavicular, infraclavicular, and axillary blocks.
- Ultrasound guidance has allowed clinicians to visualize the needle position in real time in relation to the various structures. It has proven especially useful in patients with anatomical variations.

1 Brachial Plexus Blocks

Overview

Bedside analgesia of the upper limb can be achieved by blocking the brachial plexus at different stages along its course. The four most common approaches used are interscalene, supraclavicular, infraclavicular, and axillary blocks. Ultrasound guidance has allowed clinicians to visualize the needle position in real time in relation to the various structures. It has proven especially useful in patients with anatomical variations [1]. The purpose of this chapter is to review the pertinent clinical anatomy of the brachial plexus as well as the ultrasound-guided techniques for the most common approaches used to block it. Will also focus on risks and possible

J. M. Hanna · R. N. Saad (✉)
Henry Ford Health, One Ford Place, Detroit, MI, USA
e-mail: JHANNA14@HFHS.ORG; rsaad2@hfhs.org

D. Souza et al. (eds.), *Bedside Pain Management Interventions*,
https://doi.org/10.1007/978-3-031-11188-4_52

complications that could arise during the performance of such blocks with the intention to anticipate and hopefully avoid them.

2 Common Indications and Contraindications

Interscalene block provides analgesia from the distal extent of the clavicle, shoulder joint, and proximal humerus [2]. Supraclavicular brachial plexus block provides analgesia from the mid-humerus to the fingertips. Infraclavicular brachial plexus block provides analgesia from mid-humerus to the fingertips. This block typically spares the intercostobrachial nerve.

Contraindications for Interscalene block include pulmonary disease, heart disease, cellulitis/abscess over the site of injection, patient refusal, and allergy to the local anesthetic. Morbid obesity may be a relative contraindication as respiratory insufficiency can result in hemi-diaphragmatic paralysis. As for supraclavicular and infraclavicular blocks, avoid if the patient has cellulitis and/or abscess over the site of injection. In the case of the supraclavicular block, in particular, use caution in patients with poor pulmonary reserve, as an accidental pneumothorax may significantly worsen their respiratory status (example: known pneumonia on the contralateral side).

3 Clinical Anatomy of the Brachial Plexus

The brachial plexus is a network of nerve fibers that supply the skin and musculature of the upper limb. It begins in the root of the neck, passes through the axilla, and runs through the entire upper extremity. The plexus is formed by the anterior rami of cervical spinal nerves C5, C6, C7 and C8, and the first thoracic spinal nerve, T1. The brachial plexus is divided into five parts; roots, trunks, divisions, cords and branches (see Fig. 1).

Roots

The roots of the brachial plexus are formed by the anterior rami of spinal nerves C5-T1 (the posterior divisions innervate the skin and musculature of the intrinsic back muscles). After their formation, these nerves pass between the anterior and middle scalene muscles to enter the base of the neck.

Trunks

At the base of the neck, the roots of the brachial plexus converge to form three trunks. These structures are named by their relative anatomical location: Superior trunk—combination of C5 and C6 roots. Middle trunk—continuation of C7. Inferior

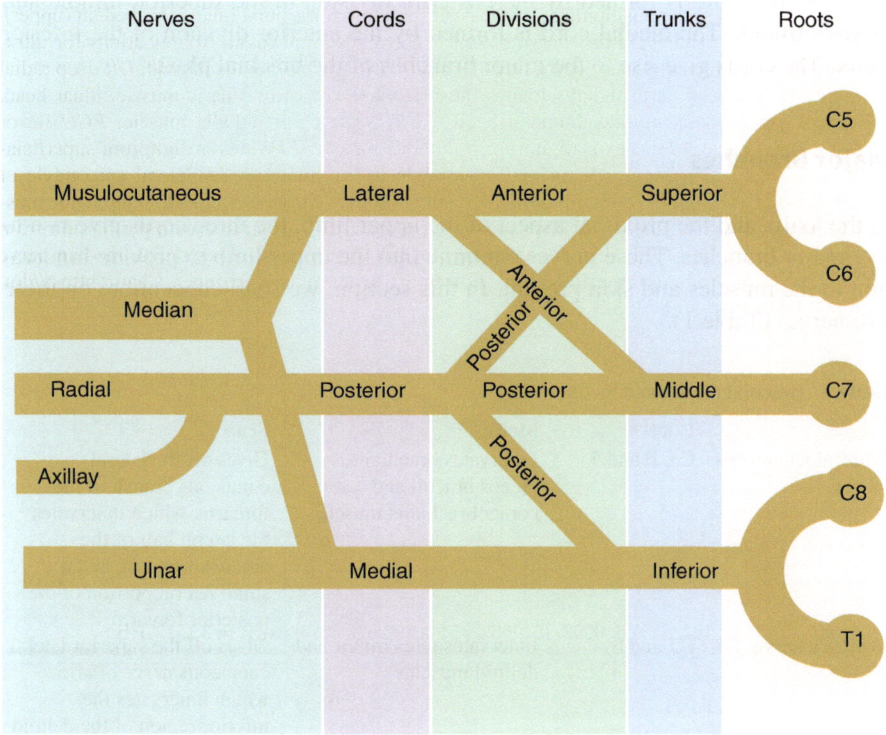

Fig. 1 Brachial plexus diagram, as labeled

trunk—combination of C8 and T1 roots.The trunks traverse laterally, crossing the posterior triangle of the neck.

Divisions

Each trunk divides into two branches within the posterior triangle of the neck. One division moves anteriorly (toward the front of the body) and the other posteriorly (towards the back of the body). Thus, they are known as the anterior and posterior divisions. We now have three anterior and three posterior nerve fibers. These divisions leave the posterior triangle and pass into the axilla. They recombine into the cords of the brachial plexus.

Cords

Once the anterior and posterior divisions have entered the axilla, they combine together to form three cords, named by their position relative to the axillary artery. The lateral cord is formed by the anterior division of the superior and middle trunks

The posterior cord is formed by the posterior division of the superior, middle and inferior trunks. The medial cord is formed by the anterior division of the inferior trunk. The cords give rise to the major branches of the brachial plexus.

Major Branches

In the axilla and the proximal aspect of the upper limb, the three cords give rise to five major branches. These nerves continue into the upper limb to provide innervation to the muscles and skin present. In this section, we shall concentrate on these five nerves (Table 1).

Table 1 Brachial plexus and its branches

Nerve	Roots	Motor	Sensory
Musculocutaneous nerve	C5, 6 and 7	Innervates brachialis, biceps brachii and coracobrachialis muscles	Gives off the lateral cutaneous branch of the forearm, which innervates the lateral half of the anterior forearm, and a small lateral portion of the posterior forearm
Axillary nerve	C5 and 6	Innervates teres minor and deltoid muscles	Gives off the superior lateral cutaneous nerve of arm, which innervates the inferior region of the deltoid
Median nerve	C6-T1. (Also contains fibers from C5 in some individuals)	Innervates most of the flexor muscles in the forearm, the thenar muscles, and the two lateral lumbricals associated with the index and middle fingers	Gives off the palmar cutaneous branch, which innervates the lateral part of the palm, and the digital cutaneous branch, which innervates the lateral three and a half fingers on the anterior (palmar) surface of the hand
Radial nerve	C5-T1	Innervates the triceps brachii, and the muscles in the posterior compartment of the forearm (which are primarily, but not exclusively, extensors of the wrist and fingers)	Innervates the posterior aspect of the arm and forearm, and the posterolateral aspect of the hand
Ulnar nerve	C8 and T1	Innervates the muscles of the hand (apart from the thenar muscles and two lateral lumbricals), flexor carpi ulnaris and medial half of flexor digitorum profundus	Innervates the anterior and posterior surfaces of the medial one and half fingers, and associated palm area

Anatomic Variations

There are many variations in the anatomy of the brachial plexus and in the course of the terminal nerves and vascular elements [3]. The plexus may include anterior rami from C4 to C8 ("prefixed") or, less commonly, from C5 to T2 ("postfixed"). The presence of the connective tissue sheath that invests the plexus at various regions are controversial. A continuous, tubular sheath has been shown unlikely, especially in the axillary region. A more convoluted and septated structure may be the cause of nonuniform distribution of local anesthetic in many cases, which supports the findings that multiple injection techniques may be superior [4] C5 and/or C6 nerve roots may traverse either through or anterior to the anterior scalene muscle [5]. In many cadaver specimens, no inferior trunk exists [6]. A single cord or a pair of cords may develop. It has been observed that no discrete posterior cord forms in some cases, with the posterior divisions diverging to form terminal nerves. The terminal nerves may lie in various relations to the axillary vessels. The musculocutaneous nerve may fuse to or have communications with the median nerve, which can result in the absence of the former from within the coracobrachialis muscle. Communication between the median and ulnar nerves in the forearm are common, with the median nerve replacing the innervation to various muscles normally supplied by the ulnar nerve [7]. There may also be variations with respect to the vessels within the arm, with aberrant formations including double axillary veins, high origin of the radial artery, and double brachial arteries.

Peripheral Nerve Ultrasound Imaging

Peripheral nerves have a fascicular or "honeycomb" echotexture [8]. This consists of the mixture of nerve fiber (hypoechoic) and connective tissue (hyperechoic) content within the nerve. Because there is little connective tissue within more central nerves (e.g., the cervical ventral rami of the brachial plexus), these nerves have a monofascicular or oligofascicular appearance on ultrasound scans. Nerves that are surrounded by hypoechoic muscle are usually easier to visualize than nerves that are surrounded by hyperechoic fat because the nerve borders are more evident. Peripheral nerves have a complex architecture. The connective tissue content and fascicle count of peripheral nerves vary directly. That is, the amount of connective tissue is more abundant in multifascicular nerves. The connective tissue within nerves protects the fascicles from injury. Therefore, monofascicular nerves are more vulnerable to damage. High ultrasound frequencies (10–15 MHz) provide better resolution of nerve fascicles. Short-axis sliding (sliding the transducer along the known nerve path with the nerve viewed in short axis) is a powerful technique not only to identify small nerves with ultrasound but also assess the longitudinal distribution of local anesthetic along the nerve.

4 Equipment and Supplies

The same equipment is basically needed for all approaches to brachial plexus block: High frequency (more than 10 MHz) linear ultrasound probe, Chlorhexidine 2% or povidone iodine skin disinfectant solution, Local anesthetic; for longer duration blocks bupivacaine 0.5% or ropivacaine 0.5%, for shorter blocks lidocaine 2% or mepivacaine 1.5%, A 10–20 mL syringe with extension tubing, Short bevel block needle (10 cm, 22–18 gauge), Sterile ultrasound probe cover, Sterile ultrasound gel and Standard vitals monitoring equipment (NIBP, rhythm monitoring, +/− pulse oximetry).

5 Interscalene Block

Interscalene block is indicated mostly for surgical anesthesia to the shoulder, upper arm, and forearm but is often insufficient for the hand [9]. It frequently spares C8 and T1 fibers, which innervate the ulnar border of the forearm. Low interscalene block (below C6) may provide sufficient anesthesia and analgesia for procedures on the lower arm. The landmarks of the block are Sternal head of the sternocleidomastoid muscle, Clavicular head of the sternocleidomastoid muscle, Upper border of the cricoid cartilage and Clavicle. The patient is positioned supine, with their head slightly rotated to the contralateral side. The head-of-bed elevation should be about 45°. The semi sitting (beach-chair) position helps comfort the patient, lowers the arm by gravity, and brings the plane of imaging closer to the plane of the display. The interscalene groove lies immediately behind the lateral border of the clavicular head of the sternocleidomastoid muscle at the level of the cricoid cartilage (C6). The operator stands either at the head or at the side of the bed, depending on the side of the block and the handedness of the operator. Prepare the needle insertion site and other applicable skin areas with an antiseptic solution. Maintain sterility of the US probe with a standard sleeve cover or transparent dressing.

Begin by scanning anteriorly at the cricoid cartilage level (C6) with movement from anterior and medial to posterior and lateral toward the interscalene groove, other option is to scan proximally from the supraclavicular fossa to the interscalene location. At the supraclavicular fossa, the brachial plexus (trunks/divisions) can be seen in short axis as a tightly enclosed cluster (i.e., honeycomb-like), superior and lateral to the subclavian artery. After tracing the nerves in a proximal fashion toward the interscalene groove, the nerve structures (roots/trunks) are visualized in a sagittal oblique section as three (usually) or up to five round or oval-shaped hypoechoic structures lying between the scalenus anterior and medius muscles (see Figs. 2, 3, and 4).

C8 and T1 roots may be difficult to identify because of their depth. Infiltrate the skin at the determined needle insertion site with local anesthetic. 22-gauge, insulated 50-mm echogenic needle is introduced in plane to the probe and advanced to a maximum of 3 cm for most patients. The needle is moved from lateral to medial

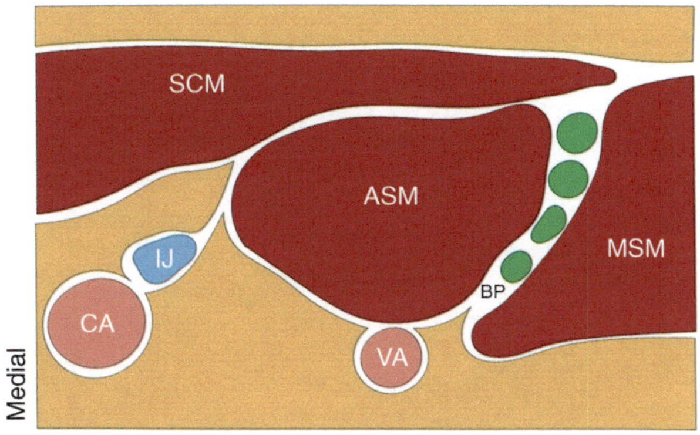

Fig. 2 Ultrasound-guided interscalene block diagram. *IJ* internal jugular vein, *CA* carotid artery, *VA* vertebral artery, *SCM* sternocleidomastoid muscle, *ASM* anterior scalene muscle, *MSM* middle scalene muscle, *BP* brachial plexus

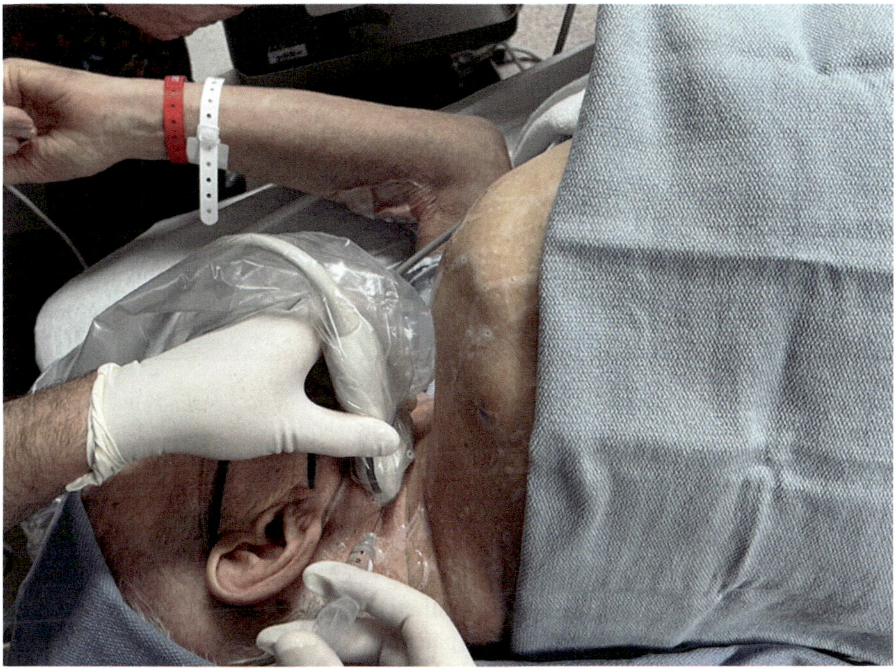

Fig. 3 Patient and transducer orientation, needle trajectory as seen

(still slightly caudad) to first pass through the scalenus medius muscle before entering the interscalene groove. It is recommended to use normal saline to enable further nerve localization. The needle tip should be positioned adjacent to the components of the brachial plexus for injection within the interscalene groove. Most authors recommend a multiple injection technique to ensure complete plexus anesthesia. With this approach the initial aim of the needle is deep (under the more caudal elements of the plexus) so that the brachial plexus rises closer to the skin

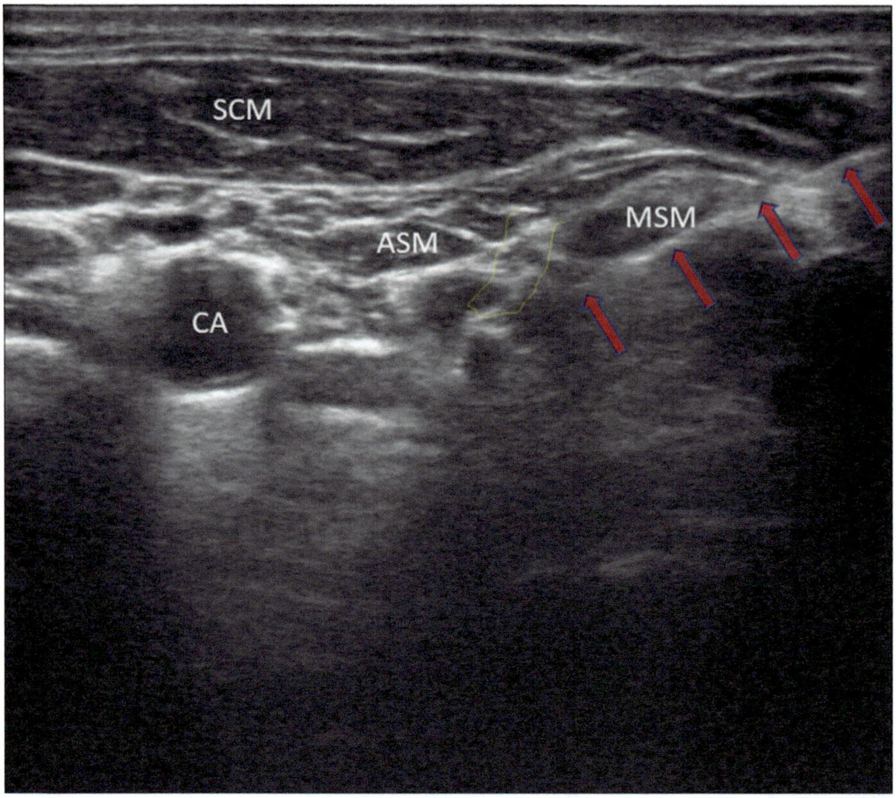

Fig. 4 Ultrasound-guided interscalene block. Red arrows point to the needle. Yellow line—brachial plexus, *CA* carotid artery, *SCM* sternocleidomastoid muscle, *ASM* anterior scalene muscle, *MCM* middle scalene muscle

surface with the injection of local anesthetic. This makes the subsequent needle passes easier to perform. Inferior trunk sparing occurs less often with this multiple injection ultrasound technique. Local anesthetic distention in this compartment can be seen by US as a hypoechoic (fluid) expansion. If a continuous block is indicated, the bevel of the introducing needle should be directed laterally. Placement of a stimulating catheter may be aided by dilating the perineural space with D5W, which will allow the user to monitor the catheter's advancement to a location where motor response is maintained at <0.5 mA. Securing catheters in the freely mobile neck is a challenge. Some prefer to secure the catheter by tunneling 3–4 cm below the skin by passing it back through an intravenous catheter that has been introduced subcutaneously near the entry site. Despite the fact that subarachnoid or intraneural injection can occur even when the threshold current is >0.4 mA, it is advisable to avoid injecting when the current responses are less than 0.4 mA. During OOP US-guided technique, angling the needle more than 45° should be avoided as the needle may be inserted too deep and directed toward the spinal cord.

Complications

Complications from this approach are related to the structures located in the vicinity of the tubercle. The cupola of the lung is close, particularly on the right side, and can be contacted if the needle is directed too far caudally. Pneumothorax should be considered if cough or chest pain is produced while exploring for the nerve. If the needle is allowed to pass directly medially, it may enter the intervertebral foramen, and injection of local anesthetic may produce spinal or epidural anesthesia. The vertebral artery passes posteriorly at the level of the sixth vertebra to lie in its canal in the transverse process that can be seen as a pulsatile structure deep to the plexus; direct injection into this vessel can rapidly produce central nervous system toxicity and convulsions. Careful aspiration and incremental injections are important to help avoid both of these potential problems. Even with appropriate injection, local anesthetic solution can spread to contiguous nerves. It may produce cervical plexus block, including motor fibers to the diaphragm. Horner's syndrome is common because of spread to the sympathetic chain. Neuropathy of the C6 root is a potential problem because the needle may unintentionally pin the nerve root against the tubercle and predispose to intraneural injection.

6 Supraclavicular Block [10]

The supraclavicular block targets the trunks and/or divisions of the brachial plexus, depending on the location of the injection site and the patient's anatomy. Landmarks and positioning is similar to the interscalene block. The probe is first placed in a coronal oblique plane just above the upper border of the clavicle. Start scanning from lateral to medial until the subclavian artery is identified. Dorsal and ventral rotations of the probe may be necessary to optimize imaging. Transducer rotation clockwise often facilitate best imaging of the tissue space (sheath) containing the plexus. With the subclavian artery in the middle of the Ultrasound screen (anechoic, hypodense, pulsatile and round, can be verified with color doppler), the plexus enclosed within the brachial plexus sheath (cluster of hypoechoic "grape-like" structures surrounded by a hyperechoic lining) is located superolateral to the artery with the first rib (hyperechoic line with dorsal shadowing) noted under the neurovascular bundle. The anechoic subclavian vein may be seen inferomedial to the artery. Infiltrate the skin at the determined needle insertion site with local anesthetic (see Fig. 3).

A 22-gauge, insulated 50-mm echogenic needle or less is inserted immediately above the clavicle and introduced in plane to the probe and advanced from lateral to medial with a slight cephalad angle. The brachial plexus is very shallow at this location, typically 1–3 cm; therefore, inclination of the needle should be equally shallow. Consider the use normal saline to help with nerve localization (Hydro-localization). Consider the usage of additional monitor to prevent intraneural injection by having the threshold stimulation >0.2 mA. Best to deposit local anesthetic next to the nerve structures immediately lateral to the subclavian artery on top of the first rib. Typically, 20–25 mL of local anesthetic is required for adequate block. It has been suggested that lower volumes can be used in older patients. The ultrasound-guided continuous supraclavicular block is in many ways similar to the technique used for interscalene catheter placement. The goal is to place the catheter within the vicinity of the trunks and divisions of the brachial plexus adjacent to the subclavian artery. The needle is typically inserted in plane from the lateral-to-medial direction so that the tip is just posterior to the brachial plexus sheath. The needle is then advanced to pierce the sheath, followed by catheter placement.

Complications

The greatest risk of the block is pneumothorax given that the cupola of the lung lies just medial to the first rib. Overall, Pneumothorax is a rare but possible complication, typically delayed rather than immediate, therefore, it is important to keep the needle tip visible at all times. The risk of pneumothorax increases in: Right sided block, as the cupola of the lung is higher on that side as well as in tall, thin patients. The neck is a highly vascular area, and care must be exercised to avoid needle placement or injection into the vascular structures (subclavian artery, dorsal scapular artery, suprascapular artery and the transverse cervical artery). The use of color Doppler before needle placement and injection is highly recommended. The inability to initiate injection with an opening injection pressure of less than 15 psi may signal an intrafascicular injection.

7 Infraclavicular Block

This approach targets the cords of the brachial plexus [11–13]. The landmarks of this block is mainly the medial aspect of the coracoid process. The patient is placed in the supine position with the head turned to the opposite side. The arm may be to the patient's side or in the abduction position. Immediately medial and inferior to the coracoid process, position the transducer in a parasagittal plain to visualize a short-axis view of the brachial plexus cords and axillary artery and vein. The pectoralis major and minor muscles are superficial to the abovementioned neurovascular bundle. The axillary vein lies medial and caudad to the artery. The lateral cord of the plexus is easily visualized. The medial cord lies between the axillary artery and vein, and the posterior cord can be deep to the axillary artery (see Fig. 4).

Another advantage of using ultrasound is to account for anatomic variations. The skin is infiltrated with local anesthetic. A 22-gauge 50 mm echogenic needle is inserted cephalad to the probe and is then advanced caudally and posteriorly at approximately 30° to the skin, with the goal being to place the needle and visualize local anesthetic spread posterior to the axillary artery next to the posterior cord. Repositioning the needle may be required if inadequate spread is noted around the

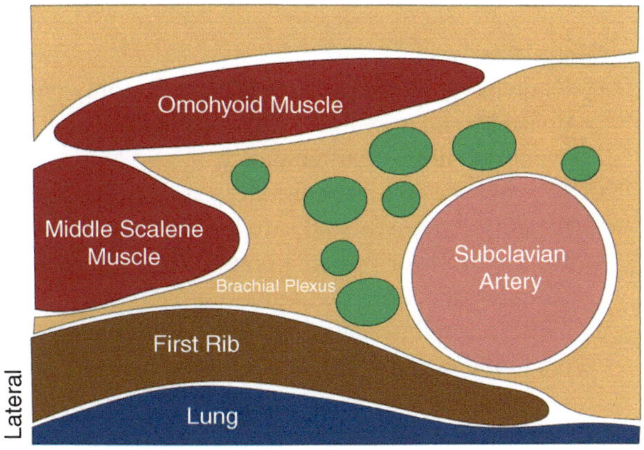

Fig. 5 Ultrasound-guided supraclavicular block diagram, as labeled

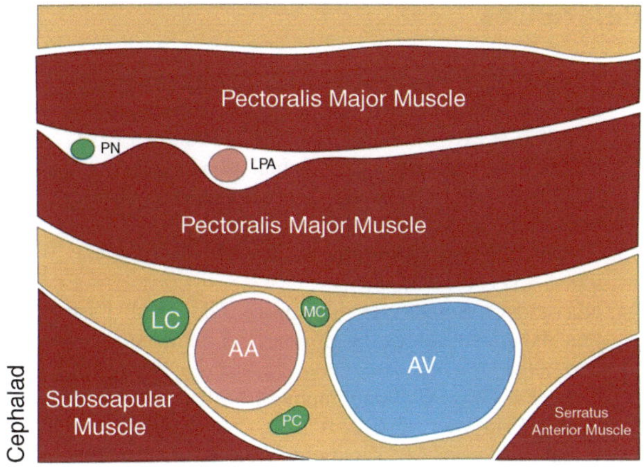

Fig. 6 Ultrasound-guided infraclavicular block diagram, as labeled. *AA* axillary artery, *AV* axillary vein, *PN* pectoral nerve, *LC* lateral cord, *MC* medial cord, *BC* posterior cord

lateral and medial cords with the initial needle placement. The technique is similar to block under ultrasound visualization. One technical aspect, though, is sometimes the catheter may be adjacent to one cord and not provide adequate coverage with small volume infusions. Increasing the volume or injecting boluses may sometimes improve coverage of the distribution of the other cords (Figs. 5 and 6).

Complications

Greatly reduced by the use of real time ultrasound and needle visualization at all times. Intravascular puncture and injection is a documented risk. Pneumothorax risk is decreased by lateral needle placement. Lower risk of phrenic nerve blockade and stellate ganglion block compared to interscalene and supraclavicular approaches.

Clinical Pearls

- Knowledge of the Brachial plexus anatomy and possible anatomical variations is mandatory to effectively and safely perform upper extremity blocks even with ultrasound guidance.
- Appropriate patient positioning and scanning techniques are helpful in performing successful and safe blocks.
- Be watchful for possible complications/side effects, like accidental intravascular injection, blocking of adjacent nerve structure (example: phrenic nerve or stellate ganglion) and/or unintended organ injury (for instance pneumothorax mainly with supraclavicular block).

References

1. Mian A, Chaudhry I, Huang R, Rizk E, Tubbs RS, Loukas M. Brachial plexus anesthesia: a review of the relevant anatomy, complications, and anatomical variations. Clin Anat. 2014;27(2):210–21. https://doi.org/10.1002/ca.22254.
2. Pester JM, Varacallo M. Brachial plexus block techniques. [Updated 13 Feb 2019]. In: StatPearls. Treasure Island, FL: StatPearls Publishing; 2019. https://www.ncbi.nlm.nih.gov/books/NBK470213/.
3. Barash P. Clinical Anesthesia. 7th ed. Philadelphia: Wolters Kluwer. 2013, p. 951. ISBN 978-1-4511-4419-2.
4. Klaastad O, Smedby O, Thompson GE, et al. Distribution of local anesthetic in axillary brachial plexus block: a clinical and magnetic resonance imaging study. Anesthesiology. 2002;96:1315–24.
5. Kessler J, Gray AT. Sonography of scalene muscle anomalies for brachial plexus block. Reg Anesth Pain Med. 2007;32:172–3.
6. Uysal II, Seker M, Karabulut AK, et al. Brachial plexus variations in human fetuses. Neurosurgery. 2003;53:676–84.
7. Amoiridis G. Median–ulnar nerve communications and anomalous innervation of the intrinsic hand muscles: an electrophysiological study. Muscle Nerve. 1992;15:576–9.
8. Gray A. Atlas for ultrasound-guided regional anesthesia. Third Edition, Chapter 18, Peripheral nerves. 2019. ISBN 9780323512107.
9. Barash P. Clinical Anesthesia. 7th ed. Philadelphia: Wolters Kluwer 2013, p. 960. ISBN 978-1-4511-4419-2.
10. Barash P. Clinical Anesthesia. 7th ed. Philadelphia: Wolters Kluwer 2013, p. 961. ISBN 978-1-4511-4419-2.
11. Barash P. Clinical Anesthesia 8th ed. Philadelphia: Wolters Kluwer. 2017, p. 970–72. ISBN 978-1-4963-3700-9.
12. Bonnel F. Microscopic anatomy of the adult human brachial plexus: an anatomical and histological basis for microsurgery. Microsurgery. 1984;5:107–18.
13. Brull R, McCartney CJ, Chan VW. A novel approach to infraclavicular brachial plexus block: the ultrasound experience. Anesth Analg. 2004;99:950–1.

Further Reading

Clinical anesthesia (Barash). 7th ed. Philadelphia: Wolters Kluwer. p. 951, 960–61.
Clinical anesthesia (Barash). 8th ed. Philadelphia: Wolters Kluwer; 2017. p. 970–72.

Axillary Nerve Block

Elizabeth A. Scholzen and Kristopher M. Schroeder

Essential Concepts

- Axillary nerve block, when combined with suprascapular nerve block, can provide adequate analgesia for shoulder surgery without concern for phrenic nerve involvement.
- Axillary nerve blockade can be performed at the bedside for procedures related to the deltoid in the emergency department and is technically less complex than performing a brachial plexus block for the same procedure.
- Axillary nerve blockade is well tolerated and easy to perform with ultrasound guidance or nerve stimulation.

1 Axillary Nerve Block

Overview

The axillary nerve branches off of the posterior cord of the brachial plexus before traversing through the quadrangle space and along the posterior aspect of the humerus. It provides sensory to the deltoid as well as the glenohumeral joint meaning that it can be used for both analgesia of the shoulder and the deltoid and can be used for surgeries related to either.

E. A. Scholzen · K. M. Schroeder (✉)
Department of Anesthesiology, University of Wisconsin School of Medicine and Public Health, University of Wisconsin, Madison, WI, USA
e-mail: naab@wisc.edu; kmschro1@wisc.edu

D. Souza et al. (eds.), *Bedside Pain Management Interventions*,
https://doi.org/10.1007/978-3-031-11188-4_53

Indications and Contraindications

- Axillary nerve blockade may be utilized for anesthesia/analgesia in the setting of surgical procedures involving the deltoid such as deltoid abscess incision and drainage that may be performed in the emergency department. Deltoid abscesses are most commonly encountered in the setting of intravenous drug abuse. Axillary nerve blockade provides analgesia in the distribution required for proximal deltoid abscess I&D. However, anterior abscess extension towards the axilla may not be adequately anesthetized with an axillary nerve block and supplemental local anesthetic administration may be required [1].
- Axillary nerve blockade combined with suprascapular nerve blockade may be utilized as an alternative to a brachial plexus block for shoulder surgery. While interscalene blockade may be considered the "gold standard" for the provision of analgesia following surgical procedures of the shoulder, this technique can be associated with a number of potential undesirable outcomes including phrenic nerve blockade, vascular puncture, pulmonary injury and Horner's syndrome. The risk of these complications can be minimized with the provision of axillary and suprascapular nerve blocks. It is important to remember that the combination of these blocks does not provide as complete analgesia when compared to an interscalene block and it is unlikely that these techniques will provide surgical anesthesia and additional analgesics may be required in the immediate post-operative period [2]. Contrainidications include patient refusal, infection at the injection site, axillary lymphadenopathy, and severe coagulopathy.

Clinical Anatomy

The axillary nerve is a branch of the brachial plexus off the posterior cord of the plexus; encompassing fibers from C5 and C6 nerve routes (Fig. 1). An infraclavicular ultrasound image of the brachial plexus demonstrates the three cords (medial, lateral, and posterior) surrounding the axillary nerve (Fig. 2). The nerve then travels to the axilla posterior to the axillary artery and exits the axilla through the quadrangular space (Table 1, Fig. 3). It then wraps around the humerus where it divides into its terminal branches [3]. See Fig. 4 for sensory innervation of the arm.

- Posterior terminal branch: Sensory innervation of the skin over the deltoid as well as motor to the posterior deltoid and the teres minor muscles.
- Anterior terminal branch: Sensory innervation through cutaneous branches to the anterior and lateral shoulder and motor innervation to the anterior deltoid
- Articular branch: Innervation of the glenohumeral joint

Equipment and Supplies

Axillary nerve blocks are easily performed at the bedside in the emergency department or in the preoperative area. Typically, a 100 mm insulated, short bevel needle

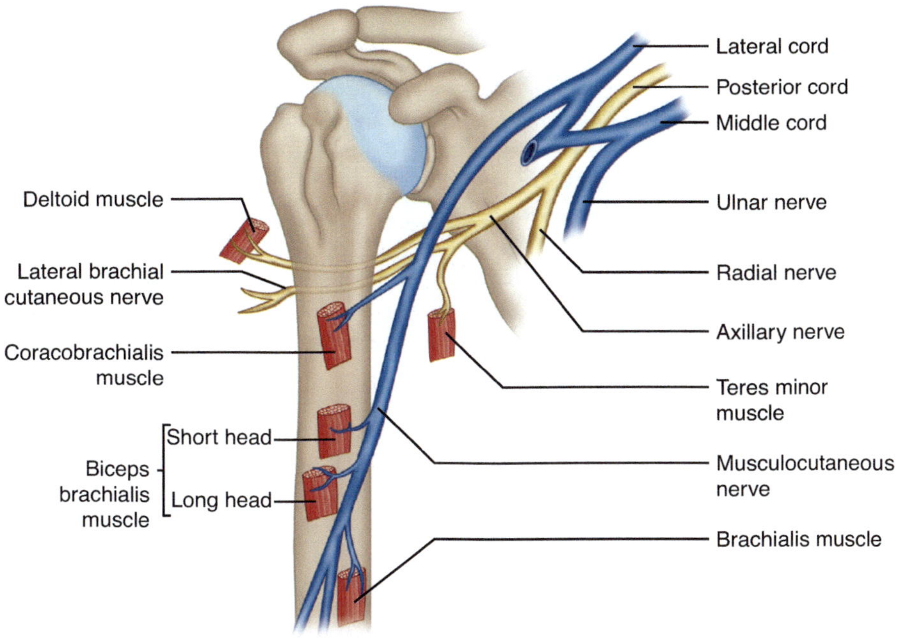

Fig. 1 Take off of axillary nerve from the posterior cord

is used with or without nerve stimulation. Ten to fifteen milliliters of 0.25% bupivacaine with 2.5 mcg/mL epinephrine is typically injected following the use of subcutaneous lidocaine for cutaneous infiltration (Table 2).

Axillary Nerve Block Technique

The axillary nerve is best blocked after it exits the quadrangle space and runs along the posterior aspect of the humerus. Blocking the nerve more distally prevents accidental intraarticular injection. The block is generally performed with the patient in the seated position with the targeted arm positioned at their side.

In a landmark based approach, the point of needle insertion is determined by identifying the cross section between a horizonal and vertical plane. The horizonal plane is determine by palpating the acromion process and the inferior aspect of the scapula and drawing a line between the two. The midway point of this line is the horizonal plane for the block. The vertical plane is determined by palpating the acromion process again and drawing a vertical line from this point vertically down the back of the humerus. The needle insertion point is at the intersection of these two lines [4].

A 100 mm insulated short bevel needle is inserted perpendicular to the skin and directed anteriorly. Motor stimulation of the anterior deltoid indicates appropriate

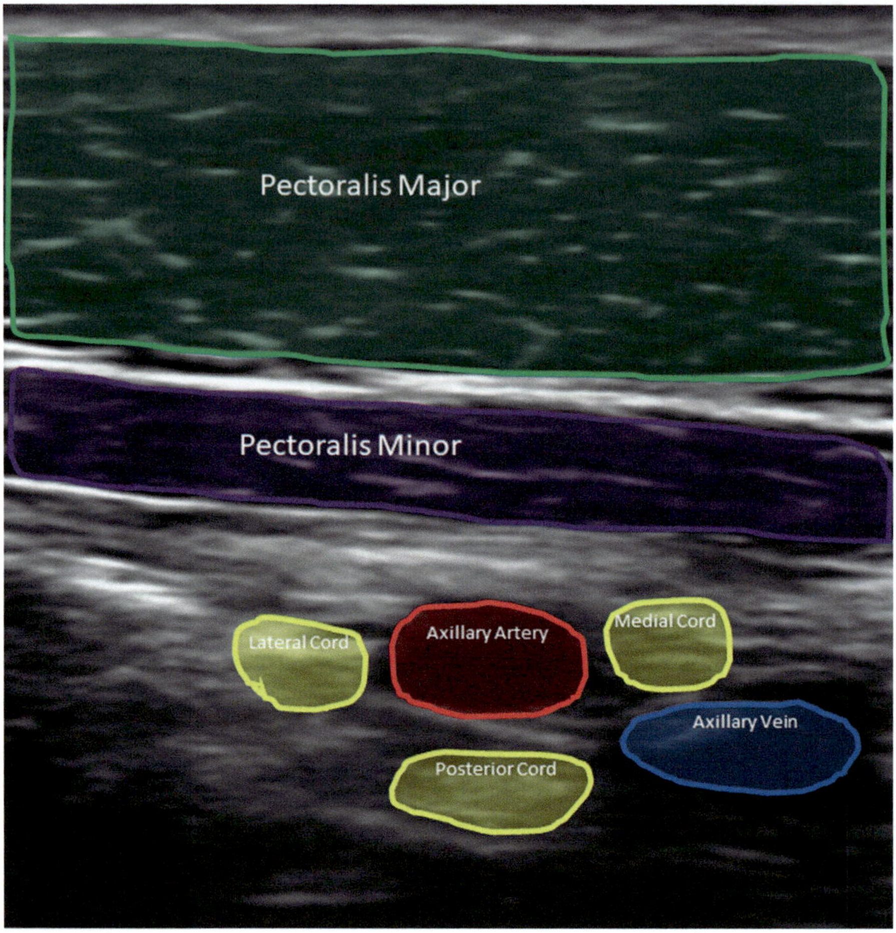

Fig. 2 Infraclavicular ultrasound image of the brachial plexus outlining the three cords of the brachial plexus

Table 1 Borders of quadrangular space

Superior	Teres minor
Inferior	Teres major
Lateral	Neck of the humerus
Medial	Triceps
Anterior	Subscapularis

localization of the axillary nerve. In the event that motor stimulation of the deltoid muscle is unable to be accomplished, the needle can be slowly redirected in the vertical plane until the anterior deltoid is stimulated. Once the location of the nerve is identified, 10–15 mL of 0.5% bupivacaine with 2.5 mcg/mL epinephrine is injected.

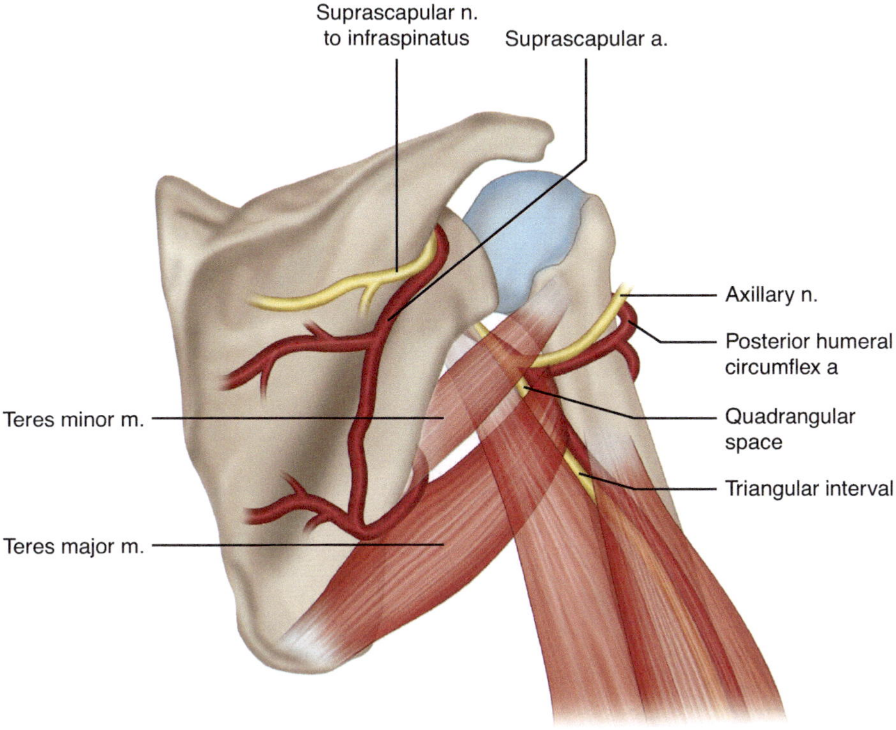

Fig. 3 Axillary nerve exits through the quadrangle space

Ultrasound Technique

Ultrasound guided axillary nerve blockade is best performed with the patient either sitting or in the lateral decubitus position with the targeted arm against the side of the patient's body. A high-frequency, linear ultrasound probe is placed on the humerus, see Fig. 5. On ultrasound, the deltoid muscle is visualized superficial to the nerve while the teres minor and triceps muscles will be visible on either side of the nerve. The posterior circumflex humeral artery is visualized posterior to the humerus. The axillary nerve may be visualized adjacent to the artery but this may not be a reliable finding in all patients. See Fig. 6. If uncertainty exists regarding nerve location on ultrasound imaging, simultaneous nerve stimulation may provide a dual-endpoint for nerve localization.

Potential Complications and Adverse Effects

This procedure is generally well tolerated. However, as with any procedure, risks are ever-present for any interventional procedure. In select patients, the posterior

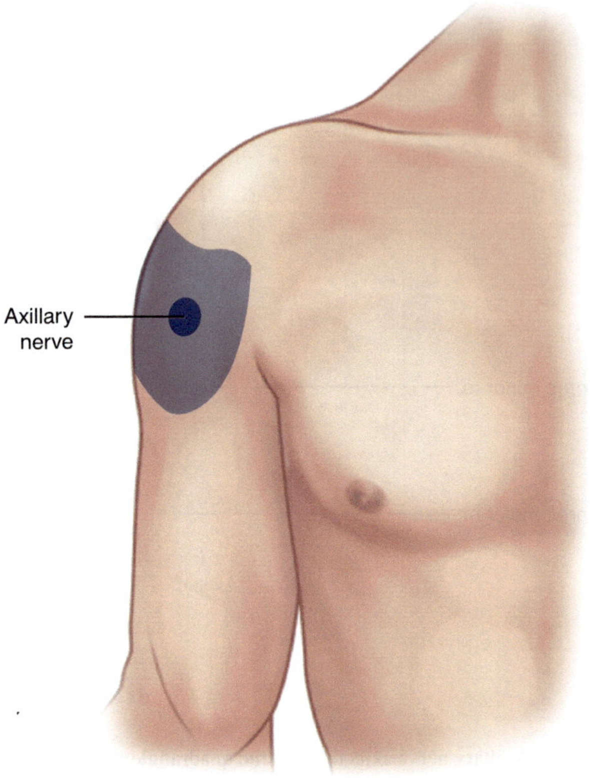

Fig. 4 Sensory innervation of the axillary nerve

Table 2 Required supplies for axillary nerve blocks

Syringe	20 mL syringe
Needle	100 mm insulated short bevel needle
Anesthetic	0.25% bupivacaine with 1:200,000 epinephrine

circumflex humeral artery may travel near the axillary nerve and therefore there is a risk of arterial injury or intraarterial injection. This risk may be significantly minimized through the utilization of ultrasound guidance [5]. The majority of complications related to axillary nerve block are not specific to the axillary nerve but rather apply to all peripheral nerve blocks [6] (Table 3) (C. L. Jeng, December 2010).

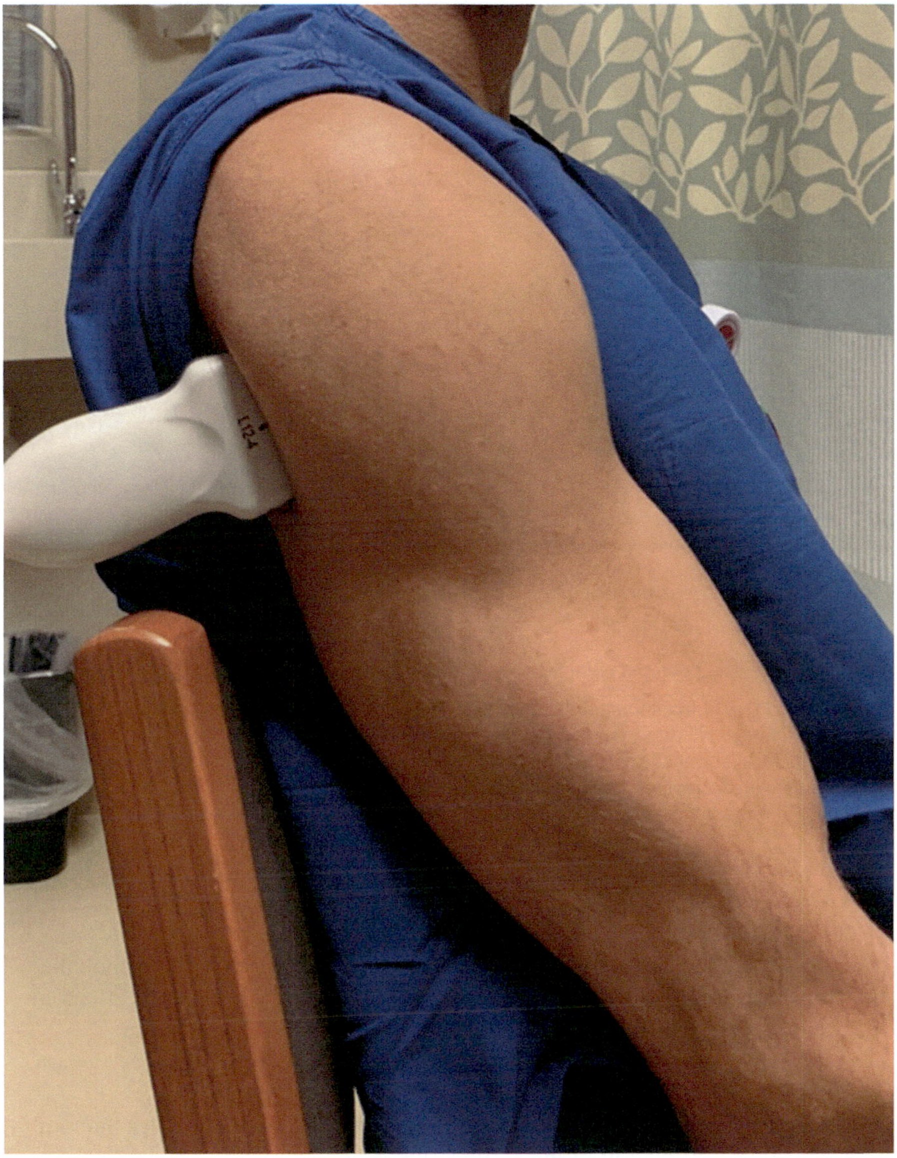

Fig. 5 Ultrasound position for obtaining axillary artery picture

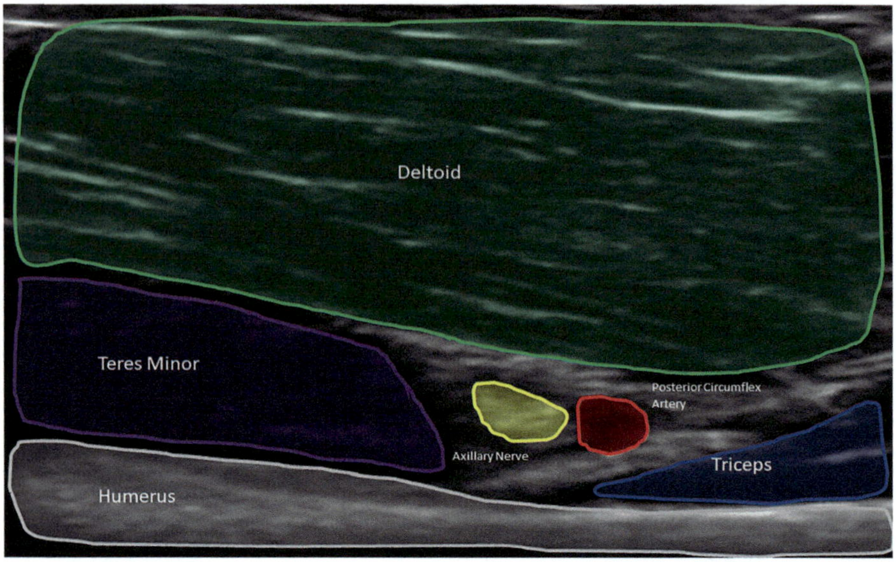

Fig. 6 Axillary artery on ultrasound

Table 3 Additional potential complications and adverse effects. References

• Increased risk of hematoma in patients with acquired or inherent coagulopathies
• Nerve damage via direct needle trauma or intraneural injection
• Risk of local anesthetic systemic toxicity (LAST) similar to all regional anesthesia procedures with accidental intravascular injection
• Anaphylaxis reaction to the local anesthetic used

Clinical and Technical Pearls

- Axillary and suprascapular nerve blocks are usually performed simultaneously to provide shoulder analgesia in patients with contraindications to interscalene blockade.
- Axillary nerve blocks can be easily performed in the emergency department for bedside procedures involving the deltoid.
- Attention should be paid to the location of the posterior circumflex humeral artery and utilization of ultrasound guidance may reduce the risk of inadvertent vascular puncture.

References

1. Lyons C, Herring AA. Ultrasound-guided axillary nerve block for ED incision and drainage of deltoid abscess. Am J Emerg Med. 2017;35(7):1032.e3–7.
2. Dhir S, Sondekoppam RV, Sharma R, Ganapathy S, Athwal GS. A comparison of combined suprascapular and axillary nerve blocks to interscalene nerve block for analgesia in arthroscopic shoulder surgery: an equivalence study. Reg Anesth Pain Med. 2016;41(5):564–71.
3. Jones O. The axillary nerve. Teach Me Anatomy; 2018.
4. Price DJ. The shoulder block: a new alternative to interscalene brachial plexus blockade for the control of postoperative shoulder pain. Anaesth Intensive Care. 2007;35:575–81.
5. Kim ED, Baek JW, Kim JS, Oh SA, Kim YH. Ultrasound-guided block of the axillary nerve: a prospective, randomized, single-blind study comparing interfascial and perivascular injections. Pain Physician. 2019;22(4):369–76.
6. Jeng CL, Torrillo TA, Rosenblatt MA. Complications of peripheral nerve blocks. Br J Anaesth. 2010;105(S1):i97–i107.

Further Reading

Peng P, Finlayson R, Lee SH, Bhatia A, editors. Ultrasound for interventional pain management: an illustrated procedural guide. 1st ed. New York: Springer Science; 2020. p. 1–377.

Bedside Pectoralis Minor and Scalene Muscles Injections

Reza Salajegheh, Logan D. Kinch, and Cody C. Rowan

Essential Concepts

- Ultrasound-guided Pectoralis Minor and Scalene Injections serve as potential diagnostic tools in the discovery of Neurogenic Thoracic Outlet Syndrome (NTOS) and Pectoralis Minor Syndrome
- Along with physical therapy, these procedures may also serve as potential therapeutic modalities in the treatment of NTOS.
- Goals of treatment with Pectoralis Minor and Scalene injections may be to interrupt a symptomatic flare, as part of maintenance therapy, or as a precursor to potential definitive surgical correction.
- The mechanism of action is unknown but is thought to involve relaxation of the musculature, resulting in alleviation of the neurogenic compression.
- Pain/symptomatic relief should be rapid (determination of relief should occur within the same visit) and may last hours, to days, to weeks, to months.
- Lateral pectoral nerve, located between pectoralis minor and pectoralis major muscles can be injected for relief of otherwise unexplained anterior shoulder pain.

R. Salajegheh (✉)
Department of Anesthesiology and Pain Medicine, University of Virginia Medical Center, Charlottesville, VA, USA

OrthoVirginia, Lynchburg, VA, USA
e-mail: Reza.Salajegheh@OrthoVirginia.com

L. D. Kinch
Department of Anesthesiology and Pain Medicine, University of Virginia Medical Center, Charlottesville, VA, USA
e-mail: LDK6GV@hscmail.mcc.virginia.edu

C. C. Rowan
Department of Pain Medicine, Northeast Georgia Physicians Group, Dawsonville, GA, USA
e-mail: CCR8EZ@hscmail.mcc.virginia.edu

D. Souza et al. (eds.), *Bedside Pain Management Interventions*,
https://doi.org/10.1007/978-3-031-11188-4_54

1 Bedside Pectoralis Minor and Scalene Muscles Injections

Overview

- Thoracic outlet syndrome is a controversial diagnosis in the evaluation of neck, shoulder, and upper extremity pain and paresthesias. Originally introduced in 1956, the term "Thoracic Outlet Syndrome" (TOS) was coined to describe neurovascular compression within the thoracic outlet as a possible cause for these symptoms [1]. The two primary subtypes of TOS include neurogenic thoracic outlet syndrome (NTOS) which will be the focus of this chapter and vascular thoracic outlet syndrome. Greater than 90% of cases of TOS are considered to be neurogenic in origin, and though sometimes categorized separately. Pectoralis Minor Syndrome does fall under this umbrella as well [2, 3]. Neurogenic TOS is further divided into "Disputed" or "True"; where true NTOS is defined as having objective diagnostic findings while disputed NTOS lacks these [2]. Indeed, an advantage of pectoralis minor and scalene muscles injections is that they may help to shift more cases from the "disputed", to the "true" subcategory. Along with physical therapy, these procedures may also serve as potential therapeutic modalities in the treatment of NTOS.

2 Indications and Contraindications

Neurogenic TOS is thought to be due to compression of brachial plexus structures within the interscalene triangle, the costoclavicular space, or the retropectoralis minor (subpectoralis) space [2]. This can be due to trauma, repetitive use, or congenital anatomic abnormalities [4]. Any circumstance that results in inadequate volume or reduced compliance of the thoracic outlet can cause neurogenic TOS, but the presence of these factors does not always prove symptomatic. Why this is the case is unclear, but it has contributed to the controversy surrounding the diagnosis. One explanation is the possibility of a double crush scenario, where nerve compression may remain subclinical unless it occurs at two or more sites [5]. In any case, a diagnosis of NTOS should be one of exclusion as provocative testing has proven to have a high false-positive rate [6]. If TOS is suspected, every effort should be made to confirm the diagnosis and treat conservatively, and pectoralis/scalene injections are a tool to that end (Tables 1, 2, and 3). The lateral pectoral nerve can be typically found in the fascial plane between pectoralis minor and pectoralis major muscles. A blockade of this nerve can be used for the relief of otherwise unexplained anterior shoulder pain.

Common indications for this procedure include neurogenic thoracic outlet syndrome. The procedure can be diagnostic or therapeutic. Common contraindications include infection at the injection site or systemic infection, known side effects or allergy to injectate, and patient refusal. Anticoagulation, including iatrogenic, or platelet dysfunction, including iatrogenic, are typically not considered to be contraindications.

Table 1 Symptomatology of neurogenic thoracic outlet syndrome (NTOS)

• Numbness or paresthesias in upper extremity
• Pain in neck, shoulder, or upper extremity
• Often unilateral, but can present bilaterally
• Occipital headaches
• Cold intolerance (sympathetically mediated rather than vascular source)
• Diminished dexterity

Table 2 Clinical tests for neurogenic thoracic outlet syndrome

• Elevated arm stress
• Supraclavicular pressure
• Cyriax release
• Upper limb tension
• Cervical rotation lateral flexion

Table 3 Other diagnoses to consider that may have similar symptomatology

Rule out other causes:
• Cervical radiculopathy
• Rotator cuff injury
• Peripheral nerve injury/impingement
• Psychological conditions
• CNS conditions such as CVA or MS

3 Clinical Anatomy

As mentioned, the "thoracic outlet" is comprised of three relevant spaces: the interscalene triangle, the costoclavicular space, and the retropectoralis minor (subpectoralis) space. The interscalene triangle is comprised of the anterior scalene muscle (anteriorly), the middle scalene muscle (posteriorly), and the medial surface of the first rib (inferiorly) (Fig. 1).

The retropectoralis minor space is comprised of the coracoid process superiorly, the pectoralis minor anteriorly, and ribs two through four posteriorly [2]. It is the interaction of the subclavian artery, vein, and brachial plexus with the described anatomy above that determines the subtype of TOS, as well as helps to guide the diagnostic and therapeutic course. Specifically, with NTOS, brachial plexus compression can occur between the anterior and middle scalene muscles, or as it passes below the pectoralis minor. This can be observed with the brachial plexus structures observed between the scalene musculature on ultrasound but is less obvious with the pectoralis minor (Fig. 2). The lateral pectoral nerve can be typically found in the fascial plane between pectoralis minor and pectoralis major muscles.

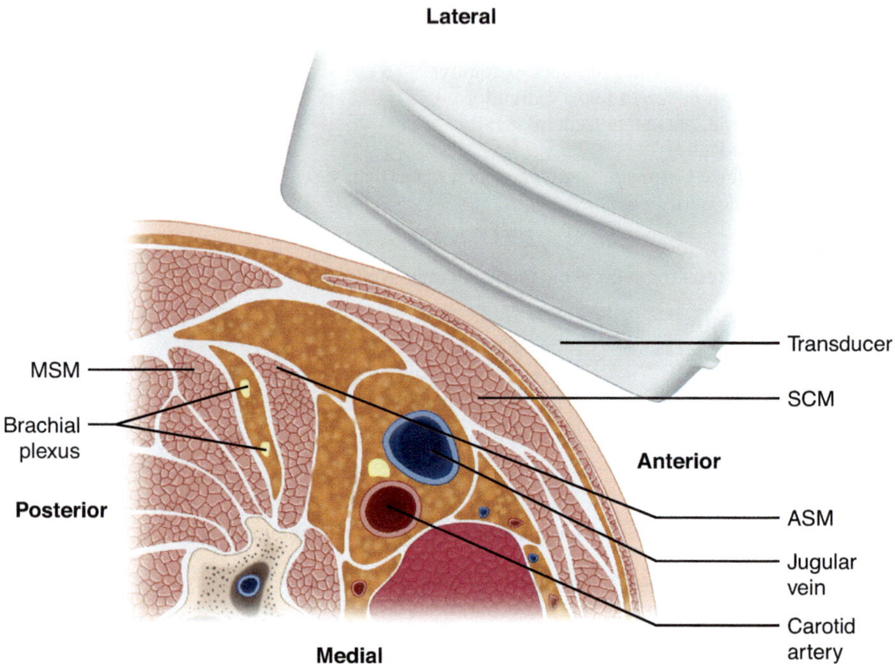

Fig. 1 Cross-sectional anatomy schematic. *ASM* anterior scalene muscle, *MSM* middle scalene muscle, *SCM* sternocleidomastoid muscle

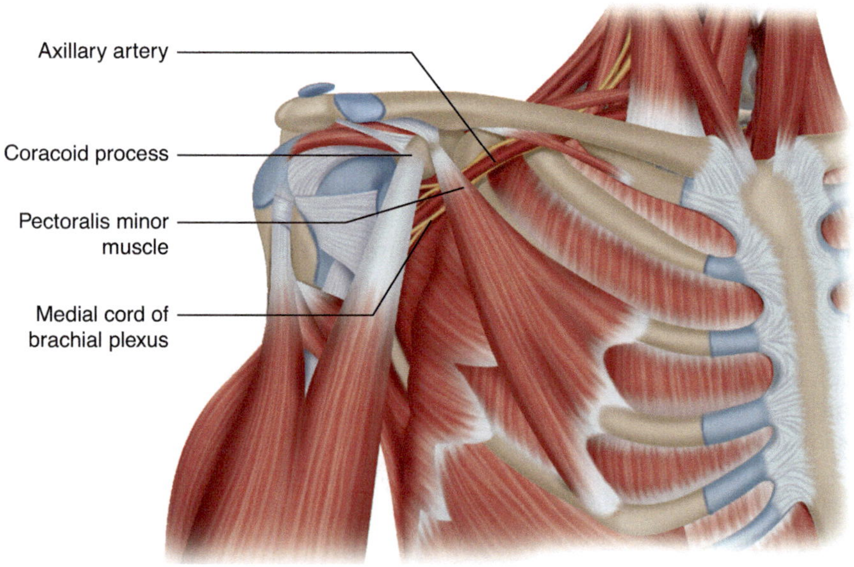

Fig. 2 Pectoralis minor muscle, anatomy schematic, as labeled

4 Equipment and Supplies

Anterior and middle scalene intramuscular injections can readily be performed at the bedside. Alcohol (or betadine in those allergic) based skin prep will be necessary for appropriate skin sterilization. A linear high-frequency ultrasound probe with sterile probe cover is utilized for identifying target muscles, critical structures, and needle guidance. A small syringe with local anesthetic (lidocaine), attached to a small gauge needle will be needed to attain cutaneous anesthesia. A 22–25 G needle, typically 1.5 for scalene injections, and up to 3.5 in. for pectoralis minor muscle injections, will be needed for in-plane advancement to the target tissue. A larger syringe with an anesthetic or an anesthetic and steroid combination will be needed for deposition of injectate at the target site(s). Similarly, ultrasound-guided pectoralis minor intramuscular injections are also straightforward and may utilize the same set of the equipment described above. Adjustments in needle size and ultrasound probe of choice may be required depending on patient body habitus (Table 4).

5 Anterior and Middle Scalene Injections

While these injections can be potentially performed utilizing landmarks we do not recommend that. The anterior and middle scalene intramuscular injections can be completed utilizing a similar view and approach as an interscalene nerve block. Patient placed semi-recumbent with head turned towards the contralateral shoulder. Perform a sterile wide prep over the neck and supraclavicular area (Fig. 3).

Utilizing a linear, high-frequency probe, identify the subclavian artery and associated brachial plexus. Track the brachial plexus cephalad until nerve roots C5–7 are identified between the anterior and middle scalene muscles (Fig. 4).

Maintain awareness of major vascular structures such as the carotid artery and internal jugular. Provide local anesthetic with approximately 1 ml of 1% lidocaine with a small gauge needle. Utilizing preferably an echogenic b-bevel needle, advance with an in-plane approach into the anterior and/or middle scalene muscle body. This is an intramuscular injection only, use caution to avoid deposition of local anesthetic outside of the muscle around the brachial plexus as this can create

Table 4 Equipment/medications needed for the procedure

Syringe	3 ml and 5–10 ml syringe
Needle	25–27 gauge or smaller for skin wheal 22–25 gauge 1.5 in. needle (may need 3.5 in. needle for pectoralis minor injection)
Local anesthetic	0.25–0.5% bupivacaine or 0.2–0.5% Ropivacaine 1–2% lidocaine (for skin wheal)
Corticosteroid	Triamcinolone 40–80 mg (*t*1/2 life: 18–36 h) Methylprednisolone 40–80 mg (*t*1/2 life: 18–36 h) Betamethasone 6–12 mg (*t*1/2 life: 36–54 h) Dexamethasone 4–10 mg (*t*1/2 life: 36–54 h)

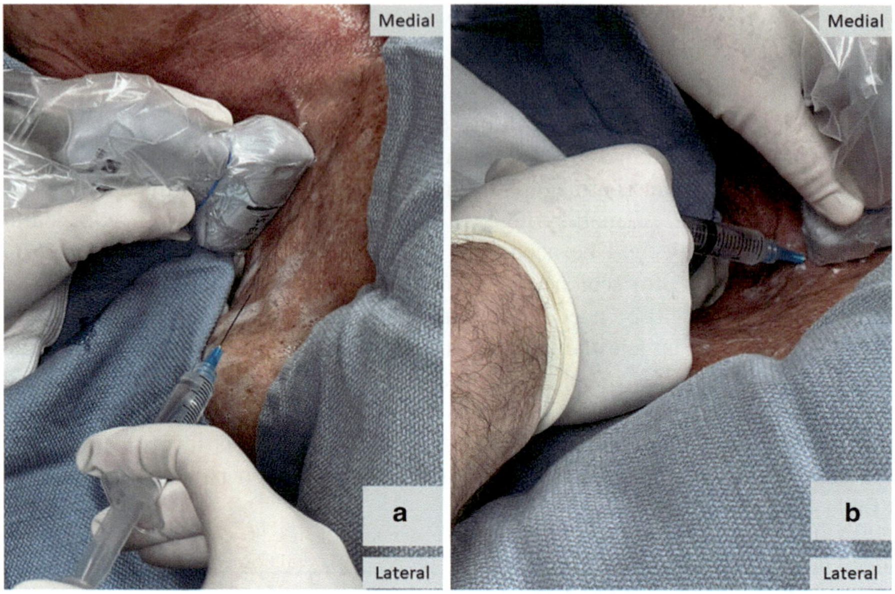

Fig. 3 Anterior scalene muscle injection. The patient positioning and ultrasound transducer orientation (**a**) and needle direction (**b**) are presented

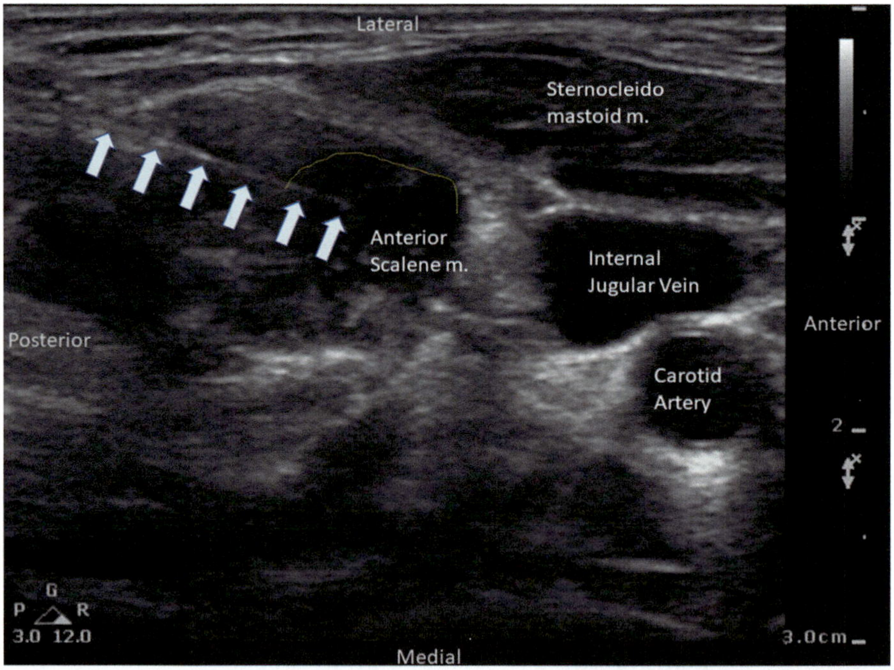

Fig. 4 Ultrasonogram identifying target structures as labeled. Blue arrows point towards the needle advanced towards the anterior scalene muscle. The yellow line indicates the local anesthetic volume injected into the muscle

a false positive diagnostic and therapeutic response. For small or thin muscles, this may require repositioning needle into multiple locations within the muscle belly to prevent extravasation that can occur with a single large depot (or if patient has multiple trigger points, may target these specifically). Utilize Doppler as needed to avoid these vascular structures.

6 Pectoralis Minor Injection

Similar to the previous procedure, the pectoralis minor muscle or tendon sheath injection can be performed using landmarks. We do not recommend this approach. Below were present ultrasound-guided pectoralis minor injection. Pectoralis minor intramuscular injections can be performed with the patient in supine or semi-recumbent position with the ipsilateral arm at the patient's side or abducted to the side (Fig. 5).

With the probe oriented in a cephalad to caudad direction, or lateral to medial direction, identification of the pectoralis minor can be achieved deep to the pectoralis major and superficial to the serratus anterior (Fig. 6). The typical volume of local anesthetic injected is 2–4 ml.

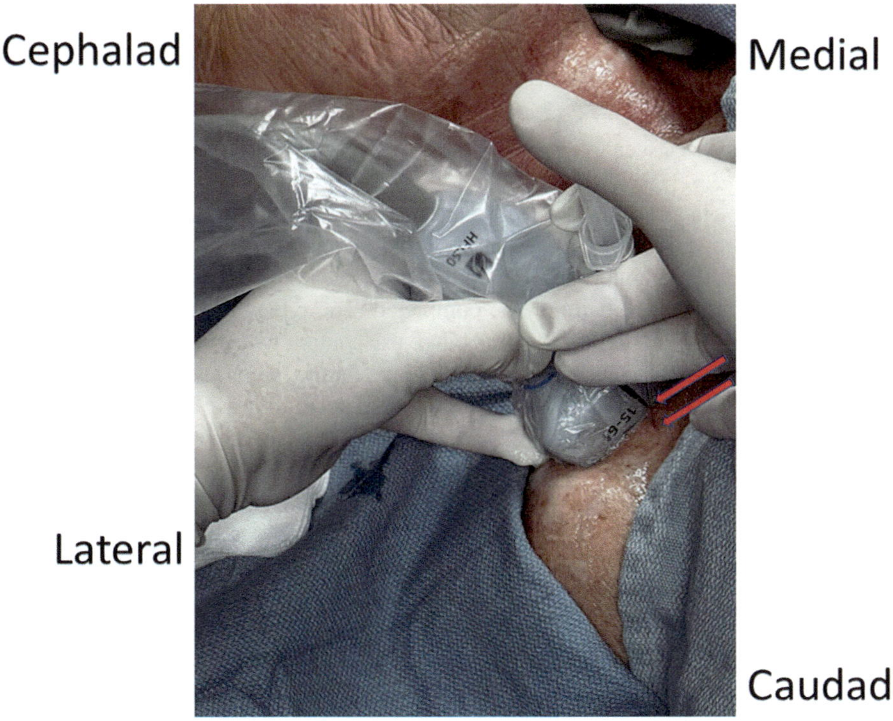

Fig. 5 Pectoralis minor muscle injection. The patient positioning and ultrasound transducer orientation. Red arrows point towards the needle

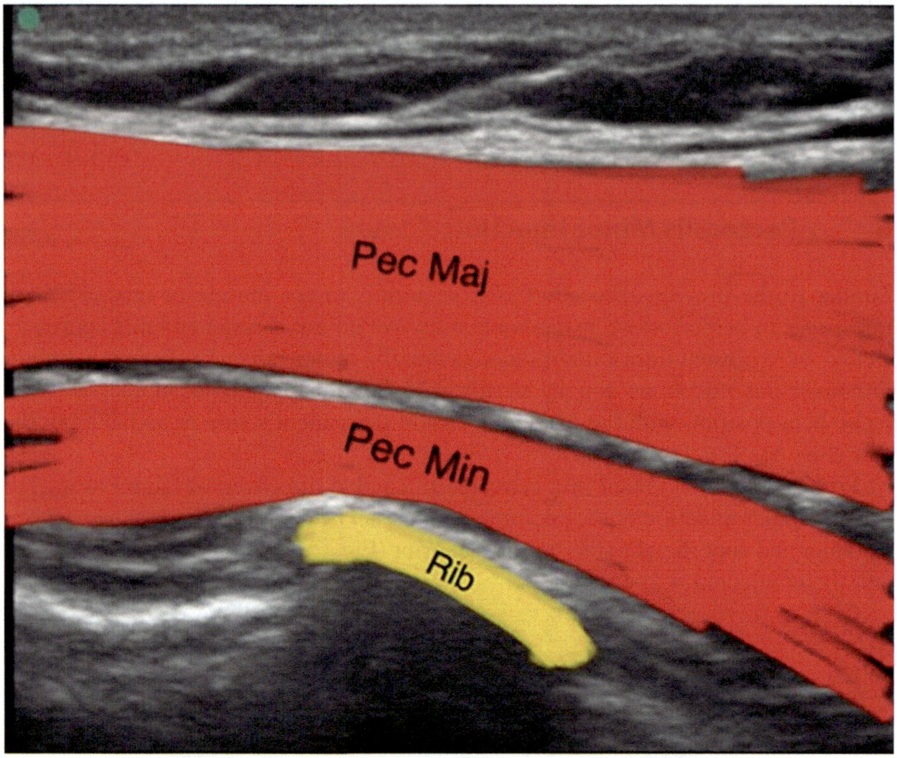

Fig. 6 Cross-sectional anatomy schematic on the ultrasonogram, as labeled

Following sterile prep and skin wheal anesthetic, in-plane advancement of an echogenic or nonechogenic needle under ultrasound guidance with a high-frequency linear probe is conducted until placement is within the muscle body. Injection of anesthetic or anesthetic/steroid mixture can now be completed. The typical volume of local anesthetic injected is 2–4 ml. during this procedure use caution to avoid placement of local anesthetic within the fascial plane between the pectoralis major and minor as this can result in a false positive procedure unless the lateral pectoral nerve is targeted (Fig. 7).

For small or thin muscles, this may require repositioning the needle into multiple locations within the muscle belly to prevent extravasation that can occur with a single large depot (or if patient has multiple trigger points, may target these specifically). Moreover, given the close proximity to the pleura, needle visualization during advancement is vital to avoid causing a pneumothorax.

7 Potential Complications and Adverse Effects

Pectoralis minor and scalene injections are ultrasound guided intramuscular injections, and as such similar to trigger point injections, they are considered generally safe and well tolerated. However, as with any interventional procedure, there is

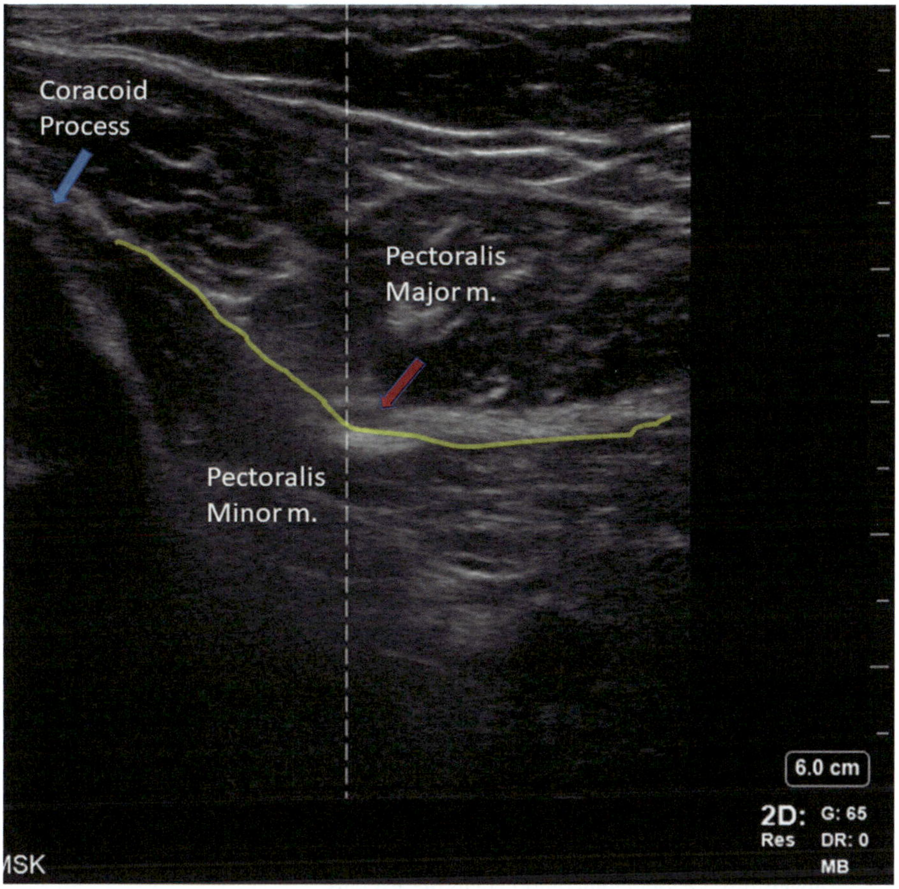

Fig. 7 Ultrasonogram identifying target structures. Blue arrow points towards the coracoid process, the site of attachment of pectoralis minor muscle. Dashed line represents needle trajectory. The needle shaft is not seen as the injection performed using out of plane technique. However, the position of the injectate around the lateral pectoral nerve is visible (red arrow). Injection of local anesthetic around this nerve can lead to false-positive results of the diagnostic injection but can be used as a technique to alleviate otherwise unexplained anterior shoulder pain

the risk of bleeding or hematoma formation (particularly in anti-coagulated patients), infection or abscess formation, nerve injury (plexus injury given the anatomic proximity) or injury of other nearby structures, allergic reactions or intolerance to the substances injected. The anatomy and needle trajectory of the pectoralis minor injection lends itself to the possibility of lung injury or pneumothorax. There is also the risk of temporary phrenic nerve blockade with scalene injections. Discomfort at the injection site or worsening of usual pain symptoms may occur. It is of particular importance to be cautious in patients with atypical anatomy—such as that with prior pectoralis injury, or atypical course of brachial plexus (Table 5).

Table 5 Additional potential complications and adverse effects

• Though unlikely with volume of local anesthetic utilized and with ultrasound guidance, but due to proximity of vascular structures, clinician should be vigilant about signs and treatment of local anesthetic systemic toxicity (LAST).
• Risks should be weighed against benefits in the pregnant patient, particularly with utilization of steroid, though not administered systemically or chronically, there may be a weak association with oral cleft, gestational diabetes, or other complications [7, 8].
• There is the potential for sympathetic blockade and resultant Horner's syndrome given the proximity of the stellate ganglion and other sympathetic structures.
• Caution should be taken in the diabetic patient if utilizing steroid and baseline glucose levels should be determined.
• Though unlikely, anaphylaxis can occur with exposure to local anesthetics or due to preservatives within steroid injectate.
• Caution should be taken in the COPD patient given the risk for pneumothorax and phrenic nerve blockade.

Clinical and Technical Pearls

- Meticulous care should be taken to prevent spread of local anesthetic onto the brachial plexus, as this would diminish the diagnostic value of the intramuscular injection
- Though controversial, to reduce the potential for procedural placebo effect, injection should not be considered to have diagnostic value without a minimum 60% (but ideally 80%) reduction in pain and symptomatology [9].
- Extra caution should be taken in patients with chronic obstructive pulmonary disease, given their increased risk of pneumothorax, but also due to the potential for phrenic nerve block with scalene injection.
- Though unlikely with US guidance and with the volume of local anesthetic use, proximity to arterial structures should warrant extra vigilance for the possibility of local anesthetic systemic toxicity.
- When combined with physical therapy, these injections can form the basis of maintenance or potentially curative treatment. But if they fail to provide prolonged relief, they can provide diagnostic value for potential surgical treatment.

References

1. Peet RM, Hendricksen JD, Anderson TP, Martin GM. Thoracic outlet syndrome: evaluation of a therapeutic exercise program. Proc Mayo Clin. 1956;31:281–7.
2. Hooper TL, Denton J, Mcgalliard MK, Brismée J-M, Sizer PS. Thoracic outlet syndrome: a controversial clinical condition. Part 1: anatomy, and clinical examination/diagnosis. J Manual Manipul Ther. 2010;18(2):74–83.
3. Sanders RJ. Pectoralis minor syndrome. In: Illig K, Thompson R, Freischlag J, Donahue D, Jordan S, Edgelow P, editors. Thoracic outlet syndrome. London: Springer; 2013.
4. Lee GW, Kwon YH, Jeong JH, Kim JW. The efficacy of scalene injection in thoracic outlet syndrome. J Korean Neurosurg Soc. 2011;50(1):36.

5. Wood VE, Biondi J. Double-crush nerve compression in thoracic-outlet syndrome. J Bone Joint Surg. 1990;72(1):85–7.
6. Nord KM, Kapoor P, Fisher J, Thomas G, Sundaram A, Scott K, et al. False positive rate of thoracic outlet syndrome diagnostic maneuvers. Electromyogr Clin Neurophysiol. 2008;48:67–74.
7. Skuladottir H, Wilcox AJ, Ma C, Lammer EJ, Rasmussen SA, Werler MM, et al. Corticosteroid use and risk of orofacial clefts. Birth Defects Res A Clin Mol Teratol. 2014;100(6):499–506.
8. Yildirim Y, Tinar S, Oner RS, Kaya B, Toz E. Gestational diabetes mellitus in patients receiving long-term corticosteroid therapy during pregnancy. J Perinat Med. 2006;34(4):280–4. https://doi.org/10.1515/JPM.2006.053.
9. Finniss D, Nicholas M, Brooker C, Cousins M, Benedetti F. Magnitude, response, and psychological determinants of placebo effects in chronic low-back pain. Pain Rep. 2019;4(3):e744.

Further Reading

Benzon HT, Rodes ME, Chekka K, Malik K, Pearce WH. Scalene muscle injections for neurogenic thoracic outlet syndrome: case series. Pain Pract. 2011;12(1):66–70.

Freischlag J, Orion K. Understanding thoracic outlet syndrome. Scientifica. 2014;2014:1–6.

Humphries M, Pekurovsky A, Salhan N, Sheth S, Demesa C. IP155. Ultrasound-guided pectoralis minor muscle block to aid diagnosis of neurovascular pectoralis minor syndrome. J Vasc Surg. 2016;63(6)

Sanders RJ, Annest SJ. Pectoralis minor syndrome: subclavicular brachial plexus compression. Diagnostics. 2017;7(3):46.

Elbow Joint, Intra-articular Injections

Bryant W. Tran, Michael R. Buxhoeveden, and Timothy T. Wills

Essential Concepts

- Intra-articular injections for the elbow are performed to provide pain relief for rheumatoid arthritis, degenerative joint disease, or crystal arthropathies.
- The injection is typically performed by landmark technique.
- Elbow intra-articular injections are easy to perform, well-tolerated, and have few side effects.
- Transient resolution of pain with elbow injections occurs but long-term pain relief for months to years has not been demonstrated.

1 Intra-articular Elbow Injection

Overview

The intra-articular elbow injection is performed to provide pain relief and reduce inflammation, with the goal of improving functional status for the patient. This procedure should be considered after non-invasive interventions have been utilized, such as multimodal medication therapy with acetaminophen and Non-Steroidal Anti-inflammatory Drugs, physical therapy, and heat and ice application. As a bedside procedure, elbow intra-articular injections are easy to perform, well-tolerated, and have few side effects. Although the use of ultrasound is gaining popularity with

B. W. Tran (✉) · M. R. Buxhoeveden · T. T. Wills
Department of Anesthesiology, Virginia Commonwealth University Medical Center, Richmond, VA, USA
e-mail: bryant.tran@vcuhealth.org; michael.buxhoeveden@vcuhealth.org; timothy.wills@vcuhealth.org

D. Souza et al. (eds.), *Bedside Pain Management Interventions*, https://doi.org/10.1007/978-3-031-11188-4_55

periarticular elbow injections, literature does not support the use of ultrasound technique for injection within the elbow joint [1]. Alternative medications such as hyaluronic acid are also not indicated [2].

2 Indications and Contraindications

A summary of the procedure, indications, techniques, and contraindications is presented in Table 1.

3 Clinical Anatomy

The needle approach into the elbow joint capsule can be determined by identifying the lateral epicondyle, olecranon process, and the radial head. These osseous structures can be palpated superficially. Labeled anatomy is shown in Figs. 1 and 2.

4 Equipment and Supplies

In addition to alcohol or chlorhexidine sterile preparation, sterile gloves, and sterile towels, a summary of necessary equipment is presented in Table 2. Ultrasound machine is optional.

5 Intra-articular Elbow Injection, Landmark Technique

The procedure is performed with the patient in the sitting position. Position the arm on a table with the lateral portion of the arm exposed and the elbow flexed at 45°. The olecranon process, lateral epicondyle, and the radial head form a triangle that provides a target for needle insertion (Fig. 3) [3]. Outlining this triangle with a surgical marker is optional. Insert the needle in the middle of the "triangle" and direct toward the medial epicondyle. Advance the needle until clear fluid is aspirated. Aspiration of clear fluid indicates adequate needle position in the joint capsule. The medication can then be injected. If bone is contacted, withdraw and redirect.

Table 1 Intra-articular elbow injections for management of elbow pain

Procedure	Indications	Technique	Contraindications
Intra-articular elbow injection	Rheumatoid arthritis, degenerative joint disease, crystal arthropathy	Landmark	Patient refusal, active joint infection, cellulitis, systemic infection

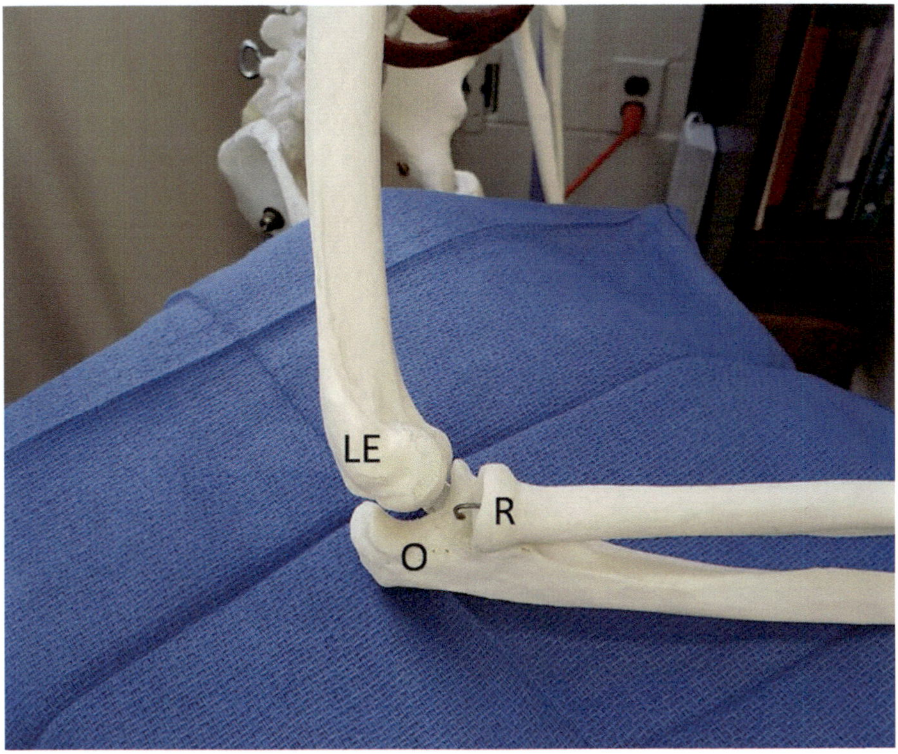

Fig. 1 Labeled anatomy of the elbow joint with respect to osseous structures. *LE* lateral epicondyle, *R* radial head, *O* olecranon

6 Ultrasound Technique

Ultrasound technique is not preferred for this procedure due to poor acoustic windows of the injection target. Although ultrasound has been used for elbow joint aspiration in the setting of pathologic fluid collection, the literature does not yet support this technique for the elbow joint [4].

7 Potential Complications and Adverse Effects

Elbow intra-articular injections are easy to perform and well-tolerated. Reported side effects for intra-articular elbow injections have not been reported but a number of side effects from periarticular injections have been reported [5]. Possible side effects are listed below.

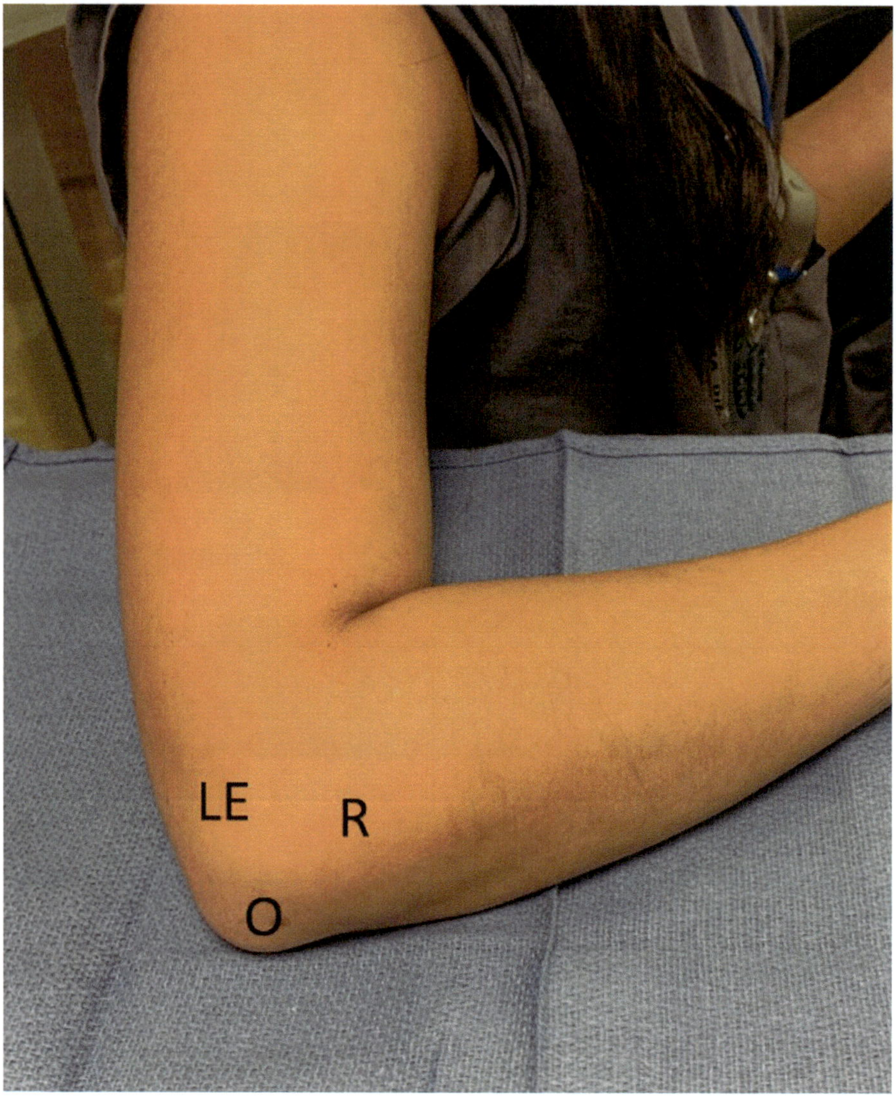

Fig. 2 Labeled surface anatomy of the elbow joint. *LE* lateral epicondyle, *R* radial head, *O* olecranon

Table 2 Necessary equipment for intra-articular elbow injection

Syringe	Needle	Anesthetic	Corticosteroid
5 cc, sterile, Luer lock tip	25 gauge, 1–1.5 in.	3–5 mL 1% lidocaine, 0.25% bupivacaine, 0.25% ropivacaine, or equivalent strength	1–2 mL betamethasone (6 mg/mL) or 1–2 mL methylprednisolone (40 mg/mL)

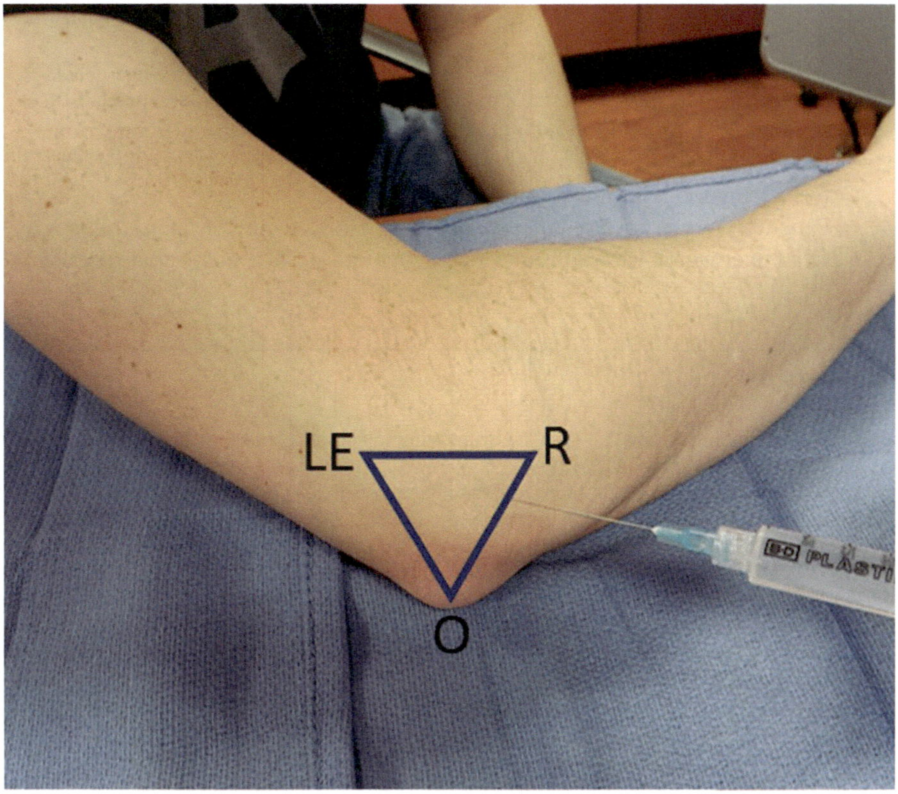

Fig. 3 Labeled surface anatomy of the elbow joint. The middle of the triangle that connects the relevant structures represent the ideal entry point for needle insertion. *LE* lateral epicondyle, *R* radial head, *O* olecranon

Procedure-related [6]
Anxiety
Discomfort
Minor skin infection
Bruising
Glucocorticoid-associated toxicity [6].
Post-injection flare
Facial flushing
Local skin or fat changes
Osteonecrosis
Cartilage damage
Systemic effects
Bleeding
Allergic reaction

Clinical and Technical Pearls

- Aspiration of clear fluid is the standard for confirmation of adequate needle position. Therefore, landmark technique is likely to be faster and more accurate than ultrasound technique for the elbow intra-articular injection.
- Prior local infiltration of the skin with 1% lidocaine may decrease discomfort during the joint injection.
- Patient expectations are important. As an isolated intervention, transient relief over weeks to months may occur, but long-term relief is not expected.

References

1. Daley EL, Bajaj S, Bisson LJ, Cole BJ. Improving injection accuracy of the elbow, knee, and shoulder. Am J Sports Med. 2011;39(3):656–62.
2. Van Brakel RW, Eygendaal D. Intra-articular injection of hyaluronic acid is not effective for the treatment of post-traumatic osteoarthritis of the elbow. Arthroscopy. 2006;22(11):1199–203.
3. Cardone DA, Tallia AF. Diagnostic and therapeutic injection of the elbow region. Am Fam Physician. 2002;66(11):2097–100.
4. Reijinierse M, Miller TT. Video: musculoskeletal ultrasound imaging of the elbow: part 2, pathology. AM J Roentgenol. 2013;200(6):W645.
5. Brinks A, Koes BW, Volkers AC, Verhaar JA, Bierma-Zeinstra SM. Adverse effects of extra-articular corticosteroid injections: a systematic review. BMC Musculoskelet Disord. 2010;11:206.
6. Roberts WN, Hauptman HW. Joint aspiration or injection in adults: complications. In UpToDate, Curtis MR (Ed.), UpToDate, Waltham, MA. Accessed 10 Nov 2019.

Further Reading

Cheng J, Abdi S. Complications of joint, tendon, and muscle injections. Tech Reg Anesth Pain Manag. 2007;11(3):141–7.

Periarticular Elbow Interventions

Bryant W. Tran, Michael R. Buxhoeveden,
and Timothy T. Wills

Essential Concepts

- Periarticular elbow injections are performed to relieve pain associated with lateral epicondylitis, medial epicondylitis, and olecranon bursitis.
- Side effects have been reported and studied but the incidence is low.
- Evidence shows short term efficacy with corticosteroids and other medications, such as hyaluronic acid, prolotherapy, sclerosing therapy, and orthobiologics [1].
- Resolution of pain with elbow injections may occur for approximately 2–4 weeks but long-term pain relief after months to years has not been demonstrated [2].
- Landmark technique and ultrasound technique have a similar accuracy rate [3].

1 Periarticular Elbow Interventions

Overview

Lateral epicondylitis, often referred to as "tennis elbow," is the most common ailment that warrants evaluation for periarticular elbow injection. Along with medial epicondylitis, these conditions typically develop after repetitive motions produce

B. W. Tran (✉) · M. R. Buxhoeveden · T. T. Wills
Department of Anesthesiology, Virginia Commonwealth University Medical Center, Richmond, VA, USA
e-mail: bryant.tran@vcuhealth.org; michael.buxhoeveden@vcuhealth.org; timothy.wills@vcuhealth.org

D. Souza et al. (eds.), *Bedside Pain Management Interventions*,
https://doi.org/10.1007/978-3-031-11188-4_56

chronic degenerative changes along the tendons surrounding the epicondyles. Olecranon bursitis can occur after repetitive trauma or as a result of swelling associated with rheumatoid arthritis [4]. Non-invasive treatment should be considered first, which includes multimodal medication therapy, physical therapy, or bracing.

Indications and Contraindications

A summary of the procedure, indications, techniques, and contraindications is presented in Table 1.

Clinical Anatomy

The relevant anatomy includes the lateral epicondyle, medial epicondyle, olecranon process, and radial head. These osseous structures can be palpated superficially and visualized by ultrasound. Pertinent anatomy is shown in Figs. 1, 2, and 3.

Equipment and Supplies

In addition to alcohol or chlorhexidine sterile preparation, sterile gloves, and sterile towels, a summary of necessary equipment is presented in Table 2. Ultrasound machine is optional [4]. The authors use a linear probe with a frequency bandwidth of 13–6 MHz and scan depth of 6 cm. The width of the transducer should allow for easy needle entry using an in-plane technique.

2 Periarticular Elbow Interventions, Landmark Technique

Lateral Epicondyle Injection

The patient can be seated in a chair with their elbow flexed on a flat surface (Fig. 4). The lateral epicondyle will be palpable. The needle will be directed towards the lateral epicondyle, and if the needle tip contacts os, the needle can be withdrawn 1–2 mm to allow space for local anesthetic injection. The injection target should match with the focal area that the patient reports as most bothersome.

Table 1 Periarticular elbow injections for management of elbow pain

Procedure	Indications	Technique	Contraindications
Lateral epicondyle injection	Lateral epicondylitis	Landmark or ultrasound	Patient refusal, active joint infection, cellulitis, systemic infection
Medial epicondyle injection	Medial epicondylitis	Landmark or ultrasound	Patient refusal, active joint infection, cellulitis, systemic infection
Olecranon bursa injection	Olecranon bursitis	Landmark or ultrasound	Patient refusal, active joint injection, cellulitis, systemic infection

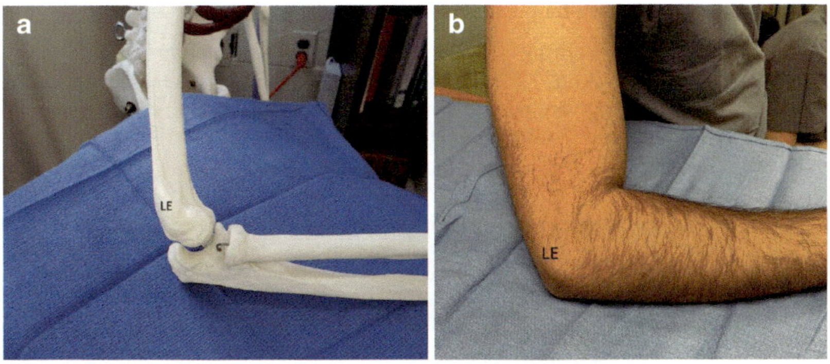

Fig. 1 (**a**) Lateral epicondyle labeled on a skeleton model. *LE* lateral epicondyle. (**b**) Lateral epicondyle labeled with surface anatomy. *LE* lateral epicondyle

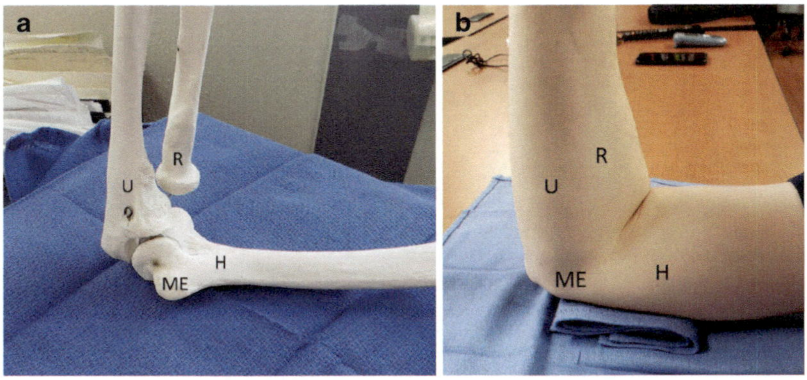

Fig. 2 (**a**) Medial epicondyle labeled on a skeleton model. *ME* medial epicondyle, *U* ulna, *R* radius, *H* humerus (distal). (**b**) Medial epicondyle labeled with surface anatomy. *ME* medial epicondyle, *U* ulna, *R* radius, *H* humerus (distal)

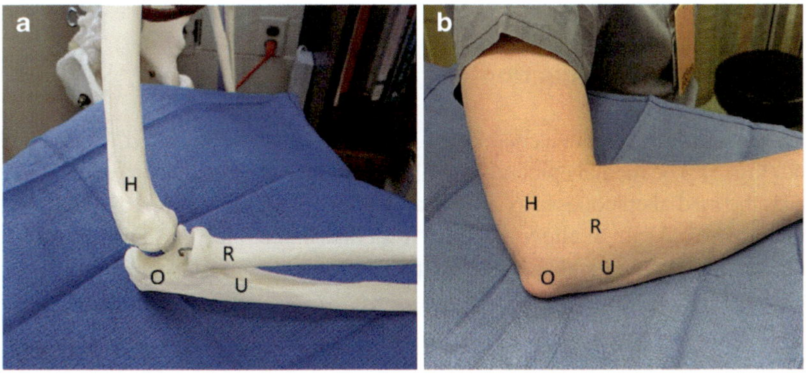

Fig. 3 (**a**) Olecranon labeled on a skeleton model. *O* olecranon, *H* humerus (distal), *R* radius, *U* ulna. (**b**) Olecranon labeled with surface anatomy. *O* olecranon, *H* humerus (distal), *R* radius, *U* ulna

Table 2 Necessary equipment for periarticular elbow injection

Syringe	Needle	Anesthetic	Corticosteroid
5 cc, sterile, Luer lock tip	25 gauge, 1 in.	2–3 mL 1% lidocaine, 0.25% bupivacaine, 0.25% ropivacaine, or equivalent strength	1 mL betamethasone (6 mg/mL) or 1 mL methylprednisolone (40 mg/mL)

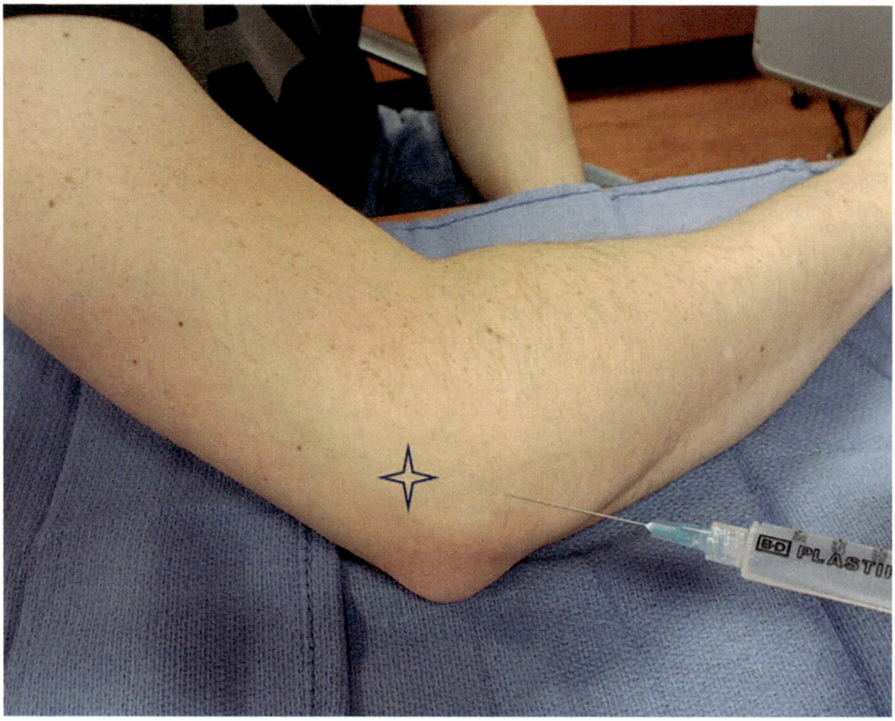

Fig. 4 Lateral epicondyle injection via landmark approach. Stellate mark—injection site over lateral epicondyle

Medial Epicondyle Injection

The patient can be seated in a chair. Their arm will need to be abducted with their elbow flexed (Fig. 5). The medial epicondyle will be palpable. The needle entry will be directed towards the medial epicondyle as shown, and if the needle tip contacts os, the needle can be withdrawn 1–2 mm to allow space for local anesthetic injection. The injection target should match with the focal area that the patient reports as most bothersome.

Olecranon Bursa Injection

The patient will be in prone position on the examination table with the arm abducted and the elbow flexed (Fig. 6). The olecranon will be palpable and if the bursa is inflamed, there may be protrusion from the skin. The needle will be directed

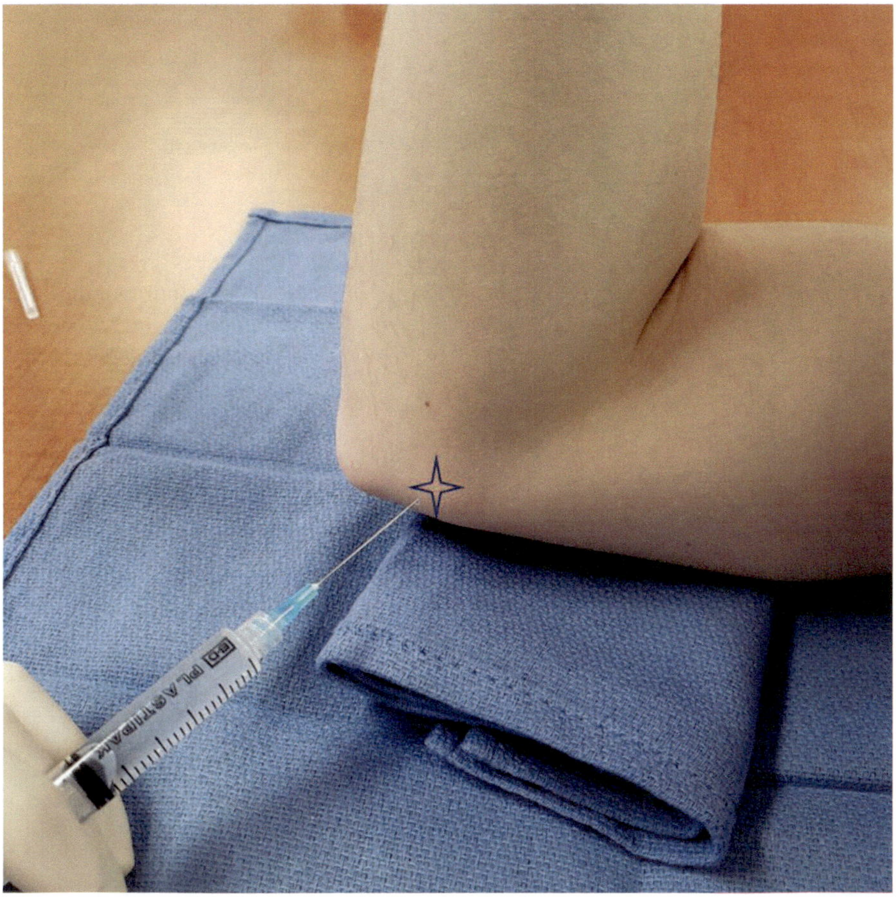

Fig. 5 Medial epicondyle injection via landmark approach. Stellate mark—injection site over medial epicondyle

towards the focal point where the patient reports as most tender. If the needle tip contacts os, the needle can be withdrawn 1–2 mm to allow space for local anesthetic injection.

3 Ultrasound Technique

Generally, there are no major vascular or neural structures to avoid for these bedside interventions. The needle trajectory should allow for needle visualization via ultrasound and with an in-plane approach [5].

Lateral Epicondyle Injection

Similar to landmark technique, the patient will be seated with their arm on a flat surface and elbow flexed (Fig. 7a). The ultrasound probe will be oriented in a

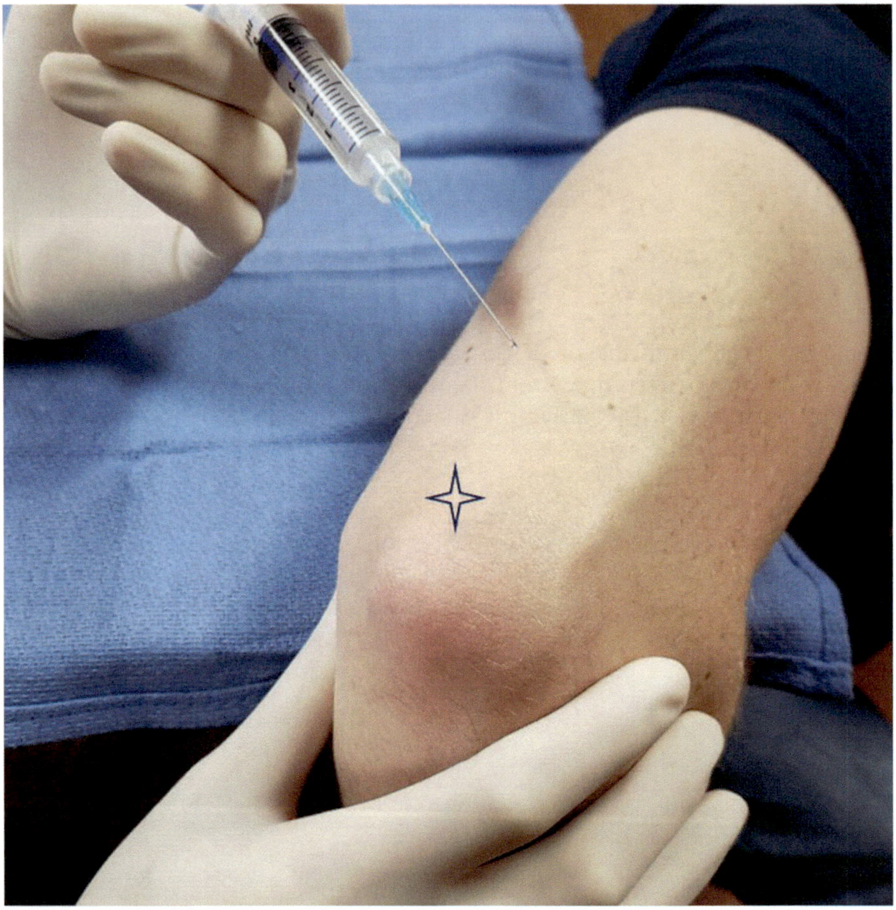

Fig. 6 Olecranon bursa injection via landmark approach. Stellate mark—injection site over olecranon bursa

longitudinal plane. Relevant ultrasound anatomy includes the lateral epicondyle and radial head (Fig. 7b). The needle will be directed toward the lateral epicondyle, and if the needle tip contacts os, the needle can be withdrawn 1–2 mm to allow space for local anesthetic injection.

Medial Epicondyle Injection

The patient will lie either supine or in semi-sitting position on an examination table. Their arm will need to be abducted with their elbow flexed on a flat surface (Fig. 8a). The ultrasound probe will be oriented in a longitudinal plane. Relevant ultrasound anatomy only shows the medial epicondyle, which will be shaped like a trapezoid (Fig. 8b). The needle will be directed toward the superficial border of the medial epicondyle, and if the needle tip contacts os, the needle can be withdrawn 1–2 mm to allow space for local anesthetic injection.

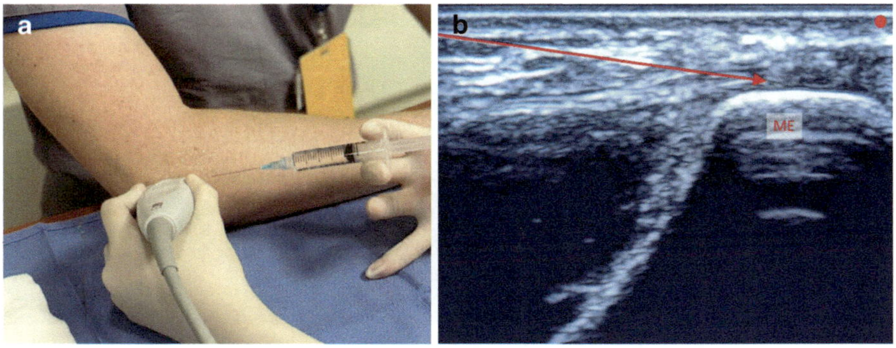

Fig. 7 (**a**) Needle approach for lateral epicondyle injection with ultrasound guidance. (**b**) Corresponding ultrasound image for lateral epicondyle injection. The red arrow represents the proposed needle approach via in-plane technique. Red dot = Proximal; *LE* lateral epicondyle, *R* radial head

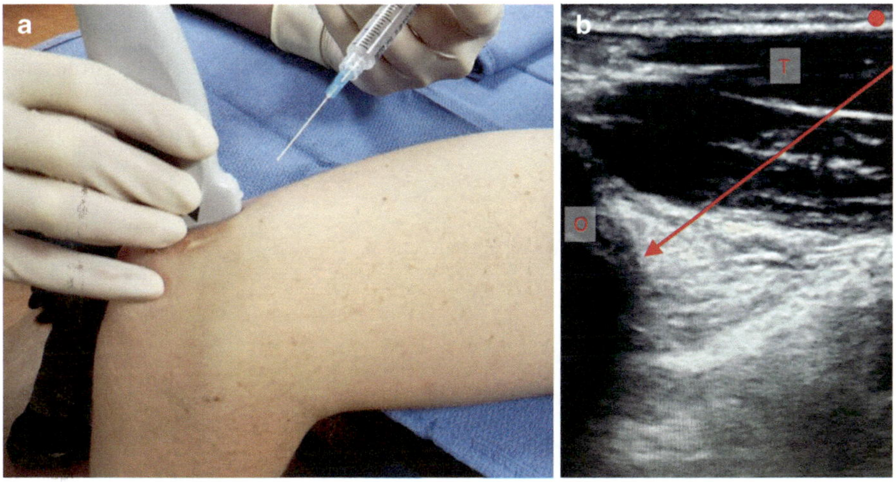

Fig. 8 (**a**) Needle approach for medial epicondyle injection with ultrasound guidance. (**b**) Corresponding ultrasound image for medial epicondyle injection. The red arrow represents the proposed needle approach via in-plane technique. Red dot = Proximal; *ME* medial epicondyle

Olecranon Bursa Injection

The patient will be in the prone position on the examination table with the arm abducted and the elbow flexed on the edge of a flat surface (Fig. 9a). The olecranon will be palpable and if the bursa is inflamed, the bursa may protrude from under the skin. The ultrasound probe will be oriented in a longitudinal plane. Relevant ultrasound anatomy only shows the olecranon and the triceps muscle (Fig. 9b). The needle will be directed towards an area adjacent to the olecranon and deep to the triceps muscle. An inflamed bursa may be visible in the ultrasound image as a dark hypoechoic pocket of fluid. If the needle tip contacts os, the needle can be withdrawn 1–2 mm to allow space for local anesthetic injection.

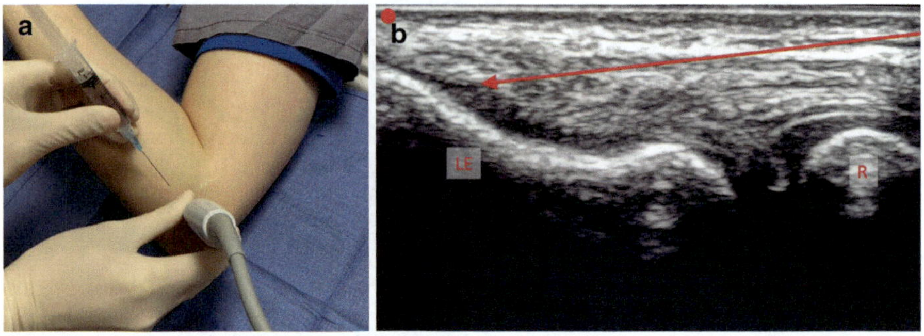

Fig. 9 (**a**) Needle approach olecranon bursa injection with ultrasound guidance. (**b**) Corresponding ultrasound image for olecranon bursa injection. The red arrow represents the proposed needle approach via in-plane technique. Red dot = Proximal; *O* olecranon, *T* triceps muscle

4 Potential Complications and Adverse Effects

Elbow periarticular injections are easy to perform and well-tolerated. Side effects from periarticular injections have been reported and studied [6]. Possible side effects are listed below.

Procedure-Related [7]

- Anxiety
- Discomfort
- Minor skin infection
- Bruising

Glucocorticoid-Associated Toxicity [7]

- Post-injection flare
- Facial flushing
- Local skin or fat changes
- Osteonecrosis

Clinical and Technical Pearls

- In addition to landmark palpation or ultrasound visualization, the optimal injection target may be determined by asking the patient to point to the area that is most tender or bothersome.
- Prior local infiltration of the skin with 1% lidocaine may decrease discomfort during the joint injection

- Patient expectations are important. As an isolated intervention, transient relief over weeks to months may occur, but long-term relief is not expected.
- Ultrasound transducers that are too large or wide may impede needle entry and make the procedure more difficult. The authors recommend a small flat probe with a bandwidth of 13–6 MHz and maximum scanning depth of 6 cm.

- Cartilage damage
- Systemic effects
- Bleeding
- Allergic reaction

References

1. Krogh TP, Bartels EM, Ellingsen T, et al. Comparative effectiveness of injection therapies in lateral epicondylitis: a systematic review and network meta-analysis of randomized controlled trials. Am J Sports Med. 2013;41(6):1435–46.
2. Coombes BK, Bisset L, Brooks P, et al. Effect of corticosteroid injection, physio- therapy, or both on clinical outcomes in patients with unilateral lateral epicondylalgia: a randomized controlled trial. JAMA. 2013;309(5):461–9.
3. Lopes RV, Furtado RN, Parmigiani L, et al. Accuracy of intra-articular injections in peripheral joints performed blindly in patients with rheumatoid arthritis. Rheumatology (Oxford). 2008;47(12):1792–4.
4. Cardone DA, Tallia AF. Diagnostic and therapeutic injection of the elbow region. Am Fam Physician. 2002;66(11):2097–100.
5. Sussman WI, Williams CJ, Mautner K. Ultrasound-guided elbow procedures. Phys Med Rehabil Clin N Am. 2016;27:573–87.
6. Brinks A, Koes BW, Volkers AC, Verhaar JA, Bierma-Zeinstra SM. Adverse effects of extra-articular corticosteroid injections: a systematic review. BMC Musculoskelet Disord. 2010;11:206.
7. Roberts WN, Hauptman HW. Joint aspiration or injection in adults: complications. In UpToDate, Curtis MR (Ed.), Waltham, MA. Accessed 10 Nov 2019.

Further Reading

Cheng J, Abdi S. Complications of joint, tendon, and muscle injections. Tech Reg Anesth Pain Manag. 2007;11(3):141–7.

Ulnar, Median, Radial, and Antebrachial Cutaneous Nerve Blocks

Tina M. Dailey and Mayur Vallabhaneni

Essential Concepts

- Nerve blocks of the arm, forearm, and wrist can be crucial techniques for both the treatment of acute or chronic pain of various etiologies.
- These procedures can be used perioperatively for surgical procedures involving the forearm, wrist, and hand.
- They can be used for analgesia for injuries, or manipulations, including but not limited to fracture reduction or laceration repair.
- These blocks can be easily performed at the bedside.

1 Introduction

Nerve blocks of the arm and wrist can be crucial techniques for both the treatment of acute/chronic pain as well as in preparation for surgical procedures and hand injuries, including but not limited to fracture reduction or laceration repair. This makes upper extremity nerve blocks quite effective and they have the ability to target specific nerves and dermatomes as needed. While single nerve blocks may suffice in pain control, injuries often traverse multiple dermatomes and may require multiple nerve blocks. The nerves of interest in this chapter are the ulnar, median,

T. M. Dailey (✉)
Elite Spine & Pain Center, Frederick, MD, USA

University of Virginia, Charlottesville, VA, USA

M. Vallabhaneni
University of Virginia, Charlottesville, VA, USA

D. Souza et al. (eds.), *Bedside Pain Management Interventions*,
https://doi.org/10.1007/978-3-031-11188-4_57

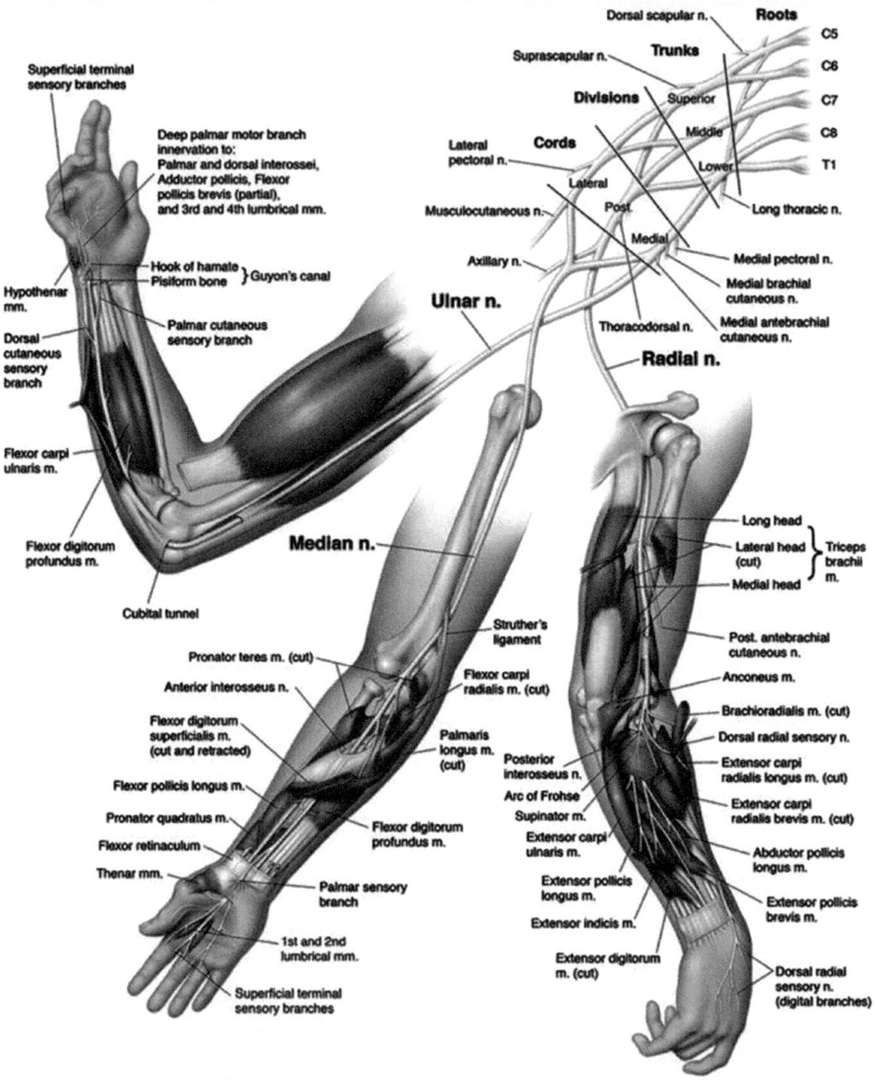

Fig. 1 Peripheral nerves of the upper extremity. Peripheral nerves of the upper extremity. A summary view of the brachial plexus organization and the paths of the ulnar, radial, and median nerves. The site of each plane transition, identified as where the nerves pierce through or traverse *above* or *below* a given anatomic structure, along the respective nerve's course is represented. Reprinted with permission from Stromberg JA, Isaacs J. (2015) Nerve anatomy and diagnostic evaluation. In: Abzug J, Kozin S, Zlotolow D. (eds) The pediatric upper extremity. Springer, New York, NY. https://doi.org/10.1007/978-1-4614-8515-5_23

radial, and antebrachial cutaneous nerves. Each nerve originates from the brachial plexus and courses through the arm, elbow, forearm, and hand across various anatomical landmarks [1, 2] (Fig. 1).

Fig. 2 Dermatomal distribution of the nerves over the palmar surface of the hand, as labeled

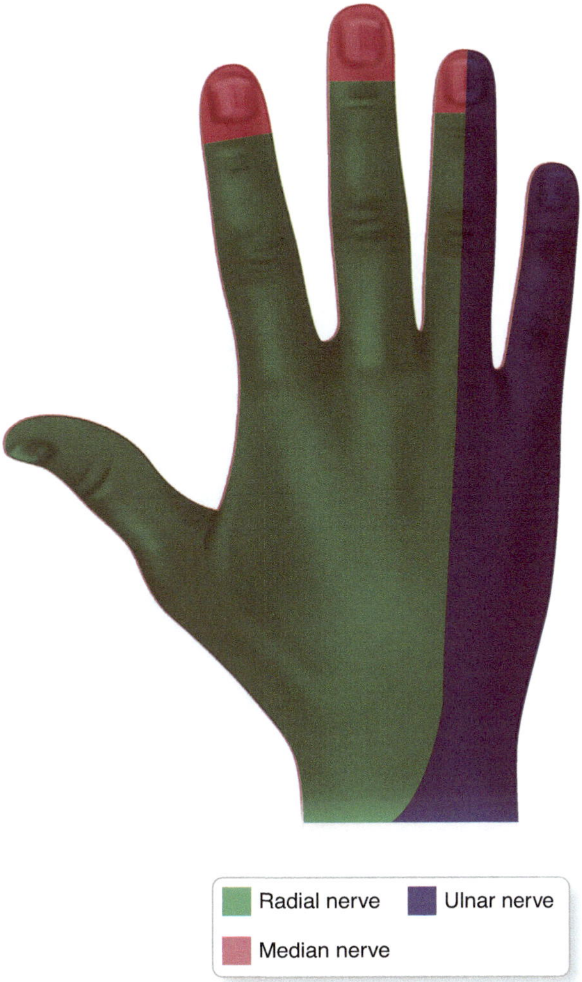

The arm and hand are supplied by multiple nerves with well-defined dermatomal distributions (Figs. 2 and 3) [1, 2].

The elbow and wrist are particularly well-suited to nerve blocks as the nerves often travel superficially in these locations with easily identifiable landmarks that can be palpated and used to guide treatment. Ultrasound can also be used for the identification of the nerves and can guide the proper placement of the needle and anesthetic, even in areas without obvious landmarks.

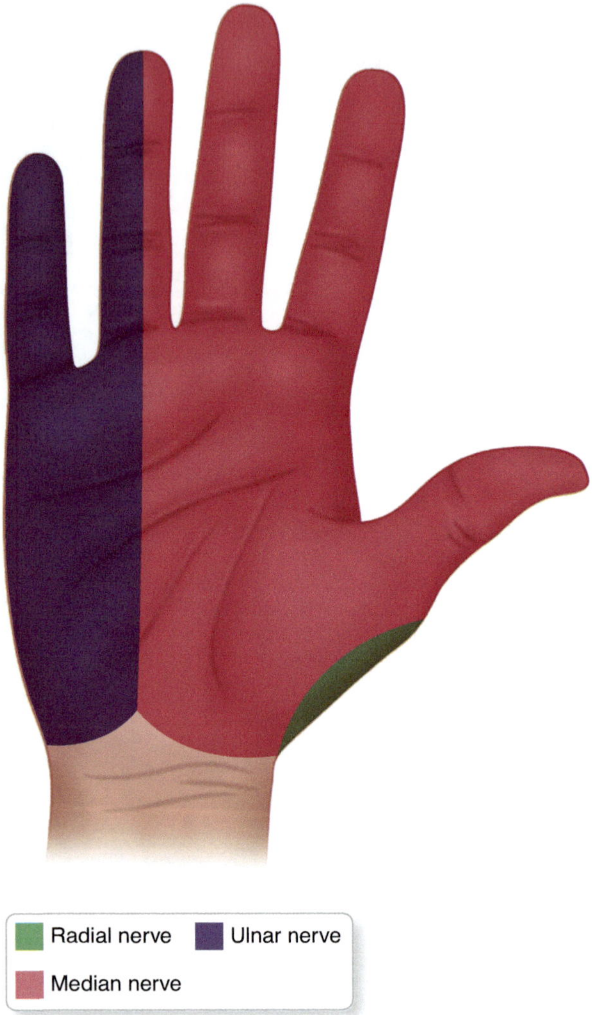

Fig. 3 Dermatomal distribution of the nerves over the dorsal surface of the hand, as labeled

2 Common Indications and Contraindications

Each nerve block is indicated based on the location of injuries and the corresponding dermatomal distribution of each specific nerve. A nerve block can be used for multiple reasons, including procedures such as laceration repairs or finger reductions, or acute pain relief for injuries including fractures, lacerations, or burns. Contraindications include skin or soft tissue infection over injection site, allergy or intolerance to the injectate, or its components, patient refusal, injuries presenting with vascular compromise or potential for compartment syndrome, patients with pre-existing or post-traumatic neurapraxia. Coagulopathy, including iatrogenic coagulopathy, and platelet dysfunction, are generally not considered contraindications.

3 Equipment and Supplies

- Ultrasound with linear transducer at frequency between 8–14 MHz, sterile sleeve, gel
- 3–5 ml of local anesthetic: Bupivacaine 0.5% for long-acting blocks, lidocaine 2% for short-acting blocks
- 25 G needle for skin anesthesia
- 5–10 ml syringe
- 21–25 gauge needle
- Chlorhexidine or iodopovidone for skin sterilization

4 General Approach

For each nerve, it can be helpful to palpate specific landmarks and then use these landmarks as a guide for ultrasound evaluation. After first identifying the nerve, it is prudent to follow its course until an optimal location is determined. This would ideally be in a place where the nerve is relatively superficial and has adequately separated from other neurovascular structures. Important general practices include the following: initial sterilization, sterile technique with sterile gel and ultrasound cover, slow injection of anesthetic, Intravenous (IV) access in case of negative reaction; continuous monitoring, and aspiration prior to injection to evaluate for intravascular placement are recommended. If there is significant pain or resistance with injection, this may indicate intraneural injection, which would require repositioning of the needle.

Ulnar Nerve Block

Indications

- Pain or procedures involving the fifth finger, fifth metacarpal
- Injuries involving the ulnar region of the hand
- Combined with median nerve block for procedures involving the fourth finger

Clinical Anatomy

The ulnar nerve originates as a terminal branch of the medial cord, with innervation from nerve roots C8, T1, and occasionally C7. It starts anteriorly along the axilla and teres major and travels down the upper arm medially with the brachial artery. It subsequently pierces through the intermuscular septum and travels between the septum and the medial head of the triceps. As the ulnar nerve approaches the elbow, it starts to travel posteriorly until it courses behind the medial epicondyle of the humerus. The nerve is particularly accessible as it travels behind the medial epicondyle [2]. After passing posteriorly to the medial epicondyle, the ulnar nerve enters the forearm by passing between the flexor carpi ulnaris and flexor digitorum profundus (Fig. 4).

As it approaches the wrist, the ulnar nerve starts to travel superficially and enters the hand between the pisiform and the hook of the hamate [1, 2].

On its route through the arm, the ulnar nerve has articular branches at the elbow and muscular branches that innervate the flexor carpi ulnaris and the medial half of the flexor digitorum profundus. The sensory component of the ulnar nerve consists

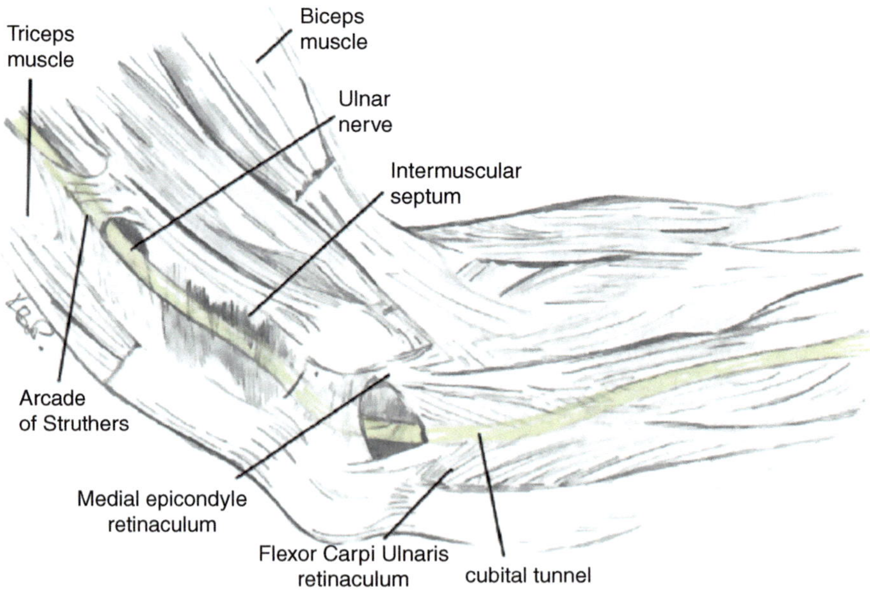

Fig. 4 Ulnar nerve anatomy

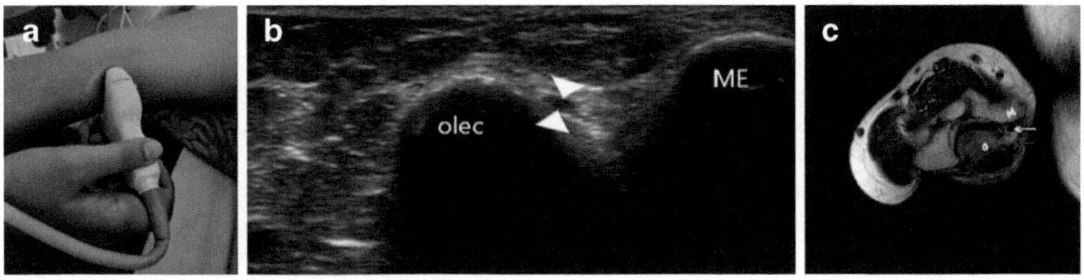

Fig. 5 Probe position, Ultrasonography, probe position, and MRI showing ulnar nerve at the distal forearm. (**a**) Probe position for localization of the ulnar nerve at the elbow. (**b**) The nerve (arrowhead) is localized in its short axis within the cubital tunnel between the medial epicondyle (ME) and olecranon process (olec). (**c**) MR image showing the normal ulnar nerve (yellow arrow) in the cubital tunnel: medial epicondyle (M) and olecranon process (O) forming the medial and lateral walls, Osborne's ligament (red arrow) forming the roof and the floor being formed by the joint capsule of elbow and the medial collateral ligament (red arrowhead). Reprinted with permission from Agarwal A, Chandra A, Jaipal U, et al. Imaging in the diagnosis of ulnar nerve pathologies—a neoteric approach. *Insights Imaging* 10, 37 (2019). https://doi.org/10.1186/s13244-019-0714-x

of three branches, the palmar cutaneous branch, the dorsal cutaneous branch, and the superficial cutaneous branch. These sensory nerves give innervation to the medial hand, fifth finger, and the medial half of the fourth finger [1, 2] (Figs. 1 and 2).

Procedural Technique

Elbow/Antecubital Fossa

Start with the patient's arm supinated with the elbow flexed between 45 and 90°. At the elbow, the ulnar nerve travels in the cubital tunnel between the olecranon and the medial epicondyle (Fig. 5). This is a good location to place the ultrasound probe to initially identify the nerve. The nerve is located deep to the two heads of the flexor carpi ulnaris. While the ulnar nerve can be blocked in the cubital tunnel, there is a theoretical concern of nerve compression in the tight cubital tunnel space [3, 4]. As such, after finding the nerve, follow its course proximally to the distal upper arm or further to the mid-arm, where the nerve should be superficially located. The nerve has a characteristic "honey comb" appearance (Figs. 5 and 6).

Insert the needle from the ulnar aspect of the transducer, and inject 3–5 cc of local anesthetic [5].

Forearm

Start with the patient's arm abducted and the hand in supination on a flat surface. Place the transducer over the medial wrist crease. After identifying the ulna and ulnar nerve, the ulnar artery should be lateral to it, just deep to the flexor carpi ulnaris muscle. From the wrist to the mid-forearm, the ulnar nerve travels medially to the artery. Make sure to follow the nerve proximally until it separates adequately from the ulnar artery. An ulnar approach with the needle under ultrasound minimizes the chance of arterial puncture [5, 6] (Fig. 7).

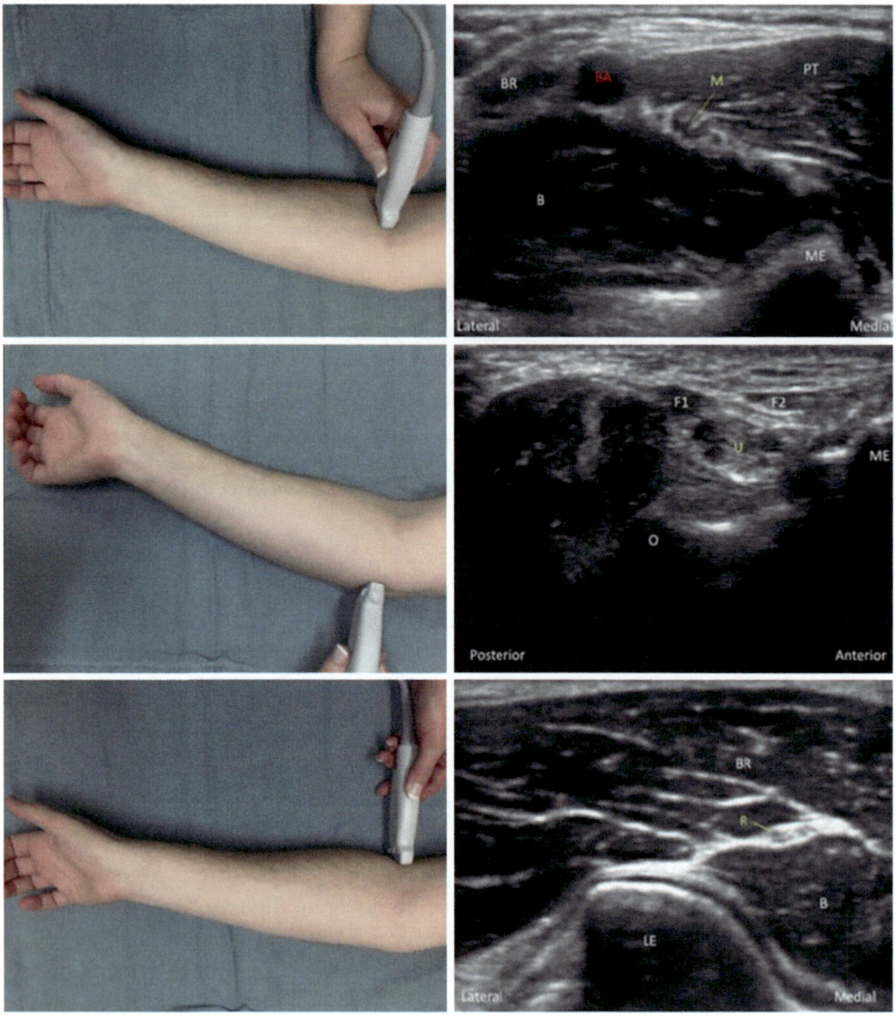

Fig. 6 Ultrasound probe positioning and the corresponding ultrasound image for median (upper), ulnar (middle), and radial (lower) nerve blocks at the antecubital fossa. Abbreviations for ultrasound images. *B* brachialis muscle, *BA* brachial artery, *BR* brachioradialis muscle, *DR* deep radial nerve, *ECRL* extensor carpi radialis longus muscle, *F1* flexor carpi ulnaris muscle, ulnar head, *F2* flexor carpi ulnaris muscle, humeral head, *FCR* flexor carpi radialis muscle, *FCU* flexor carpi ulnaris muscle, *FDP* flexor digitorum profundus muscle, *FDS* flexor digitorum superficialis muscle, *M* median nerve, *ME* medial epicondyle of the humerus, *LE* lateral epicondyle of the humerus, *O* olecranon of the humerus, *PT* pronator teres muscle, *R* radius, *S* supinator muscle, *SR* superficial radial nerve, *U* ulnar nerve, *UA* ulnar artery. Reprinted with permission from Sachse, K., Allen, B. (2022). Upper extremity blocks: wrist blocks: ulnar, radial, median nerve blocks. In: Banik RK (eds) Anesthesiology in-training exam review. Springer, Cham. https://doi.org/10.1007/978-3-030-87266-3_25

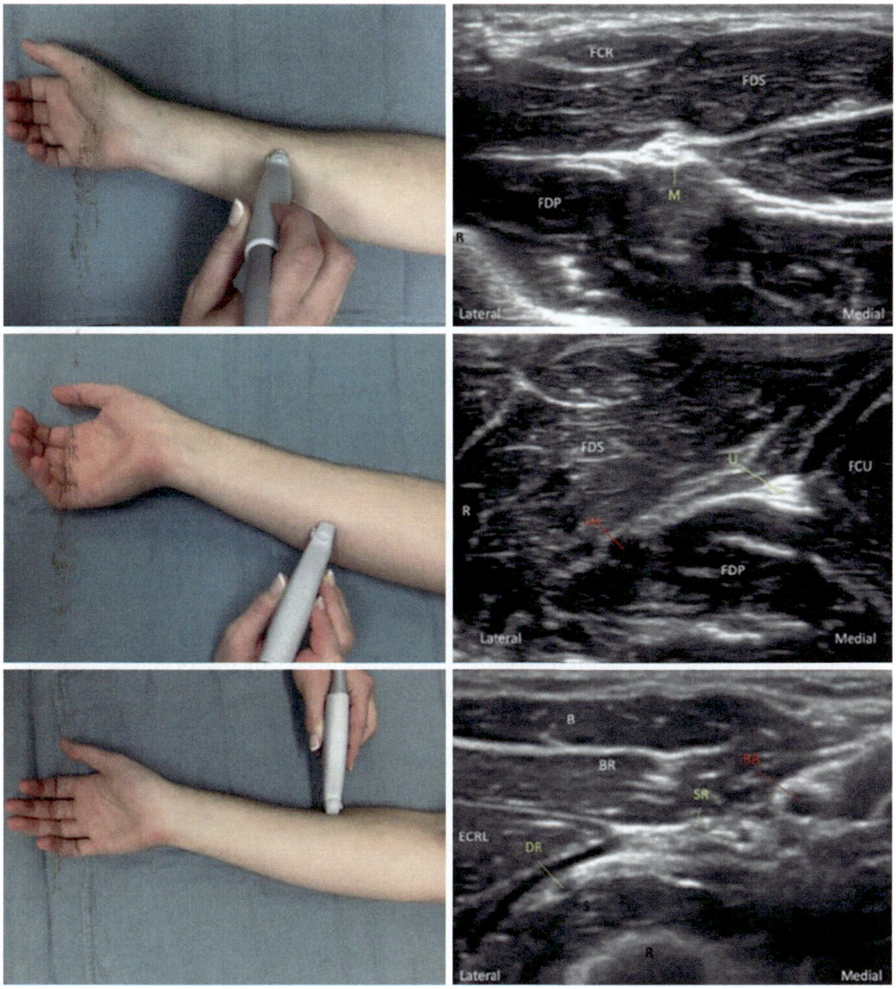

Fig. 7 Ultrasound probe positioning and the corresponding ultrasound image for median (upper), ulnar (middle), and radial (lower) nerve blocks at the mid-forearm. Abbreviations for ultrasound images. *B* brachialis muscle, *BA* brachial artery, *BR* brachioradialis muscle, *DR* deep radial nerve, *ECRL* extensor carpi radialis longus muscle, *F1* flexor carpi ulnaris muscle, ulnar head, *F2* flexor carpi ulnaris muscle, humeral head, *FCR* flexor carpi radialis muscle, *FCU* flexor carpi ulnaris muscle, *FDP* flexor digitorum profundus muscle, *FDS* flexor digitorum superficialis muscle, *M* median nerve, *ME* medial epicondyle of the humerus, *LE* lateral epicondyle of the humerus, *O* olecranon of the humerus, *PT* pronator teres muscle, *R* radius, *S* supinator muscle, *SR* superficial radial nerve, *U* ulnar nerve, *UA* ulnar artery. *Reprinted with permission from* Sachse K, Allen B (2022). Upper extremity blocks: wrist blocks: ulnar, radial, median nerve blocks. In: Banik RK (eds) Anesthesiology in-training exam review. Springer, Cham. https://doi.org/10.1007/978-3-030-87266-3_25

With this approach, the needle is advanced posterior to the flexor carpi ulnaris muscle from the medial side. This approach also gives easy access to the dorsal cutaneous branch of the ulnar nerve, which provides innervation to the dorsal ulnar hand. After blocking the ulnar nerve, the needle can then be guided anterior to the flexor carpi ulnaris, and local anesthetic can be delivered to block the dorsal branch [4].

Median Nerve Block

Indications

- Pain or procedures involving the first to third fingers, as well as the radial half of the palm
- Combined with ulnar nerve block for procedures involving the fourth finger

Clinical Anatomy

The median nerve originates from a lateral root (C6, C7) and medial root (C8, T1), which merge to form the median nerve lateral to the axillary artery. The nerve then travels lateral and parallel to the brachial artery until the cubital fossa, where it crosses anterior to the artery and lies medial to it within the fossa (Fig. 3).

The nerve leaves the cubital fossa between the heads of the pronator teres and travels between the flexor digitorum superficialis and flexor digitorum profundus. This route keeps the nerve in the midline of the forearm. As it approaches the wrist, the median nerve becomes more superficial prior to entering the carpal tunnel deep to the flexor retinaculum. As the nerve is both midline and more superficial, this is an ideal target location [1, 2].

On its route through the arm, the median nerve does not give off any significant branches, with the exception of articular branches to the elbow. In the forearm, it gives off the anterior interosseous nerve (supplies the deep forearm flexors) and the palmar cutaneous branch proximal to the flexor retinaculum. The palmar cutaneous branch supplies the central palm, while the median nerve branches distal to the carpal tunnel. These branches provide sensory innervation to the palmar surface, the first three digits, lateral half of the fourth digit, and the dorsal, lateral surface of the first four digits (Figs. 1 and 2) [1, 2].

Procedural Technique

Antecubital Fossa/Elbow

Blocking the median nerve at the elbow provides better paralysis than at the wrist, as this also includes the anterior interosseous nerve before it branches. Start with the arm extended, externally rotated, elbow flexed at approximately 45°. Within the antecubital fossa, the median nerve travels medially to the brachial artery. Place the high-frequency linear ultrasound transducer where the brachial pulse can be palpated. Ultrasound should show the nerve just medial to the artery. Insert the needle medial to the probe, and inject approximately 3–5 ml local anesthetic after placing the needle tip at the base of the nerve [4, 7] (Fig. 6). Spread should be noted circumferentially around the nerve.

Midforearm

Blocking the median nerve at the wrist provides the same analgesia as at the elbow but without the associated paralysis of the forearm muscles. Start with the arm and hand supinated, with the ultrasound transducer at the volar wrist crease. The ultrasound image should show several hyperechoic structures that are a combination of tendons and the median nerve, making initial identification difficult. The best way to locate the median nerve is to travel proximally with the transducer to the mid-forearm, where the tendons become muscle, and the nerve is easier to identify. It is recommended to block the nerve in the mid-forearm, where it can be easily distinguished from the surrounding anatomy [4, 7]. The median nerve in this location is located deep to the flexor digitorum superficialis and superficial to the flexor digitorum profundus. An in plane or out of plane technique can be utilized. Inject approximately 3–5 ml of LA around the nerve (Fig. 7).

Radial Nerve Block

Indications

- Pain or procedures involving the lateral hand, dorsal first to third fingers.

Clinical Anatomy

The radial nerve originates from the posterior cord (C5-T1) of the brachial plexus. It enters the arm medial to the humerus, anterior to the long head of the triceps. The nerve then travels across the humerus shaft within the radial groove, which is approximately halfway down the humerus. At the lateral edge of the humerus, it continues to travel inferiorly between the between the brachial and brachioradialis muscles.

It then travels anterior to the lateral epicondyle, where it subsequently divides into deep and superficial branches. The deep branch contains the motor fibers of the radial nerve, while the superficial branch exclusively carries the sensory fibers of the hand. The superficial branch travels laterally to the radial artery, deep to the brachioradialis along the forearm. It pierces the deep fascia of the forearm, and continues anteriorly to the anatomic snuff box. The branch becomes more superficial prior to entering the wrist and is more accessible for blocks [1, 2] (Fig. 8).

On its route through the arm, the radial nerve first gives motor innervation to the medial and long head of the triceps. As it passes through the radial groove, it gives off another branch to the lateral head of the triceps, along with the posterior cutaneous nerve of the forearm. The posterior cutaneous nerve supplies sensory innervation from the posterior forearm to the wrist. The radial nerve splits into two terminal branches at the lateral epicondyle, the superficial and deep branches of the radial nerve. The deep branch (posterior interosseous nerve) supplies motor innervation

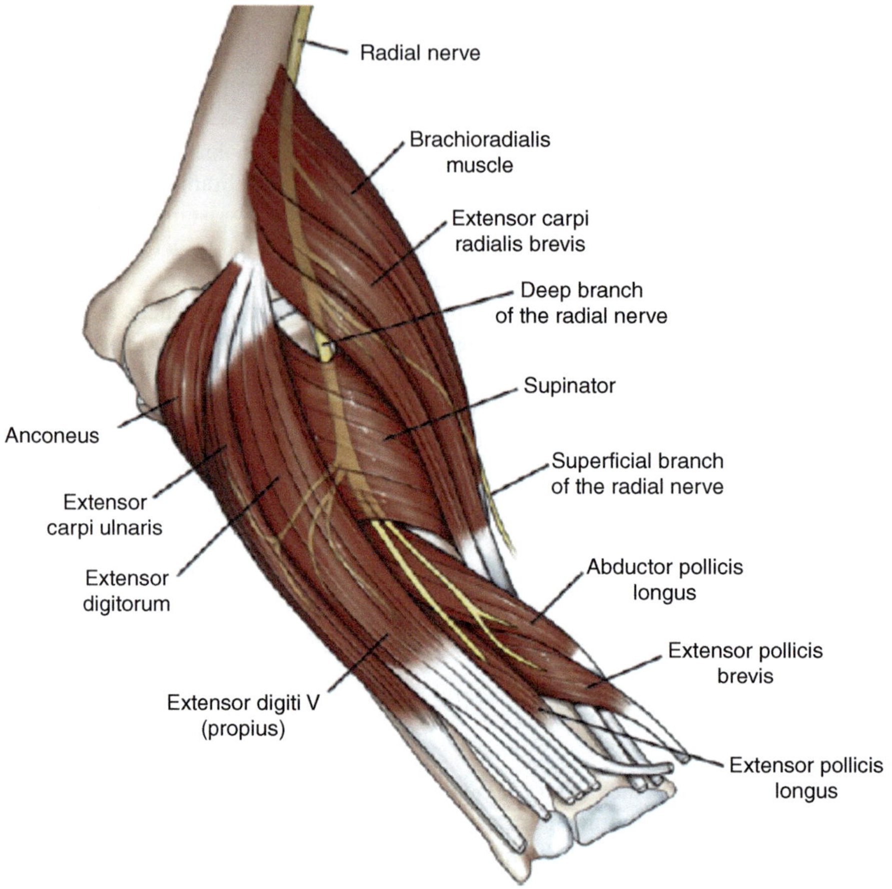

Fig. 8 Anatomy of the radial nerve at the elbow. Reprinted with permission from Vögelin E, Bignion D, Leclère F, Andrea C, PierLuigi B, Guglielmo L (2020) Radial nerve entrapment at the elbow. In: Bain G, Eygendaal D, van Riet R (eds) Surgical techniques for trauma and sports related injuries of the elbow. Springer, Berlin. https://doi.org/10.1007/978-3-662-58931-1_104

to the posterior forearm muscles. The superficial branch supplies sensory innervation to the lateral 2/3rds of the dorsal hand, the dorsum of the thumb, dorsum of proximal 1/2 of index finger, radial and proximal half of the long finger (Figs. 1 and 2) [1, 2].

Procedural Technique

Elbow/Antecubital Fossa

Start with the arm abducted at 45°, with the hand resting on the abdomen. Place the transducer on the anterolateral distal arm, 3 cm proximal to the elbow crease. At this location, the radial nerve travels between the brachioradialis and brachialis muscles. With the nerve dividing distal to the elbow, a nerve block in this area guarantees a complete blockade of the entire nerve. This site is also preferred, as there are no other neurovascular structures in the immediate vicinity. With the ultrasound probe held transversely, introduce the needle from the lateral side of the probe and inject approximately 5 ml of LA at the base of the nerve [8] (Fig. 6).

Forearm

The superficial radial nerve is often difficult to visualize at the wrist thus it is often recommended to find the nerve near the mid-forearm. Start by tracing the nerve from the lateral epicondyle into the lateral forearm where it divides into superficial and deep branches (Fig. 7). From here follow the superficial branch distal to the division. At this location it can be seen just lateral to the radial artery. An in plane or out of plane technique can be used. The skin can be localized and 3–5 ml of LA injected around the nerve (Fig. 7).

Antebrachial Cutaneous Nerve Block

Indications

- Injuries of the forearm
- AV fistula creation

Clinical Anatomy

There are two antebrachial cutaneous nerves, one medial and one lateral. The medial cutaneous nerve originates from the medial cord of the brachial plexus (C8-T1) and descends the medial arm, where it divides into a volar and dorsal nerve halfway down the arm. These two nerves provide sensory innervation to the medial forearm. The lateral cutaneous nerve is the terminal branch of the musculocutaneous nerve (C5-C7), which travels alongside the axillary artery and then laterally between the biceps brachii and brachialis muscles (Fig. 9).

Approximately 2 cm proximal to the elbow, it gives off its final motor branch to the biceps brachii and subsequently continues as the lateral antebrachial cutaneous nerve. At the elbow, the lateral cutaneous nerve branches into volar and dorsal branches, which supply sensory innervation to the lateral forearm (Figs. 1 and 2) [1, 2].

Procedural Technique

When performing a forearm block, unless it is an obvious medial or lateral injury, it is usually necessary to perform both a lateral and medial cutaneous nerve block. Start with the patient supine, with the arm externally rotated and abducted to 90°. Place the transducer over the midline, medial arm, and identify the biceps brachii muscle, brachial artery, median nerve, basilic vein. The medial cutaneous branch should be

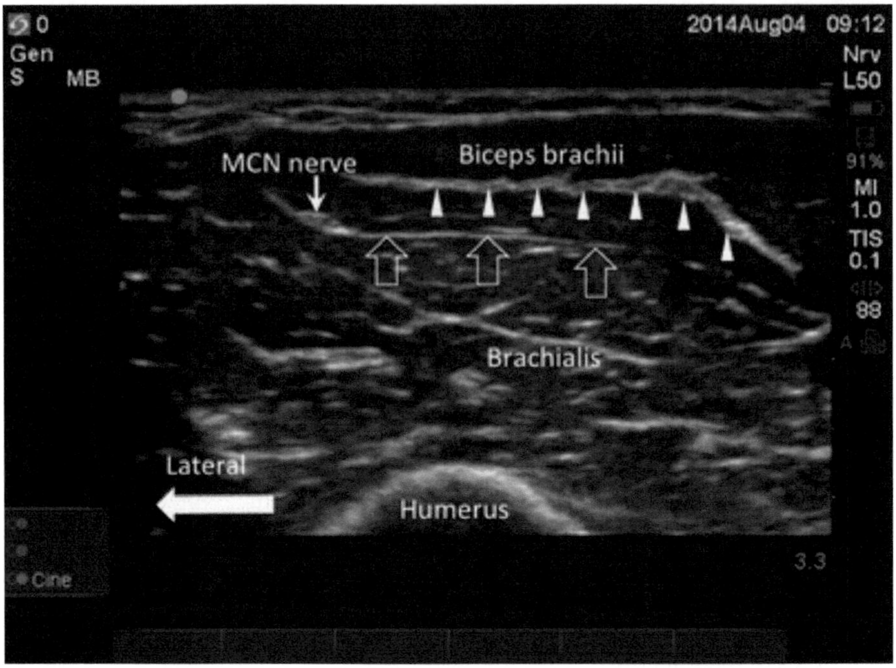

Fig. 9 Sonogram of the cutaneous branch of musculoskeletal nerve. At distal one third of the arm, the nerve is consistently in the fascia plane between the biceps brachii and brachialis muscles (*void arrows*). The fascia plane between these two muscles can be difficult to be visualized because of anisotropy, and tilting the ultrasound until the plane is clearly seen is crucial. Some practitioners may mistake the tendon (*arrowheads*) of the biceps brachii as the fascia plane. Reprinted with permission from Jankovic D, Peng P (2015) Peripheral nerve blocks in the elbow region. In: Regional nerve blocks in anesthesia and pain therapy. Springer, Cham. https://doi.org/10.1007/978-3-319-05131-4_34

found lateral to the basilic vein (which is the most superficial structure), where it can then be followed distally to its branching point. The nerve should separate from the basilic vein during its course and can be safely blocked after separation [9].

For the lateral cutaneous nerve, start with the patient supine, the arm abducted, and the elbow extended. The transducer should be placed on the medial arm just proximal to the elbow. Identify the biceps brachii aponeurosis and the biceps tendon. The nerve is lateral to the tendon and can be followed distally, where it becomes more superficial prior to dividing into its volar and dorsal branches. This is an ideal area to perform the block [9].

5 Potential Adverse Events and Complications

Complications are rare. They include bleeding, infection, injury to the nerves, and local anesthetic toxicity (LAST). The risk of LAST is relatively low given the low volume utilized in these blocks [10].

Clinical Pearls

- Do not hesitate to perform multiple nerve blocks as needed to obtain adequate analgesia. Although the dermatomal distribution of the nerves is generally well-defined, there is still significant overlap that may necessitate multiple blocks.
- Ultrasound should always be used initially to identify the nerve and important neurovascular structures around it. Ultrasound should also be used during the procedure to guide the needle to increase efficacy and decrease complications.

References

1. Moore KL, et al. Upper limb. In: Clinically oriented anatomy. 7th ed. Dordecht: LWW; 2013. p. 688–784.
2. Baglien P, Varacallo M. Anatomy, shoulder and upper limb, cutaneous innervation. In: StatPearls [Internet]. Treasure Island, FL: StatPearls Publishing; 2019. [Updated 22 Jul 2019].
3. Pester JM, Varacallo M. Ulnar nerve block techniques. In: StatPearls [Internet]. Treasure Island, FL: StatPearls Publishing; 2019. [cited 30 Nov 2019]. https://www.ncbi.nlm.nih.gov/books/NBK459208/?report=reader#!po=87.5000.
4. McMahon R, Bedforth N. Peripheral nerve block at the elbow and wrist. Cont Edu Anaest Critic Care Pain. 2007;7(2):42–4.
5. Kathirgamanathan A, French J, Foxall G, Hardman J, Bedforth N. Delineation of distal ulnar nerve anatomy using ultrasound in volunteers to identify an optimum approach for neural blockade. Eur J Anaesthesiol. 2009;26(1):43–6.
6. Varshney R, Sharma N, Malik S, Malik S. A cadaveric study comparing the three approaches for ulnar nerve block at wrist. Saudi J Anaest. 2014;8(5):25. [cited 30 Nov 2019]. https://www.ncbi.nlm.nih.gov/pmc/articles/PMC4268523/?report=reader.
7. Pester J, Varacallo M. Median nerve block techniques [Internet]. In: StatPearls [Internet]. Treasure Island, FL: StatPearls Publishing; 2019. [cited 30 Nov 2019]. https://www.ncbi.nlm.nih.gov/books/NBK459141/.
8. Durrani M, Dasgupta S. Radial nerve block [Internet]. In: StatePearls [Internet]. Treasure Island, FL: StatPearls Publishing; 2019. [cited 30 Nov 2019]. https://www.ncbi.nlm.nih.gov/books/NBK532951/#!po=70.0000.
9. Sehmbi H, Shah U, Madjdpour C, Chin K. Ultrasound guided distal peripheral nerve block of the upper limb: a technical review. J Anaest Clin Pharmacol. 2015;31(3):296. [cited 30 Nov 2019]. http://www.joacp.org/article.asp?issn=0970-9185;year=2015;volume=31;issue=3;spage=296;epage=307;aulast=Sehmbi.
10. Neal J. Cutaneous blocks for the upper extremity: textbook of regional anesthesia and acute pain management. New York: McGraw Hill; 2007. p. 467–75.

Further Reading

Chan VWS. Peripheral nerve block. In: VWS C, editor. Ultrasound imaging for regional anesthesia: a practical guide booklet, upper limb, vol. 2. Toronto Center for Ultrasound Education. 1st ed. San Diego, CA: iBook, Apple Inc.; 2013. p. 116–36.

Neal JM, Gerancher JC, Hebl JR, et al. Upper extremity regional anesthesia: essentials of our current understanding, 2008. Reg Anesth Pain Med. 2009;34(2):134–70.

Sohoni A, Nagdev A, Takhar S, Stone M. Forearm ultrasound-guided nerve blocks vs landmark-based wrist blocks for hand anesthesia in healthy volunteers. Am J Emerg Med. 2016;34(4):730–4. https://doi.org/10.1016/j.ajem.2016.01.020.

Carpal and Cubital Tunnel Injections

Ankur A. Patel, Neal Rakesh, and Navdeep S. Jassal

Essential Concepts

- Carpal Tunnel Syndrome (CTS) and Cubital Tunnel Syndrome (CuTS) are common peripheral nerve entrapment syndromes commonly due to mechanical or systemic etiologies.
- When evaluating for median and ulnar nerve compression, physical examination and electrodiagnostic imaging can help rule out other pathologies.
- Carpal and cubital tunnel injections are a safe and effective diagnostic and therapeutic modality for patients with persistent, mild to moderate pain and paresthesia due to median or ulnar nerve pathology, that has poorly responded to conservative modalities.
- This intervention can be easily performed at the bedside by landmark or ultrasound-guided technique and is typically well tolerated by patients.

A. A. Patel · N. Rakesh
Department of Physical Medicine and Rehabilitation, New York-Presbyterian Hospital, Columbia University Medical Center/Weill Cornell Medical Center, New York, NY, USA
e-mail: anp9251@nyp.org; ner9038@nyp.org

N. S. Jassal (✉)
Department of Neurology/Pain, University of South Florida College of Medicine, Tampa, FL, USA

Spine and Pain Institute of Florida, Lakeland, FL, USA

Lakeland, FL, USA
e-mail: DrJassal@spiflorida.com

D. Souza et al. (eds.), *Bedside Pain Management Interventions*,
https://doi.org/10.1007/978-3-031-11188-4_58

1 Carpal Tunnel Injection

Overview

Carpal Tunnel Syndrome (CTS) presents as a constellation of signs and symptoms brought on by compression of the median nerve as it travels through the carpal tunnel. It is the most common entrapment neuropathy with an estimated lifetime risk of 10% and is the most expensive upper extremity musculoskeletal disorder in the United States [1, 2]. CTS classically presents with intermittent pain or paresthesia at the wrist and/or in the distribution of the median nerve, including the palmar surface of the first three digits and the radial half of the fourth digit. Progression of the syndrome can lead to motor involvement and often presents as weakness of the hand, particularly the thenar muscles, resulting in the inability to open jars or dropping objects. Often times symptoms are more prevalent at night, resulting in nocturnal awakening. It may present bilaterally; however, the dominant hand is often affected first.

Indications and Contraindications

Etiologies of CTS can be divided into mechanical or systemic causes. Mechanical causes commonly present due to repetitive wrists movements, including keyboard typing, playing the piano, or use of vibratory tools, which cause swelling of the flexor tendon membrane, resulting in median nerve compression. Common systemic causes include diabetes, hypothyroidism, congestive heart failure, renal failure, rheumatoid arthritis, and pregnancy [3]. A complete diagnostic workup including ruling out systemic causes is imperative.

CTS is a clinical diagnosis requiring a thorough history and physical examination, including motor and sensory examination of the cervical spine, shoulder, elbow, and wrist. Provocative tests (Table 1 [4, 5] and Figs. 1, 2 and 3) may reproduce symptoms in the form of pain and/or paresthesia in the median nerve distribution and may be helpful in narrowing the diagnosis, although some of these tests have poor specificity. It is important to note that a normal physical examination does

Table 1 Description of provocative tests for carpal tunnel syndrome with corresponding sensitivities and specificities

Provocative test	Description	Sensitivity	Specificity
Carpal compression test [3]	Placing both thumbs over the transverse carpal ligament and applying direct pressure for 30 s. Wrist should be in neutral position	87%	90%
Phalen's test [4]	Maximal wrist flexion with holding the dorsal surfaces of the hand together for 60 s	85%	89%
Tinel's test [4] (of the wrist)	Percussing over the transverse carpal ligament	67%	68%

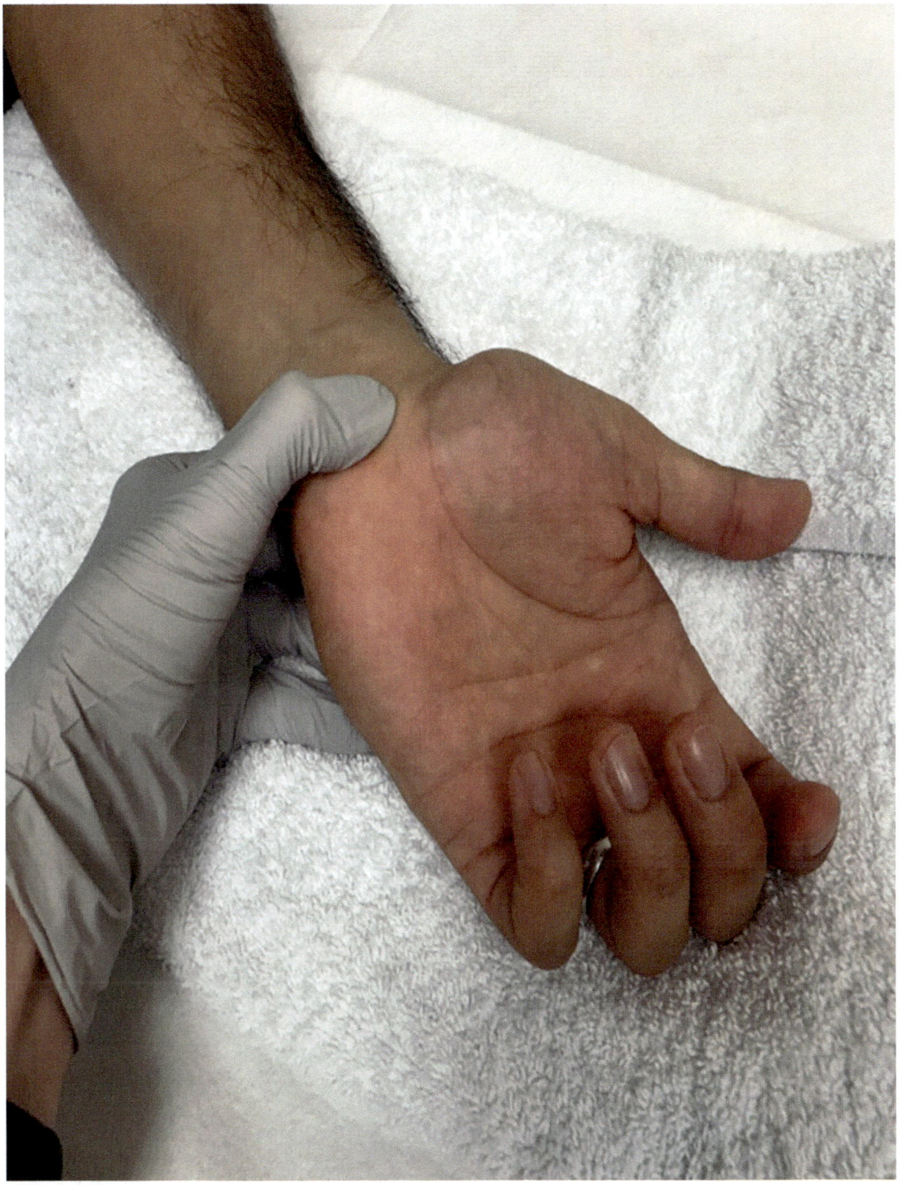

Fig. 1 Tinel's sign of the wrist

not rule out CTS and if there is a high clinical suspicion, electrodiagnostic studies including electromyography (EMG) and nerve conduction studies (NCS) should be done to confirm or rule out the diagnosis.

Patients with mild to moderate symptoms of CTS that are refractory to conservative management, such as activity modification, splinting and treatment of underline

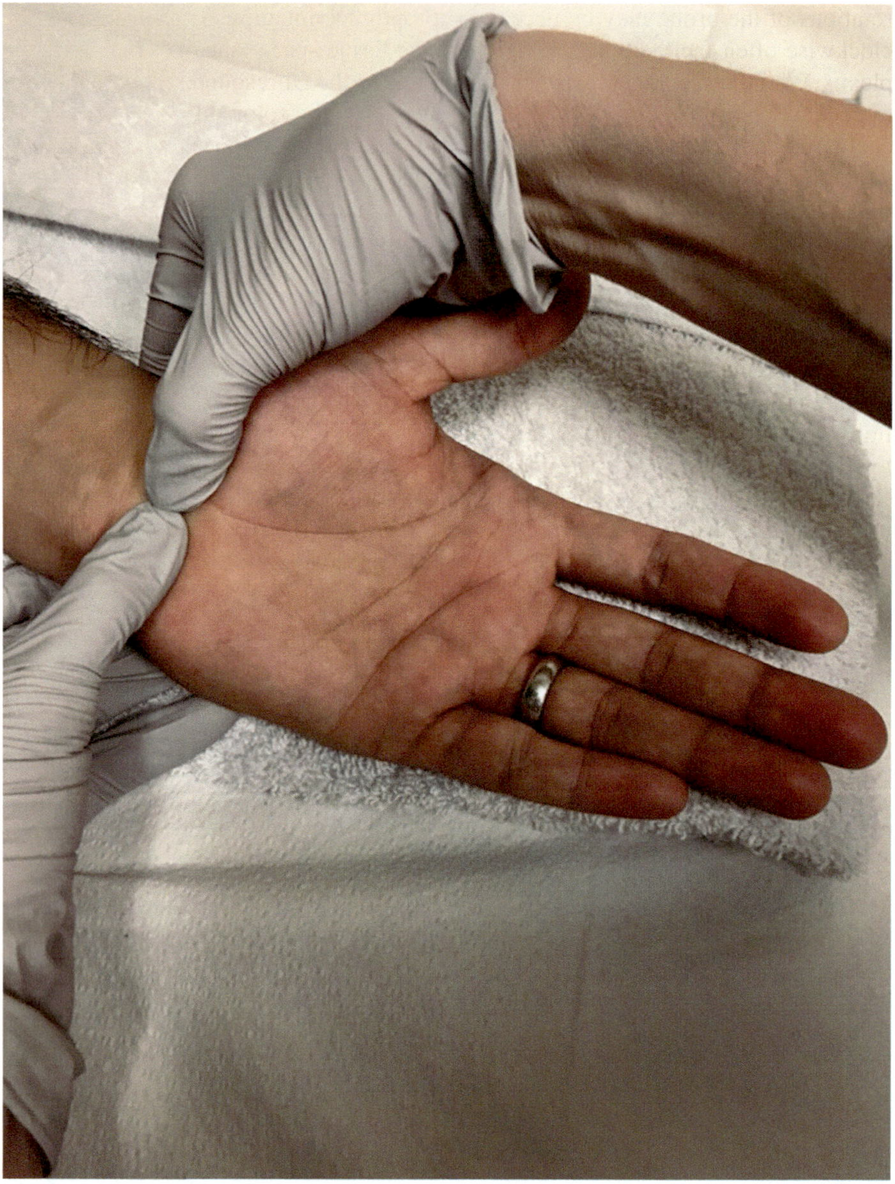

Fig. 2 Carpal compression test

systemic etiology, should be considered for carpal tunnel injection with a combination of corticosteroid and local anesthetic. Prior to proceeding, the indications and contraindications should be reviewed to ensure the patient is an appropriate candidate (Table 2).

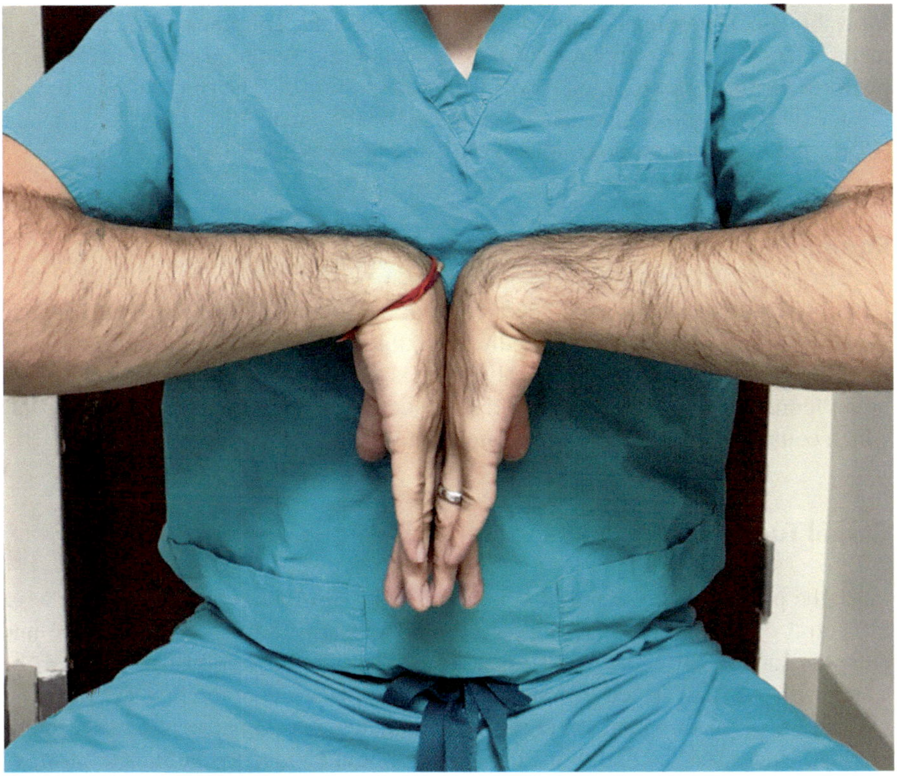

Fig. 3 Phalen's test

Table 2 Indications and contraindications for carpal tunnel injection

Indications	Contraindications	
• Management of wrist and hand pain due to median nerve compression that is refractory to conservative treatment options	Relative: • Uncontrolled diabetes • Use of anticoagulants • Coagulopathies • Systemic infection	Absolute: • Patient refusal • Local injection at the site of injection • Local malignancy • History of allergic reaction to injectate

Clinical Anatomy

The carpal tunnel is an osseofibrous canal located on the volar aspect of the wrist. The tunnel is formed by two layers: a carpal arch and flexor retinaculum, also known as the transverse carpal ligament. The carpal arch forms a concave surface that is composed of the carpal bones. The pisiform and hamate form the medial proximal to distal aspect, respectively, of the carpal arch, and the scaphoid and trapezium form the lateral proximal to distal aspect, respectively. The transverse carpal ligament extends from the tubercle of the trapezium and scaphoid to the hamate and pisiform forming the so called "roof" of the carpal tunnel. The carpal tunnel houses the median nerve and nine tendons, including the flexor digitorum superficialis (FDS), flexor digitorum profundus (FDP), and flexor pollicis longus (PFL).

Equipment and Supplies

Carpal tunnel injection is easily performed at bedside with landmark or ultrasound guidance. Using a 25–27 gauge needle, a mixture of local anesthetic and corticosteroid is injected into carpal tunnel (Table 3). It is advised that injectate amount should be no more than 2–3 cc due to the risk of increased pressure in the tunnel space, which could further worsen compression symptoms.

Carpal Tunnel Injection, Landmark Technique

Place the patient in the seated or supine position with forearm supinated and wrist in neutral or slight extension. Palpate the flexor carpi radialis (FCR) tendon and palmaris longus (PL) tendon, if present. To identify the tendons, the PL can be tested with the wrist flexed in combination with opposition of the first and fifth digits. The site of injection, lateral to the PL tendon at the proximal wrist crease, can be marked. Under sterile conditions, the needle should be inserted at the site of injection at 35–45° angle (Fig. 4). The injector can instruct the patient to slowly flex and extend his/her fingers to ensure the needle is not through the tendon. Once the needle tip is at midpoint of the flexor retinaculum, aspirate prior to slowly injecting to ensure needle is not inadvertently placed in a vascular structure.

Carpal Tunnel Injection, Ultrasound Technique

Alternatively, an ultrasound guidance technique can be utilized for this procedure. For this technique, place the patient in a seated or supine position with the forearm supinated and wrist in neutral or slight extension. Palpate and identify the scaphoid and pisiform bone. Place the high frequency linear ultrasound transducer just

Table 3 Required supplies for carpal tunnel injection

Syringe	3 cc
Needle	25 or 27 gauge 1.5–2 in.
Ultrasound probe	High-frequency linear probe (10 MHz)
Anesthetic	0.25–0.5% bupivacaine 1–2% lidocaine
Corticosteroid	Particulate or non-particulate steroid

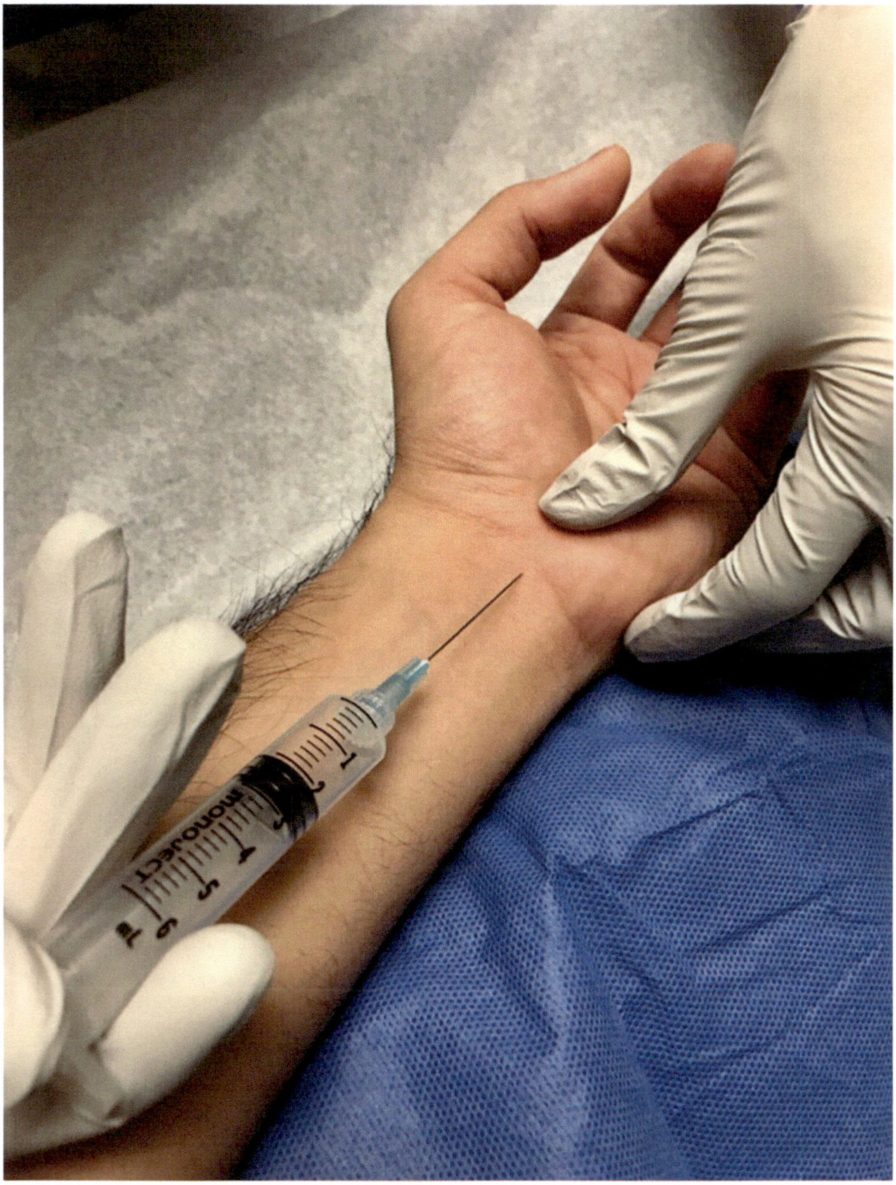

Fig. 4 Landmark guided injection of the carpal tunnel

proximal to the pisiform and scaphoid bones (Fig. 5) and scan distally until the structures of carpal tunnel are visualized, including the median nerve, FDP, FDS, and FPL. Once the structures are identified in a transverse view, either an in-plane or out-of-plane technique can be used for the injection (Fig. 6). For the in-plane

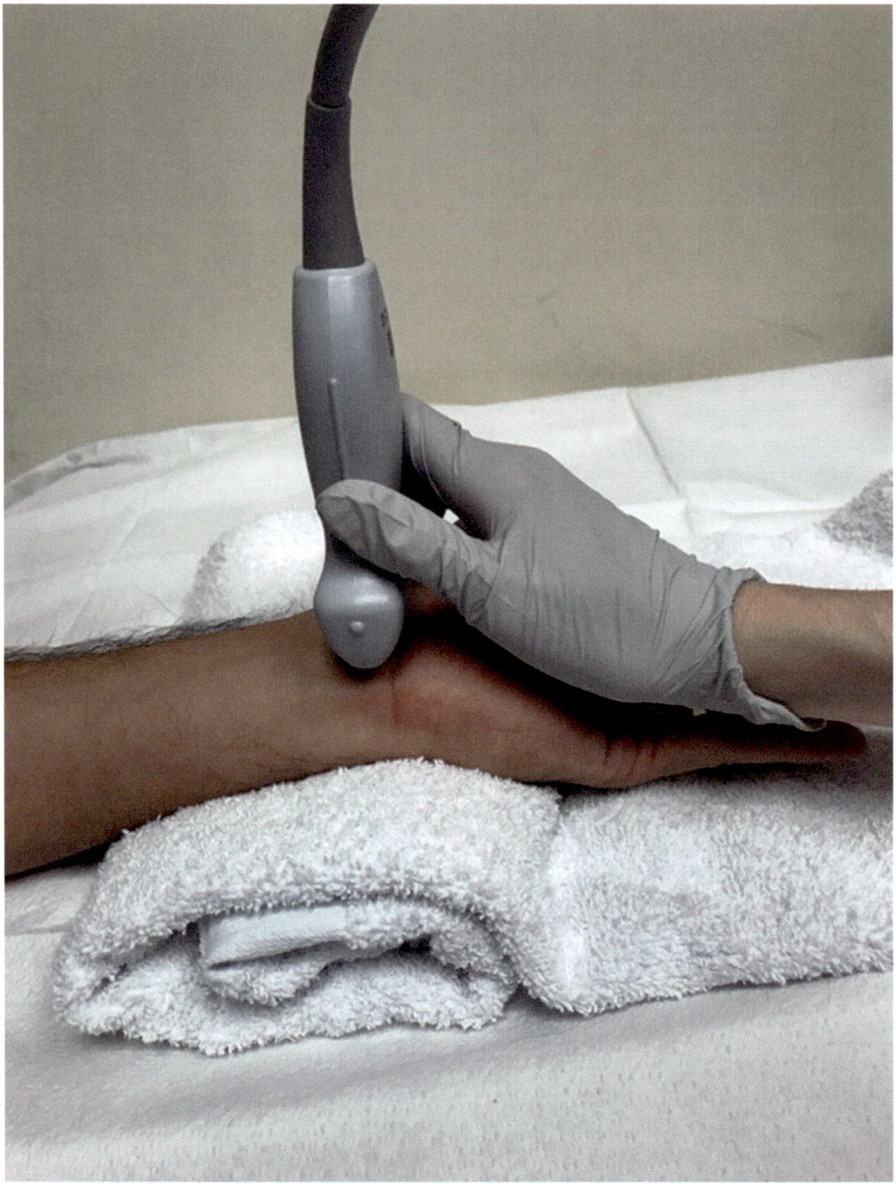

Fig. 5 Ultrasound probe placement in transverse view for carpal tunnel injection

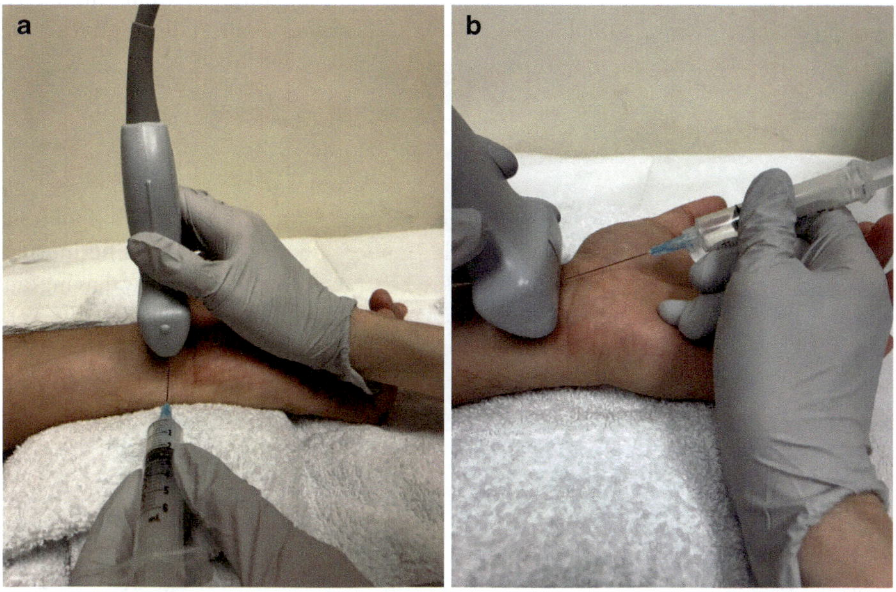

Fig. 6 (**a**) Needle trajectory for in-plane (IP) ultrasound guided carpal tunnel injection. (**b**) Needle trajectory for out-of-plane (OP) ultrasound guided carpal tunnel injection

approach, under sterile conditions, the needle is inserted on the radial aspect and advanced until it's in proximity of the median nerve. A lateral to medial approach is recommended due to the close proximity of ulnar artery and vein, medially. Once the needle tip is within the tunnel and adjacent to the median nerve, slowly inject and visualize the flow. Alternatively, an out-of-plane approach can be performed. Under sterile conditions, the needle is inserted midline of the probe adjacent to the median nerve. Once the tip of the needle is visualized, the injectate is slowly injected and flow is visualized (Fig. 7).

Potential Complications and Adverse Effects

Although this procedure is generally well tolerated by patients, it is important to be aware of potential complications and adverse effects. With the landmark approach, there is a higher risk of neurovascular damage due to the lack of direct visualization. Key structures that can be injured with this approach include the median nerve, ulnar artery, ulnar vein and/or tendons. When possible, ultrasound guidance should be utilized to mitigate injury to neurovascular structures. Even with ultrasound guidance, it is important injectors accurately define the patient's anatomy prior to proceeding with an injection and adapt the approach appropriately to decrease risk of injury.

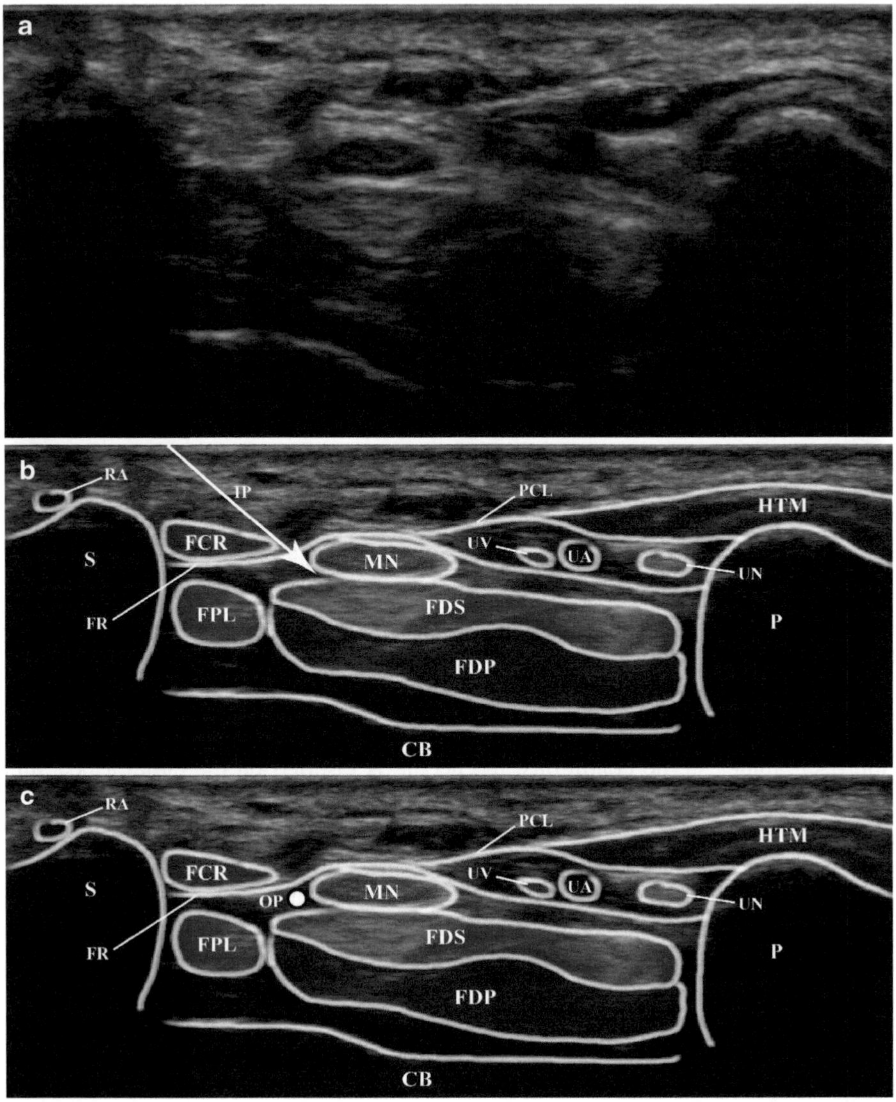

Fig. 7 (**a**) Ultrasound image of the carpal tunnel in transverse view. (**b**) Labeled ultrasound image of in-plane (IP) carpal tunnel injection. (**c**) Labeled ultrasound image of out-of-plane (OP) carpal tunnel injection. *CB* carpal bones, *FCR* flexor carpal radialis, *FDP* flexor digitorum profundus, *FDS* flexor digitorum superficialis, *FPL* flexor pollicis longus, *FR* flexor retinaculum, *HTM* hypothenar muscle, *MN* median nerve, *P* pisiform, *PCL* palmar carpal ligament, *RA* radial artery, *S* scaphoid, *UA* ulnar artery, *UN* ulnar nerve, *UV* ulnar vein

Clinical and Technical Pearls

- Carpal tunnel injection is a safe and effective diagnostic and therapeutic intervention that can be done at bedside.
- A comprehensive physical examination with diagnostic imaging and electrodiagnostic testing is imperative when evaluating patients with median nerve dysfunction, as other pathologies can mimic CTS.
- With the landmark approach, there is higher risk for neurovascular injury, especially in patients who do not have a PL tendon. When possible, ultrasound-guided approach should be utilized.
- Amount of injectate should be limited to 2–3 cc to prevent further compression of the median nerve.

2 Cubital Tunnel Injection

Overview

Cubital Tunnel Syndrome (CuTS) presents due to compression of the ulnar nerve as it travels through the cubital tunnel at the elbow. It is the second most common peripheral nerve entrapment and initially presents with intermittent pain or paresthesia at the palmar and dorsal surface of the medial half of the fourth digit, the entirety of the fifth digit, and the associated medial section of the hand [6]. As the disease process progresses, patients may experience weakness in the ulnar innervated intrinsic hand muscles, which may lead to froment's sign, pronounced flexion of the distal thumb with resistance, and wartenberg's sign, resting unopposed abduction of the fifth digit. In severe cases, atrophy of the intrinsic hand muscles is noted. Although the most common site of ulnar nerve entrapment is the cubital tunnel, clinicians should rule out other sites of entrapment prior to proceeding with a cubital tunnel injection.

Indications and Contraindications

At the elbow region, the ulnar nerve is subjected to compression at five different sites: the arcade of Struthers, medial intermuscular septum, medial epicondyle, cubital tunnel, and deep flexor pronator aponeurosis [7]. The cubital tunnel is the most common site of compression of the ulnar nerve, which results in CuTS. Similar to CTS, CuTS is commonly due to mechanical etiologies, such as repetitive and prolonged elbow flexion particularly against a hard surface, which increases intraneural pressure of the ulnar nerve. During elbow flexion, the ulnar nerve is stretched and the cross-sectional area of the cubital tunnel is decreased resulting in increased intraneural pressure by up to 20-folds [8]. Patients who are at increased risk for CuTS include those with existing ulnar nerve subluxation, obesity, arthritis, previous upper extremity fractures or dislocations, and/or space occupying lesions such as cysts or tumors.

When evaluating for CuTS, an in-depth history and physical examination is vital to rule out other causes of ulnar mononeuropathy including brachial plexopathy or C8 radiculopathy. Positive provocative maneuvers, such as Tinel's sign at the wrist and elbow flexion test, may increase clinical suspicion (Table 4 and Figs. 8 and 9); however, electrodiagnostic testing is recommended to confirm the diagnosis, as well as differentiate from other clinically overlapping pathologies [9]. If there is concern for anatomical variations or space occupying lesions, ultrasound and magnetic resonance imaging can be performed to better aid in clinical evaluation.

The initial management of mild to moderate symptoms of CuTS include education, pain/inflammation reduction, and rehabilitation. Corticosteroid injections can

Table 4 Description of provocative tests for cubital tunnel syndrome

Provocative test	Description
Elbow flexion test	Full elbow flexion, forearm supination and wrist extension for up to 3 min
Tinel's test (of the elbow)	Percussing over the cubital tunnel

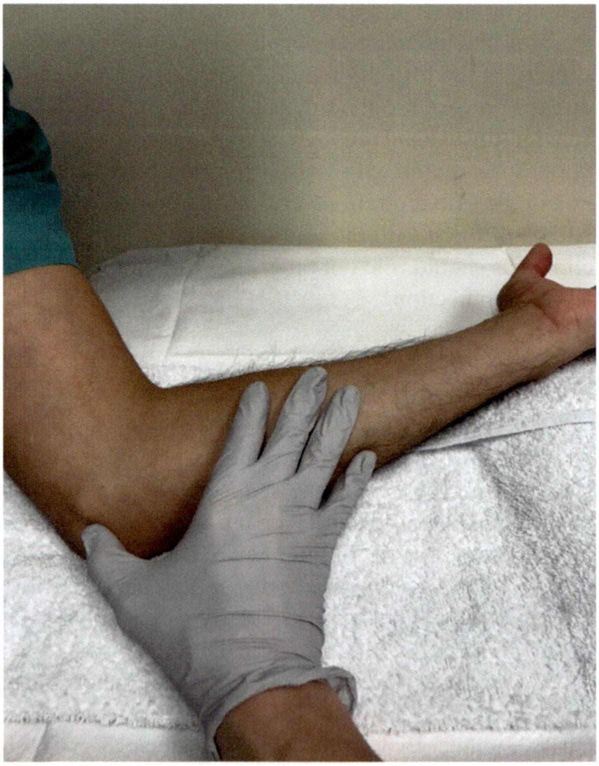

Fig. 8 Tinel's sign of the elbow

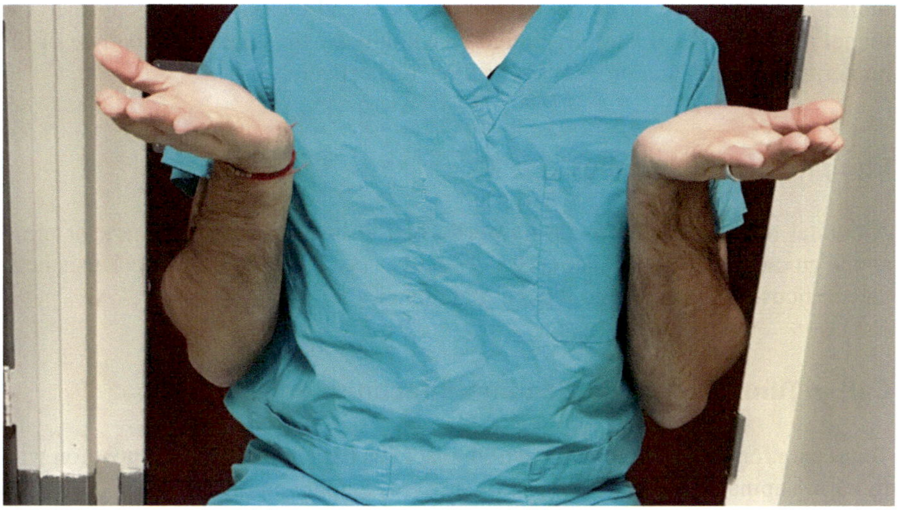

Fig. 9 Elbow flexion test

Table 5 Indication and contraindications for cubital tunnel injection

Indications	Contraindications	
• Management of elbow and hand pain due to ulnar nerve compression at the site of the cubital tunnel that is refractory to conservative treatment options	Relative: • Uncontrolled diabetes • Use of anticoagulants • Coagulopathies • Systemic infection	Absolute: • Patient refusal • Local injection at the site of injection • Local malignancy • History of allergic reaction to injectate

be considered in select patients who have not found symptomatic relief from other therapies, including but not limited to, activity modification and splinting. Prior proceeding, the indications and contraindications should be reviewed to ensure patient is appropriate candidate (Table 5).

Clinical Anatomy

Derived from the anterior rami of C8 and T1 spinal nerves, the ulnar nerve travels in the upper arm along the brachial artery and median nerve to the midpoint of the upper arm where it pierces the arcade of Struthers down into the retrocondylar groove at the elbow. Once exiting the groove, the ulnar nerve passes under the humeroulnar arcade into the cubital tunnel.

The roof of the cubital tunnel is crafted by Osborne's ligament/fascia, which spans from humeroulnar arcade proximally and between the humeral and ulnar heads of the flexor carpi ulnaris (FCU) muscle distally. The floor of the cubital tunnel is made of the medial collateral ligament and the elbow joint capsule. The tunnel is medially and laterally bound proximally by the medial epicondyle of the humerus and olecranon process of the ulna, respectively.

Equipment and Supplies

A cubital tunnel injection is easily performed at bedside with landmark or ultrasound guidance (Table 6). Using a 25–27 gauge needle, a mixture of local anesthetic and corticosteroid is injected into cubital tunnel.

Carpal Tunnel Injection, Landmark Technique

To prepare for a cubital tunnel injection, place the patient in the seated position with forearm supinated and rested on a flat surface. Palpate and identify the olecranon process and medial epicondyle. Between these two bony landmarks lies the ulnar nerve within the cubital tunnel and the target injection site is 1–2 cm distally from the bony landmarks. Under sterile conditions, the needle is inserted at 35–45° angle and advanced proximally between the olecranon process and medial epicondyle (Fig. 10). Once the needle tip is in the desired location, aspirate prior to slowly injecting to ensure needle is not inadvertently placed in a vascular structure.

Carpal Tunnel Injection, Ultrasound Technique

Place the patient in the seated position with the arm in forced internally rotation, elbow flexed to 90°, and hand resting on a flat surface. Palpate and identify the olecranon process and medial epicondyle. Although the cubital tunnel can be evaluated in the transverse and longitudinal views, the transverse view approach is described in this chapter. Place the high-frequency linear ultrasound transducer in the transverse plane proximal to the medial epicondyle and scan distally to identify the structures of the cubital tunnel including the ulnar nerve, medial epicondyle, olecranon process, ulnar and humeral head of the FCU, and Osborne's ligament/fascia (Fig. 11). Once the structures are identified, an in-plane approach is utilized (Fig. 12). Under sterile condition, the needle is inserted medially, advanced until the tip is adjacent to the

Table 6 Required supplies for cubital tunnel injection

Syringe	3 cc
Needle	25 or 27 gauge 1.5–2 in.
Ultrasound probe	High-frequency linear probe (10 MHz)
Anesthetic	0.25–0.5% bupivacaine 1–2% lidocaine
Corticosteroid	Particulate or non-particulate steroid

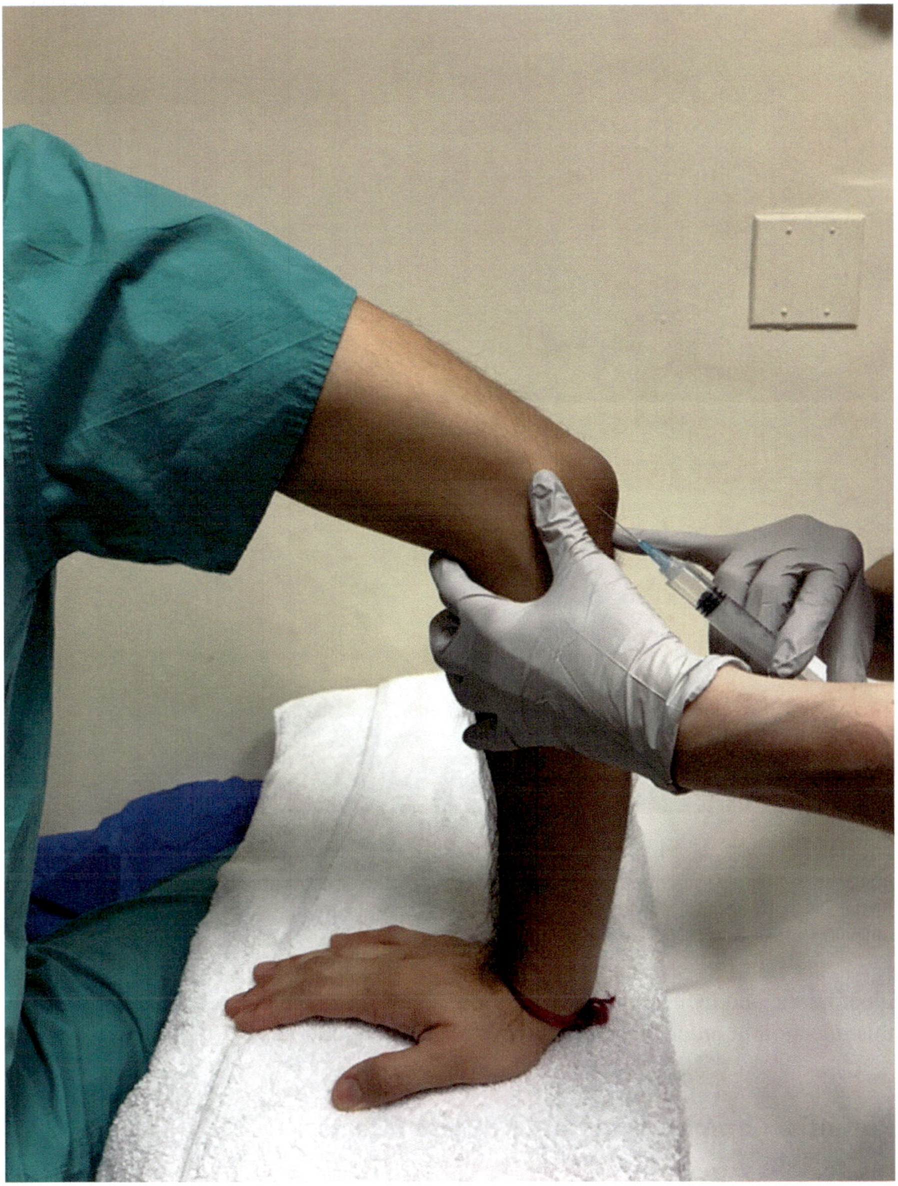

Fig. 10 Landmark guided injection of the cubital tunnel

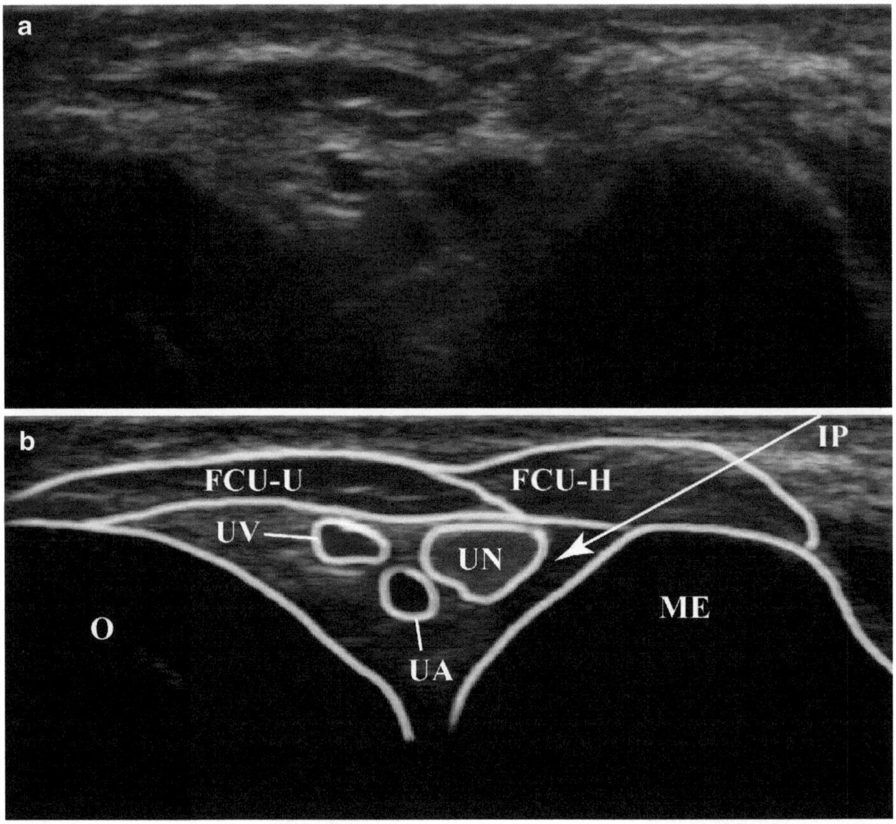

Fig. 11 (**a**) Ultrasound image of the cubital tunnel in transverse view. (**b**) Labeled ultrasound image of in-plane (IP) cubital tunnel injection. *FCU-H* flexor carpi ulnaris, humeral head, *FCU-U* flexor carpi ulnaris, ulnar head, *ME* medial epicondyle of the humerus, *O* olecranon process of the ulnar, *UA* ulnar artery, *UN* ulnar nerve, *UV* ulnar vein

ulnar nerve, and then slowly injected. The medial to lateral approach is preferred for this injection in order to avoid injury to ulnar artery and vein.

Potential Complications and Adverse Effects

Cubital tunnel injections, guided by either the landmark or ultrasound techniques, are generally well tolerated by patients. However, it is important to be aware of potential complications and adverse effects. Since there is no real-time imaging guidance with the landmark approach, there is a higher risk of neurovascular damage. Key structures that may be injured are the ulnar artery and ulnar nerve. The ultrasound technique mitigates the injury to these key structures and allows for a more targeted injection.

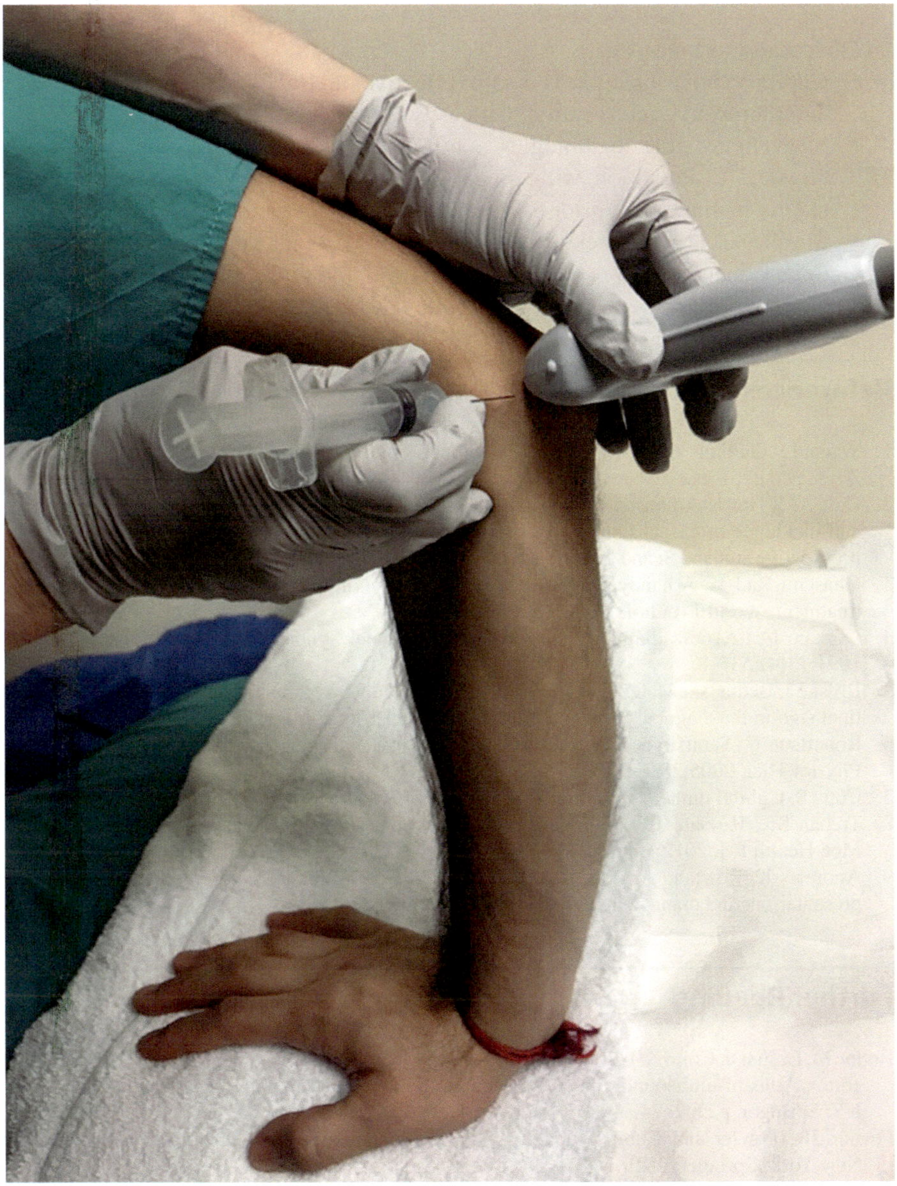

Fig. 12 Ultrasound probe placement in transverse view and needle trajectory for in-plane (IP) cubital tunnel injection

Clinical and Technical Pearls

- Cubital tunnel injection is a safe, effective, and well tolerated diagnostic and therapeutic intervention that easily can be done at bedside.
- Since many other pathologies may present like CuTS, a comprehensive physical examination with diagnostic imaging and/or electrodiagnostic testing is imperative prior to proceeding with a cubital tunnel injection.
- Similar to carpal tunnel injection, the amount of injectate should be limited to less than 3 cc to prevent further compression of the ulnar nerve.

References

1. Wang L. Guiding treatment for carpal tunnel syndrome. Phys Med Rehabil Clin N Am. 2018;29(4):751–60.
2. Dale AM, Harris-Adamson C, Rempel D, Gerr F, Hegmann K, Silverstein B, et al. Prevalence and incidence of carpal tunnel syndrome in US working populations: pooled analysis of six prospective studies. Scand J Work Environ Health. 2013;39(5):495–505.
3. Ghasemi-Rad M. A handy review of carpal tunnel syndrome: from anatomy to diagnosis and treatment. World J Radiol. 2014;6(6):284–300.
4. Durkan JA. A new diagnostic test for carpal tunnel syndrome. J Bone Joint Surg Am. 1991;73(4):535–8.
5. Brüske J, Bednarski M, Grzelec H, Zyluk A. The usefulness of the phalen test and the hoffmann-tinel sign in the diagnosis of carpal tunnel syndrome. Acta Orthop Belg. 2002;68(2):141–5.
6. Robertson C, Saratsiotis J. A review of compressive ulnar neuropathy at the elbow. J Manip Physiol Ther. 2005;28(5):345.
7. Cutts S. Cubital tunnel syndrome. Postgrad Med J. 2007;83(975):28–31.
8. Trehan SK, Parziale JR, Akelman E. Cubital tunnel syndrome: diagnosis and management. Med Health R I. 2012;95(11):349–52.
9. Andrews K, Rowland A, Pranjal A, Ebraheim N. Cubital tunnel syndrome: anatomy, clinical presentation, and management. J Orthop. 2018;15(3):832–6.

Further Reading

Bodor M, Lesher J, Colio S. Ultrasound-guided hand, wrist, and elbow injections. In: Narouze SN, editor. Atlas of ultrasound-guided procedures in interventional pain management. New York, NY: Springer. p. 307–24.

Fowler JR, Fowler JR. Cubital tunnel syndrome: diagnosis, management and rehabilitation. New York: Springer; 2019.

Lin E, Aligene K, Kirschner J. Elbow. In: Atlas of ultrasound guided musculoskeletal injections. New York, NY: Springer; 2016. p. 35–46.

Luchetti R. Carpal tunnel syndrome. Berlin: Springer; 2007.

Peng P. Carpal tunnel injection. In: Regional nerve blocks in anesthesia and pain therapy. New York, NY: Springer; 2015. p. 441–3.

Singh V, Ericson WB. Median nerve entrapments. In: Peripheral nerve entrapments. Cham: Springer International; 2016. p. 369–82.

Singh V, Trescot A. Ulnar nerve entrapments. In: Peripheral nerve entrapments. Cham: Springer International; 2016. p. 383–96.

Spinner D, Rosado M. Wrist and hand. In: Albrecht E, editor. Atlas of ultrasound guided musculo-skeletal injections. New York, NY: Springer; 2016. p. 47–59.

Bedside Injections for Wrist Pain

Eric M. Stockwell and Harlan B. Stern

Essential Concepts

- De Quervain's disease first extensor compartment injections are increasingly a first line and superior treatment compared with conservative medical management
- Radiocarpal joint injections are an effective therapeutic tool in treating a variety of painful etiologies including inflammatory arthritis, osteoarthritis, posttraumatic arthritis, and overuse
- Goals of injections for De Quervain's Disease and the radiocarpal joint include long-term relief and to prevent pain recurrence and additional management
- Ganglion cyst aspirations are indicated in the management of pain and for decompression of a vessel or nerve
- Pain relief is often rapid, and the duration of therapeutic benefit may last days to months.

Eric M. Stockwell is first author.

E. M. Stockwell (✉)
Louisiana State University Health Sciences Center, New Orleans, LA, USA
e-mail: estoc1@lsuhsc.edu

H. B. Stern
Ochsner Clinic, LA, USA

D. Souza et al. (eds.), *Bedside Pain Management Interventions*,
https://doi.org/10.1007/978-3-031-11188-4_59

1 Bedside Injections for De Quervain's Disease

Overview

De Quervain's Disease (DQD) is a mechanical irritation of the tendons within the first dorsal extensor compartment on the radial side of the wrist [1]. The two tendons within this compartment are of the abductor pollicis longus (APL) and the extensor pollicis brevis (EPB) (Fig. 1).

It is characterized by pain, swelling, and tenderness with an incidence of 0.5% in men and 1.3% in women [2]. Treatment modalities can be grouped into conservative medical management (CMM), including medications, splints, & injections; and surgical interventions, including surgical release. Ultrasound-guided corticosteroid injection of the first extensor compartment are increasingly being recognized as a superior of CMM [3].

Indications and Contraindications

De Quervain's Disease may appear with repetitive thumb extension and abduction causing ulnar deviation occurring in activities such as hammering and skiing. It may also appear under hormonal influence such as in post-partum patients. DQD

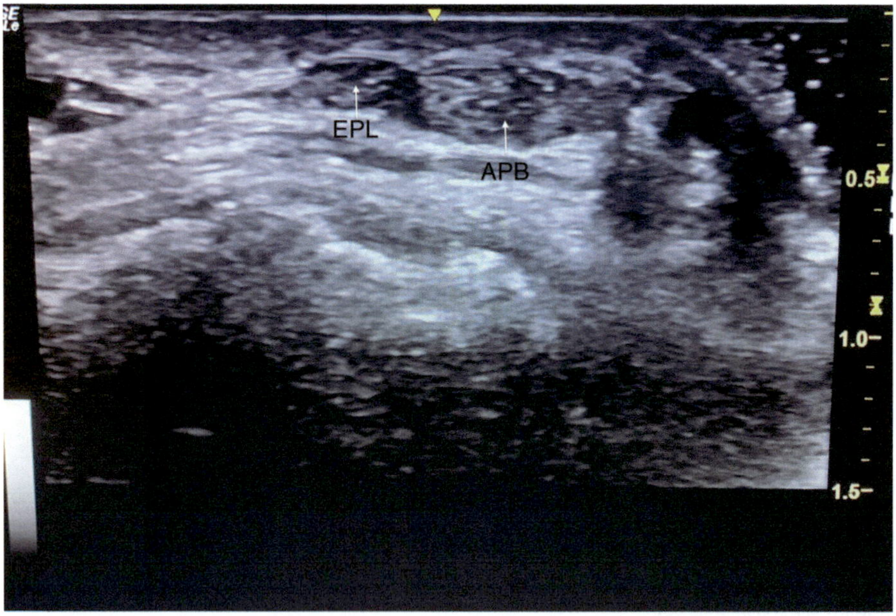

Fig. 1 Abductor pollicis longus and the extensor pollicis brevis tendons within the first extensor compartment. Ultrasonogram. *APL* abductor pollicis longus, *EPB* extensor pollicis brevis

arises when degenerative changes occur within the first extensor compartment causing tenosynovitis of the APL and EPB. It is a clinical diagnosis based on history and physical exam findings that include local tenderness and swelling of the radial wrist, as well as positive Finkelstein's test. The Finkelstein test is performed by holding the distal tip of the patient's thumb and adducting and pronating it over the palm to elicit their pain. The diagnosis is easily confirmed by ultrasound having a sensitivity of 100% and a specificity of 96% [2]. Ultrasound imaging of the tendons within the extensor compartment will show thickening of the synovium (Fig. 2a).

Common contraindications include infection at the injection site, intolerance or allergy to injectate, including steroids, and patient refusal. Anticoagulation, including iatrogenic, and platelet dysfunction, including iatrogenic, are not considered to be a contraindication for these injections.

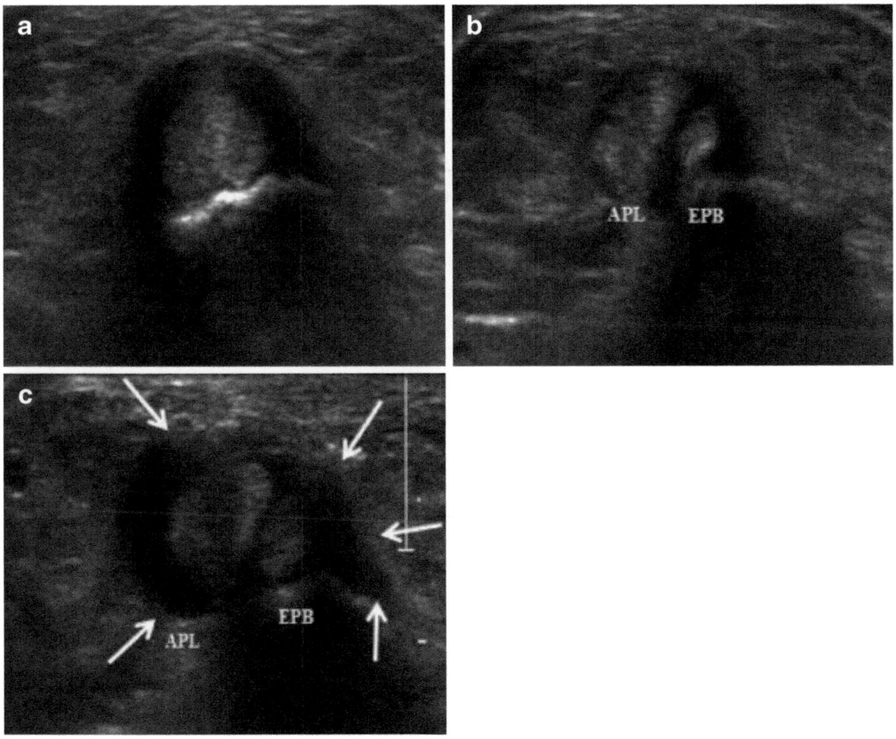

Fig. 2 (**a**) Thickening of the synovium within the first extensor compartment. Ultrasonogram. Hypoechoic area represents thickened synovium. (**b**) "Complete" compartmentalization of the abductor pollicis longus and extensor pollicis brevis in distinct compartments ultrasonogram. *APL* abductor pollicis longus, *EPB* extensor pollicis brevis. (**c**) Hypoechoic appearance of a septum between the adductor pollicis longus and extensor pollicis brevis tendons ultrasonogram. Arrows indicate hypoechoic appearance of the septum between the APL and EPB. *APL* abductor pollicis longus, *EPB* extensor pollicis brevis

Clinical Anatomy

The first dorsal extensor compartment is the most laterally located tendon compartment of the wrist. The compartment is lateral to the metacarpal bones and distal radial bone. Two tendons course through this compartment: abductor pollicis longus (APL) and the extensor pollicis brevis (EPB). There are three anatomical variations practitioners should be aware of due to their suspected influence on failure rates associated with corticosteroid injection to this compartment [3]. These variations relate to compartmentalization of the APL and EPB tendons. With "complete" compartmentalization we find the APL and EPB in distinct compartments. "Incomplete" compartmentalization has the APL and EPB in a shared compartment at the distal radius but in separate compartments more distally. Finally, there may be no compartmentalization when the tendons share a compartment. As described below, it is recommended that practitioners identify these compartments on ultrasound to guide technique (Fig. 2b).

Equipment and Supplies

This procedure can be performed at the bedside and in an office setting. It is recommended that practitioners use ultrasound (US) to confirm correct needle placement and adjust technique based on anatomical variation (Table 1).

Landmark Technique

Landmark-based technique can be used for these injections. However, as mentioned above, we do not recommend it because the ultrasonography allows confirming needle placement, adjusting the injection technique to anatomical variations, potentially decreasing the chance of unintentional vascular or neural injury, and possibly improving patient satisfaction. The same concerns about a blind injection are relevant to the other procedures described in this chapter. Therefore, we proceeded with describing only the ultrasound-guided technique.

Table 1 Equipment and supplies

Syringe	3 or 5 ml
Needle	25, 27, 30 gauge 1/2 to 1 in.
Anesthetic	0.5 mL 1–2% lidocaine 0.5 mL 0.25–0.5% bupivacaine 0.5 mL lidocaine/bupivacaine combination
Corticosteroid	Triamcinolone 20–40 mg (*t*1/2 life: 18–36 h) Methylprednisolone 40–80 mg (*t*1/2 life: 18–36 h)

Ultrasound-Guided Technique

In a clean fashion, begin by placing US probe on wrist to obtain a transverse view of the first extensor compartment, visualizing the two tendons (Fig. 3).

Scan the probe proximally and distally to identify whether the tendons have complete, distal incomplete, or no sub-compartmentalization. If there is no sub-compartmentalization, then the medication is injected in their common compartment. If incomplete compartmentalization is seen, then it is recommended to inject the medication within the proximally located shared compartment; to allow medication to diffuse distally within the separate compartments. Finally, if complete compartmentalization is seen then inject half of the prepared medication into each distinct compartment [4]. Figure 2c demonstrates the hypoechoic appearance of a septum between the tendons.

Potential Complications and Adverse Effects

The complication rate is extremely low and nearly all complications are self-limiting; requiring no medical intervention [5]. In addition to common complications such as bleeding or infection, patients may report mild paresthesia in the distribution of the radial nerve. Mild local depigmentation may occur as a result of superficially located steroid. Additionally, practitioners should be vigilant of allergic reactions to both steroid or local anesthetic.

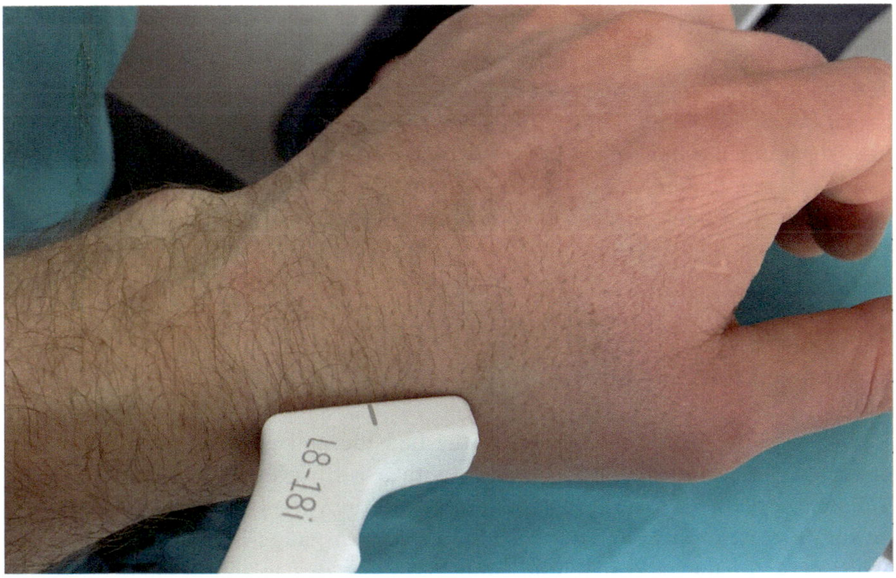

Fig. 3 Probe orientation and US image for first extensor compartment injection

2 Bedside Radiocarpal Joint Injection

Overview

Radiocarpal (RC) joint injection serves as a useful therapeutic tool in the management of painful conditions of the RC joint.

Indications and Contraindications

In patients that fail conservative management, RC joint injection is indicated for painful conditions due to inflammatory arthritis, osteoarthritis, posttraumatic arthritis, and overuse [6, 7]. Analysis of aspired effusion may be part of the diagnostic workup for inflammatory arthropathies. Pain at the RC joint can be predisposed from prior scaphoid fractures. Aging, genetics, gender, BMI, and daily use can all be factors in the development of RC joint pain. Pain usually manifests in the wrist with restrictions of wrist flexion and extension, and can also be accompanied by mild swelling and weakness [8, 9].

Common contraindications include infection at the injection site, intolerance of allergy to injectate, including steroids, and patient refusal. Anticoagulation, including iatrogenic, and platelet dysfunction, including iatrogenic, are not considered to be a contraindication for these injections.

Clinical Anatomy

The radiocarpal joint is composed of the distal radius and the proximal row of three carpal bones: scaphoid, lunate, and triquetrum. The triangular fibrocartilage complex separates the radioulnar joint, and the scapholunate and lunotriquetral ligaments separate the midcarpal joints. The wrist joint is not one compartment due to various divisions, but there is a communicating synovial cavity. The radiocarpal joint communicates with the pisiform-triquetral joint in approximately 75% of cases [10, 11].

Equipment and Supplies

This procedure can be performed at the bedside and in an office setting. The patient is placed in a seated position with a fully pronated forearm. Lister's Tubercle is palpated. The skin at the dorsum of the wrist is prepped with antiseptic solution. After localization of the RC joint, a 25-gauge 1-in. needle is inserted at the level of the radioscaphoid joint and advanced to the periosteum of the underlying distal radius. The needle is guided into the joint cavity until fluid flows freely. Steroid and local anesthetic are injected; please refer to Table 1 for specific volumes. After negative aspiration is confirmed, the solution is injected [12].

Ultrasound-Guided Technique

After prepping the skin with antiseptic, a high-frequency linear-array transducer is situated using a dorsal approach and longitudinal planes. The transducer should be translated with Lister's Tubercle in the center. The transducer should be rotated 90° into the anatomic sagittal plane for a long-axis view. In this position, it should be possible to visualize the distal radius, lunate, and capitate. The transducer can be rotated to ensure that the needle is placed between the second and third extensor compartments (separated by Lister's Tubercle). The needle is inserted in-lane distal-to-proximal trajectory at 45° to the transducer (Fig. 4).

A few millimeters distal to the joint is the optimum placement to avoid the dorsal lip of the radius [13]. Joint effusions, thickening of the synovium, articular space narrowing, osteophyte formation, and cortical irregularities are all common ultrasound findings.

Potential Complications and Adverse Effects

The complication rate is extremely low. The region of the scapholunate ligament should be avoided due to potential ligamentous damage. In addition to common complications such as bleeding or infection, patients may report mild paresthesia in the distribution of the radial nerve. In addition, mild depigmentation and allergic reactions as described in the initial section are potential complications. Two weeks of relative rest may be advised with splinting to protect the joint [13] (Fig. 5).

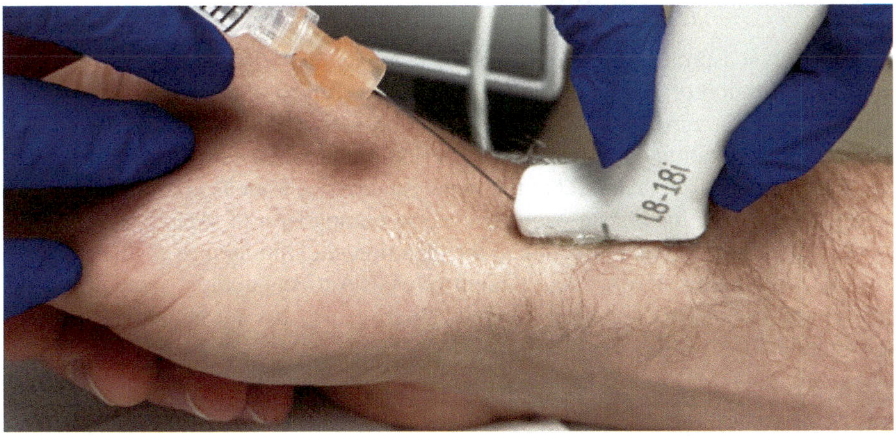

Fig. 4 Probe orientation and US image for radiocarpal joint injection

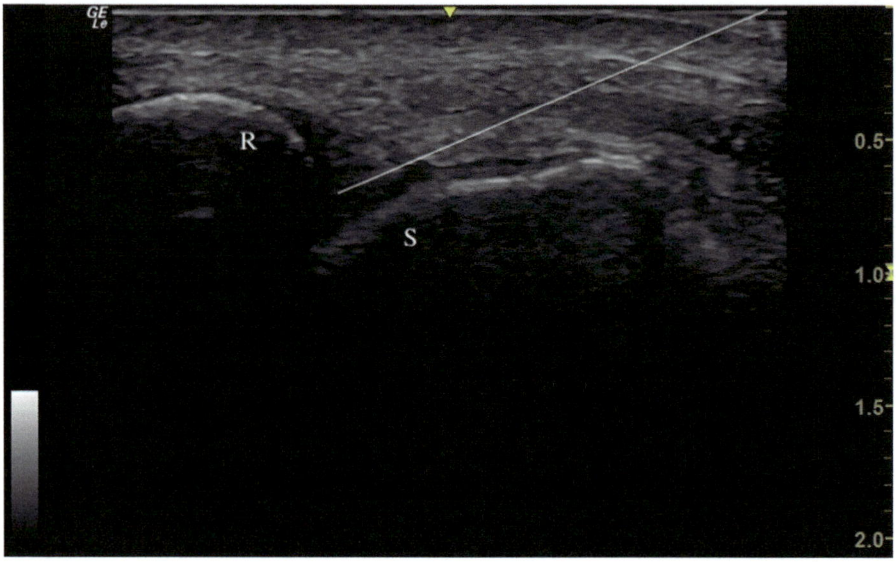

Fig. 5 Ultrasound image for radiocarpal injection. Ultrasonogram. *R* radius, *S* scaphoid

3 Bedside Ganglion Cyst Aspirations

Overview

Ganglion cyst aspiration serves as a useful therapeutic tool at the bedside and in an office setting.

Indications and Contraindications

Ganglion cyst aspiration is indicated in the management of pain and less frequently in decompression of a vessel or nerve. The cyst is typically a swelling in conjunction with a joint capsule or tendon sheath. The cystic lesions are filled with fluid from the degeneration of periarticular or peritendinous soft tissues [6, 7]. They typically occur on the dorsal aspect of the wrist. Recurrence after aspiration is common, and surgery has a lower rate of recurrence in comparison to aspiration. Common contraindications include infection at the injection site, intolerance of allergy to the injectate, including steroids, and patient refusal. Anticoagulation, including iatrogenic, and platelet dysfunction, including iatrogenic, are not considered to be a contraindication for these injections.

Clinical Anatomy

Surrounding anatomical structures should be considered with respect to the cyst location. The majority of ganglia are at the dorsum of the wrist superficial to the scapholunate ligament. Volar ganglia originate from the scaphotrapezium joint; they are located on the radial side and may displace the radial artery or the superficial sensory branch of the radial nerve. Vascular structures should be located with doppler imaging.

Equipment and Supplies

It is recommended that practitioners use ultrasound to confirm correct needle placement and adjust technique based on anatomical variation. For dorsal ganglia, the patient is placed in a seated position with a fully pronated forearm. The skin surrounding the cyst is prepped with antiseptic solution. After localization of the cyst with transducer, a 16-gauge 1-in. needle is inserted at an approximately 45° to the transducer. A 16-gauge needle is often necessary due to the high viscosity of aspirated material, but the needle size will also depend on the size and location of the cyst. Adequate time should be given between anesthetic injection and aspiration due to the high pain with wrist injections. Local anesthetic, and less frequently steroids, may be injected if there is wrist pain and/or synovitis near the cyst; please refer to Table 1 for specific volumes.

Ultrasound-Guided Technique

After prepping the skin with antiseptic, a high-frequency linear-array transducer is situated typically using a dorsal approach and longitudinal planes. Hockey-stick transducers are ideal for aspiration to have adequate space for placement of the needle. The transducer should be translated to place the cyst in the center of the transducer. The needle is inserted at 45° to the transducer to enter the body of the cyst (Fig. 6) [6].

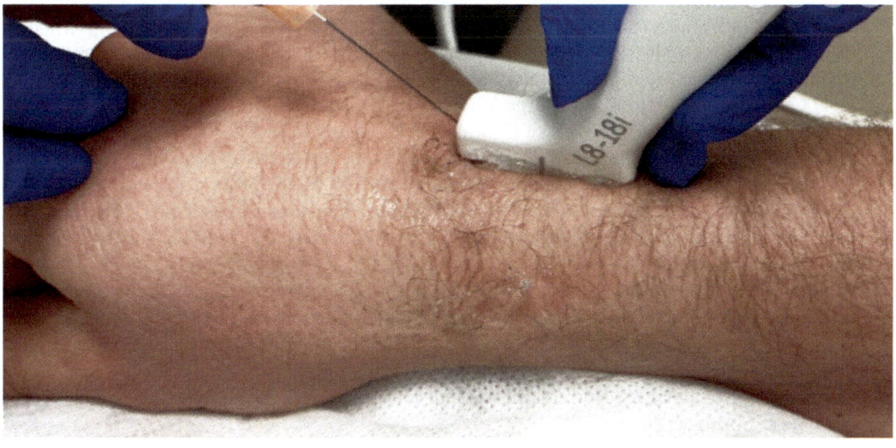

Fig. 6 Probe orientation and US image for the wrist ganglion cyst aspiration

Potential Complications and Adverse Effects

The complication rate is low and nearly all complications are self-limiting. In addition to common complications such as bleeding or infection, mild local depigmentation and allergic reactions are less common complications. Well-defined lesions may present as anechoic or hypoechoic with posterior enhancement close to a joint or tendon sheath, which should be avoided when possible. US guidance is advantageous for aspiration of multiloculated ganglia [6].

Clinical and Technical Pearls

- For optimal positioning during RC joint injections, a pillow or rolled towel should be placed under the forearm to obtain slight wrist flexion.
- The needle is guided into the ganglion cyst until fluid flows freely. If fluid does not flow freely, the contents can be liquefied with injection of normal saline.
- Patient should be informed with the possibility of developing of lipodystrophy with use of steroids or punctate scars especially with repeated blocks.
- Meticulous attention should be paid to an immunocompromised patient to prevent development of infections. Although it is rare, early detection is imperative to prevent deleterious fatal consequences.
- Extra caution must be taken in patients on anticoagulation. Patients should be observed for at least 15 min after the injection.

References

1. Wagner ER, Gottschalk MB. Tendinopathies of the forearm, wrist, and hand. Clin Plast Surg. 2019;46:317–27. https://doi.org/10.1016/j.cps.2019.02.005.
2. Hajder E, de Jonge MC, van der Horst CMAM, Obdeijn MC. The role of ultrasound-guided triamcinolone injection in the treatment of De Quervain's disease: treatment and a diagnostic tool? Chir Main. 2013;32:403–7. https://doi.org/10.1016/j.main.2013.09.002.
3. Bing J-H, Choi S-J, Jung S-M, Ryu D-S, Ahn J-H, Kang C-H, et al. Ultrasound-guided steroid injection for the treatment of de Quervain's disease: an anatomy-based approach. Skelet Radiol. 2018;47:1483–90. https://doi.org/10.1007/s00256-018-2958-9.
4. Ippolito JA, Hauser S, Patel J, Vosbikian M, Ahmed I. Nonsurgical treatment of De Quervain tenosynovitis: a prospective randomized trial. Hand (New York, NY). 2020;15:215–9. https://doi.org/10.1177/1558944718791187.
5. Huisstede BM, Gladdines S, Randsdorp MS, Koes BW. Effectiveness of conservative, surgical, and postsurgical interventions for trigger finger, Dupuytren disease, and De Quervain disease: a systematic review. Arch Phys Med Rehabil. 2018;99:1635–1649.e21. https://doi.org/10.1016/j.apmr.2017.07.014.
6. Spinner DA, Kirschner JS, Herrera JE. Atlas of ultrasound guided musculoskeletal injections. New York: Springer; 2014.

7. Resteghini P. Diagnostic musculoskeletal ultrasound and guided injection: a practical guide. New York: Thieme; 2018.
8. Geissler WB, Burkett JL. Ligamentous sports injuries of the hand and wrist. Sports Med Arthrosc Rev. 2014;22:39–44. https://doi.org/10.1097/JSA.0000000000000013.
9. Tagliafico A, Rubino M, Autuori A, Bianchi S, Martinoli C. Wrist and hand ultrasound. Semin Musculoskelet Radiol. 2007;11:95–104. https://doi.org/10.1055/s-2007-1001875.
10. Theumann NH, Pfirrmann CWA, Chung CB, Antonio GE, Trudell DJ, Resnick D. Pisotriquetral joint: assessment with MR imaging and MR arthrography. Radiology. 2002;222:763–70. https://doi.org/10.1148/radiol.2223010466.
11. Pessis E, Drapé J-L, Bach F, Feydy A, Guerini H, Chevrot A. Direct arthrography of the pisotriquetral joint. Am J Roentgenol. 2006;186:800–4. https://doi.org/10.2214/AJR.04.1640.
12. Colio SW, Smith J, Pourcho AM. Ultrasound-guided interventional procedures of the wrist and hand: anatomy, indications, and techniques. Phys Med Rehabil Clin N Am. 2016;27:589–605. https://doi.org/10.1016/j.pmr.2016.04.003.
13. Malfair D. Therapeutic and diagnostic joint injections. Radiol Clin N Am. 2008;46:439–53. https://doi.org/10.1016/j.rcl.2008.02.007.

Further Reading

Spinner DA, Kirschner JS, Herrera JE. Atlas of ultrasound guided musculoskeletal injections. New York: Springer; 2014.

Bedside Injections for Hand Pain: Trigger Finger, Digital Nerve Blocks, Intra-Articular Injections

Jason Christopher Gremillion, Yashar Eshraghi, Gassan Chaiban, and Maged Guirguis

Essential Concepts

- Injections for hand pain are often performed in the peri-operative setting or in the office for chronic inflammatory conditions. While classically performed by anatomical landmarks, ultrasound guidance is becoming increasingly popular.
- Corticosteroid injections for trigger finger are typically efficacious in symptom relief. Approximately 57% of patients will have resolution of their symptoms with one injection, and 86% of patients with a second injection. Resolution of symptoms often lasts longer than 12 months in 50% of patients.
- Digital nerve blocks are typically performed for emergent repair of a finger injury or postoperative pain control. Epinephrine has largely been proven to be safe to use in these injections.

1 Hand Pain, Overview

Chronic hand and wrist pain are common symptoms among the general population with a reported incidence of 5–26% depending on the diagnostic criteria and duration of symptoms [1]. While the etiology of hand pain can vary widely, injections

J. C. Gremillion (✉)
Louisiana State University Health Sciences Center, New Orleans, LA, USA
e-mail: jgrem3@lsuhsc.edu; jgremillion@spinediagnostic.com

Y. Eshraghi · G. Chaiban · M. Guirguis
Ochsner Clinic, New Orleans, LA, USA
e-mail: yashar.eshraghi@ochsner.org; gassan.chaiban@ochsner.org; maged.guirguis@ochsner.org

D. Souza et al. (eds.), *Bedside Pain Management Interventions*,
https://doi.org/10.1007/978-3-031-11188-4_60

for hand pain are often performed in the peri-operative setting or in the office for chronic inflammatory conditions. The etiology of hand pain is often diagnosed by history and physical examination with little imaging needed. Most patients with chronic hand pain present to their primary care physician and are treated with conservative measures, including physical therapy, bracing/splinting, topical agents, and nonsteroidal anti-inflammatory drugs (NSAIDS) [2]. Injections performed in the hand for chronic pain are often secondary to osteoarthritis or other degenerative joint diseases. Osteoarthritis of the hand is noted to have a prevalence of 13–26% in the general population [3]. Additionally, recent trauma or unusual and increased manual activity can lead patients to seek a physician.

While injections performed for hand pain have not been as rigorously studied compared to other anatomical locations such as the hip or knee, they are still routinely performed by various physicians. Common steroids used in hand injections include betamethasone, methylprednisolone, and triamcinolone. Many practitioners prefer water-soluble steroids as they are less likely to cause depigmentation. While all the injections described below are relatively safe and easy to perform, there are some general contraindications and risks. Contraindications include local infection of the targeted area, systemic infection, and allergic reaction, or contraindication to local anesthetics or steroids. Patients on anticoagulation therapy typically do not have to stop their medications as there is often little bleeding and compression of bleeding vessels is easy to perform, but this decision is at the discretion of the physician. General risks include bleeding, swelling, infection, damage to the surrounding vessels, musculature, and nerves, and allergic reaction [4].

2 Injections for Trigger Finger

Overview

Stenosing tenosynovitis, more commonly known as trigger finger, describes inflammation of the flexor digitorum superficialis or flexor pollicis longus caused by compression from the heads of the metacarpal bones.

Indications and Contraindications

The most common site of obstruction is the first annular pulley (A-1). Most cases are idiopathic, but patients can present with a history of strenuous manual activity or trauma to the hand. The prevalence of trigger finger is estimated to be 3% in the general population [5]. The ring finger and the thumb are the most affected digits. Trigger finger symptoms have an increased incidence in the dominant hand, children, the sixth decade of life, and patients with rheumatoid arthritis or diabetes [6]. Patients often report pain localized to the distal palm, sleep disturbances, and the affected finger "catching" or remaining in the flexed position. Pain is worsened with repeated use.

While conservative measures are typically first-line treatment, the response to corticosteroid injection is usually significant. Up to 57% of patients will have resolution of their symptoms with one injection, and 86% of patients with a second. Resolution of symptoms often lasts longer than 12 months in 50% of patients. This injection can be repeated up to every 6 weeks with a maximum of three injections [7].

Contraindications are similar for the injections in this chapter thus are discussed in the overview.

Clinical Anatomy

The primary target for the injection is the tendon sheath of the flexor digitorum superficialis (or the flexor pollicis longus for the thumb) as it transverses the metacarpal head. This location most often corresponds to the location of the A-1 pulley. Ultrasound can be used to identify the tendon sheath by placing the probe transversely just proximal to the metacarpophalangeal joint. The tendon sheath should be identified as a hypoechoic circle surrounding the hyperechoic tendon.

Equipment and Supplies

This procedure can be performed at the bedside and in an office setting (Table 1). Ultrasound can be utilized to visualize the tendon and the affected sheath as well as to avoid any vascular structures.

Landmark Technique

With the patient in the supine or seated position, the arm is adducted, and the hand is placed flat on a sterile drape with the palmar surface of the hand facing upwards. After sterilely prepping the hand, the metacarpal head and the metacarpophalangeal joint of the affected digit are identified, and a 1 in., 25-G needle is inserted just proximal to the joint space at a 45° angle to the skin, parallel to the path of the tendon. The needle is advanced through the subcutaneous tissues into the tendon sheath (Fig. 1). Aspiration with the syringe should be performed, followed by soft injection of the syringe's contents. If there is significant resistance to injection, the

Table 1 Required supplies for trigger finger injection

Syringe	3 or 5 mL
Needle	25 or 27 gauge 1/2–1 in.
Anesthetic	1 mL 1% lidocaine 1 mL 0.25% bupivacaine
Corticosteroid	Methylprednisolone 40 mg (t1/2 life: 18–36 h)

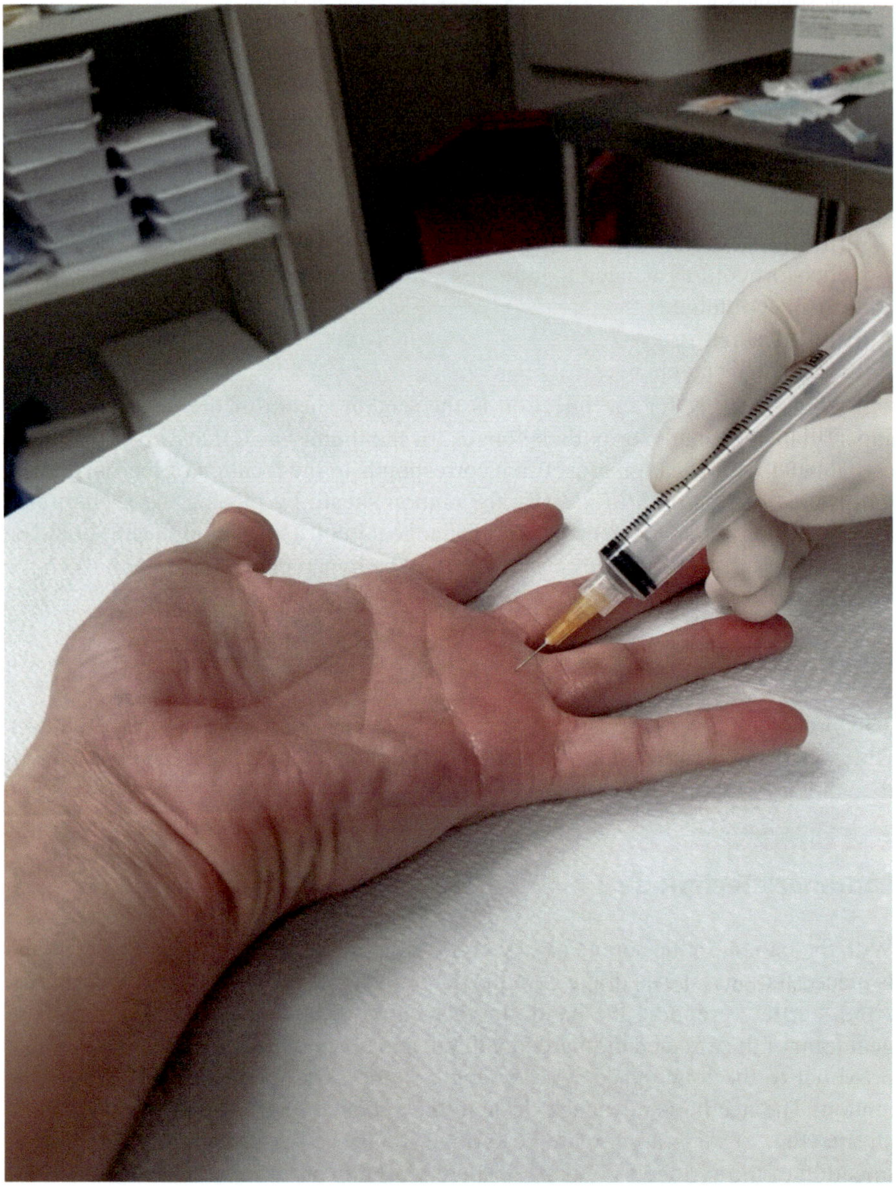

Fig. 1 Positioning for landmark trigger finger injection

needle is likely in the tendon or contacting bone and should be withdrawn until the contents can be easily injected. Injectate solutions are commonly 1 mL of steroid (40 mg methylprednisolone or 3 mg of betamethasone) with 1–2 mL of a local anesthetic [8].

Ultrasound Technique

After positioning and prepping the hand similarly to the landmark technique, a high-frequency linear probe is placed in the transverse position just proximal to the metacarpophalangeal joint. Using the ultrasound, the tendon sheath should be identified as a hypoechoic circle surrounding the hyperechoic tendon. In this view, the A1 pulley may be visualized as a hyperechoic structure due to hypertrophy and inflammation. A 1-inch, 22-G needle should be inserted out-of-plane and 5 mm proximal to the probe at a 45° angle to the skin, parallel to the course of the tendon. The needle should be advanced until it is visualized in the tendon sheath (Figs. 2, 3 and 4). After negative aspiration, the contents should be softly injected. Under direct visualization, the contents should spread within the tendon sheath with little resistance to injection [9].

Potential Complications and Adverse Effects

The complication rate is extremely low and nearly all complications are self-limiting, requiring no medical intervention. The most common complications include bleeding, swelling, local infection of the injection site, or mild paresthesia along the targeted digit. Mild local depigmentation may occur as a result of superficially located steroid. The most serious complication is tendon rupture if the flexor tendon is injected directly. This can be avoided by using ultrasound or retracting a few millimeters if the patient experiences significant pain with injection. Additionally, practitioners should be vigilant of allergic reactions to both steroid or local anesthetic.

Evidence for Trigger Finger Injections

In a Cochrane Review performed in 2009 by Peters-Veluthamaningal et al. two randomized controlled trials (RCT's) were analyzed with a total of 63 participants: 34 allocated to corticosteroids and lidocaine, and 29 allocated to lidocaine alone. Corticosteroid injection with lidocaine was more effective than lidocaine alone for treatment success at 4 weeks. The number needed to treat was cited as 3 [10]. In a retrospective review by Grandizio et al. in 2017, the authors reviewed 264 patients who received one to two injections at the A-1 pulley for trigger finger. A successful injection was defined as an injection that resulted in over 1 year of relief. The overall success of corticosteroid injection was 84% with 16% of patients requiring surgical release of the A-1 pulley. Single injection efficacy was 49%, and second injection efficacy was 68% [7].

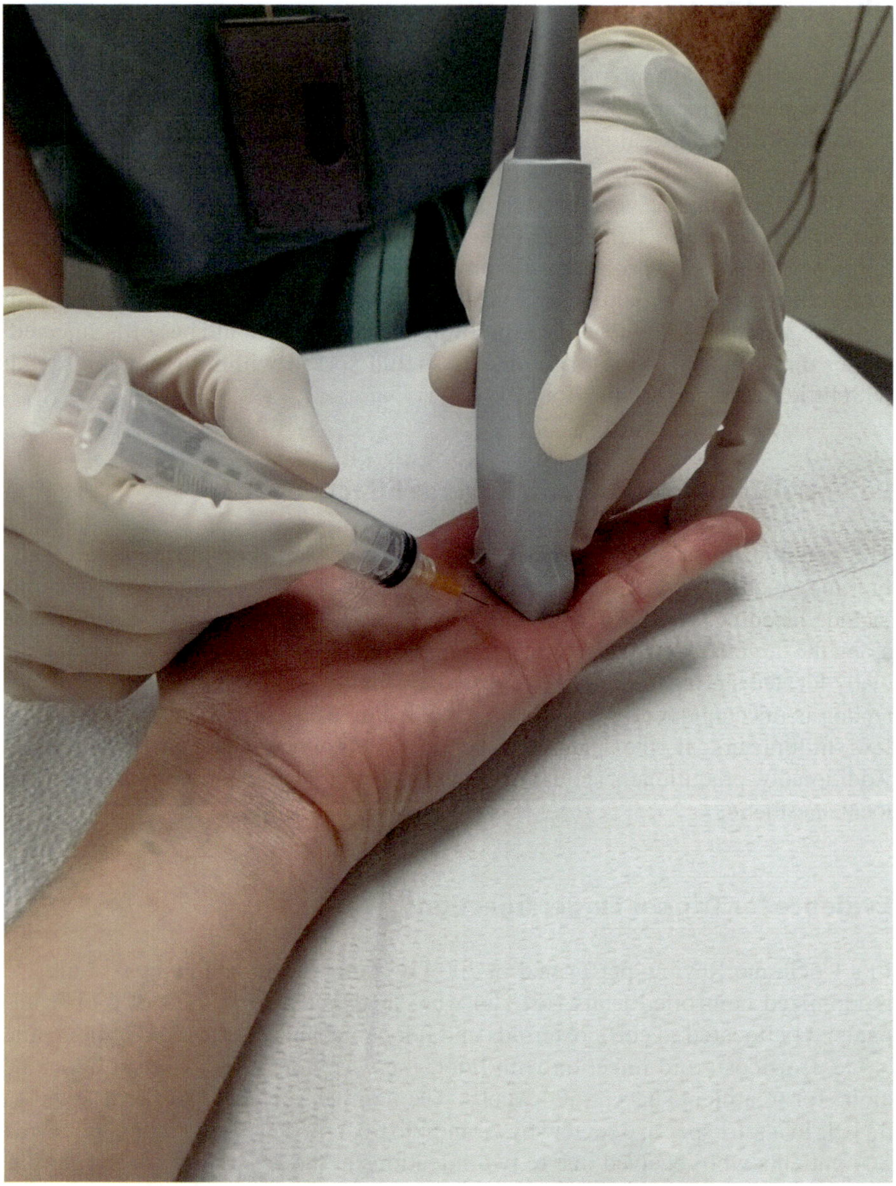

Fig. 2 Ultrasound position for trigger finger position, out-of-plane approach

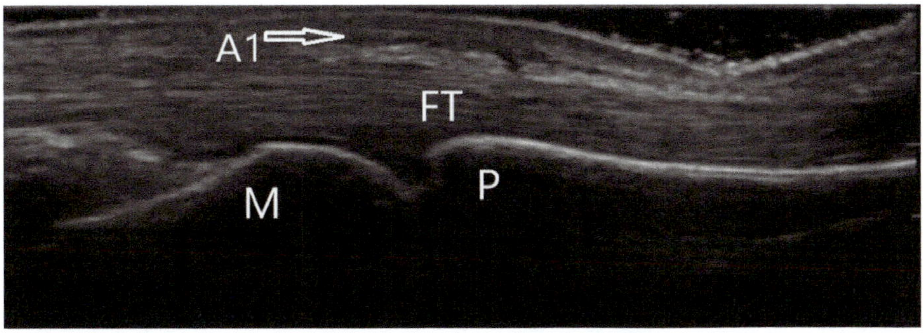

Fig. 3 Longitudinal ultrasound image of trigger finger injection. *A1* A1 Pulley, *FT* flexor tendon, *M* metacarpal head, *P* proximal phalanx

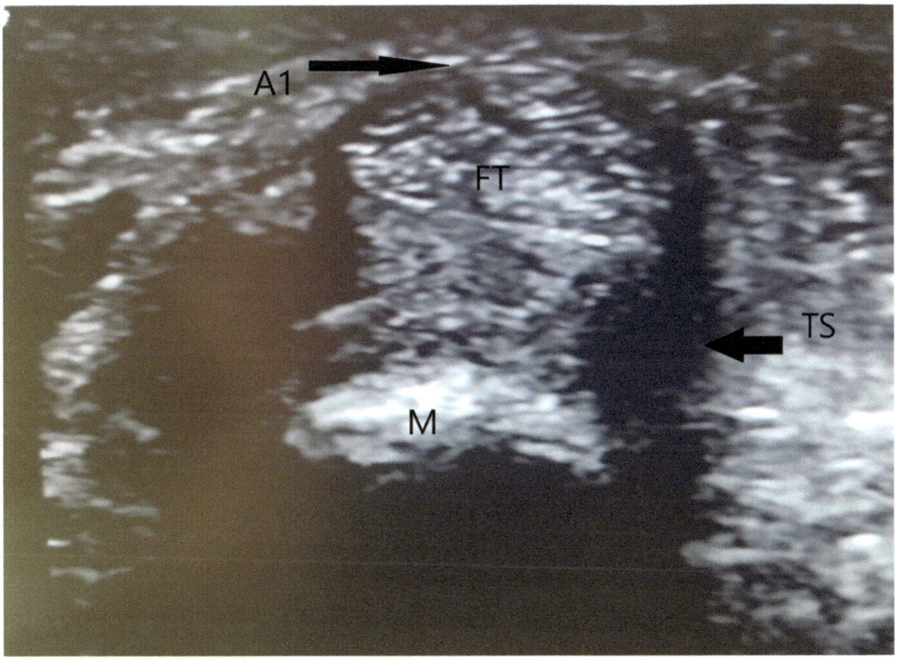

Fig. 4 Transverse ultrasound image of trigger finger injection. *A1* A1 Pulley, *FT* flexor tendon, *M* metacarpal head, *TS* tendon sheath

3 Injections for Dupuytren's Contracture

Overview

Dupuytren's contracture describes the progressive fibrosis of the palmar fascia leading to "puckering" of the palmar tissue and formation of nodules along the palmar fascia. As the disease progresses, these nodules form longitudinal cords along the

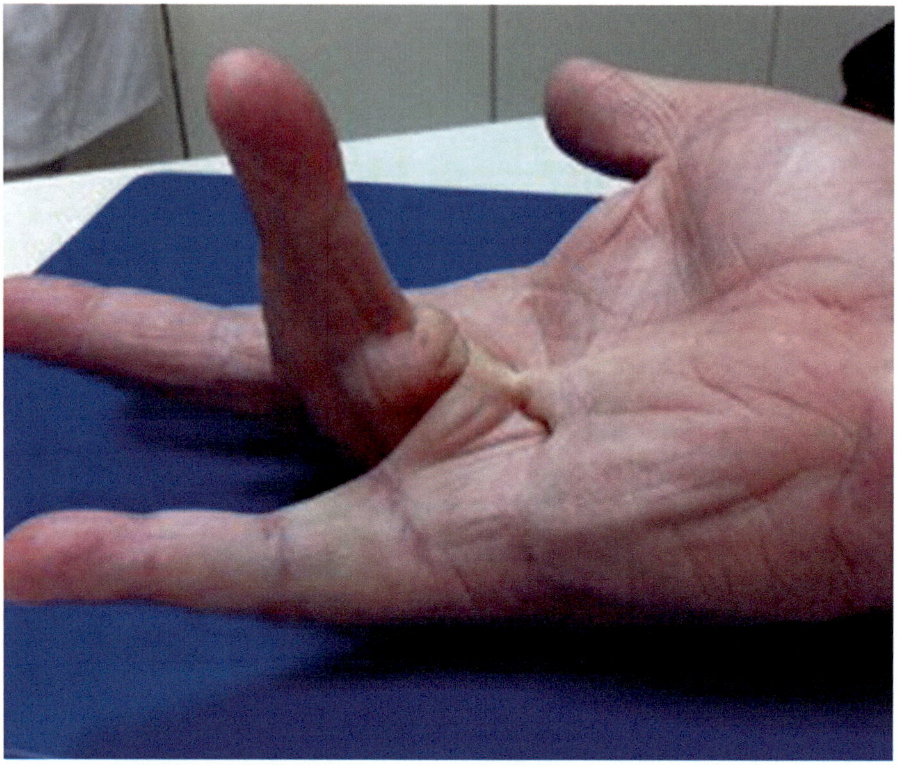

Fig. 5 Dupuytren's contract of the fourth digit. (Image Courtesy of American Academy of Orthopedic Surgeons)

palmar fascia resulting in loss of extension at the metacarpophalangeal (MCP) joint and proximal interphalangeal (PIP) joint (Figs. 5 and 6). While these bands typically begin along the palmar fascia, they can form along the digital fascia and the dorsum of the hand at later stages [11]. Patients often report stiffness and difficulty with finger extension as the disease progresses. While the initial nodules can be painful, the cords seen in the latter stages of the disease are often painless [12].

Indications and Contraindications

Risk factors for Dupuytren's contractures include male sex, age >50 years, Northern European descent, family history of Dupuytren's contracture, diabetes mellitus, tobacco use, alcohol use, and careers with excessive manipulation of the hands. Contractures occur more frequently on the fourth and fifth digit [11]. There are currently several interventional procedures for Dupuytren's contractures including steroid injection, needle aponeurotomy, collagenase injection, and surgical fasciotomy. There is still debate regarding the best algorithm for deciding a treatment modality, but typically patients with mild to moderate disease (MCP contracture less than 40°

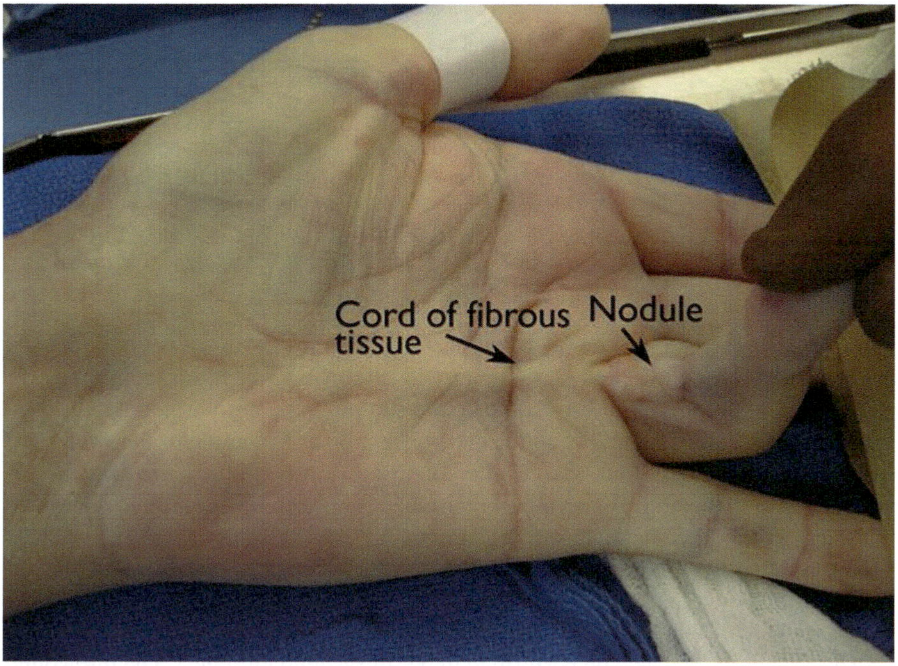

Fig. 6 Dupuytren's contract of the fourth digit. (Image Courtesy of American Academy of Orthopedic Surgeons)

or PIP contracture less than 20°) can be managed with activity modification and steroid injection, while more severe disease may require surgical release or collagenase injection. Steroids, local anesthetic, or collagenase solutions may all be injected using the techniques below [12].

Contraindications are similar for the injections in this chapter thus are discussed in the overview.

Clinical Anatomy

Nodules and cords typically form along the palmar fascia over the metacarpophalangeal (MCP) joint and proximal interphalangeal (PIP) joint. While these bands typically begin along the palmar fascia, they can form along the digital fascia and the dorsum of the hand at later stages.

Equipment and Supplies

This procedure can be performed at the bedside and in an office setting (Table 2). Ultrasound can be utilized to visualize the tendon and Dupuytren's lesions as well as to avoid any vascular structures.

Table 2 Required supplies for Dupuytren's contracture injection

Syringe	3 mL
Needle	25 or 27 gauge 1/2–1 in.
Anesthetic	1 mL 1–2% lidocaine
Corticosteroid	Methylprednisolone 40 mg (t1/2 life: 18–36 h) OR Triamcinolone 60 mg (t1/2 life: 18–36 h)
Collegenase *Clostridium histolyticum*	0.58 mg per cord if lysis is desired

Injection Technique

With the patient in the supine or seated position and the arm in adduction, the hand is positioned flat on the procedural table with the palmar surface facing upwards. After sterilely prepping the hand, palpate the symptomatic cord or nodule. A 25-G, 1-in. needle is inserted parallel to the cord or nodule at 45° angle to the skin, typically just lateral of midline. The needle is advanced through the subcutaneous tissues and into the lesion. While initial resistance to injection is common, continued resistance could be indicative of the needle being directly against bone. The needle should be slightly withdrawn, and injection can be resumed. Common steroid injection solutions include 1 mL of 40 mg methylprednisolone or 60 mg triamcinolone acetonide with 1–2 mL of local anesthetic [13].

This injection may also be performed under ultrasound guidance. The ultrasound may be placed either longitudinally or transversally to the nodule or cord. The palmar aponeurosis should appear as a thin hyperechoic structure running ventral to the thicker and slightly more hyperechoic tendon. After the hand is prepped, a 25-G, 1-inch needle should be advanced in-plane until it is identified in the lesion. The injectate solution should spread along the path of the lesion [14].

Potential Complications and Adverse Effects

The complication rate is extremely low and nearly all complications are self-limiting, requiring no medical intervention. The most common complications include bleeding, swelling, or local infection of the injection site. Mild local depigmentation may occur as a result of superficially located steroid. The most serious complication is tendon rupture if the affected tendon is injected directly. This can be avoided by using ultrasound or retracting a few millimeters if the patient experiences significant pain with injection.

Evidence for Dupuytren's Contracture Injections

While reoccurrence of disease is common no matter what treatment modality is chosen, both steroid and collagenase injections are common treatments for Dupuytren's contractures. In a study by Ketchum et al. 63 patients with Dupuytren's nodules in early stages of disease underwent a series of triamcinolone acetonide injections. 62

of the patients experienced visible regression of disease with softening and flattening of the nodules. Overall, the study reported an average of 3.2 injections per nodule and 97% of patients experiencing softening and flattening of nodules. Approximately half of these patient had reoccurrence at the 1-year mark [15].

In a study by Hurst et al. 308 patients with joint contractures of 20° or more at the MCP or PIP were randomly assigned to receive up to three injections of collagenase *Clostridium histolyticum* (at a dose of 0.58 mg per injection) or placebo in the contracted collagen cord at 30-day intervals. Overall, the range of motion in the joints was significantly improved after injection with collagenase as compared with placebo (from 43.9° to 80.7° vs. from 45.3° to 49.5°, $P < 0.001$). Response rates were better in patients with less severe contractures [16]. In a retrospective study by Zhou et al. 130 patients were identified that underwent either needle aponeurotomy ($n = 46$) or collagenase injections ($n = 84$). While both interventions were successful in symptom relief, no technique was proven superior in improvement in contractures at the MCP or PIP. No serious adverse effects occurred in either of the two treatment groups [17].

4 Injections for Digital Nerve Block

Overview

Digital nerve blocks are performed by a variety of providers often for emergent repair of a finger injury (lacerations, removal of nails, tendon ruptures, fractures, etc.) or postoperative pain control. Less commonly, the block can be performed to alleviate neuropathies from overuse of the digits or entrapment injuries [18].

Indications and Contraindications

As noted above indications for digital nerve block include emergent repair of finger injuries and to provide analgesia postoperatively or for neuropathic finer pain. Contraindications include compromised digit circulation, allergy to local anesthetic, or infection at the injection site.

Clinical Anatomy

The common digital nerves arise from either the median or ulnar nerves, with the thumb receiving some fibers from the radial nerve. They divide into two common palmar digital nerves typically at the level of the metacarpal bones. They are accompanied by the digital arteries as the run along either side of the flexor tendon close to the palmar surface. While the proper palmar digital nerves supply most of the innervation to the digit, they also send off a dorsal branch at the level of the MCP that supplies innervation to the dorsal proximal phalanx.

There are three major techniques for performing the digital nerve block as discussed below.

Equipment and Supplies

This procedure can be performed at the bedside and in an office setting (Table 3). Ultrasound can be utilized to visualize the digital nerves and vasculature. When comparing different anesthetic solutions, 0.5% bupivacaine provides a long period of analgesia at approximately 24.9 h. Comparatively, 2% lidocaine with epinephrine (1:100,000) provides 10.4 h, and 2% lidocaine without epinephrine provides 4.9 h [19].

Traditional Technique With and Without Ultrasound

With the patient in the supine or seated position, the hand is positioned flat on the procedural table with the dorsal surface facing upwards. After the hand is sterilely prepped, a 27-G, 1-in. needle is inserted into the subcutaneous tissues of the web space of the targeted digit just distal to the MCP at a 90° angle to the skin. After negative aspiration, 2–3 mL of preservative-free local anesthetic is injected. The same injection is then performed on the other side of the targeted digit (Fig. 7).

This technique can also be performed with ultrasound guidance. With the patient in the supine or seated position, the hand is positioned flat on the procedural table with the palmar surface facing upwards. A linear probe is placed transversely along the digit just distal to the MCP. The flexor tendon is often easily identified as a circular, hypoechoic structure. The digital artery is often identified as a pulsating structure on either side, just lateral to the tendon. The digital nerve should be just ventral to the digital artery in this position. After the hand is sterilely prepped, a 27-G, 1-in. needle is inserted on the proximal side of the probe in an out-of-plane approach. The needle is advanced until it is just adjacent to the digital nerve (Figs. 8 and 9). After negative aspiration, 1–2 mL of preservative-free local anesthetic is injected. Repeat this same injection on the other side of the digit [20].

While the bilateral technique is described above, if anesthesia of just one side of the digit is needed, a unilateral injection may be performed. If this injection is being performed for a neuropathy, one ml of 40 mg/mL of methylprednisolone may be injected.

Table 3 Required supplies for digital nerve block

Syringe	5 mL
Needle	25 or 27 gauge 1/2–1 in.
Anesthetic	2–3 mL 0.5% Bupivacaine OR 2–3 mL 2% Lidocaine with epinephrine OR 2–3 mL 2% Lidocaine
Corticosteroid	Methylprednisolone 40 m (t1/2 life: 18–36 h) if for neuropathy

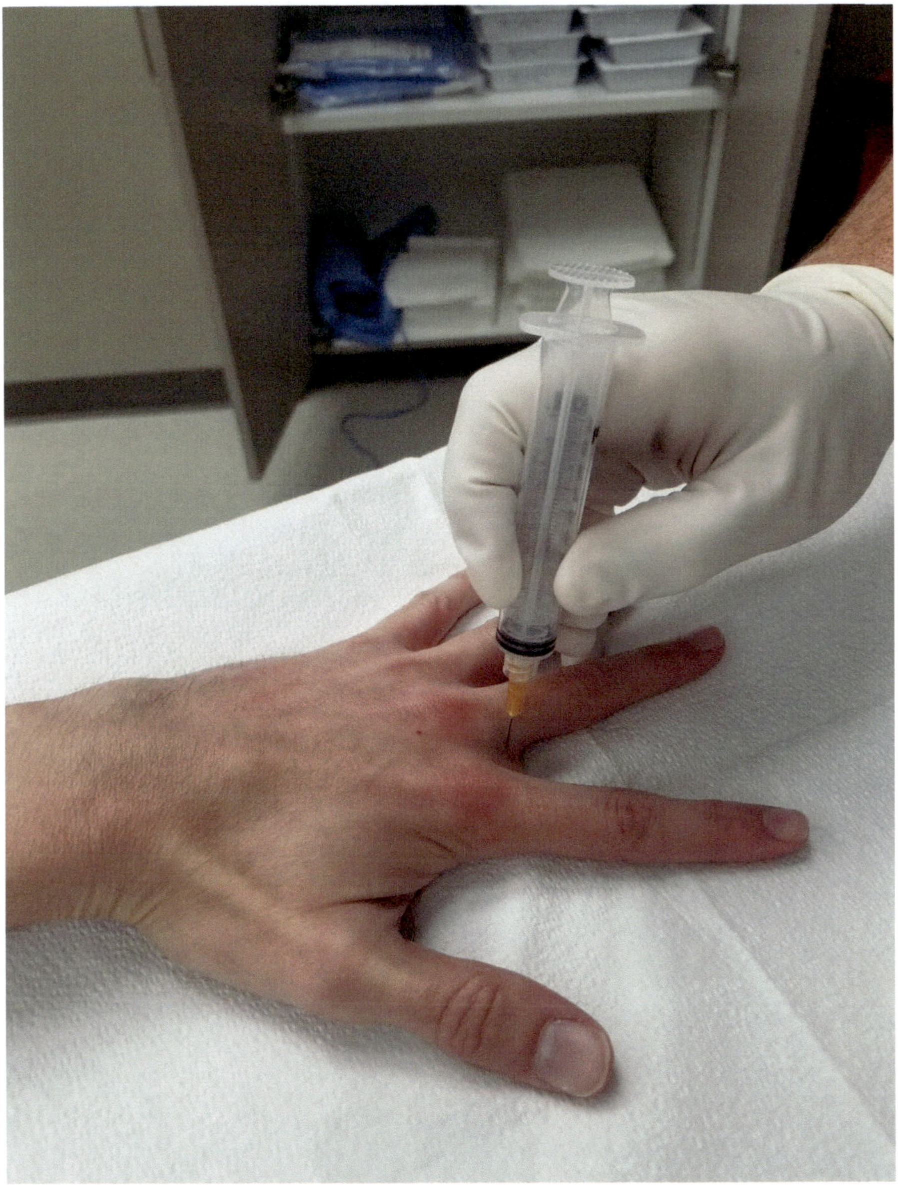

Fig. 7 Positioning for landmark traditional nerve block

Transthecal Technique

The transthecal technique provides anesthesia to the affected digit by infusing the flexor tendon sheath with local anesthetic. The hand is positioned flat on the procedural table with the palmar surface facing upwards. The flexor tendon is identified just proximal to the proximal digital crease. After the hand is sterilely prepped, a

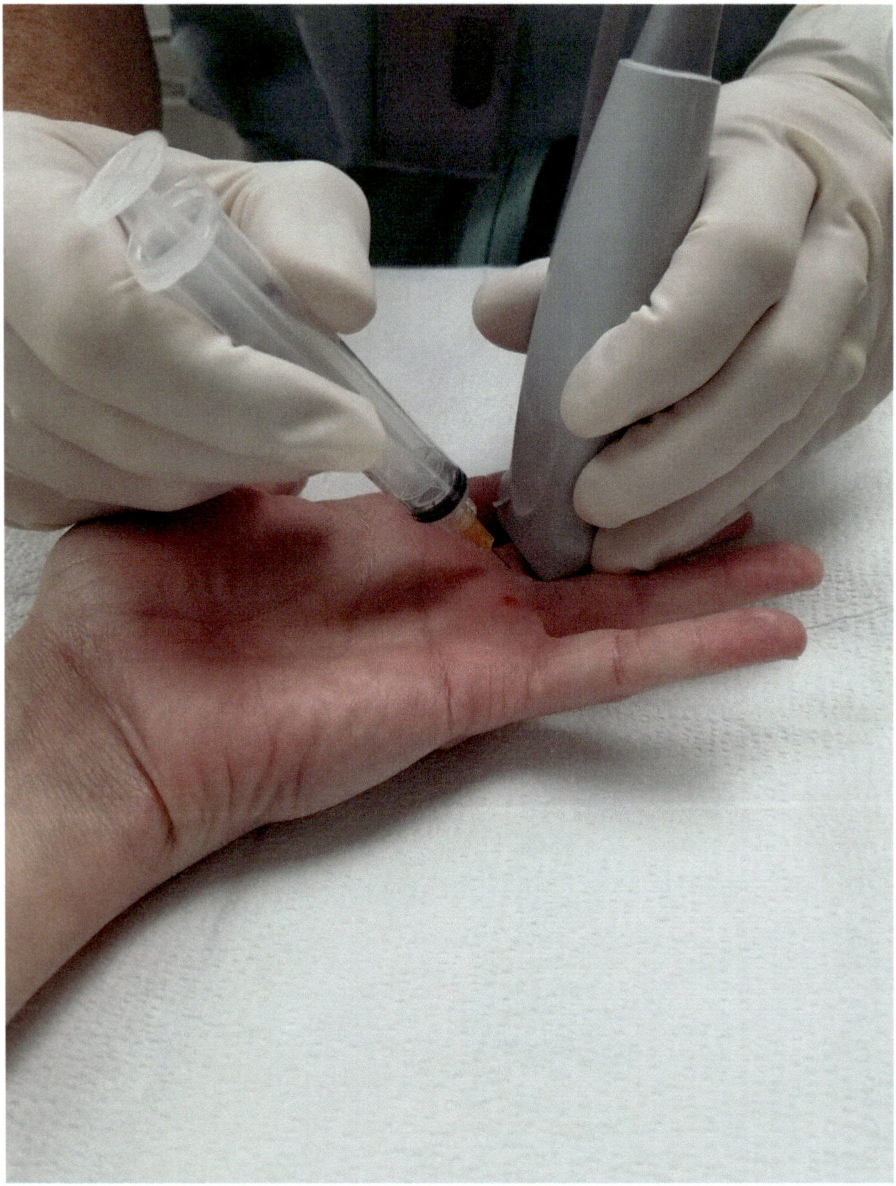

Fig. 8 Ultrasound position for digital nerve block, out-of-plane approach

27-G, 1-in. needle is directed distally at a 45° angle to the skin at this level. The needle is advanced through the subcutaneous tissues and into the flexor tendon sheath (Fig. 10). After aspiration, 2 mL of local anesthetic may be injected [21]. Ultrasound can be used to identify the tendon and tendon sheath, as described in the trigger finger injection technique section.

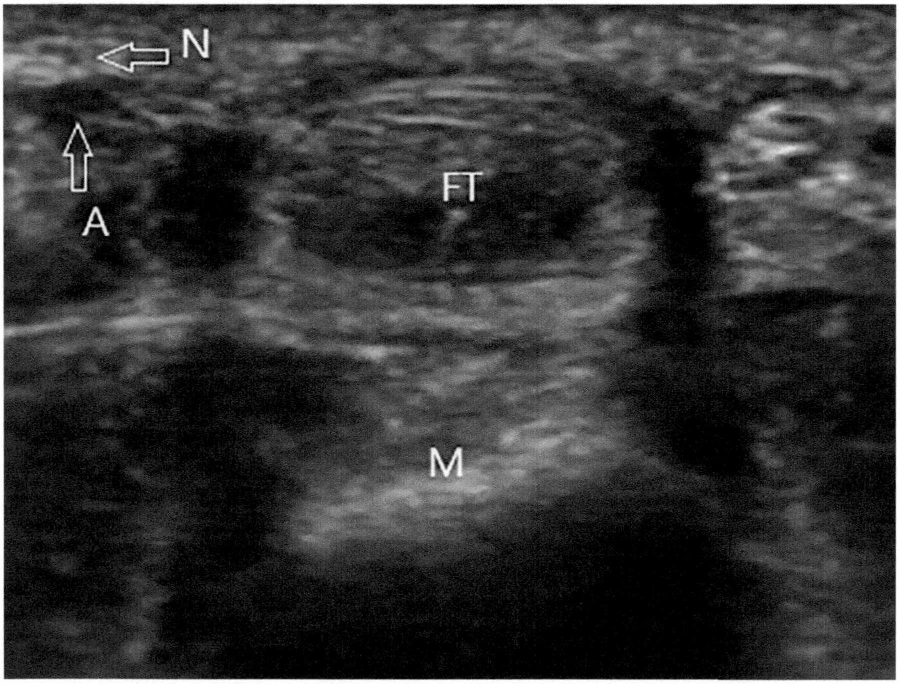

Fig. 9 Transverse ultrasound image of digital nerve block. *FT* flexor tendon, *M* metacarpal head, *A* digital artery, *N* digital nerve

Subcutaneous Technique

The subcutaneous technique involves injecting local anesthetic into the subcutaneous tissues of the targeted finger and then massaging the tissues so that the medication spreads toward the digital nerves and tendon sheath. Unlike the other two techniques, this technique rarely provides adequate anesthesia to the dorsum of the proximal phalanx.

The hand is positioned flat on the procedural table with the palmar surface facing upwards. After the hand is sterilely prepped, a 27-G, 1-in. needle is directed distally into the proximal digital crease at a 45° angle to the skin. The needle is advanced into the subcutaneous tissue. After negative aspiration, 2 mL of local anesthetic is injected (Fig. 11). With sterile gloves, the local anesthetic is massaged into to the tissues and distally for 30–40 s [22].

Potential Complications and Adverse Effects

The complication rate is extremely low and nearly all complications are self-limiting, requiring no medical intervention. The most common complications include bleeding, swelling, or local infection of the injection site, and mild

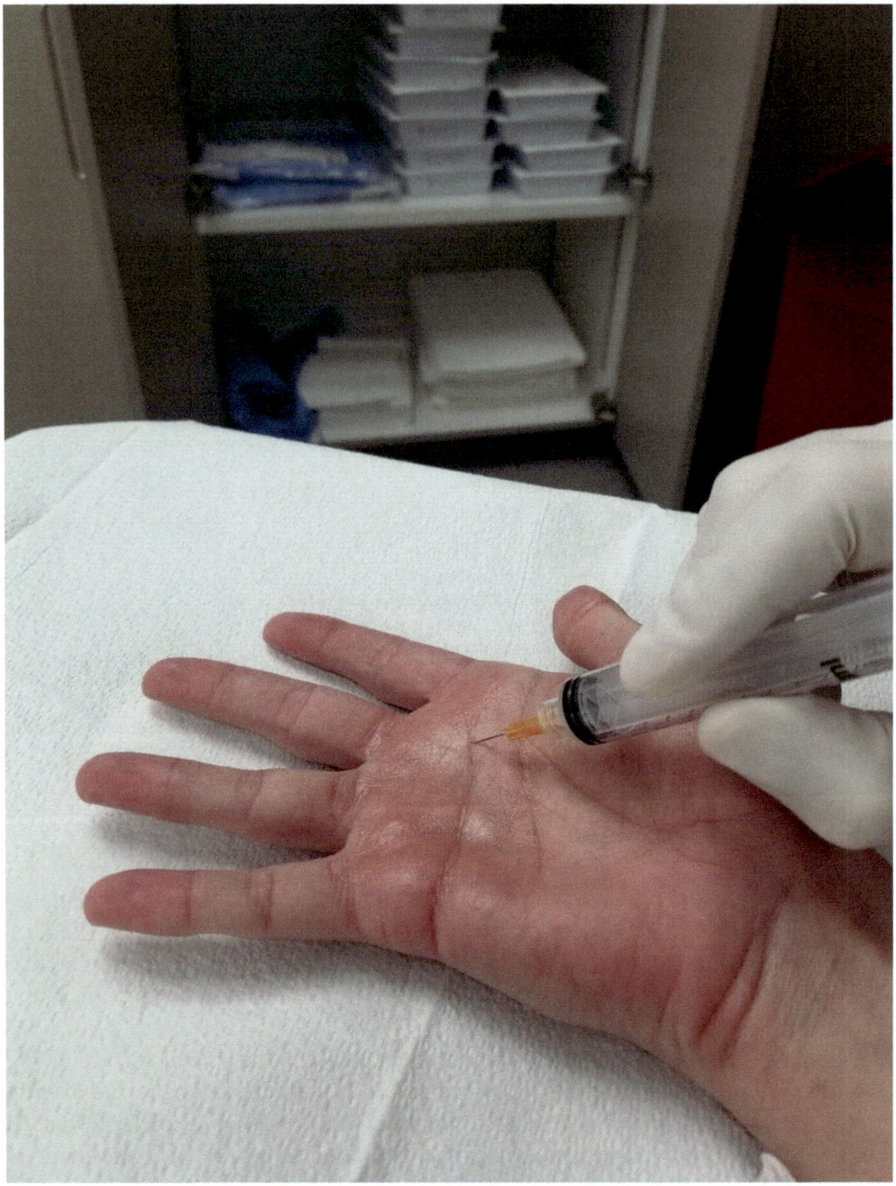

Fig. 10 Positioning for landmark transthecal digital nerve block

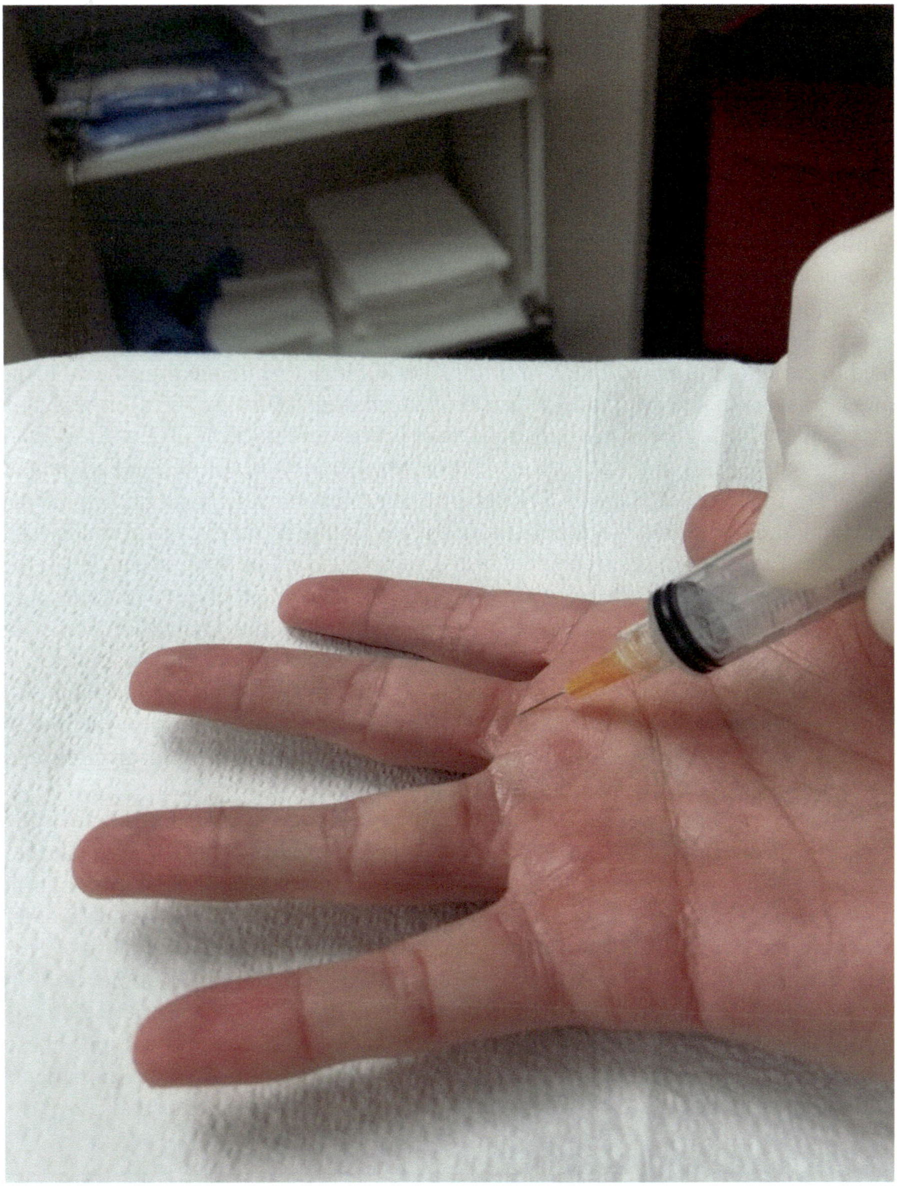

Fig. 11 Positioning for landmark subcutaneous digital nerve block

paresthesia if the nerve is contacted. There is potential for tissue necrosis if an epinephrine solution is injected intravascularly which is discussed below in the "Choice of Technique and Injectate" section.

Choice of Technique and Injectate

While all three techniques mentioned above are relatively easy to perform and provide consistent analgesia of the targeted digit, there have been several studies reviewing pain with injection and pain at the site of injection with these different approaches. In one RCT performed by Kerimidas et al. 104 patients were randomized to either a traditional block or a transthecal block. While the transthecal technique was associated with quicker onset of anesthesia (100 s vs. 165 s), it was also associated with higher visual analogue pain scores on injection (3.2 vs. 1.6), and approximately 50% of those patients receiving the transthecal injection had pain at the site of injection 24 h after it was performed. Comparatively, none of the patients receiving the traditional block had injection-site pain at 24 h [23]. Additionally, the transthecal injection has a hypothetical risk of tendon rupture with injection.

In a meta-analysis performed by Yin et al. comparing all three techniques, the traditional and subcutaneous techniques had similar onset of analgesia, pain with injection, and post-operative pain at the injection site. Of note, the subcutaneous technique was less likely to cover the dorsal proximal phalanx compared to the other two techniques. While the transthecal technique was noted to have the fastest onset of analgesia, it was also associated with increased pain with injection and postoperative pain at the injection site [22].

While epinephrine was initially avoided in digital nerve blocks due to a fear that the vasoconstriction of digital arteries could lead to tissue necrosis, epinephrine-containing local anesthetic solutions are becoming increasingly more common in digital nerve blocks. In a meta-analysis of 9 review articles, 18 RCT's, and 18 other articles there were no reports of digital necrosis or gangrene from epinephrine. This included both 1:100,000 and 1:200,000 epinephrine containing solutions used in approximately 2797 digital nerve blocks. Furthermore, the vasoconstrictive effects from digital nerve blockade appear to resolve in less than 90 min. Despite these findings, it is advised that epinephrine-containing solutions are avoided in patients with peripheral vascular disease or who have a high risk of tissue necrosis [24].

5 Intra-articular Injections of the Hand

Overview

Intra-articular injections of the carpometacarpal (CMC) and interphalangeal joints are commonly performed procedures for arthritis secondary to various etiologies (osteoarthritis, rheumatoid arthritis, post-traumatic arthritis, etc.) as well as collagen disorders.

Indications and Contraindications

Symptomatic osteoarthritis of the hand is common in the elderly with a prevalence of 13% in men and 26% in women [25]. The CMC joint of the thumb is cited as the most affected joint. Glucocorticoids and hyaluronic acid (HA) are the two substances most commonly injected into these joints with trials for other injectates like infliximab and glucose.

Contraindications are similar for the injections in this chapter thus are discussed in the overview.

Equipment and Supplies

This procedure can be performed at the bedside and in an office setting (Table 4). Ultrasound can be utilized to visualize the targeted joint and surrounding structures.

Injection Technique

With the patient in the supine or seated position and the arm fully adducted, the hand is positioned flat on a procedural table with the dorsum of the hand facing upwards. The joint is then palpated; traction may be placed on the targeted digit as to open the joint space. Similarly, flexion and extension of the joint may help identify the joint space. After the hand is prepped, a 25-G, 1-in. needle is introduced into the midline of the joint space at a 90° angle to the skin if possible (significant degenerative disease may make this approach impossible and a shallower angle may be needed). The needle is then advanced through the subcutaneous tissues, joint capsule, and into the joint space (Fig. 12). The needle may have to be redirected if bone is contacted. If resistance to injection is met, then the needle is likely in a tendon and should be advanced slightly. Once in the joint space, 1 mL of local anesthetic and 1 mL of 40 mg methylprednisolone is injected [26]. This injection may be aided by ultrasound guidance by placing the ultrasound longitudinally along the joint line and identifying the joint space. The needle may then be introduced either out-of-plane or in-plane directed toward the synovial membrane until the needle enters the joint space (Figs. 13 and 14).

Table 4 Required supplies for intra-articular hand injection

Syringe	3 mL
Needle	25 or 27 gauge 1/2–1 in.
Anesthetic	1 mL 1–2% lidocaine
Corticosteroid	Methylprednisolone 40 mg (t1/2 life: 18–36 h)

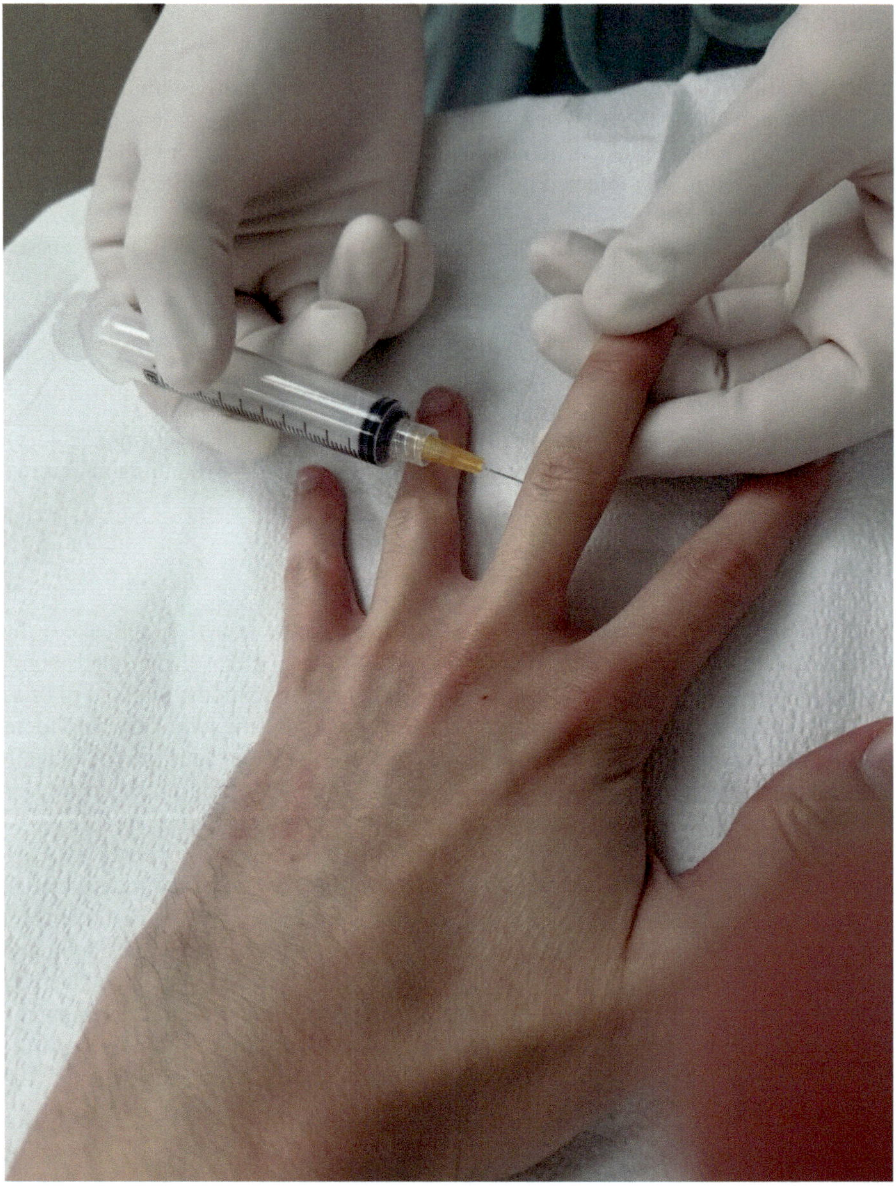

Fig. 12 Positioning for landmark intra-articular PIP injection

Evidence for Intra-articular Injection

While intra-articular injections remain common, efficacy and long-term results are still debated. In a meta-analysis by Kroon et al. 13 RCT's comparing glucocorticoid or HA injections vs. placebo injections in the CMC or interphalangeal joints were analyzed. Glucocorticoid and HA injections had no increased risks and similar

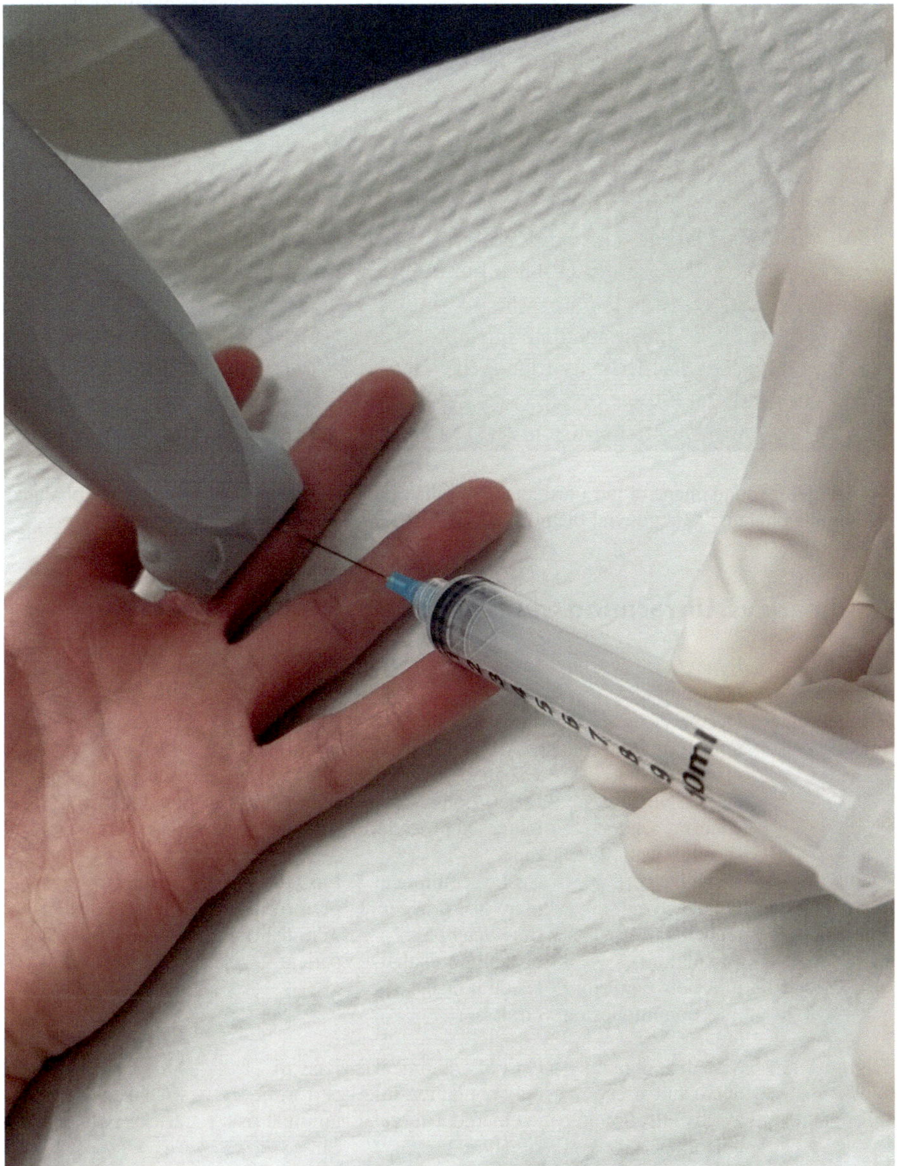

Fig. 13 Ultrasound position for intra-articular PIP injection, out-of-plane approach

safety profiles to placebo. Glucocorticoid and HA injections on the CMC joints generally showed a decrease in pain and swelling compared to placebo, but these results were not statistically significant. One trial did find that glucocorticoid injections of the interphalangeal joints resulted in statistically significant pain relief at the 12-week mark compared to placebo [27].

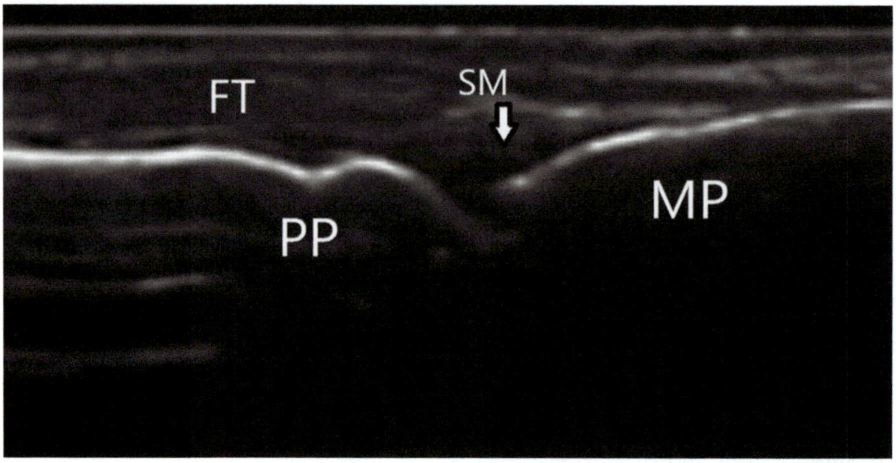

Fig. 14 Ultrasound image of intra-articular PIP injection. *FT* flexor tendon, *PP* proximal phalanx, *MP* middle phalanx, *SM* synovial membrane

Landmark vs. Ultrasound Guidance

Procedure	Benefits of ultrasound	Limitations of ultrasound	Benefits of landmark	Limitations of landmark
Trigger finger injection	Decrease chance of tendon rupture, can visualize tendon and vasculature, confirms tendon sheath injection	Cost of equipment, may be difficult to visualize pulley if hypertrophy is mild, increased procedure time	Can be performed quickly with minimal risk to patient	Unable to visualize if injectioning into tendon or vasculature
Dupuytren's contracture injection	Visualize cord or nodule, avoid tendon and vasculature injection, confirms injection into lesion	Cost of equipment, increased procedure time, may be difficult to visualize lesion if disease is mild	Easy to perform with minimal risk to patient	Unable to visualize lesion, unable to visualize if injection is into tendon or vasculature
Digital nerve block	Visualize digital nerve and artery, avoids injection into tendon	Cost of equipment, may not be feasible in emergent surgical situation	Easy to perform, minimal risk, can be performed in emergent situations	Unable to visualize digital artery and nerve
Intra-articular injections	Visualize joint space, confirms intra-articular injection	Cost of equipment, difficult to visualize joint in advanced disease	Can be performed quickly with minimal risk to patient	Unable to visualize joint space

Clinical and Technical Pearls

- While injections of the hand are typically safe and easy to perform, relative risks must be discussed with patients when compared to conservative treatment.
- Ultrasound guidance during trigger finger injection can help identify the A-1 pulley and may prevent patient pain by avoiding insertion of the needle into the flexor tendon.
- While no universally agreed upon algorithm exists for the treatment of Dupuytren's contractures, corticosteroid and hyaluronic acid injections can provide significant relief of symptoms mild to moderate disease (MCP contracture less than 40° or PIP contracture less than 20°).
- While transthecal digital nerve blockade has the fastest onset of analgesia and requires only one injection, it is also associated with increased pain on injection and post-operative pain at the site of injection.
- While potentially hazardous in patients with peripheral vascular disease, epinephrine-containing local anesthetic solutions appear to be safe to use in digital nerve blocks.

References

1. Nicholls EE, et al. Factors associated with the severity and progression of self-reported hand pain and functional difficulty in community-dwelling older adults: a systematic review. Musculoskeletal Care. 2012;10(1):51–62.
2. Huisstede BM, et al. Effectiveness of conservative, surgical, and postsurgical interventions for trigger finger, Dupuytren disease, and de Quervain disease: a systematic review. Arch Phys Med Rehabil. 2018;99(8):1635–49.
3. Kelley BP, Shauver MJ, Chung KC. Management of acute postoperative pain in hand surgery: a systematic review. J Hand Surg Am. 2015;40(8):1610–9.
4. Tallia AF, Cardone DA. Diagnostic and therapeutic injection of the wrist and hand region. Am Fam Physician. 2003;67(4):745–50.
5. Ryzewicz M, Wolf JM. Trigger digits: principles, management, and complications. J Hand Surg Am. 2006;31(1):135–46.
6. Saldana MJ. Trigger digits: diagnosis and treatment. J Am Acad Orthop Surg. 2001;9(4):246–52.
7. Grandizio LC, et al. Predictors of recurrence after corticosteroid injection for trigger digits. Hand. 2017;12(4):352–6.
8. Waldman SD. Flexor digitorum superficialis and profundus injection for tendonitis and trigger finger. In: Atlas of pain management injection techniques E-Book. Amsterdam: Elsevier Health Sciences; 2016. p. 296–300.
9. Bodor M, Flossman T. Ultrasound-guided first annular pulley injection for trigger finger. J Ultrasound Med. 2009;28(6):737–43.
10. Peters-Veluthamaningal C, et al. Corticosteroid injection for trigger finger in adults. Cochrane Database Syst Rev. 2009;1:CD005617.
11. Gudmundsson KG, Jónsson T, Arngrímsson R. Guillaume Dupuytren and finger contractures. Lancet. 2003;362(9378):165–8.
12. Shih B, Bayat A. Scientific understanding and clinical management of Dupuytren disease. Nat Rev Rheumatol. 2010;6(12):715.

13. Waldman SD. Dupuytren contracture injection. In: Atlas of pain management injection techniques E-Book. Amsterdam: Elsevier Health Sciences; 2016. p. 325–7.
14. Bianchi S, Martinoli C, Abdelwahab IF. High-frequency ultrasound examination of the wrist and hand. Skeletal Radiol. 1999;28(3):121–9.
15. Ketchum LD, Donahue TK. The injection of nodules of Dupuytren's disease with triamcinolone acetonide. J Hand Surg Am. 2000;25(6):1157–62.
16. Hurst LC, et al. Injectable collagenase *Clostridium histolyticum* for Dupuytren's contracture. N Engl J Med. 2009;361(10):968–79.
17. Zhou C, et al. Collagenase *Clostridium histolyticum* versus limited fasciectomy for Dupuytren's contracture: outcomes from a multicenter propensity score matched study. Plast Reconstr Surg. 2015;136(1):87–97.
18. Deniel A, et al. Entrapment and traumatic neuropathies of the elbow and hand: an imaging approach. Diagn Interv Imaging. 2015;96(12):1261–78.
19. Thomson CJ, Lalonde DH. Randomized double-blind comparison of duration of anesthesia among three commonly used agents in digital nerve block. Plast Reconstr Surg. 2006;118(2):429–32.
20. Waldman SD. Digital nerve block of the fingers. In: Atlas of pain management injection techniques E-Book. Amsterdam: Elsevier Health Sciences; 2016. p. 334–6.
21. Chiu DTW. Transthecal digital block: flexor tendon sheath used for anesthetic infusion. J Hand Surg Am. 1990;15(3):471–3.
22. Yin ZG, et al. A comparison of traditional digital blocks and single subcutaneous palmar injection blocks at the base of the finger and a meta-analysis of the digital block trials. J Hand Surg. 2006;31(5):547–55.
23. Keramidas EG, et al. Comparison of transthecal digital block and traditional digital block for anesthesia of the finger. Plast Reconstr Surg. 2004;114(5):1131–4.
24. Ilicki J. Safety of epinephrine in digital nerve blocks: a literature review. J Emerg Med. 2015;49(5):799–809.
25. Qin J, et al. Lifetime risk of symptomatic hand osteoarthritis: the Johnston County Osteoarthritis Project. Arthritis Rheumatol. 2017;69(6):1204–12.
26. Gray RG, Tenenbaum J, Gottlieb NL. Local corticosteroid injection treatment in rheumatic disorders. In: Seminars in arthritis and rheumatism., vol. 10. Philadelphia: WB Saunders; 1981.
27. Kroon FPB, et al. Intra-articular therapies in the treatment of hand osteoarthritis: a systematic literature review. Drugs Aging. 2016;33(2):119–33.

Further Reading

Gil JA, Hresko AM, Weiss AC. Current concepts in the management of trigger finger in adults. J Am Acad Orthop Surg. 2020;28(15):e642–50. https://doi.org/10.5435/JAAOS-D-19-00614.

Botulinum Toxin Injections for Muscle Spasticity

Geoffrey R. Smith, Chelsea D. Frost, and Andrea T. Aguirre

Essential Concepts

- Intramuscular botulinum toxin injections targeting specific muscles can be effective for treating spasticity-associated pain in the upper and lower limbs.
- Spasticity is necessarily associated with an upper motor neuron injury or lesion.
- The mechanism of action of botulinum toxin involves a dose-dependent degree of paralysis of the injected muscle, and attention must be paid to avoiding adverse function effects from this paralysis.
- Goals of treating spasticity must be weighed against the potential benefits of maintaining spasticity.
- Pain relief is often dependent on the paralyzing effect of botulinum toxin on the target muscle which takes 1–4 weeks to achieve its full effect and must be repeated every 3–4 months to maintain the paralyzing effect.

1 Botulinum Toxin Injections for Upper and Lower Limb

Overview

Intramuscular botulinum toxin injection causes a degree of paralysis of the injected muscle, which can be useful for treatment of spasticity-associated pain [1]. Spasticity is necessarily associated with a lesion of upper motor neurons [1], so an associated brain or spinal cord pathology must be identified. Spasticity can involve involuntary

G. R. Smith (✉) · C. D. Frost · A. T. Aguirre
Department of Physical Medicine and Rehabilitation, University of Virginia, Charlottesville, VA, USA
e-mail: gs4gd@virginia.edu

D. Souza et al. (eds.), *Bedside Pain Management Interventions*,
https://doi.org/10.1007/978-3-031-11188-4_61

velocity-dependent increase in tone with muscle stretch, as well as spasms [2]. Botulinum toxin injections can be beneficial for focal, temporary treatment of spasticity and require repeat injections every 3–4 months to maintain the paralyzing effect [1]. Peak therapeutic effect occurs 1–4 weeks post-injection [3]. To minimize risks and optimize accuracy, injections are given with guidance via electrical stimulation, electromyography, and/or ultrasound [1]. Three types of botulinum toxin are FDA-approved for spasticity management, including onabotulinumtoxinA, abobotulinumtoxinA, and incobotulinumtoxinA (upper limb only) [3–5]; each has specific FDA-approved doses for specific muscles (Tables 1 and 2). Other spasticity treatment methods include stretching, bracing, oral or intrathecal medications, or surgical interventions.

Indications and Contraindications to Botulinum Toxin Injections

Spastic muscles can contribute to pain directly as myalgia, or indirectly by altering biomechanics with associated musculoskeletal pain [1]. However, spasticity can be beneficial for function, and botulinum toxin-associated paralysis can lead to further dysfunction [1]; if there are concerns about functional sequelae of treatment, coordinate care with a physiatrist. Spasticity is part of an upper motor neuron syndrome and should be distinguished from other causes of increased muscle tone. In contrast

Table 1 FDA-approved botulinum toxin dosing for the management of upper limb spasticity [3–5]

Injection	OnabotulinumtoxinA	AbobotulinumtoxinA	IncobotulinumtoxinA
Adductor pollicis	20 units 1 site	N/A	5–30 units 1 site
Biceps brachii	100–200 units Divided at 4 sites	200–400 units 1–2 sites	50–200 units 1–4 sites
Brachialis	N/A	200–400 units 1–2 sites	25–100 units 1–2 sites
Brachioradialis	N/A	100–200 units 1–2 sites	25–100 units 1–2 sites
Flexor carpi radialis	12.5–50 units 1 site	100–200 units 1–2 sites	25–100 units 1–2 sites
Flexor carpi ulnaris	12.5–50 units 1 site	100–200 units 1–2 sites	20–100 units 1–2 sites
Flexor digitorum profundus	30–50 units 1 site	100–200 units 1–2 sites	25–100 units 2 sites
Flexor digitorum superficialis	30–50 units 1 site	100–200 units 1–2 sites	25–100 units 2 sites
Flexor pollicis brevis	N/A	N/A	5–30 units 1 site
Flexor pollicis longus	20 units 1 site	N/A	10–50 units 1 site
Pronator quadratus	N/A	N/A	10–50 units 1 site
Pronator teres	N/A	100–200 units 1 site	25–75 units 1–2 sites

Table 2 FDA-approved botulinum toxin dosing for the management of lower limb spasticity [3, 4]

Injection	OnabotulinumtoxinA	AbobotulinumtoxinA
Gastrocnemius (medial and lateral heads)	75 units per head 3 sites per head	100–150 units per head 1 site per head
Flexor digitorum longus	50 units 2 sites	130–200 units 1–2 sites
Flexor hallucis longus	50 units 2 sites	70–200 units 1–2 sites
Soleus	75 units 3 sites	330–500 units 3 sites
Tibialis posterior	75 units 3 sites	200–300 units 2 sites

Table 3 Upper limb spasticity patterns [2]

Spasticity pattern	Muscles involved
– Pronated flexed elbow	– Biceps brachii – Brachialis – Brachioradialis – Pronator teres
– Flexed wrist	– Flexor carpi radialis – Flexor carpi ulnaris – Flexor digitorum profundus – Flexor digitorum superficialis – Flexor pollicis longus – Palmaris longus
– Thumb-in-palm	– Abductor pollicis brevis – Adductor pollicis – Flexor pollicis brevis – Flexor pollicis longus
– Clenched fist	– Flexor digitorum superficialis – Flexor digitorum profundus – Lumbricals – Interossei

to spasticity, dystonia involves involuntary muscle contractions in distinct patterns, often without a known upper motor neuron injury or lesion [6]. If the etiology of muscle hypertonicity is in question, diagnosis by either a physiatrist or neurologist prior to initiating treatment is recommended. Black Box Warnings for distant spread of toxin effect should be considered, especially in the context of respiratory impairment ([3–5], see Table 3). Contraindications include neuromuscular junction disease (e.g. myasthenia gravis) and infection at the injection site [3].

Clinical Anatomy

Upper Limb

Each botulinum toxin subtype approved for spasticity management is approved for specific muscle targets with specific doses (see Table 1). Common upper limb spasticity patterns are listed in Table 3. For the clenched fist pattern, it is important to identify the involved joints as the flexor digitorum superficialis (FDS) flexes the proximal interphalangeal joints while the flexor digitorum profundus (FDP) flexes the proximal and distal interphalangeal joints. FDS and FDP each have four separate muscle bellies that can be targeted distinctly. For ergonomic and safety reasons, the patient is placed supine with the forearm held vertically by an assistant or other safe suspension device for all upper limb injections. While single sites are described below, other injection sites can be found by moving 2–3 cm more proximal or distal along the target muscle. Given adjacent vessels and risk for systemic spread of neurotoxin, negative aspiration should always be confirmed before injecting.

Lower Limb

Each botulinum toxin subtype approved for spasticity management is approved for specific muscle targets with specific doses (see Table 2). Common lower limb spasticity patterns are listed in Table 4. The patient is placed prone with the foot and ankle hanging off the end of the examination table for all injections except for E-stim guided soleus injection (see below). While single sites are generally described below, other injection sites can be found by moving 2–3 cm more proximal or distal along the target muscle. Given adjacent vessels and risk for systemic spread of neurotoxin, negative aspiration should always be confirmed before injecting.

Equipment and Supplies

Given the ergonomic challenges of positioning spastic limbs, the risk of spasm during the procedure, and the use of guidance modalities, consider using 1–2 assistants for the procedure. Typically, a syringe with a hypodermic needle electrode (25–30 gauge for upper extremities and 22–25 gauge for lower extremities) is used to inject the reconstituted solution (Table 5). We recommend adherence to the manufacturer's instructions for storage and reconstitution of the botulinum toxin. If using onabotulinumtoxinA, the medication should be reconstituted only using preservative-free 0.9% sodium chloride [3]; a fatal case of anaphylaxis has been reported with reconstitution using lidocaine [3]. Guidance modalities such as EMG, E-stim, and/or US are recommended to localize muscle targets [1]. Consideration of ultrasound (US)

Table 4 Lower limb spasticity patterns [2]

Spasticity pattern	Muscles involved
– Equinovarus foot	– Gastrocnemius – Flexor digitorum longus – Flexor hallucis longus – Soleus – Tibialis anterior – Tibialis posterior
– Flexed knee	– Gastrocnemius – Hamstrings
– Flexed toes	– Flexor digitorum longus – Flexor hallucis longus

Table 5 Required supplies for botulinum toxin injections

Syringe	1 or 3 mL
Needle	Upper limb: 25–30 gauge, 25–50 mm length Lower limb: 22–25 gauge, 50 mm length
Reconstitution	1–2 mL preservative-free 0.9% sodium chloride
For ultrasound guidance	Upper limb: medium-frequency linear probe Lower limb: medium-frequency linear or low-frequency curvilinear probe (based on patient size)
For E-stim guidance	Hypodermic needle electrode Reference and ground surface electrodes 3–10 mAmps usually required for visible isolated target muscle stimulation
For EMG guidance	Hypodermic needle electrode Reference and ground surface electrodes Audible EMG device

guidance is especially recommended when targeting the tibialis posterior [2] or in the setting of anticoagulation [7]. To minimize bleeding risk, consider US guidance viewing the muscle and adjacent arteries in short axis with the needle inserted longitudinally [7].

Injection of Biceps Brachii, E-stim or EMG Guidance

The spastic muscle is easily palpated when the elbow is positioned at end-range of extension. The muscle is isolated between the thumb and index finger of the injector's nondominant hand and is injected with the dominant hand at sites in the middle-third of the muscle. The muscle is approached anteromedially and anterolaterally to divide the total injection amount into the two muscle bellies. Needle placement is confirmed via E-stim resulting in elbow flexion or via EMG with audible motor unit action potentials.

Injection of Biceps Brachii, Ultrasound Guidance

The US probe is placed short-axis to the anterior arm, roughly halfway between the shoulder and elbow (Fig. 1). The biceps brachii is the most anterior and superficial of the muscles visualized (Fig. 2). Needle insertion is at the discretion of the injector, based on ergonomics.

Injection of Flexor Pollicis Longus (FPL), E-stim or EMG Guidance

The injection site is 2/3 the distance from elbow to wrist on the volar aspect of the radius. The needle is inserted in a radial-to-ulnar orientation and angled deep, traveling between the radius and radial artery into the FPL (Fig. 3). Needle placement

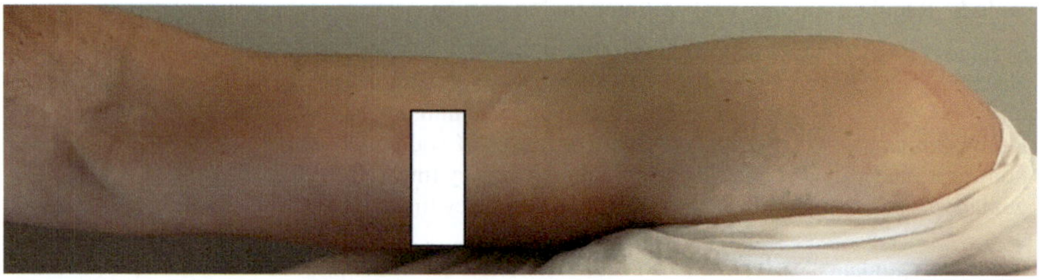

Fig. 1 Ultrasound probe placement (white box) for identification of the biceps brachii muscle

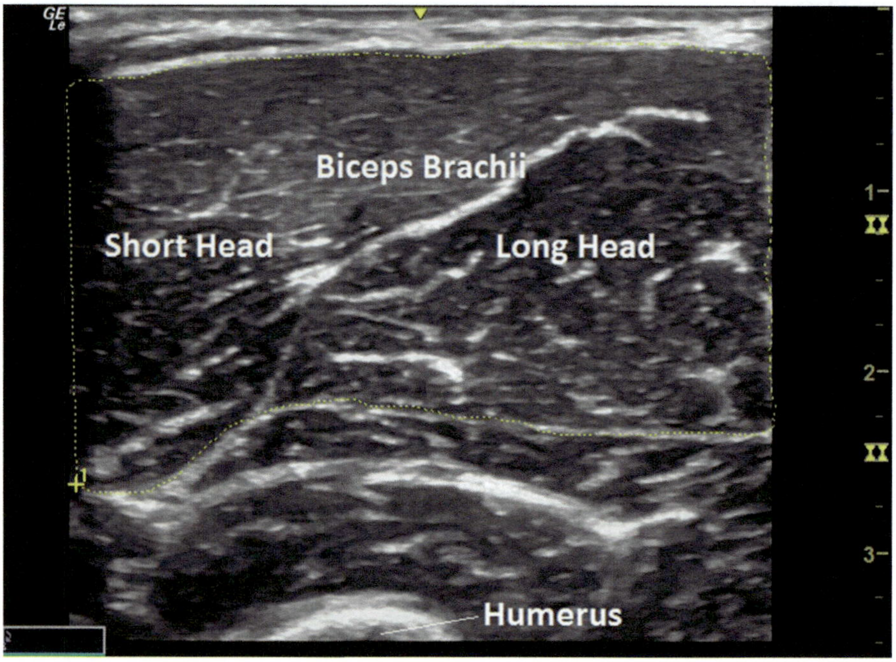

Fig. 2 Sonogram of biceps brachii; probe placement as per Fig. 1

is confirmed via E-stim resulting in isolated thumb flexion or via EMG with audible motor unit action potentials.

Injection of FPL, Ultrasound Guidance

The US probe is placed short-axis to the radius at the midpoint of the FPL (Fig. 4). Prior to needle insertion, the radial artery should be identified and avoided. The needle is inserted in a radial-to-ulnar orientation and angled deep, traveling between the radius and radial artery into the FPL (Fig. 3).

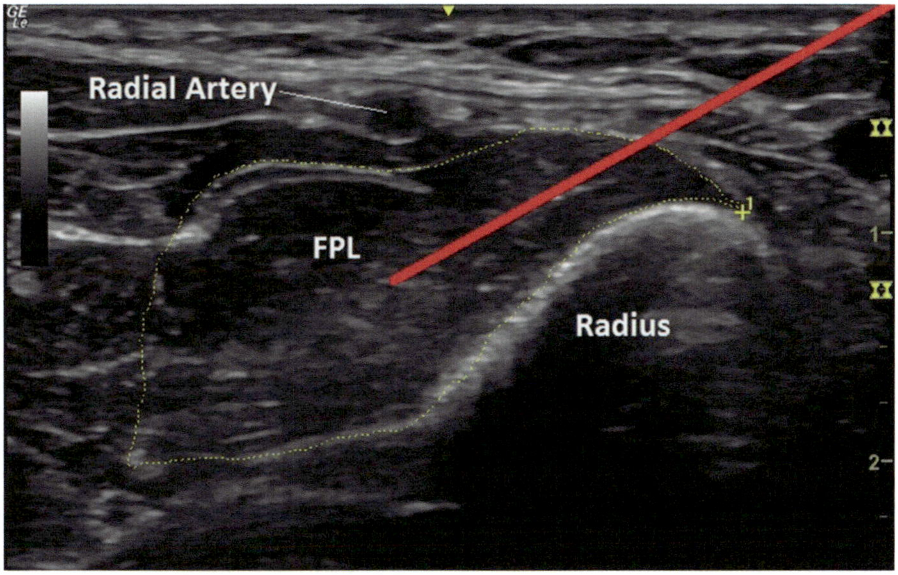

Fig. 3 Sonogram of flexor pollicis longus (red line signifies needle); probe placement as per Fig. 4

Injection of Flexor Carpi Radialis (FCR), E-stim or EMG Guidance

The injection site is 1/3 of the distance from the medial epicondyle to the distal FCR tendon at the volar wrist (Fig. 5). Needle placement is confirmed via E-stim resulting in isolated wrist flexion with radial deviation or via EMG with audible motor unit action potentials.

Injection of FCR, Ultrasound Guidance

The US probe is placed short-axis to the forearm at the FCR injection site described above (Fig. 5). FCR is the most volar and superficial of the muscles visualized (Fig. 6). Needle insertion is at the discretion of the injector, based on ergonomics.

Injection of Flexor Carpi Ulnaris (FCU), E-stim or EMG Guidance

The injection site is 1/3 of the distance from the medial epicondyle to the pisiform. Needle placement is confirmed via E-stim resulting in isolated wrist flexion with ulnar deviation or via EMG with audible motor unit action potentials.

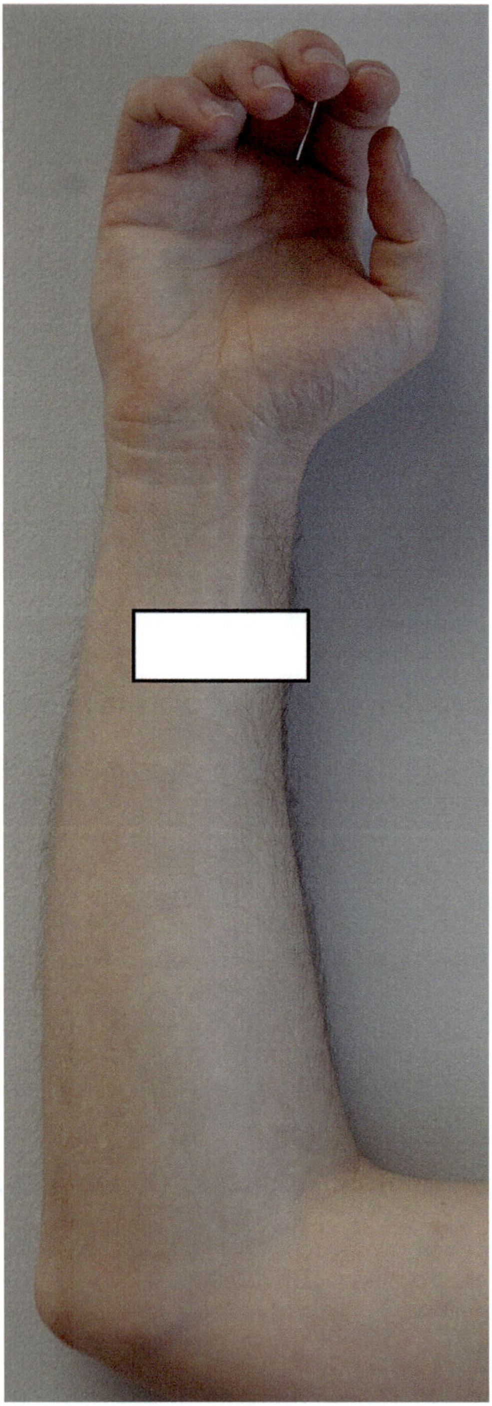

Fig. 4 Ultrasound probe placement (white box) for identification of the flexor pollicis longus muscle

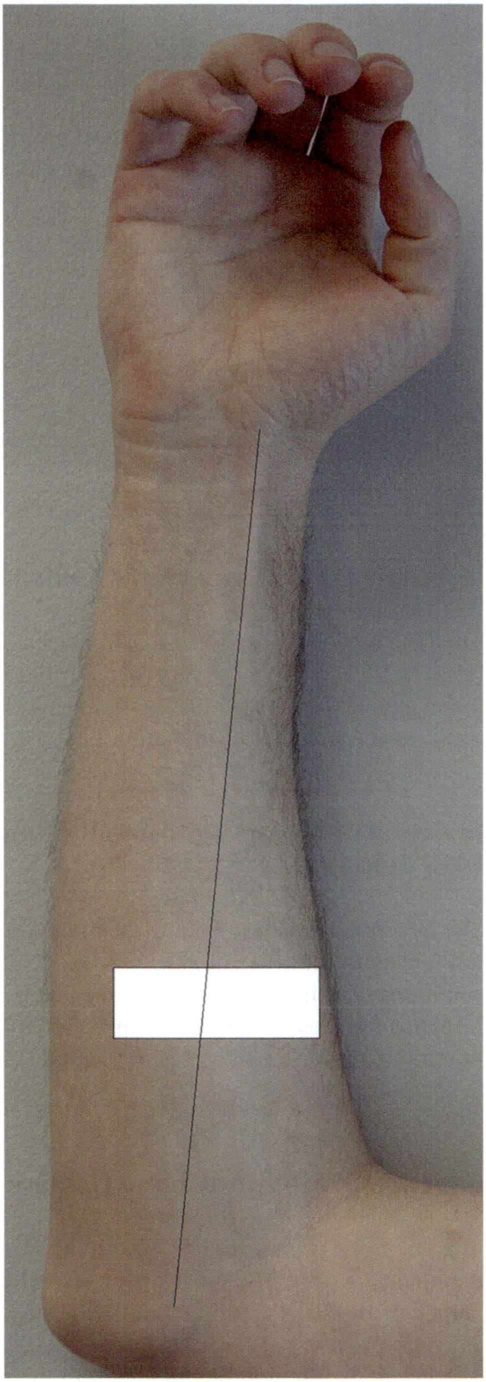

Fig. 5 Ultrasound probe placement (white box) for identification of the flexor carpi radialis muscle

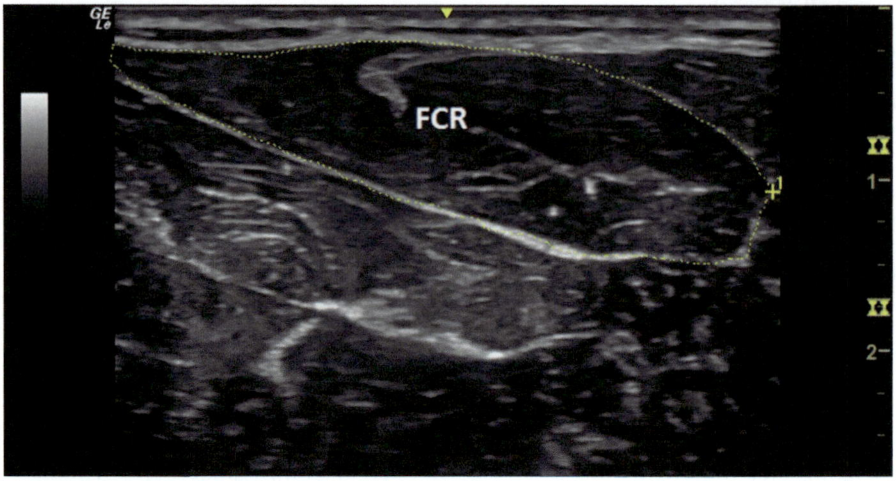

Fig. 6 Sonogram of flexor carpi radialis muscle; probe placement as per Fig. 5

Injection of FCU, Ultrasound Guidance

The US probe is placed short-axis to ulna at the FCU injection site described above (Fig. 7). FCU is the most superficial of the muscles visualized along the line from the medial epicondyle to the pisiform (Fig. 8). Needle insertion is at the discretion of the injector, based on ergonomics.

Injection of Flexor Digitorum Profundus (FDP), E-stim or EMG Guidance

The injection site is just volar to the midpoint of the ulna, aiming towards the radius. All four muscle bellies of FDP can be accessed from this site, going in order from small finger to index finger as the needle is inserted more deeply (Fig. 9). Needle placement is confirmed via E-stim resulting in isolated finger flexion (including flexion of the distal interphalangeal joint) or via EMG with audible motor unit action potentials.

Injection of FDP, Ultrasound Guidance

The US probe is placed short-axis to the volar aspect of the ulna at the midpoint of the ulna (Fig. 10). The ulnar artery should be identified. All digit-specific muscle bellies of the FDP can be identified on the US image dynamically by having an assistant passively flex and extend a specific distal interphalangeal joint (Fig. 9). The needle is inserted longitudinally to the probe into FDP as described above for E-stim/EMG guidance.

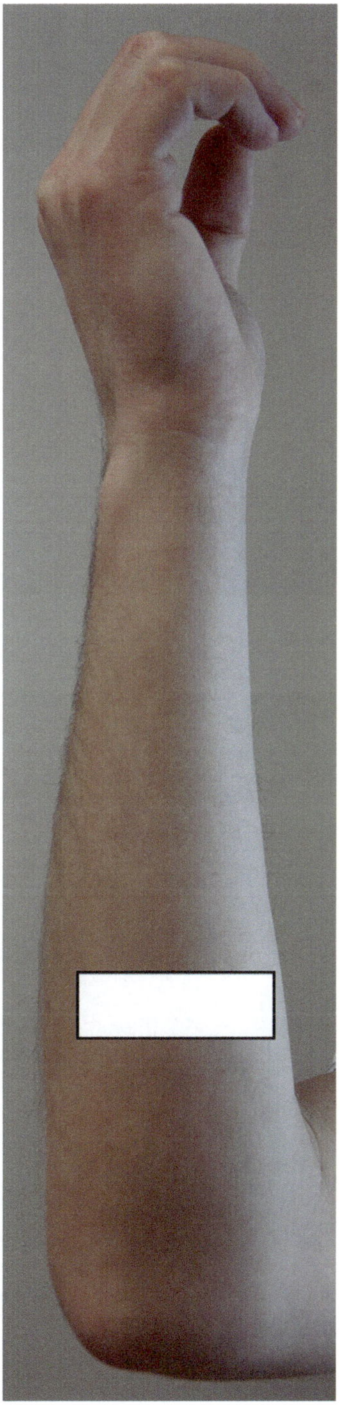

Fig. 7 Ultrasound probe placement (white box) for identification of the flexor carpi ulnaris muscle

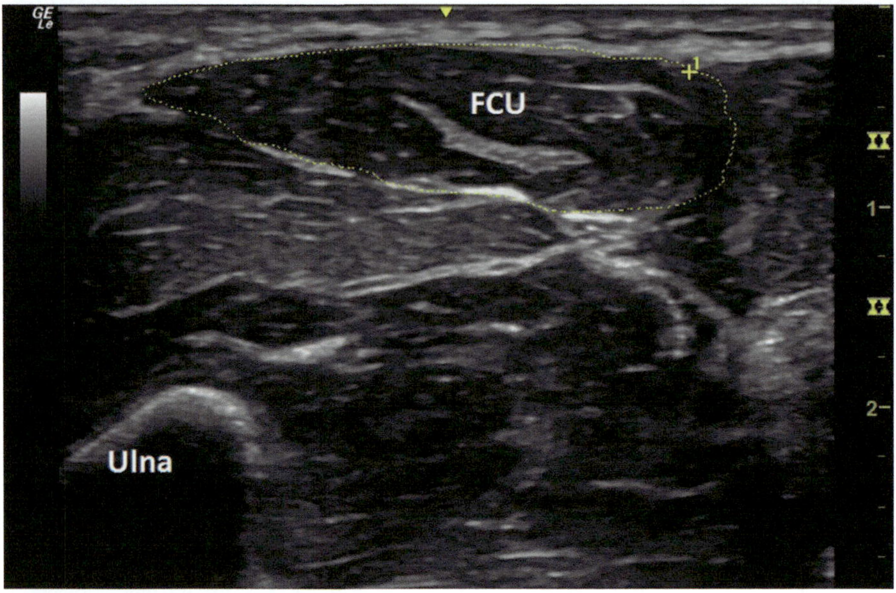

Fig. 8 Sonogram of flexor carpi ulnaris muscle; probe placement as per Fig. 7

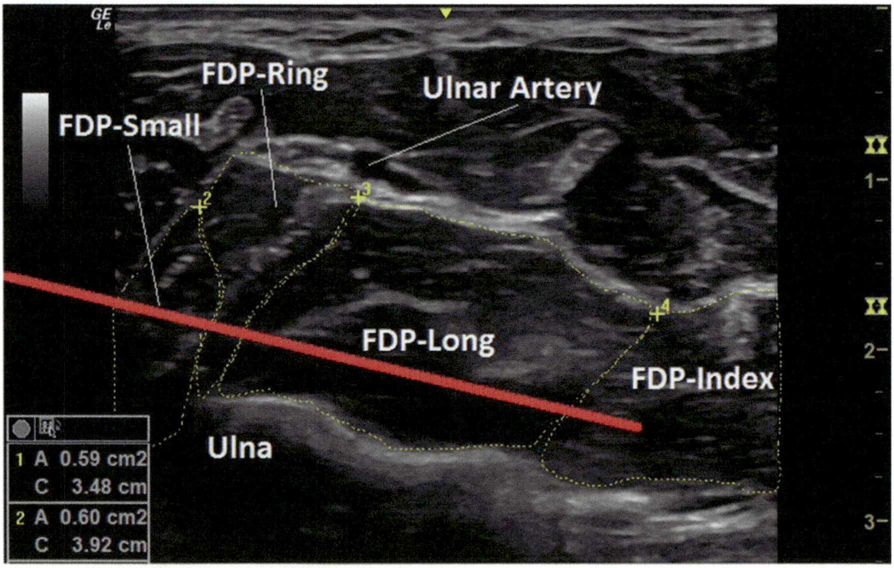

Fig. 9 Sonogram of flexor digitorum profundus (red line signifies needle); probe placement as per Fig. 10

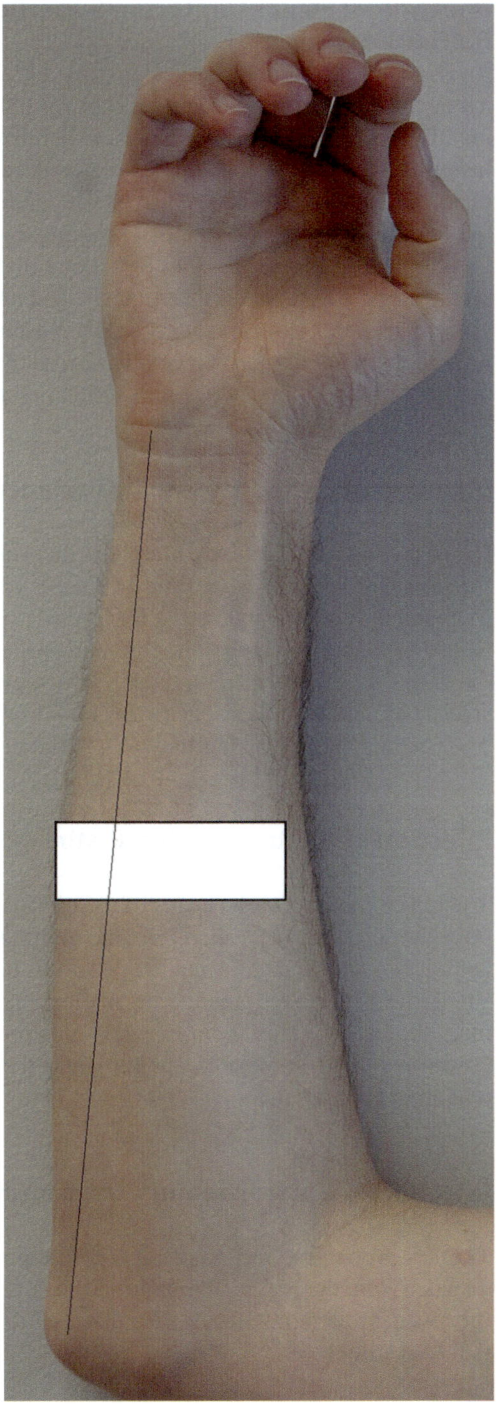

Fig. 10 Ultrasound probe placement (white box) for identification of the flexor digitorum profundus muscle

Injection of Flexor Digitorum Superficialis (FDS), E-stim or EMG Guidance

Like FDP, digit-specific muscle bellies for FDS can be targeted; unlike FDP, targeting all four FDS digit-specific muscle bellies usually requires four separate needle insertions [8]. For localization, a line is drawn from the medial epicondyle to the pisiform (Fig. 11); at the halfway point, approximately 0.5 cm radial to that line is the FDS-ring insertion site and approximately 1.5 cm radial to that line is the FDS-long insertion site. At the 3/4 point along that line, approximately 0.5 cm radial to that line is the FDS-small insertion site and approximately 1.5 cm radial to that line is the FDS-index insertion site. Needle placement is confirmed via E-stim resulting in isolated finger flexion (especially flexion of the proximal interphalangeal joint) or via EMG with audible motor unit action potentials.

Injection of FDS, Ultrasound Guidance

For FDS-ring and FDS-long muscle bellies, the US probe is placed short-axis to the forearm halfway along the line from the medial epicondyle to the pisiform; for FDS-small and FDS-index, the US probe is placed at the 3/4 point along this line (Fig. 11). The ulnar artery should be identified. All digit-specific muscle bellies of the FDS can be identified on the US image dynamically by having an assistant passively flex and extend a specific proximal interphalangeal joint (Figs. 12 and 13). The needle is inserted longitudinally to the probe in a radial-to-ulnar direction.

Injection of Gastrocnemius, E-stim or EMG Guidance

The injection sites for the heads of the gastrocnemius are in the proximal half of the posterior leg (Fig. 14). A line from the midpoint of the popliteal fossa to the Achilles tendon divides the medial and lateral heads; injections for the medial gastrocnemius should be within 3 cm medial of this line, and injections for the lateral gastrocnemius should be within 2 cm lateral of this line. Needle placement is confirmed via E-stim resulting in isolated ankle plantar flexion or via EMG with audible motor unit action potentials.

Injection of Gastrocnemius, Ultrasound Guidance

The US probe is placed short-axis to the posterior leg, approximately 1/3 of the distance from the popliteal fossa to the heel (Fig. 14). The Gastrocnemius muscle is the broad, superficial muscle visualized (Fig. 15). Needle insertion is at the discretion of the injector.

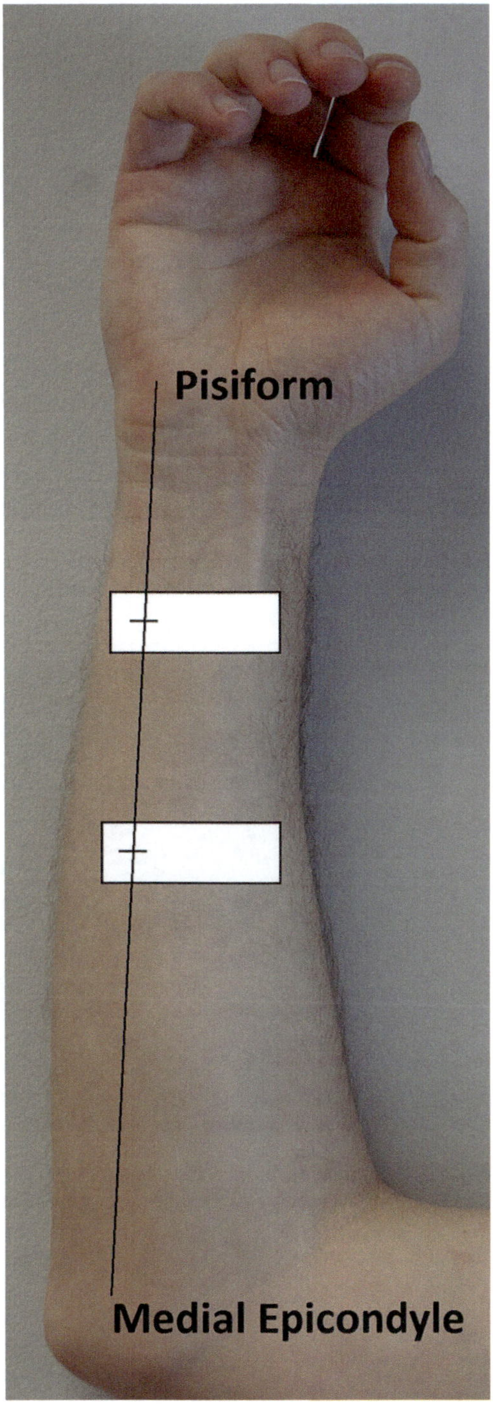

Fig. 11 Ultrasound probe placement (white box) for identification of the flexor digitorum superficialis muscle

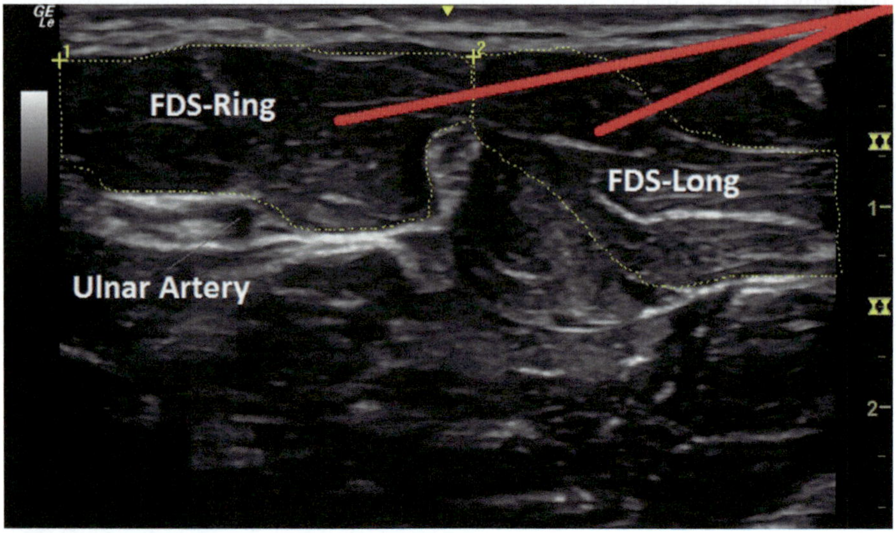

Fig. 12 Sonogram of flexor digitorum superficialis muscle bellies to the ring and long fingers (red line signifies needle); probe placement as per Fig. 11

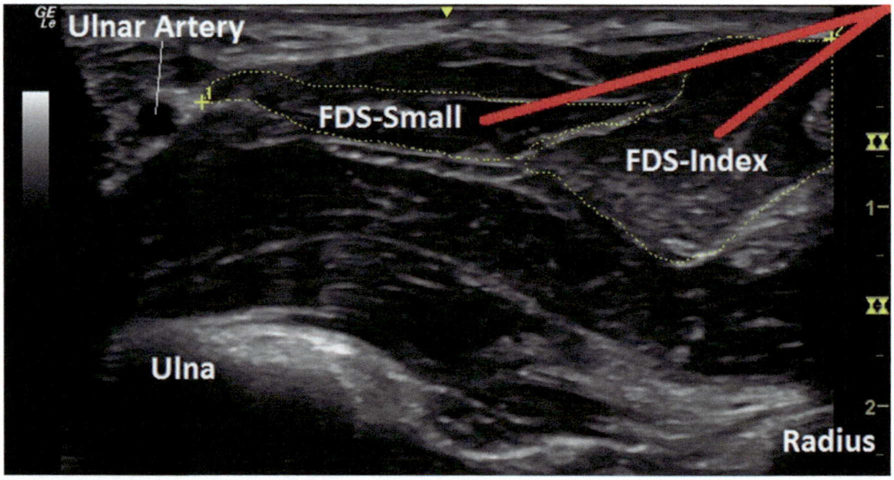

Fig. 13 Sonogram of flexor digitorum superficialis muscle bellies to the small and index fingers (red line signifies needle); probe placement as per Fig. 11

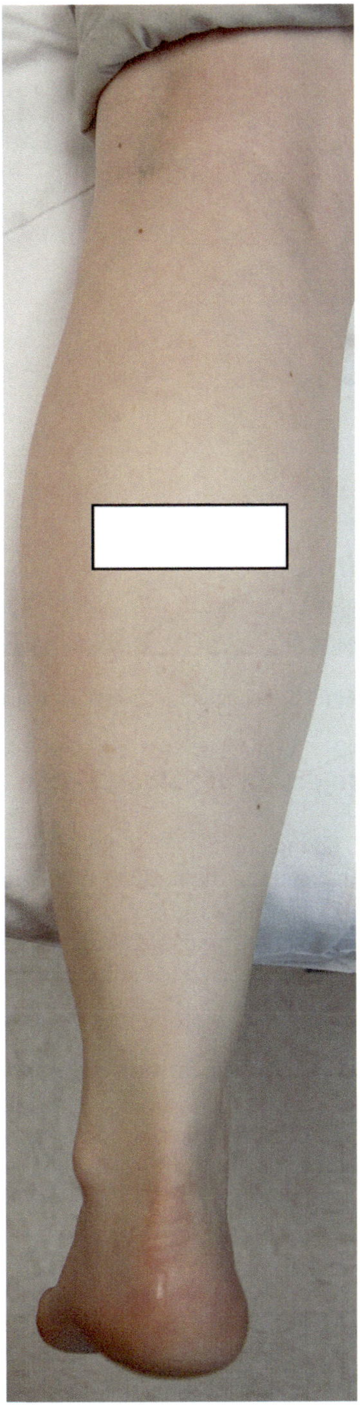

Fig. 14 Ultrasound probe placement (white box) for identification of the gastrocnemius muscle

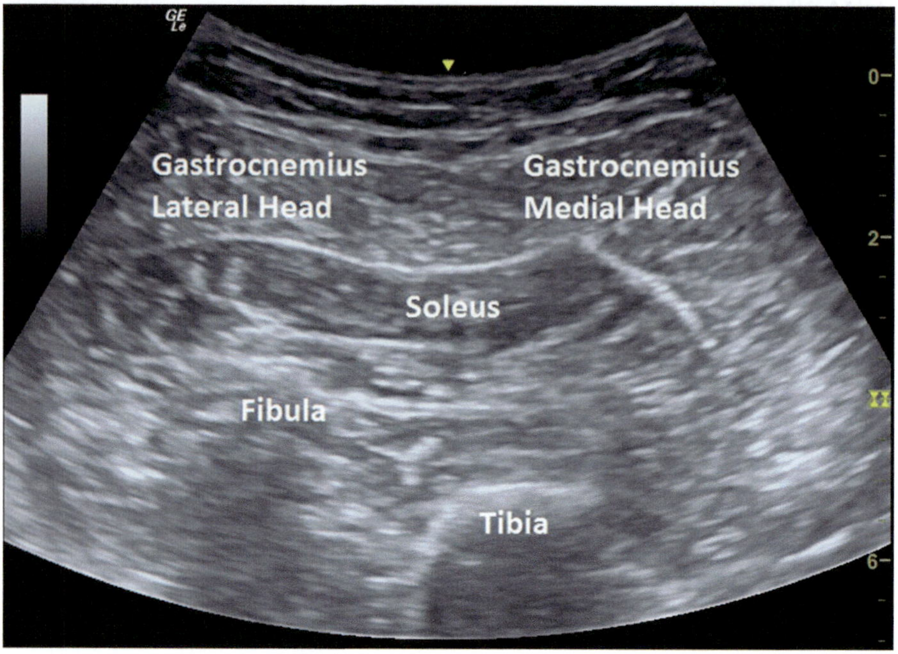

Fig. 15 Sonogram of gastrocnemius and soleus muscles; probe placement as per Fig. 14

Injection of Soleus, E-stim or EMG Guidance

The injection site for the soleus is around the halfway point between the knee and the ankle in the midline of the posterior leg, just distal to the distal edge of the gastrocnemius (Fig. 16). Needle placement is confirmed via EMG with audible motor unit action potentials or via E-stim (patient supine with knee held flexed to 90°) resulting in isolated ankle plantar flexion.

Injection of Soleus, Ultrasound Guidance

The US probe is placed short-axis to the posterior leg at the soleus injection site described above (Fig. 16). At this site and more distally, the soleus is the most superficial muscle (Fig. 17); more proximally, the soleus is located deep to the gastrocnemius (Fig. 15). Needle insertion is at the discretion of the injector.

Injection of Tibialis Posterior, E-stim or EMG Guidance

The injection site is the midpoint of the medial tibia, just posterior to the tibia and aiming towards the fibula. The needle must pass through the flexor digitorum longus

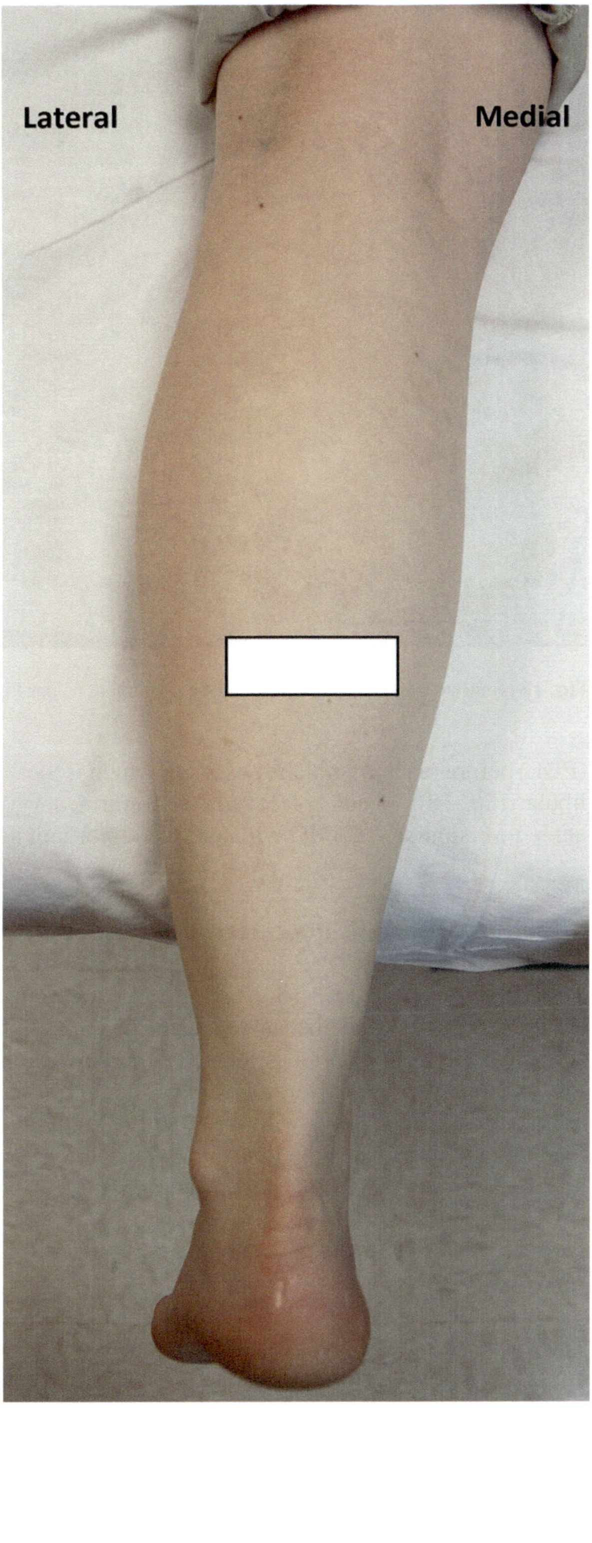

Fig. 16 Ultrasound probe placement (white box) for identification of the soleus, flexor digitorum longus, tibialis posterior, and flexor hallucis longus muscles

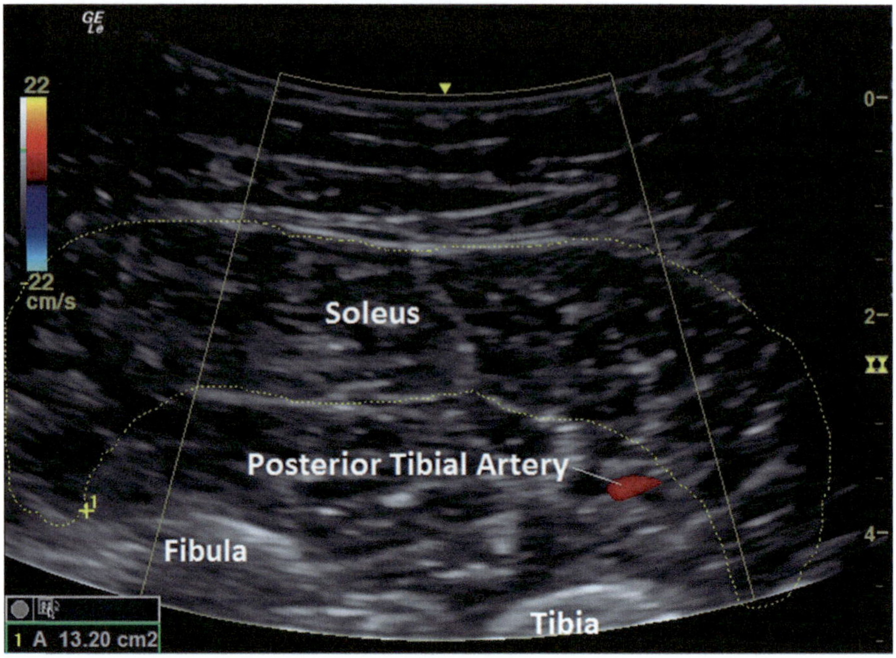

Fig. 17 Sonogram of soleus muscle; probe placement as per Fig. 16

(FDL) before reaching tibialis posterior, which is located deep between the tibia and fibula (Fig. 18). Needle placement is confirmed via E-stim resulting in isolated ankle inversion or via EMG with audible motor unit action potentials.

Injection of Tibialis Posterior, Ultrasound Guidance

The US probe is placed short-axis the posterior leg around the halfway point between the knee and the ankle, distal to the distal edge of the gastrocnemius (Fig. 16). Tibialis posterior is located deep between the tibia and fibula (Fig. 18). The location of the posterior tibial artery should be noted and avoided. Needle insertion is as described above with the E-stim/EMG guided injection, passing through the FDL and in between the tibia and the posterior tibial artery.

Injection of Flexor Digitorum Longus (FDL), E-stim or EMG Guidance

The injection site is the midpoint of the medial tibia, just posterior to the tibia and aiming towards the fibula (Fig. 18). Needle placement is confirmed via E-stim

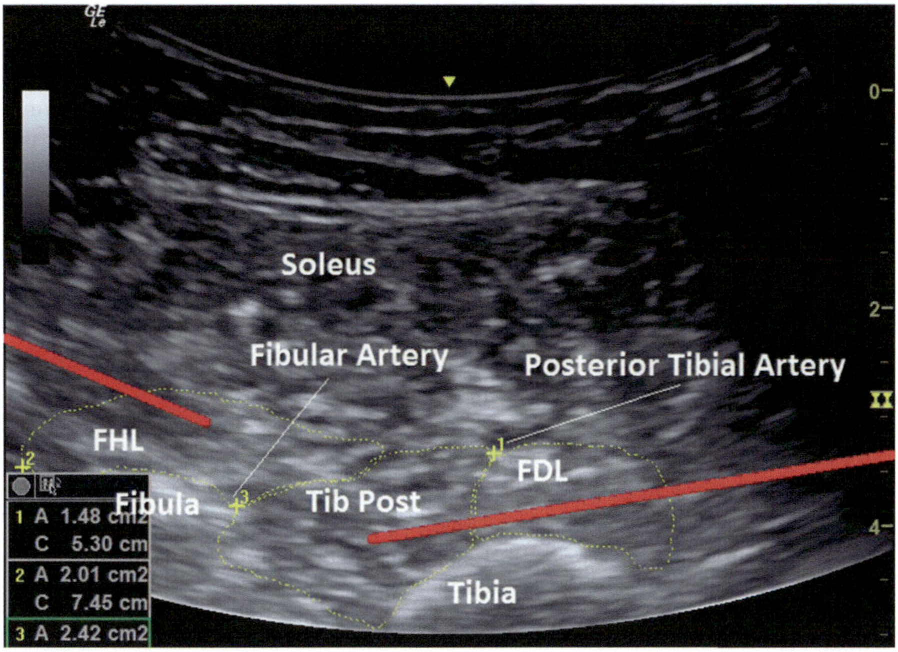

Fig. 18 Sonogram of soleus, flexor digitorum longus, tibialis posterior, and flexor hallucis longus muscles (red line signifies needle); probe placement as per Fig. 16

resulting in isolated toe flexion (exclusive of the great toe) or via EMG with audible motor unit action potentials.

Injection of FDL, Ultrasound Guidance

The US probe is placed short-axis the posterior leg around the halfway point between the knee and the ankle, distal to the distal edge of the gastrocnemius (Fig. 16). FDL is located just posterior to the tibia (Fig. 18). The location of the posterior tibial artery should be noted and avoided. Needle insertion is as described above with the E-stim/EMG guided FDL injection.

Injection of Flexor Hallucis Longus (FHL), E-stim or EMG Guidance

The injection site is the midpoint of the lateral fibula, just posterior to the fibula and aiming towards the tibia (Fig. 18). Needle placement is confirmed via E-stim resulting in isolated great toe flexion or via EMG with audible motor unit action potentials.

Injection of FHL, Ultrasound Guidance

The US probe is placed short-axis the posterior leg around the halfway point between the knee and the ankle, distal to the distal edge of the gastrocnemius (Fig. 16). FDL is located just posterior to the fibula (Fig. 18). The location of the fibular artery should be noted and avoided. Needle insertion is as described above with the E-stim/EMG guided FHL injection.

Potential Complications and Adverse Effects

Although generally well tolerated by patients, occasional adverse reactions and complications can occur which the clinician should be aware of when performing these procedures (Table 6). Generally, adverse reactions occur within the first few weeks following injection and, while generally transient, may have duration of several months or longer. Localized pain, infection, inflammation, tenderness, swelling, erythema, and/or bleeding/bruising may be associated with the injections. Symptoms associated with flu-like symptoms (e.g., nausea, fever, myalgia) have also been reported. Needle-related pain and/or anxiety may result in vasovagal responses (e.g., syncope, hypotension), which may require appropriate medical therapy [3].

Table 6 Additional potential complications and adverse effects [3]

– Spread of toxin effect *Can be observed hours to weeks after injection*	– Effects may be observed beyond the site of local injection—generalized muscle weakness, diplopia, ptosis, dysphagia, dysphonia, dysarthria, urinary incontinence, breathing difficulties
– Hypersensitivity reactions	– Anaphylaxis, serum sickness, urticaria, soft tissue edema, dyspnea
– Increased risk of clinically significant effects with pre-existing neuromuscular disorders	– Generalized muscle weakness, diplopia, ptosis, dysphonia, dysarthria, severe dysphagia, respiratory compromise
– Dysphagia and breathing difficulties	– Patients with pre-existing swallowing or breathing difficulties may be more susceptible
– Serious adverse reactions with unapproved use	– Excessive weakness, dysphagia, aspiration pneumonia *May have resulted from administration to the site of injection and/or adjacent structures*

Clinical and Technical Pearls

- Spasticity can be beneficial for function, and botulinum toxin-associated paralysis can lead to further dysfunction; if there are concerns about functional sequelae of treatment, coordinate care with a physiatrist.
- Identifying and documenting the upper motor neuron lesion causing the spasticity is necessary, including for pre-authorization and billing purposes.
- Guidance modalities (E-stim, EMG, and/or US) for botulinum toxin injections should be chosen based on the provider's comfort level with a given modality, but some type of guidance modality is recommended.
- Ergonomics for the provider for these injections, especially when using US guidance, requires significant planning to accommodate spastic posturing.
- Spasms during the procedure create unique safety challenges for all involved; the provider should plan for the patient's limb to spasm with every needle insertion and with every use of E-stim.

References

1. Brashear A. Spasticity diagnosis and management. 2nd ed. New York: Demos Medical; 2016.
2. Brashear A, Mayer NH, Pierson S, Gracies JM, Chambers HG, Pill SG, et al. Spasticity and other forms of muscle overactivity in the upper motor neuron syndrome: etiology, evaluation, management, and the role of botulinum toxin. New York: WeMove; 2008.
3. Allergen. Botox (onabotulinumtoxin A) [package insert]. Madison: Allergan USA; 2019.
4. Ipsen Biopharmaceuticals, Inc. Dysport (abobtulinumtoxin A) [package insert]. Cambridge: Ipsen Biopharmaceuticals; 2019.
5. Merz Pharmaceuticals, LLC. Xeomin (incobotulinumtoxin A) [package insert]. Raleigh: Merz Pharmaceuticals, LLC; 2019.
6. AANS. Dystonia [Internet]. 2019. https://www.aans.org/en/Patients/Neurosurgical-Conditions-and-Treatments/Dystonia. Accessed 26 Nov 2019.
7. LaVallee J, Royer R, Smith G. Prevalence of bleeding complications following ultrasound-guided botulinum toxin injections in patients on anticoagulation or antiplatelet therapy. PM R. 2017;9(12):1217–24.
8. Bickerton LE, Agur AM, Ashby P. Flexor digitorum superficialis: locations of individual muscle bellies for botulinum toxin injections. Muscle Nerve. 1997;20(8):1041–3.

Further Reading

Alter KE, Hallet M, Karp B, Lungu C. Ultrasound-guided chemodenervation procedures text and atlas. New York: Demos Medical; 2013.

Brashear A. Spasticity diagnosis and management. 2nd ed. New York: Demos Medical; 2016.

Esquenazi A, Albanese A, Chancellor MB, Elovic E, Segal KR, Simpson DM, Smith CP, Ward AB. Evidence-based review and assessment of botulinum neurotoxin for the treatment of adult spasticity in the upper motor neuron syndrome. Toxicon. 2013;67:115–28.

Part VII

Bedside Procedures for Lower Extremity Pain

Intra-Articular Hip Injections

Mohamed Attia and Mowafak Abdelghani

Essential Concepts

- Osteoarthritis of the hip is a common problem for the elderly population and increases with age. The incidence is 1 in 4 above 85 years old.
- Prior to the diagnosis of hip OA, it is important to exclude other pathologies including lumbar spine pathology and radiculopathy, patients may also present with ipsilateral knee OA in addition to hip OA due to weight bearing problems.
- Total hip replacement provides a successful intervention in end stage hip arthritis, however this is preceded with years of pain and inability to perform activities of daily living.
- At the bedside, intraarticular injections can be performed via landmark or ultrasound techniques. Ultrasound technique is thought to have less risk of adverse events.
- Complications from use of corticosteroids include accelerated osteoarthritis, subchondral insufficiency fractures, and rapid joint destruction with bone loss.

M. Attia · M. Abdelghani (✉)
Manchester University NHS Foundation Trust, Manchester, UK
e-mail: Mohamed.attia@mft.nhs.uk; Mowafak.abdelghani@mft.nhs.uk

D. Souza et al. (eds.), *Bedside Pain Management Interventions*,
https://doi.org/10.1007/978-3-031-11188-4_62

1 Intra-Articular Hip Joint Injections

Overview

Osteoarthritic pain is typically aggravated by mobility and daily activities and is often relieved by rest. The pain is usually confined to the hip joint itself, however in some patients pain can be referred the thigh [1, 2]. An atypical presentation may also include pain in the knee. Pain is usually intermittent in the early stages of the disease but becomes more frequent and severe as the disease progresses. There is a poor correlation between the severity of disease based on plain X-ray changes and symptoms of pain [1, 3].

The principal pathologic feature of OA is articular cartilage loss which is identified as reduction in joint space on plain X-ray films [4, 5]. Structural changes such as loss of joint cartilage, bone marrow lesions, synovial thickening (synovitis) and knee effusion all contribute to pain intensity. These findings are best visualized by magnetic resonance imaging which provides greater detail regarding hip joint pathology [6, 7].

Indications and Contraindications

Common indications for intra-articular hip injections include hip joint pain, inflammatory or degenerative osteoarthritis. The injections can be performed for diagnostic or therapeutic purposes [5] (Table 1).

Common contraindications include infection at the planned injection site, sepsis, allergy or intolerance to injectate or its components, and patient refusal. Coagulopathy, including iatrogenic, and platelet dysfunction, including iatrogenic, and not considered to be contraindications for intra-articular hip injections.

Table 1 Intraarticular hip injections indications and contraindications [5]

Indications	Techniques	Contraindications
1. As a diagnostic test for hip joint pain 2. To help determine the likelihood of achieving pain relief with hip arthroplasty 3. When surgical intervention is not a viable option and pain relief is desired 4. In young patient population with hip prothesis	Landmark technique Ultrasound-guided	**Absolute:** Patient refusal Systemic infection Local infection (cellulitis) at site of injection Joint fracture Prosthetic joint Coagulopathy **Relative:** Anticoagulation therapy Joint instability Poorly controlled diabetes Adjacent skin abrasions

Clinical Anatomy

The hip joint is a ball and socket diarthrodial joint with point of articulation between the head of the femur and the acetabulum of the pelvis.

The hip joint acts as the dynamic support system of the upper body and trunk while facilitating force and load transmission from the axial skeleton to the lower extremities, allowing mobility.

The hip joint receives sensory innervation from the femoral, obturator, and superior gluteal nerves. Nerve fibers of the hip capsule appear to persist or proliferate in pathological states, thus can be found in the capsular complex of individuals with OA.

The profunda femoris is a branch of the femoral artery which travels posteriorly to give rise to the medial circumflex and lateral circumflex femoral arteries which supply the head of the femur. The profunda femoris is a branch of the femoral artery which travels posteriorly. There is an additional contribution from the foveal artery (artery to the head of the femur), a branch of the posterior division of the obturator artery, which travels in the ligament of the head of the femur [2, 8, 9].

Equipment and Supplies

Intra-articular hip injections can be easily at the bedside. An antiseptic solution, typically chlorhexidine, 20–22 Gauge 3.5-in. needle, 5–10 mL syringe for injectate, mask, and sterile gloves should be typically prepared for this procedure. Local anesthetic with or without corticosteroids is typically prepared for this injection as well. Other types of injectates will be discussed further in the chapter. Normal saline or local anesthetic can be utilized for ultrasound guidance during hydrolocalization. An ultrasound unit with a high-frequency linear transducer will be typically needed (Table 2).

Landmark Technique

The landmark technique aims at piercing the hip capsule at any point on the anterolateral surface of the femoral head or neck below the acetabular rim down to the inter-trochanteric line.

Table 2 Required supplies for intraarticular hip injection

Syringe	5 or 10 mL
Needle	25 Gauge 1.5 in. needle for local anesthesia of the skin anesthesia over skin injection site 20–22 Gauge spinal needle 3.5 in.
Anesthetic	1% Lidocaine
Corticosteroid	Dexamethasone 4 mg (t1/2 life: 36–54 h) Methylprednisolone 40 mg (t1/2 life: 18–36 h)

The Lateral Approach Landmarks

The patient lies supine with the limb in neutral rotation (patella facing forward). Two points, the tip of the greater trochanter and the anterior superior iliac spine (ASIS) are marked (u shaped lines); a red line drawn between them (Fig. 1).

At the junction between the upper third and lower two-thirds of this red line lies the "soft-spot" (one can feel the anterior border of the gluteus medius); this is marked as point A (needle entry point).

The Anterior Approach Landmarks

The patient lies supine with limb in neutral position (patella facing forward). Two lines are then drawn: line 1 from the ASIS distally toward the upper pole of the patella and line 2 perpendicular to it from the tip of the greater trochanter anteriorly. The intersection point is point B which is the entry point for the anterior approach [4].

Lidocaine 1% can be used for local skin analgesia. A mixture of 6 mL is prepared in a 10 cc syringe formed of 5 mL bupivacaine 0.25% and 1 mL of 40 mg/mL of methylprednisolone if steroids are the injectate of choice or hyaluronic acid 2 mL (16 mg/2 mL) as an alternative injectate of choice.

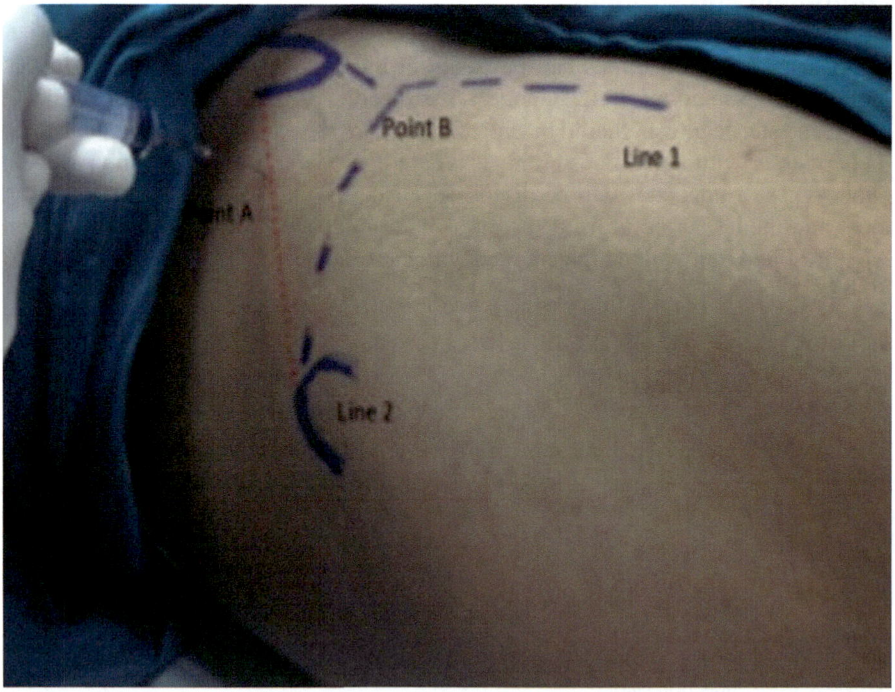

Fig. 1 Intra-articular hip injection, landmark technique. Right hip in supine position with anterolateral view. The ASIS and the greater trochanter are palpated and demarcated. Point A is the soft-spot entry point at the junction of the upper third and lower two-thirds of the imaginary line between the ASIS and tip of the greater Trochanter, point B is the meeting of both lines and is the target point in the coronal plane. Reprinted with permission from Massed and Said [4]

The lateral approach is safer in comparison to the anterior approach. A study by Kruse et al. reported that there is greater likelihood of injury to the neurovascular bundle via an anterior as opposed to lateral technique (anterior approach the needle contacted or pierced the femoral nerve 27% of the time and was within 5 mm of the nerve 60% of the time vs no needle coming within 25 mm neurovascular structures when using the lateral approach [5].

While not available at the bedside, in this case, fluoroscopy image was taken to confirm needle position with landmark technique (Fig. 2).

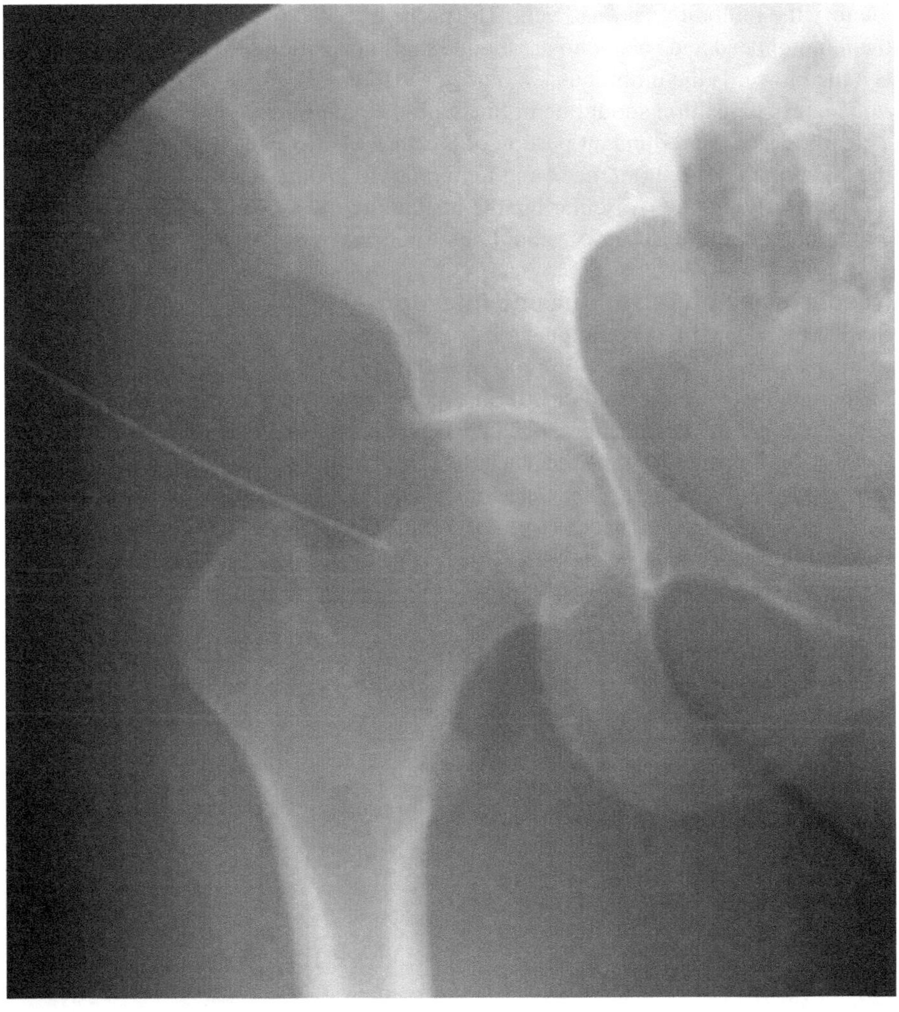

Fig. 2 Intra-articular hip injection, landmark technique. The X-ray was performed to verify the position of the needle that was advanced using landmark technique. Right hip with anterior-to-superior fluoroscopic view, showing the position of the needle under the C-arm. The needle is touching bone of the neck, which ensures that it has passed through the capsule of the hip joint. Fluoroscopic image was taken to verify the position of the needle that was originally placed using landmark technique [4]

The use of anatomic landmarks, even at the bedside, is not considered a desirable technique given the increasingly easy access to ultrasonographic guidance which can help to minimize adverse effects.

Ultrasound-Guided Technique

Ultrasound-guided technique is preferable for intra-articular hip injections. A low-frequency curvilinear probe is placed parallel to the inguinal ligament and used to identify the femoral artery and vein. The probe is then moved laterally to just above the femoral head and rotated to an oblique sagittal position so that the probe marker is aimed towards the umbilicus.

The probe position should be in line with the anterior femoral head or neck and a clear view of the redundant portion of the anterior hip capsule (anterior recess) at the junction of the femoral neck and femoral head is obtained.

The overlying neurovascular bundle containing the ascending branch of the lateral femoral circumflex artery should be visualized by color Doppler.

Needle Insertion Technique and Injection

Similar to the landmark technique, local skin analgesia is provided by injecting lidocaine 1%. A 6 mL mixture of 5 mL bupivacaine 0.25% and 1 mL of 40 mg/mL of methylprednisolone if steroids are the injectate of choice or hyaluronic acid "Synvisc" 2 mL (16 mg/2 mL) as an alternative injectate of choice is prepared in a 10 cc syringe formed. A 22-Gauge 10 mm spinal needle is used in an in-plane approach under real-time ultrasound guidance to the anterior capsular recess (Fig. 3a).

After visualizing the needle tip at the joint capsule, 1–2 mL of the solution is slowly injected under low pressure. Successful targeting of the joint space is confirmed by spread of anechoic fluid under the iliofemoral ligament within the anterior capsular recess (Fig. 3b) [6, 7].

The ultrasound-guided technique is the preferred technique for injecting hyaluronic acid to avoid extra-articular placement. The ultrasound-guided technique is likely helpful in the prevention of complications, including vascular or neural injury [8].

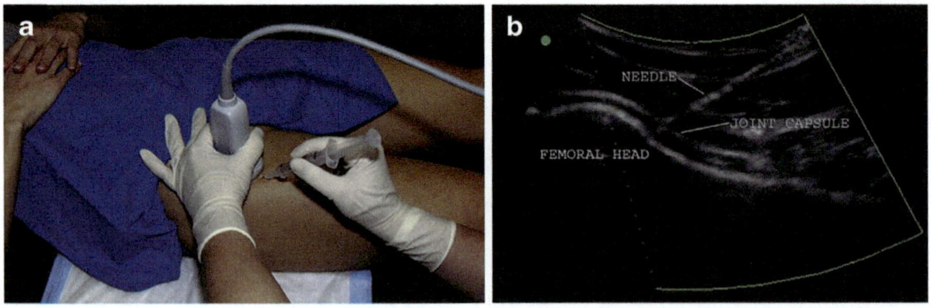

Fig. 3 Intra-articular hip injection, ultrasound-guided technique. (**a**) Proper probe positioning and in-plane needle insertion. (**b**) Depicts the needle tip entering the hip joint capsule. Reprinted with permission from Bardowski and Byrd [7]

Potential Complications and Adverse Effects

There is a significant risk for injury to the femoral nerve, femoral artery, and lateral femoral cutaneous nerve during injection of the hip joint.

There is also the potential for a high rate of extraarticular injection.

Adverse effects related to the hip joint injection include:

- Septic arthritis.
- Osteonecrosis.
- The risk of joint infection after total hip replacement.

Adverse effects related to steroid injection into the hip joint include:

- Accelerated osteoarthritis.
- Subchondral insufficiency fractures.
- Rapid joint destruction with bone loss [9].

Clinical and Technical Pearls

- A lateral approach landmark technique is considered safer than an anterior approach because it has decreased risk of injury to the femoral sheath structures.
- Ultrasound guidance is safer than landmark technique in visualizing vasculature (femoral artery, vein) and nerves (femoral nerve and lateral cutaneous nerve of the thigh) surrounding the hip joint.
- The presence of clinically suspected hip pain does not also correspond to degree of OA on radiographs.
- Avoid steroid injections 2 months prior to any planned total hip arthroplasty.
- Adequate sterile technique is essential in avoiding any joint infections post intervention.

References

1. O'Neill TW, Felson DT. Mechanisms of osteoarthritis (OA) pain. Curr Osteoporos Rep. 2018;16(5):611–6.
2. Gold M, Varacallo M. Anatomy, bony pelvis and lower limb, hip joint. Treasure Island, FL: StatPearls; 2017.
3. Lai WC, Arshi A, Wang D, Seeger LL, Motamedi K, Levine BD, Hame SL. Efficacy of intraarticular corticosteroid hip injections for osteoarthritis and subsequent surgery. Skeletal Radiol. 2018;47(12):1635–40.
4. Massed M, Said H. Intraarticular hip injection using anatomic surface landmarks. Arthrosc Tech. 2013;2(2):e147–e149.
5. Kruse DW. Intraarticular cortisone injection for osteoarthritis of the hip. Is it effective? Is it safe? Curr Rev Musculoskelet Med. 2008;1(3–4):227–33.
6. Hoeber S, Aly AR, Ashworth N, Rajasekaran S. Ultrasound-guided hip joint injections are more accurate than landmark-guided injections: a systematic review and meta-analysis. Br J Sports Med. 2016;50(7):392–6.

7. Bardowski E, Byrd JWT. Ultrasound-guided intra-articular injection of the hip: the Nashville sound. Arthrosc Tech. 2019;8(4):e383–e388.
8. Piccirilli E, Oliva F, Murè MA, Mahmoud A, Foti C, Tarantino U, Maffulli N. Viscosupplementation with intra-articular hyaluronic acid for hip disorders. A systematic review and meta-analysis. Muscles Ligaments Tendons J. 2016;6(3):293.
9. Kompel AJ, Roemer FW, Murakami AM, Diaz LE, Crema MD, Guermazi A. Intra-articular corticosteroid injections in the hip and knee: perhaps not as safe as we thought? Radiology. 2019;293(3):656–63.

Further Reading

Katz JN, Arant KR, Loeser RF. Diagnosis and treatment of hip and knee osteoarthritis: a review. JAMA. 2021;325(6):568–78. https://doi.org/10.1001/jama.2020.22171.

Lynch TS, Oshlag BL, Bottiglieri TS, Desai NN. Ultrasound-guided hip injections. J Am Acad Orthop Surg. 2019;27(10):e451–61. https://doi.org/10.5435/JAAOS-D-17-00908.

Hip: Periarticular Injections

Anita M. Lowe Taylor and Eugene Yousik Roh

Essential Concepts

- Peri-articular injections are an effective intervention used to diagnose and treat a variety of pathologies around the hip, including bursitis and minor tendinopathies.
- Ultrasound guidance improves accuracy and can help visualize and avoid neurovascular structures.
- Injections can be diagnostic (i.e. to confirm a particular structure as a pain generator), therapeutic (i.e. to reduce pain and inflammation), or a combination of both.
- Goals for therapeutic injections can include immediate and long-term pain relief, decreased reliance on systemic medications when appropriate, and improved tolerance of physical therapies.
- The mechanism of action is the result of local inhibition of the inflammatory immune response.

A. M. Lowe Taylor
Department of Physical Medicine and Rehabilitation, Stanford Healthcare, Redwood City, CA, USA
e-mail: alowe@alumni.stanford.edu

E. Y. Roh (✉)
Department of Orthopedic Surgery Sports Medicine, Stanford University, Redwood City, CA, USA
e-mail: pubeyroh@stanford.edu

D. Souza et al. (eds.), *Bedside Pain Management Interventions*,
https://doi.org/10.1007/978-3-031-11188-4_63

1 Trochanteric Bursa Injection

Overview

Greater trochanteric pain syndrome (GTPS) refers to inflammation of the trochanteric bursa and surrounding structures, including the hip abductor tendons and iliotibial band. It is one of the most common causes of lateral hip pain, occurring in an estimated 15% of adult women and 6.6% of men [1, 2]. It is characterized by lateral hip pain with ambulation and focal tenderness over the lateral hip [2]. Non-surgical treatments include non-steroidal anti-inflammatory drugs (NSAIDs) and physical therapy. Ultrasound or landmark guided corticosteroid injections into the greater trochanteric bursa can be used to reduce inflammation and pain and improve tolerance of physical therapy.

Indications and Contraindications

GTPS refers to lateral hip pain and encompasses greater trochanteric bursitis, gluteus medius and minimus tendinopathies, and external coxa saltans (i.e. snapping hip syndrome) [2]. GTPS is thought to be caused by friction of the iliotibial (IT) band over the greater trochanter of the femur, leading to microtrauma of the gluteal tendons, and weakness of the hip abductors [3]. Tightness of the IT band and osteoarthritis of the lumbar spine, hip, or knee may lead to improper biomechanics and predispose patients to the condition [1]. Corticosteroid injections reduce pain at 1 and 3 months and are indicated for patients that have failed conservative management with NSAIDs and physical therapy, have contraindications to these treatments, or who are intolerant of therapy due to pain [4]. Diagnostic injections with local anesthetic can help differentiate true weakness from pain mediated weakness (Table 1).

Common contraindications include infection at the planned injection site, or severe systemic infection, allergy or intolerance to injectate or its components, and patient's refusal. Coagulopathy, including iatrogenic, and platelet dysfunction, including iatrogenic, are typically not considered as contraindications.

Clinical Anatomy

The greater trochanter of the femur has four facets which serve as the attachment sites of the gluteus minimus (anterior facet) and gluteus medius (superior and lateral facets) tendons (Fig. 1).

Table 1 Diagnostic features of GTPS [3, 5]

A. Pain over the lateral hip
B. Tenderness to palpation over the greater trochanter of the femur
C. Pain or weakness with resisted hip abduction and external rotation
D. Ultrasound or MRI may be used to rule out alternative pathologies and evaluate for gluteus medius and/or minimus tendinopathies
E. Symptoms are not better accounted for by an alternative diagnosis

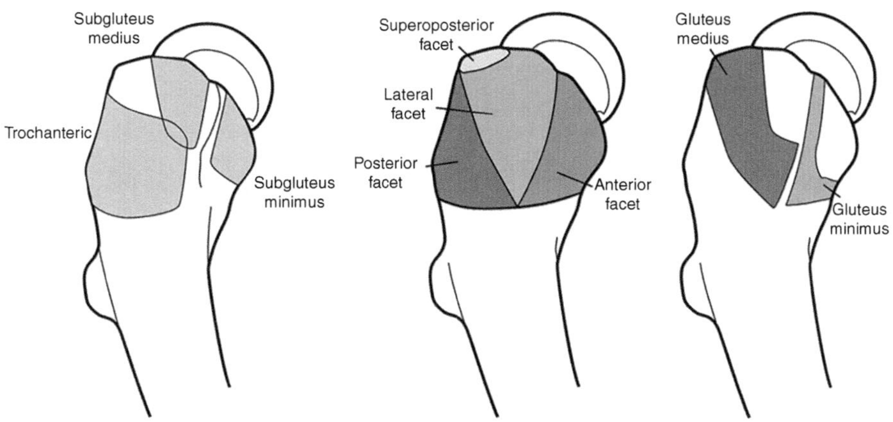

Fig. 1 Facets of the greater trochanter with gluteal muscle attachment sites and locations of the subgluteus medius, subgluteus minimus, and trochanteric bursae, as labeled. (Reprinted with permission from "Partial-Thickness Tears of the Gluteus Medius: Rationale and Technique for Trans-Tendinous Endoscopic Repair" by Benjamin G. Domb, Rima Michel Nasser, and Itamar B. Botser, 2010. Arthroscopy: The Journal of Arthroscopic & Related Surgery, volume 26, pages 1697–1705. Copyright 2010 by Elsevier)

Four bursae have been described surrounding the greater trochanter, the primary of which is the subgluteus maximus bursa [5]. The subgluteus maximus bursa demonstrates variability between subjects, but is generally located between the posterior facet and the gluteus maximus muscle [6]. The gluteus medius and minimus muscles are innervated by the superior gluteal nerve, which stems from the sacral plexus from ventral divisions of L4, L5, and S1 and are supplied by the superior gluteal artery, which accompanies the superior gluteal nerve [7].

Equipment and Supplies

Greater trochanteric bursa injections are easily performed at the bedside. Typically, a small syringe with a 22–25-gauge, 2–3.5 in. needle is utilized to inject 1–2 mL of anesthetic solution (usually 1% lidocaine or 0.5% ropivacaine) with or without a corticosteroid. Corticosteroid choices typically include 40 mg of triamcinolone, 40 mg DepoMedrol, or 6 mg of betamethasone. Injections may be performed based on landmark or ultrasound guidance (Table 2).

Greater Trochanteric Bursa Injection, Landmark Technique

The patient should be positioned on their side with the affected side upright. The bony prominence of the greater trochanter is located by palpating along the proximal aspect of the femur. This should correspond to the point of maximal tenderness. The needle is inserted perpendicular to the skin over the greater trochanter and advanced until it contacts bone, then withdrawn several millimeters. Aspirate prior to injection to ensure the needle is not intravascular [8].

Table 2 Required supplies for greater trochanteric bursa injections [26, 27]

Syringe	5 mL
Needle	22–25 gauge, 2–3.5 in.
Anesthetic	0.5% Ropivacaine 1–2% Lidocaine Or Lidocaine/bupivacaine combination: usually 1:1 ratio
Corticosteroid	Triamcinolone 20–40 mg (t1/2 life: 12–36 h), betamethasone 6 mg (t1/2 life: 36–72 h), methylprednisolone 40 mg (t1/2 life: 12–36 h)

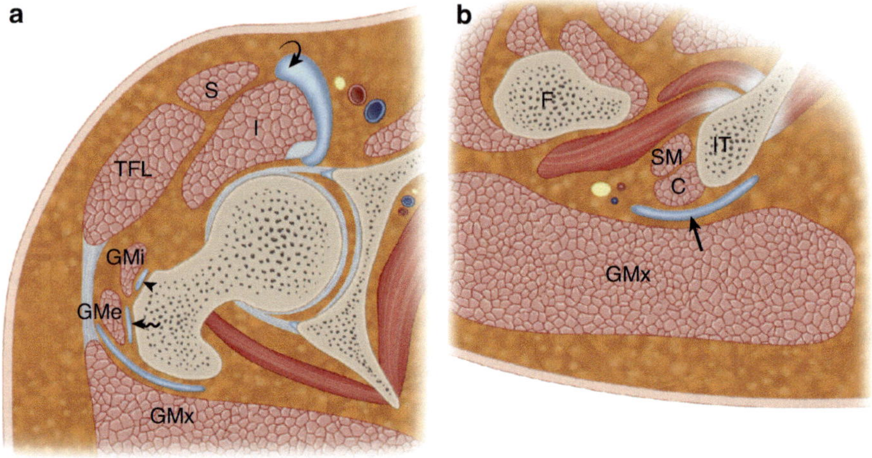

Fig. 2 Cross sectional hip anatomy. (**a**) Demonstrates the femoral head within the acetabulum with surrounding structures including the iliopsoas muscle (I) and bursa (IB), and gluteus maximus (GMax), medius (Gmed), and minimus (Gmin) muscles with their underlying bursae. (**b**) Shows the ischiogluteal bursae where it lies between the ischial tuberosity (IT), proximal hamstring insertions (H), and gluteus maximus

Ultrasound Technique

1. **Patient position**: Decubitus (side lying) with the affected side upright.
2. **Transducer type**: For normal body habitus patients, use a medium-frequency linear array. For larger body habitus patients, use a curvilinear array.
3. **Probe placement**: Position the probe in a transverse plane compared to the body. Visualize the anterior, lateral, and posterior facets of the greater trochanter, and identify the gluteus medius and minimus tendon attachments. The bursa will be slightly posterior to the border of the posterior and lateral facets.
4. **In plane**: The injection is performed in plane to visualize the needle trajectory and confirm placement within the bursa.
5. **Needle placement**: The needle should be inserted in plane (longitudinal to the transducer) using a posterior to anterior anatomical approach. The needle angle should be adjusted to ensure its trajectory towards the target, and then advanced until the target is reached (Figs. 2 and 3).

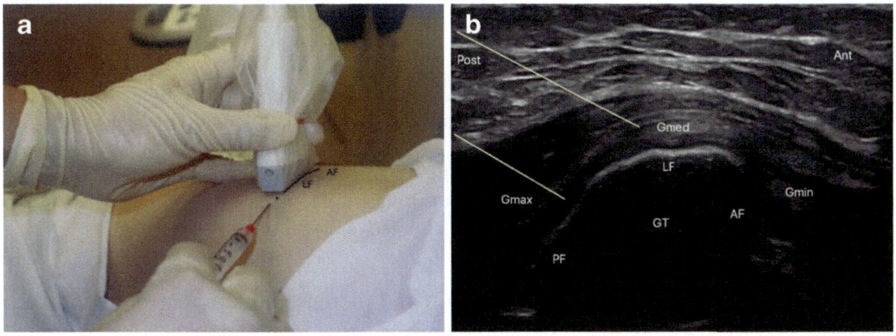

Fig. 3 (**a**) Transducer and needle position for axial greater trochanteric bursa injection. The needle is introduced in plane with the transducer from posterior to anterior. (**b**) Axial (short axis) view of the greater trochanter (GT) and surrounding structures. For greater trochanteric bursa injections, the needle (lines) is placed between the posterior facet (PF) and the gluteus maximus (Gmax). The needle is placed between the lateral facet (LF) and gluteus medius (Gmed) for subgluteus medius bursa injections, and between the anterior facet (AF) and gluteus minimus (Gmin) for subgluteus minimus injections

2 Ischial Tuberosity Injections

Ischiogluteal bursitis, also known as "weavers bottom," refers to inflammation of the ischiogluteal bursa and is characterized by pain over the ischial tuberosity from prolonged sitting on hard surfaces [9]. Pain over the ischial tuberosity may also result from proximal hamstring tendinopathies, which are often the result of repetitive stress injuries [10]. Imaging such ultrasound or magnetic resonance imaging (MRI) may be used to differentiate between these entities, determine the grade of hamstring strain if present, and rule out alternative diagnoses [9, 10]. Ultrasound guided corticosteroid injections can be used to reduce inflammation and pain and improve tolerance of physical therapy [10–12]. Injection of platelet rich plasma (PRP) for proximal hamstring tendinopathies has also been described in the literature [13].

Indications and Contraindications

Ischiogluteal bursitis is a cause of low buttock pain that results from prolonged sitting on hard surfaces, and is characterized by pain with direct pressure over the ischial tuberosity [9, 14]. Fluid in the bursa may be visualized on ultrasound or MRI, and corticosteroid injections may be used to decrease inflammation and pain.

Proximal hamstring tendinopathies result from repetitive activities and are increasingly being recognized as a source of chronic low buttock pain [10, 11]. Symptoms may be exacerbated by passive hip flexion, which stretches the hamstrings, or resisted knee flexion, which activates the hamstrings. Patients may have a positive supine plank, Puranen-Orava, or bent knee stretch test [11]. Initial treatment includes activity modification, ice, NSAIDs, and physical therapy.

Table 3 Diagnostic features of ischiogluteal bursitis and proximal hamstring tendinopathies [10, 11, 28]

A. Pain to palpation over the ischial tuberosity
B. Pain may be exacerbated by passive hip flexion or activation of the hamstring muscles with resisted knee flexion. Patients may have a positive supine plank, Puranen-Orava, or bent knee stretch test
C. Ultrasound or MRI may be used to visualize fluid in the ischial bursa, rule out alternative pathologies, and grade suspected proximal hamstring tendinopathies
D. Symptoms are not better accounted for by an alternative diagnosis

Corticosteroid injections may decrease pain and increase athletic participation, and are indicated for patients that have failed conservative management or have intolerable pain [10–12] (Table 3). Contraindications are the same as for injections described above in this chapter.

Clinical Anatomy

The ischial bursa is an inconsistent adventitious bursa located deep to the gluteus maximus muscle and superficial to the common hamstring origin over the ischial tuberosity [9, 15, 16]. It may be difficult to differentiate peritendinous edema from true bursitis. The ischial tuberosity is the proximal attachment site of the semimembranosus, semitendinosus, and long head of the biceps femoris, which act as knee flexors and hip extensors. The sciatic nerve may be identified overlying the quadratus femoris by scanning the transducer laterally [16] (Fig. 4).

Equipment and Supplies

Ischiogluteal bursa injections are easily performed at the bedside. Typically, a small syringe with a 22–25 gauge, 3.5 in. needle is utilized to inject 4 mL of local anesthetic solution and 1 mL of corticosteroid. Anesthetic solution usually consists of the local anesthetic lidocaine or bupivacaine, or a combination of the two. Injections may be performed based on landmark or ultrasound guidance (Table 4).

Ischiogluteal Bursa Injection, Landmark Technique

The patient should be positioned in a prone or decubitus position with the affected side up. Palpate the ischial tuberosity and direct the needle perpendicular to the skin towards the target. Once the needle touches bone, withdraw several millimeters to locate the bursa. Ensure that the patient is not experiencing paresthesias that might indicate contact with the sciatic nerve. If this occurs, withdraw and redirect the needle medially. Aspirate to verify that the needle is not intravascular prior to injecting. If there is resistance during injection, withdraw slightly and redirect to ensure the needle is not within a ligament or tendon.

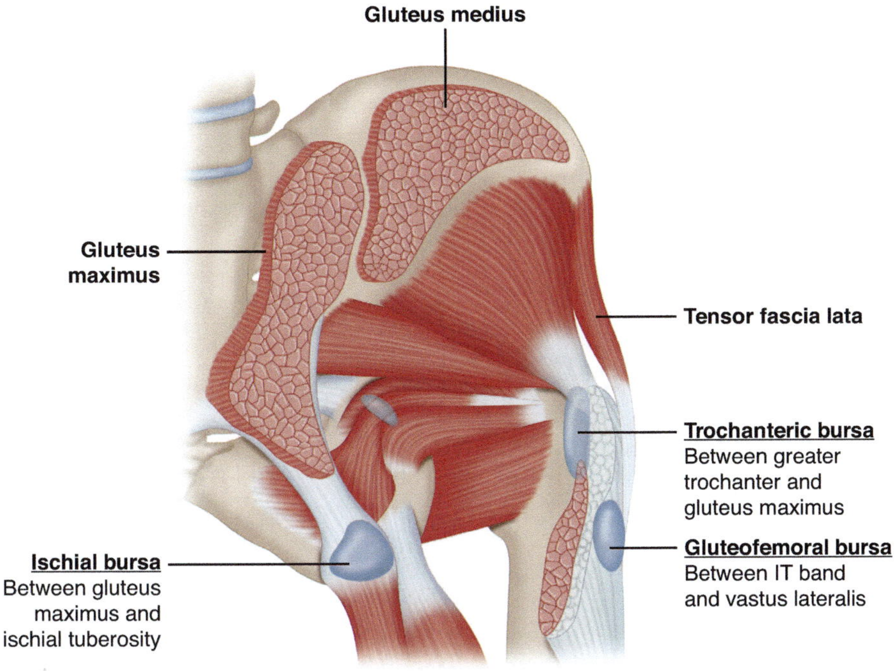

Fig. 4 Anatomy of posterior hip including the ischiogluteal and greater trochanteric bursae, as labeled. The gluteus maximus and medius muscles are retracted

Table 4 Required supplies for ischial bursa and proximal hamstring peritendinous injections [26, 27]

Syringe	5 mL
Needle	22–25 gauge 3.5 in.
Anesthetic	0.5% Ropivacaine 1–2% Lidocaine Lidocaine/bupivacaine combination: usually 1:1 ratio
Corticosteroid	Triamcinolone 20–40 mg (t1/2 life: 12–36 h), betamethasone 6 mg (t1/2 life: 36–72 h), methylprednisolone 40 mg (t1/2 life: 12–36 h)

Ultrasound Technique

1. **Patient position**: Prone or decubitus (side lying) position with the affected side up and hips and knees flexed.
2. **Transducer type**: Curvilinear array.
3. **Probe placement**: Position the probe in a transverse plane over the ischial tuberosity. Visualize for any fluid in the ischiogluteal bursa. Care should be taken to identify and avoid the sciatic nerve where it travels laterally over the quadratus femoris.

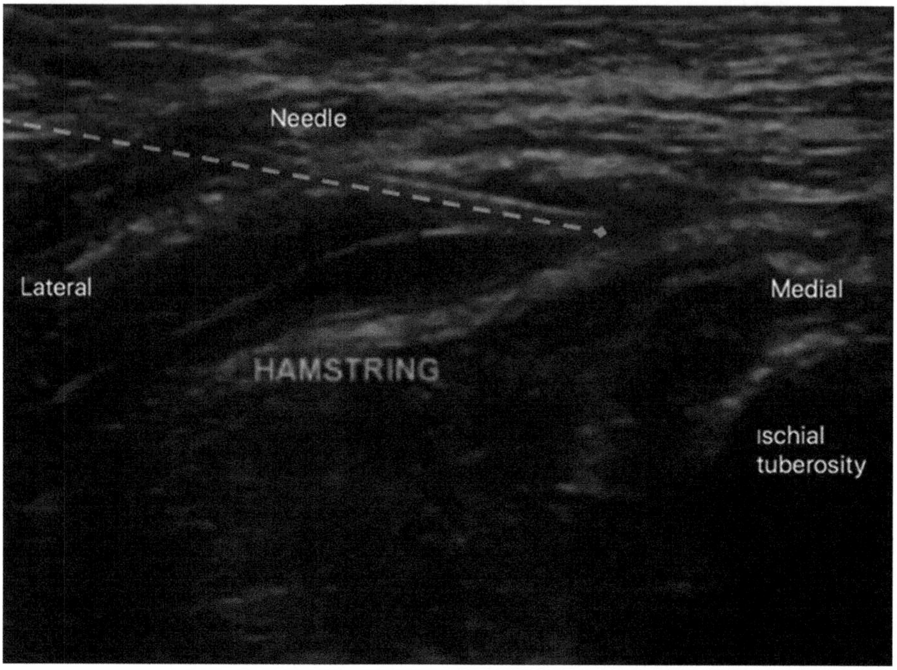

Fig. 5 Ischial tuberosity and surrounding structures. Ultrasonogram, as labeled. Ensure that the sciatic nerve is not within the needle trajectory prior to injecting. Dashed line—needle trajectory

4. **In plane**: The injection is performed in plane to visualize the needle trajectory and confirm placement within the bursa.
5. **Needle placement**: The needle should be inserted in plane (longitudinal to the transducer) using a lateral to medial or distal to proximal anatomical approach. The needle angle should be adjusted to ensure its trajectory towards the target, and then advanced until the bursa is reached (Fig. 5).

3 Iliopsoas Bursa Injections

Relatively common among athletes that perform activities with repetitive hip flexion and external rotation, iliopsoas bursitis is characterized by deep groin pain and tenderness to palpation over the iliopsoas muscle. In rare cases, a palpable mass over the femoral triangle or compressive symptoms may be present [17, 18]. Pain is exacerbated by hip extension and resisted hip flexion. Dynamic ultrasound may be used to visualize snapping of the iliopsoas tendons over adjacent structures (coxa saltans), and to evaluate for fluid in the iliopsoas bursa [19]. Non-surgical treatment includes NSAIDs and physical therapy. Ultrasound guided corticosteroid injections

Table 5 Diagnostic features of iliopsoas bursitis [18, 19]

A. Pain over the anterior groin, with or without palpable mass
B. Positive Stinchfield or Thomas test
C. Weakness of hip external rotation when the hip is in flexion
D. Positive snapping maneuver (palpable or audible snap as a flexed, abducted, and externally rotated hip is passively brought into extension)
E. Symptoms are not better accounted for by an alternative diagnosis

into the iliopsoas bursa can be used to reduce inflammation and pain and improve tolerance of physical therapy.

Indications and Contraindications

Iliopsoas bursitis may be associated with rheumatoid arthritis, acute trauma, overuse injuries, or after hip replacement. An anteriorly located prosthetic acetabular cup can create friction on the adjacent iliopsoas tendon [20]. Overuse injuries result from repetitive hip flexion with external rotation and may be caused by snapping of the iliopsoas muscle over the iliacus muscle, anterior inferior iliac spine, iliopectineal eminence, or bony ridge of the lesser trochanter [18, 20]. Infection, hardware complications, and lumbar pathology must be excluded prior to injection [20]. Corticosteroid injection may provide pain relief even in the absence of snapping tendinopathy or evidence of bursitis on ultrasound in patients clinically suspected of having iliopsoas bursitis, and are indicated for patients who have failed conservative measures [19]. Injections may provide both diagnostic and therapeutic roles prior to consideration of iliopsoas tenotomy or hip revision surgery [20] (Table 5).

Contraindications are the same as for injections described above in this chapter.

Clinical Anatomy

The tendons of the psoas and iliacus muscles merge into the iliopsoas tendon, which travels anteriorly over the hip capsule and pelvic brim before inserting anteromedially on the lesser trochanter of the femur. The iliopsoas muscle acts as a hip flexor and femur external rotator. Located between the musculotendinous junction of the iliopsoas muscle and the pelvic brim in the anterior hip, the iliopsoas bursa is the largest bursa in the body [18]. In about 14% of adults, the bursa is in continuity with the hip joint capsule [21]. The femoral neurovascular bundle lies just medial and superficial to the iliopsoas muscle and tendon, and care should be taken to avoid this structure during injections [17] (Fig. 6).

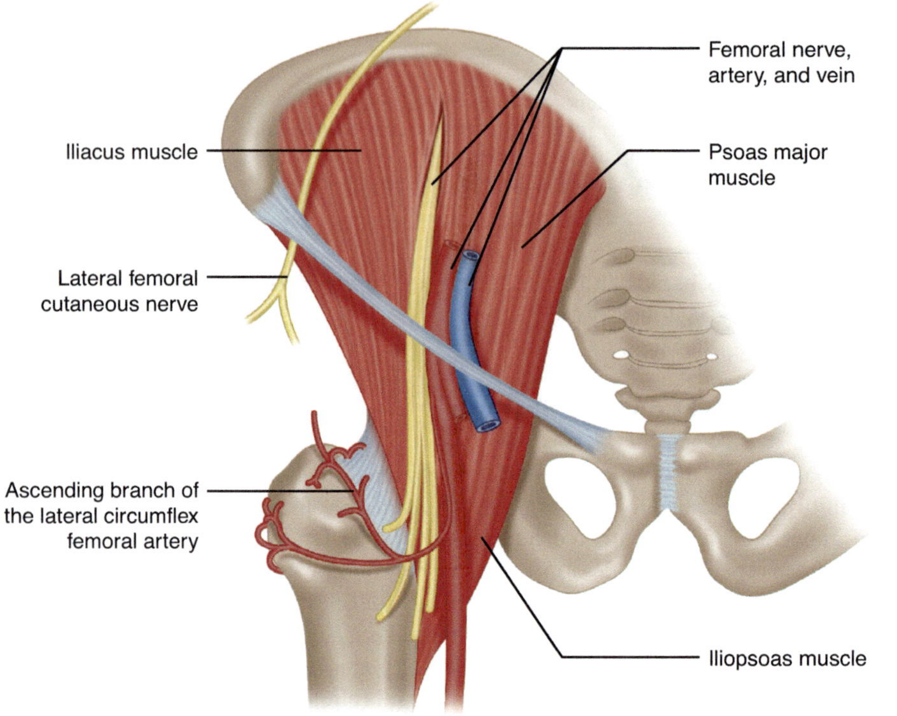

Fig. 6 Anatomy of the iliopsoas muscle and underlying bursa, as labeled. Note the proximity to the femoral neurovascular bundle

Table 6 Required supplies for iliopsoas bursa injections [26, 27]

Syringe	5 or 10 mL
Needle	25, 27 gauge 3.5 in.
Anesthetic	0.5% Ropivicaine 1–2% Lidocaine Lidocaine/bupivacaine combination: usually 1:1 ratio
Corticosteroid	Triamcinolone 20–40 mg (t1/2 life: 12–36 h), betamethasone 6 mg (t1/2 life: 36–72 h), methylprednisolone 40 mg (t1/2 life: 12–36 h)

Equipment and Supplies

Iliopsoas bursa and peritendinous injections are easily performed at the bedside. Typically, a small syringe with a 25 gauge, 3.5 in. needle is used for injection, while a 18–20 gauge needle can be used for aspiration. For injections, 3–5 mL of a local anesthetic solution (usually lidocaine or bupivacaine) can be mixed with 1 mL of corticosteroid. Ultrasound guidance can improve accuracy and ensure avoidance of the femoral vessels (Table 6).

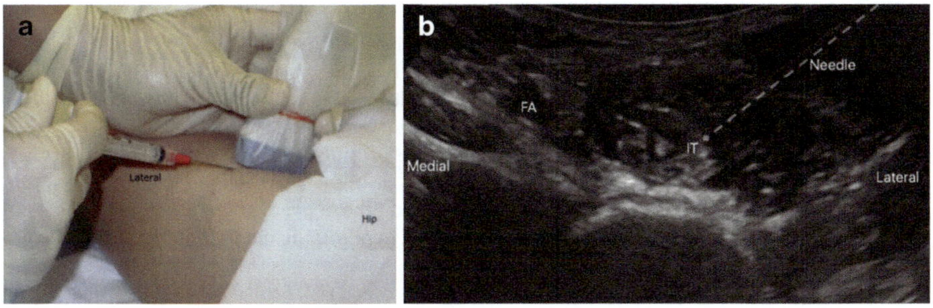

Fig. 7 (**a**) And and needle orientation for axial iliopsoas bursa injection. The needle is introduced in plane with the transducer from lateral to medial to avoid the femoral neurovascular bundle. (**b**) Axial (short axis) view of the iliopsoas tendon and surrounding structures. Ultrasonogram, as labeled. Visualize and avoid the femoral artery (FA) prior to injecting. *IT* iliopsoas tendon, dashed line—needle trajectory

Iliopsoas Bursa Injection Ultrasound Technique

Due to its deep position and proximity to the femoral vessels, ultrasound guidance is recommended for iliopsoas bursa injections.

1. **Patient position**: Supine
2. **Transducer type**: Curvilinear array
3. **Probe placement**: Position the probe in a transverse plane over the inguinal ligament just lateral to the femoral triangle. Visualize for any fluid in the bursa. Care should be taken to identify and avoid the femoral vessels and nerve where they lie medially.
4. **In plane**: The injection is performed in plane to visualize the needle trajectory and confirm placement within the bursa.
5. **Needle placement**: The needle should be inserted in plane (longitudinal to the transducer) using a lateral to medial anatomical approach (Fig. 7).

Potential Complications and Adverse Effects

Although generally well tolerated by patients, occasional complications can occur when performing peri-articular hip injections. Aside from pain and minor medication side effects, adverse events are relatively rare, and include local bleeding and infection. Medication side effects include facial flushing (up to 15%), temporary elevation of blood glucose, osteonecrosis of nearby bone, and chondrotoxicity with repeat injections (0.7–3%) [22–25].

Contraindications include allergy to corticosteroids or local anesthetics, active infection over overlying skin or soft tissues, bacteremia, and septic arthritis. Relative

Table 7 Additional potential complications and adverse effects

– Pressure should be applied to prevent hematoma production in patients with bleeding disorders or on anticoagulation. Risk of significant bleeding is low
– Patient should be warned of the risk of lipodystrophy or skin atrophy (1.5–40%), or hypopigmentation (1.3–4%) that may occur around the injection site [25]
– Patients should be counseled that there is a small risk of infection, including septic arthritis (0.01–0.03%) [22]
– Local anesthetics have been shown to have dose and time dependent chondrotoxic effects [23]. Ropivacaine 0.5% has been shown to be less chondrotoxic than 1% lidocaine or 0.5% bupivacaine [24]
– Patients receiving frequent corticosteroid injections are at risk for developing Cushing syndrome or adrenal insufficiency [29]. Injections should not be performed more frequently than every 6 weeks or more than three times per year. In addition, providers should ask about other exogenous steroid use prior to injections
– Corticosteroid side effects include temporary facial flushing (up to 15%), temporary elevation of blood glucose, osteonecrosis of nearby bone, and chondrotoxicity with repeat injections (0.7–3%) [22]. Corticosteroids have rarely been associated with tendon degeneration and rupture [25]

Clinical and Technical Pearls

- Peri-articular hip injections can be used for the diagnosis and treatment of common musculoskeletal conditions. Patient should be informed of the risks of repeated corticosteroid injections, including a small risk of chondrotoxicity and tendon rupture.
- To minimize pain and intolerance, anesthetize the dermis and subcutaneous needle track with a 27 gauge needle and 2–3 mL of local anesthetic prior to the injection. Among local anesthetics, 0.5% ropivacaine has been shown to be less chondrotoxic than other agents including lidocaine and bupivacaine.
- Sterile technique, including sterile ultrasound probe cover, ultrasound gel, gloves, and setup, is recommended to minimize infection risk.
- Avoid injecting medications in tendons, as this may lead to tendon compromise. Inject peri-tendinously when treating tendinopathies.
- Care should be taken to avoid surrounding neurovascular structures, especially the sciatic nerve with ischial tuberosity injections and the femoral neurovascular bundle with iliopsoas injections. Ultrasound can assist the clinician in visualizing and avoiding these structures.

contraindications include uncontrolled diabetes mellitus, immunocompromised patients, corticosteroid injection within the last 6 weeks, or greater than 3 corticosteroid injections within the last 12 months [22, 25].

Other important complications and relevant considerations are presented in Table 7.

References

1. Segal N, Felson D, Torner J, Zhu Y, Curtis J, Niu J, et al. Greater trochanteric pain syndrome. Arch Phys Med Rehabil. 2017;42(1):15–31.
2. Redmond J, Chen A, Domb B. Greater trochanteric pain syndrome. J Am Acad Orthop Surg. 2016;24(4):231–40.
3. Reid D. The management of greater trochanteric pain syndrome: a systematic literature review. J Orthop. 2016;13(1):15–28. https://doi.org/10.1016/j.jor.2015.12.006.
4. Barratt PA, Brookes N, Newson A. Conservative treatments for greater trochanteric pain syndrome: a systematic review. Br J Sports Med. 2017;51:97–104.
5. Williams BS, Cohen SP. Greater trochanteric pain syndrome : a review of anatomy , diagnosis and treatment. Anesth Analg. 2009;108(5):1662–70.
6. Dunn T, Heller C, McCarthy S, Dos Remedios C. Anatomical study of the "trochanteric bursa". Clin Anat. 2003;16(3):233–40.
7. Rea P. Lower limb nerve supply. In: Essential clinically applied anatomy of the peripheral nervous system in the limbs. Glaskow: Elsevier; 2015.
8. Cardone DA, Tallia AF, Johnson RW. Diagnostic and therapeutic injection of the hip and knee. Am Fam Physician. 2003;67(10):2147–52.
9. Kim S, Shin M, Kim K, Ahn J, Cho K, Chang J, et al. Imaging features of ischial bursitis with an emphasis on ultrasonography. Skeletal Radiol. 2002;31(11):631–6.
10. Zissen MH, Wallace G, Stevens KJ, Fredericson M, Beaulieu CF, Mh Z, et al. High hamstring tendinopathy: MRI and ultrasound imaging and therapeutic efficacy of percutaneous corticosteroid injection. AJR Am J Roentgenol. 2010;195:993–8.
11. Chu SK, Rho ME. Hamstring injuries in the athlete: diagnosis, treatment, and return to play. Curr Sports Med Rep. 2016;15(3):184.
12. Nicholson LT, Disegna S, Newman JS, Miller SL. Fluoroscopically guided peritendinous corticosteroid injection for proximal hamstring tendinopathy a retrospective review. Orthop J Sports Med. 2014;2:1–5.
13. Wetzel R, Patel R, Terry M. Platelet-rich plasma as an effective treatment for proximal hamstring injuries. Orthopedics. 2013;36(1):64–70.
14. Hitora T, Kawaguchi Y, Mori M, Imaizumi Y, Akisue T, Sasaki K, et al. Ischiogluteal bursitis: a report of three cases with MR findings. Rheumatol Int. 2009;29:455–8.
15. Wisniewski SJ, Hurdle M, Erickson JM, Finnoff JT, Smith J. Ultrasound-guided ischial bursa injection: technique and positioning considerations. PM&R. 2014;6(1):56–60. https://doi.org/10.1016/j.pmrj.2013.08.603.
16. Ripani M, Continenza M, Cacchio A, Barile A, Parisi A, De Paulis F. The ischiatic region: normal and MRI anatomy. Sport Inj Rehabil. 2006;46:468–75.
17. Toohey AK, Lasalle TL, Martinez S, Polisson R. Iliopsoas bursitis: clinical features, radiographic disease associations. Semin Arthritis Rheum. 1990;20(1):41–7.
18. Johnston C, Wiley P, Lindsay D, Wiseman D. Iliopsoas bursitis and tendinitis. Sports Med. 1998;25(4):271–83.
19. Blankenbaker DG, De Smet AA, Keene JS. Sonography of the iliopsoas tendon and injection of the iliopsoas bursa for diagnosis and management of the painful snapping hip. Skeletal Radiol. 2006;35:565–71.
20. Nguyen R, Roh E. Hip injections. In: Guide to musculoskeletal injections with ultrasound. Cham: Springer; 2016. p. 75–90.
21. Chandler S. The iliopsoas bursa in man. Anat Rec. 1934;58(3):235–40.
22. MacMahon P, Eustance S, Kavanagh E. Injectable corticosteroid and local anesthetic preparations: a review for radiologists. Radiology. 2009;252(3):647.
23. Kreuz P, Steinwachs M, Angele P. Single-dose local anesthetics exhibit a type-, dose-, and time-dependent chondrotoxic effect on chondrocytes and cartilage: a systematic review of the current literature. Knee Surg Sports Traumatol Arthrosc. 2018;26(3):819–30.

24. Jayaram P, Kennedy DJ, Yeh P, Dragoo J. Chondrotoxic effects of local anesthetics on human knee articular cartilage: a systematic review. PM&R. 2019;11(4):379–400.
25. Brinks A, Koes BW, Volkers ACW, Verhaar JAN, Bierma-zeinstra SMA. Adverse effects of extra-articular corticosteroid injections: a systematic review. BMC Musculoskelet Disord. 2010;11:206.
26. Best CA, Kin HBA, Bhsc AAB, Best TJ, Hamilton DA, Best CA, et al. Buffered lidocaine and bupivacaine mixture—the ideal local anesthetic solution? Plast Surg. 2015;23(2):87–90.
27. Becker DE. Basic and clinical pharmacology of glucocorticosteroids. Anesth Prog. 2013;3006(13):25–32.
28. Sherry M. Evaluation and treatment of acute hamstring strains and related injuries. Sport Phys Ther. 2012;4(2):107–14.
29. Leary J, Swislocki A. Case report hypothalamic–pituitary–adrenal suppression and iatrogenic Cushing's syndrome as a complication of epidural steroid injections. Case Rep Endocrinol. 2013;2013:617042.

Further Reading

Jacobson JA. Hip and thigh ultrasound. In: Fundamentals of musculoskeletal ultrasound. 3rd ed. Amsterdam: Elsevier; 2018. p. 223–83.

Malanga G, Mautner K. Pelvis. In: Altas of ultrasound-guided musculoskeletal injections. 1st ed. New York: McGraw Hill; 2014. p. 204–27.

Nguyen R, Roh E. Hip injections. In: Guide to musculoskeletal injections with ultrasound. Cham: Springer; 2016. p. 75–90.

Adductor Canal Block

Priyanka Singla and Paul C. DeMarco

Essential Concepts

- Saphenous nerve block in the adductor canal is an effective technique to provide analgesia for knee, foot and ankle surgeries. It also can be used for acute or chronic pain in the saphenous nerve distribution.
- It helps in early mobilization if used in the perioperative period. A major advantage of this block over other techniques that involve femoral nerve blockade is sparing motor blockade and potentially preserving quadriceps strength, thus allowing early active involvement in physical therapy and minimizing the risk of falls from imbalance postoperatively.
- Adductor canal block is technically easy to perform with ultrasound at the bedside and well-tolerated, and has relatively few side effects.

1 Saphenous Nerve Block in the Adductor Canal

Overview

The saphenous nerve (SN) provides sensory innervation to the medial aspect of the leg below the knee. This nerve can be blocked at multiple locations in the leg to provide effective analgesia for knee, lower leg, and foot/ankle surgeries. Various approaches to block this nerve above the knee include perifemoral, subsartorial, and transsartorial [1–4]. The most common and effective approach involves blocking the saphenous nerve in the adductor canal (AC). Because it is a small sensory nerve,

P. Singla · P. C. DeMarco (✉)
Department of Anesthesiology, University of Virginia, Charlottesville, VA, USA
e-mail: ps7ey@virginia.edu; pd8h@virginia.edu

D. Souza et al. (eds.), *Bedside Pain Management Interventions*,
https://doi.org/10.1007/978-3-031-11188-4_64

the SN block can be technically challenging to block well without the use of ultrasound. The AC (SN) block along with a sciatic nerve block is most commonly used to provide analgesia and surgical anesthesia for knee surgeries, surgeries on the leg such as saphenous vein stripping and foot/ankle procedures.

Indications and Contraindications

AC block is used to provide analgesia as well as anesthesia for lower extremity surgery. It also can be used for acute or chronic pain of various etiologies in the saphenous nerve distribution (Table 1). Contraindications include local or systemic infection, patient refusal, intolerance or allergy to injectate or its components. Shared decision making is required for patients with coagulopathy, including iatrogenic, and platelet dysfunction.

Clinical Anatomy

The AC is an intermuscular aponeurotic tunnel from the apex of the femoral triangle to an opening in the adductor magnus through which the femoral vessels reach the popliteal fossa [5, 6].

The boundaries of the AC include sartorius muscle anteriorly, vastus medialis muscle anterolaterally and adductor longus muscle posteromedially [5]. Contents of AC include the femoral vessels, SN, and the nerve to the vastus medialis muscle [7]. The obturator nerve may enter the distal part of the AC [7]. The SN originates from the posterior division of the femoral nerve in the femoral triangle as a sensory branch and traverses lateral to the femoral artery in the proximal AC [5, 8]. As it continues distally, the SN assumes a position anterior and then medial to the femoral artery [8]. The SN provides sensory innervation to the medial side of the leg down to the foot along with infrapatellar branches to the knee joint [9] (Fig. 1).

Table 1 Indications and contraindications to the adductor canal block

Procedure	Indications	Techniques	Contraindications
Adductor canal block	Analgesia and anesthesia for – Knee surgeries such as total knee arthroplasty – Foot and ankle surgeries – Saphenous vein stripping – Acute or chronic pain in the saphenous nerve distribution of other etiologies Diagnosis and treatment of saphenous nerve neuralgia and saphenous nerve entrapment [4]	Landmark technique Ultrasound-guided	Patient refusal Systemic or local infection Coagulopathy is a relative contraindication

Equipment and Supplies

The adductor canal block is an easy bedside procedure, most commonly done with the help of an linear (8–14 MHz) ultrasound. Typically, a small needle 25–30 gauge is used to anesthetize the skin and the tract of the block needle with 1–2% lidocaine. This is followed by insertion of the peripheral block needle under ultrasound guidance. Anesthetic solution usually consists of the local anesthetic bupivacaine or ropivacaine, with or without a corticosteroid (Table 2).

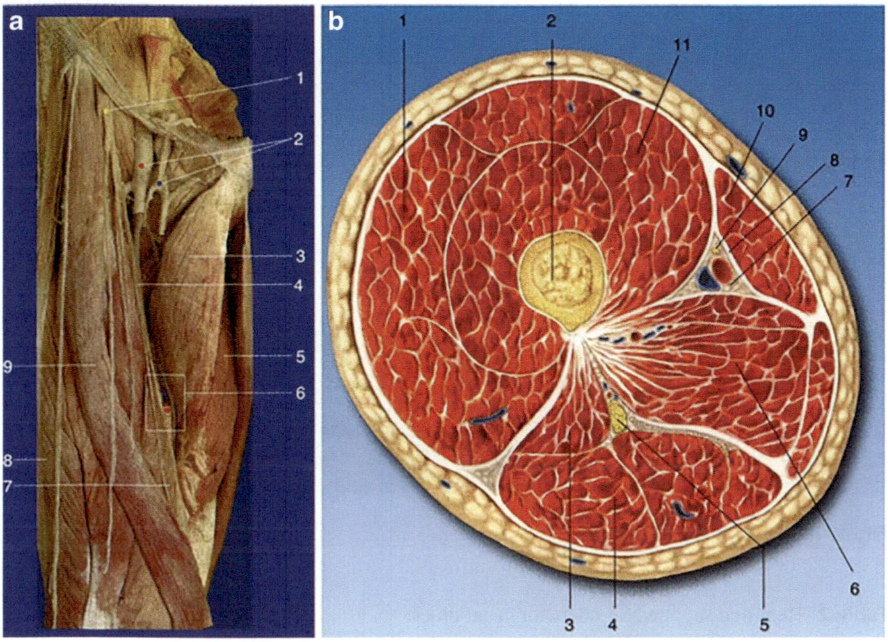

Fig. 1 Clinical anatomy, as labeled. (**a**) Dissection of front of thigh and adductor region. (*1*) Femoral nerve, (*2*) femoral artery and vein, (*3*) adductor longus muscle, (*4*) saphenous nerve, (*5*) adductor magnus muscle, (*6*) vastoadductor membrane and adductor canal with saphenous nerve and femoral artery and vein, (*7*) vastus medialis muscle, (*8*) vastus lateralis muscle, (*9*) sartorius muscle (With permission from Danilo Jankovic). (**b**) Cross-sectional depiction of the thigh. (*1*) Vastus lateralis muscle, (*2*) femur, (*3*) biceps femoris (short head), (*4*) biceps femoris (long head), (*5*) sciatic nerve, (*6*) adductor muscles, (*7*) femoral artery-nerve, (*8*) vastoadductor membrane, (*9*) saphenous nerve, (*10*) sartorius muscle, (*11*) vastus medialis muscle. (**c**) Depiction of medial thigh. (*1*) Lateral femoral cutaneous nerve, (*2*) femoral nerve, (*3*) saphenous nerve, (*4*) obturator nerve, (*5*) psoas major muscle, (*6*) vastus medialis muscle, (*7*) adductor longus muscle. (**d**) Medial view of cadaveric thigh. (*1*) Saphenous nerve (infrapatellar branch), (*2*) superior medial and inferior medial genicular arteries. (Reprinted with permission from Ghassemi J., Gray A.T. (2015) The Adductor Canal Block. In: Regional Nerve Blocks in Anesthesia and Pain Therapy. Springer, Cham. https://doi.org/10.1007/978-3-319-05131-4_63)

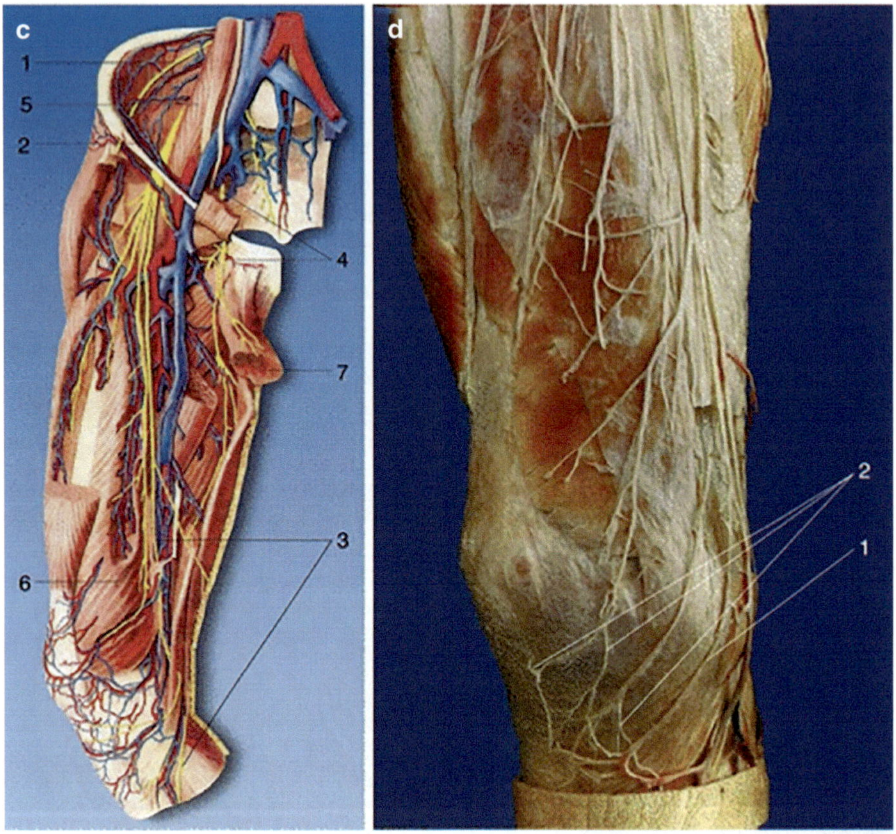

Fig. 1 (continued)

Table 2 Required supplies for adductor canal block

Syringe	10, 20 or 30 mL
Needle	80 mm 20–25 G echogenic peripheral block needle
Ultrasound	Linear transducer, sterile probe cover, sterile acoustic coupling gel
Anesthetic	0.25–0.5% Bupivacaine 0.2–0.5% Ropivacaine
Corticosteroid	Dexamethasone 4 mg

Adductor Canal Block, Landmark Technique

The landmark technique can be done blind as well as with the use of a peripheral nerve stimulator. The patient is placed in the supine position with the leg extended and elevated 5–10 cm [1]. The sartorius muscle is palpated just above the medial side of the patella [1]. The insulated needle is inserted 3–4 cm superior and 6–8 cm posterior to the superomedial border of the patella [1]. The needle is directed slightly posteriorly and caudally at an angle of 45° to a depth of 3–5 cm until a paresthesia, referred to the medial malleolus, is elicited with a nerve stimulator at 0.6 mA or less

(2-Hz frequency and 0.1-ms duration) [1]. The landmark technique can be challenging as it is not easy to palpate the sartorius muscle, especially in obese patients [5].

Ultrasound Technique

Ultrasound (US) guidance has shown to improve the success rate [9]. The patient is placed supine with the ipsilateral leg externally rotated and slightly abducted. After disinfecting the skin, a ultrasound probe can be placed over the junction of the middle and distal third of the anteromedial thigh which will enable visualization of the cross sectional view of the AC (Figs. 2 and 3).

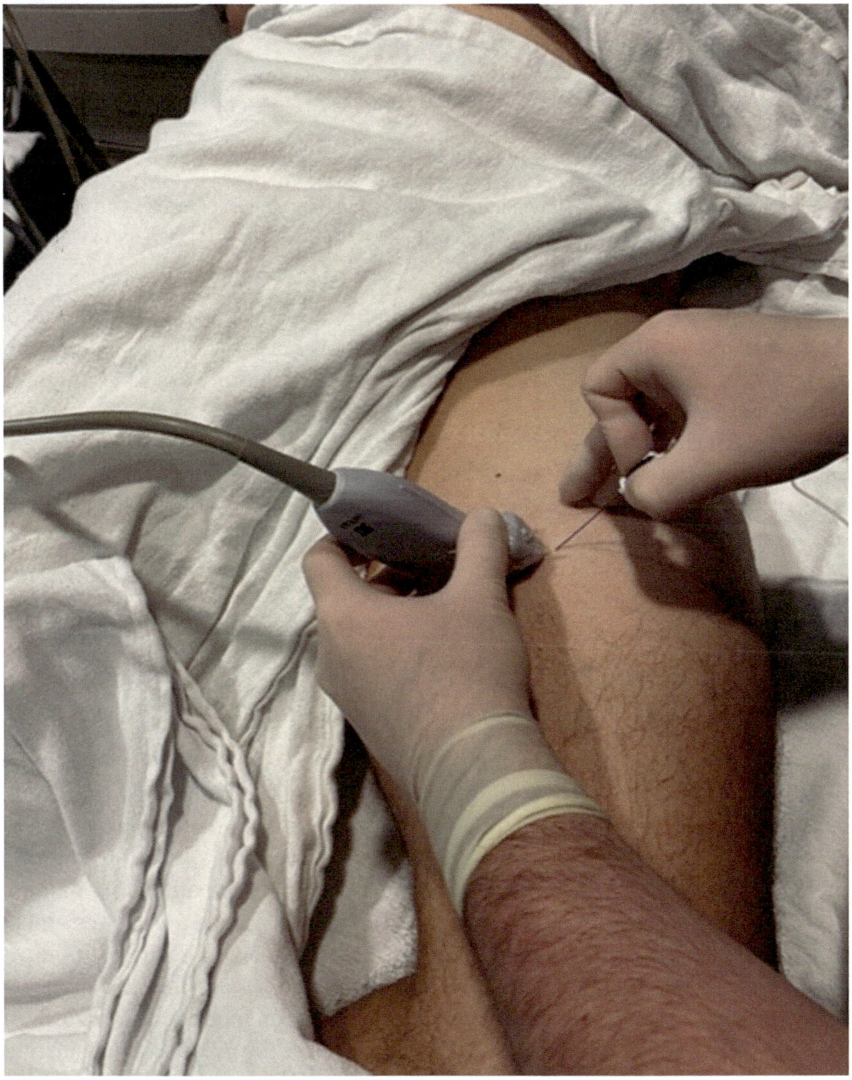

Fig. 2 Probe position (NYSORA.com)

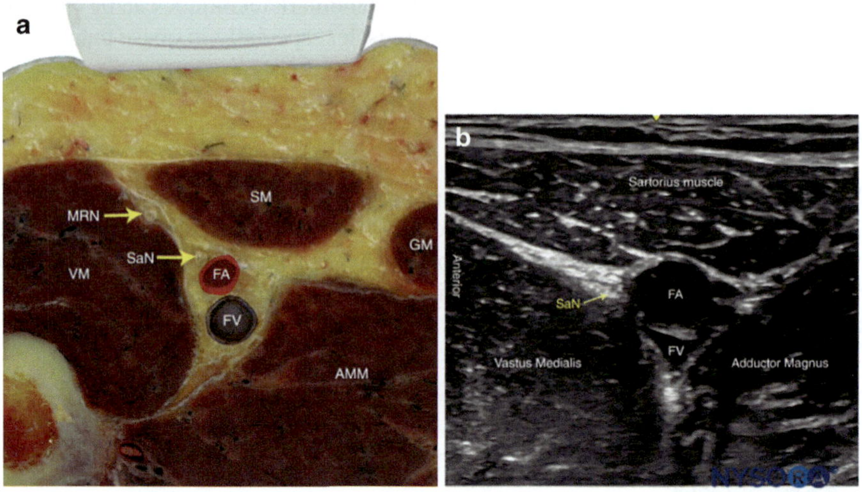

Fig. 3 Cross-sectional schematics (**a**) and ultrasound image (**b**) of the adductor canal. Target, and structures to avoid, as labeled. Saphenous nerve (SaN), sartorius muscle (SM), vastus medialis muscle (VM), femoral artery (FA), femoral vein (FV), adductor magnus muscles (AMM), gracilis muscle (GM), medial retinaclar nerve (MRN). Ultrasonogram, as labeled (NYSORA.com)

The proximal beginning of the AC is identified at the point where the medial border of the sartorius muscle intersects the lateral border of the adductor longus muscle. The distal end of the AC is identified by the femoral vessels exiting at the adductor hiatus [6].

The superficial femoral artery (SFA) is identified with color flow Doppler. After a local skin wheel with lidocaine, the block needle is inserted in plane in a lateral to medial orientation and advanced towards the SFA until the needle tip is just anterior to the artery and deep to the sartorius muscle. Spread of local anesthetic (LA) after careful aspiration should be noticed around the artery [9] (Figs. 4 and 5).

Potential Complications and Adverse Effects

AC block complications are rare. However, the clinician performing the procedure should be aware of the potential complications. Local anesthetic systemic toxicity (LAST) is a potential complication of any regional nerve block. Lower extremity blocks are often done in combination so the resultant cumulative dose of LA can predispose to LAST [8]. Symptoms can be delayed due to slow absorption of the drug [8]. It is important to monitor for metallic taste in the mouth, perioral tingling and numbness, and ringing in the ears. LAST eventually leads to seizures and cardiovascular collapse. Perioperative neurologic symptoms can occur with intrafascicular injection [8]. Particular attention should be paid to paresthesia and injection pressures. There can be prolonged saphenous distribution numbness or paresthesias (complete or patchy in nature). As with any procedure involving needles, there is a risk of bleeding and infection.

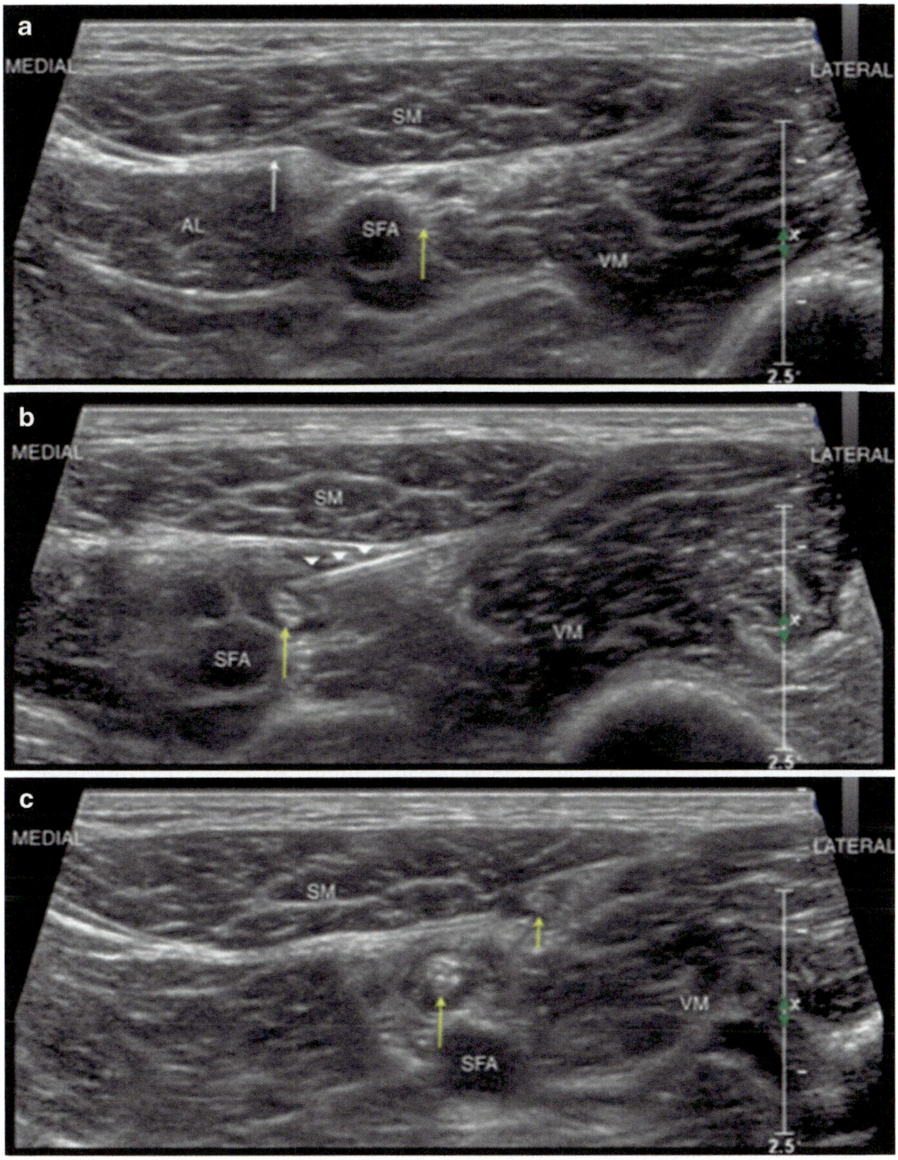

Fig. 4 Ultrasonogram, serial images demonstrating adductor canal block, as labeled. Serial sonograms demonstrating adductor canal block. Panel (**a**) baseline sonogram prior to injection (pre-scan). The saphenous nerve (*long yellow arrow*) lies deep to the sartorius muscle (*SM*) and hyperechoic vastoadductor membrane (*white arrow*) and is adjacent to the superficial femoral artery (*SFA*); adductor longus muscle (*AL*). Panel (**b**) in-plane approach to adductor canal block (the needle is shown with *white arrowheads*). Panel (**c**) distributions after injection tracked distally in the thigh demonstrating local anesthetic surrounding the saphenous (*long yellow arrow*) and infrapatellar (*short yellow arrow*) nerves. *VM* vastus medialis. (Reprinted with permission from Ghassemi J., Gray A.T. (2015) The Adductor Canal Block. In: Regional Nerve Blocks in Anesthesia and Pain Therapy. Springer, Cham. https://doi.org/10.1007/978-3-319-05131-4_63)

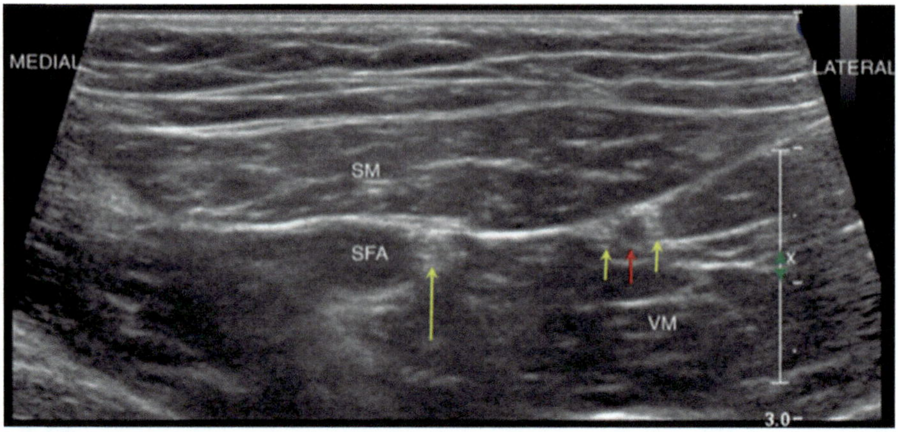

Fig. 5 Ultrasonogram, local anesthetic deposition around saphenous nerve. (Reprinted with permission from Ghassemi J., Gray A.T. (2015) The Adductor Canal Block. In: Regional Nerve Blocks in Anesthesia and Pain Therapy. Springer, Cham. https://doi.org/10.1007/978-3-319-05131-4_63)

Clinical and Technical Pearls

- Adductor canal block along with sciatic nerve block can provide adequate analgesia and anesthesia for acute and chronic pain or surgical procedures of the foot and ankle.
- Patients should be educated about possible motor weakness and mobilization with assistance after surgery.
- Avoid large volume of LA to prevent partial motor blockade from proximal spread to the femoral artery.
- The nerve block should be done with US guidance and as distal as possible in adductor canal.

References

1. Benzon HT, Sharma S, Calimaran A. Comparison of the different approaches to saphenous nerve block. Anesthesiology. 2005;102(3):633–8.
2. Mansour NY. Sub-sartorial saphenous nerve block with the aid of a nerve stimulator (letter). Reg Anesth. 1993;18(4):266–8.
3. Bouaziz H, Benhamou D, Narchi P. A new approach for saphenous nerve block (letter). Reg Anesth. 1996;21(5):490.
4. Van der Wal M, Lang SA, Yip RW. Transsartorial approach for saphenous nerve block. Can J Anaesth. 1993;40(6):542–6.
5. Manickam B, Perlas A, Duggan E, Brull R, Chan VW, Ramlogan R. Feasibility and efficacy of ultrasound-guided block of the saphenous nerve in the adductor canal. Reg Anesth Pain Med. 2009;34(6):578–80.

6. Wong WY, Bjorn S, Strid JM, Borglum J, Bendtsen TF. Defining the location of the adductor canal using ultrasound. Reg Anesth Pain Med. 2017;42(2):241–5.
7. Bendtsen TF, Moriggl B, Chan V, Pedersen EM, Borglum J. Defining adductor canal block. Reg Anesth Pain Med. 2014;39(3):253–4.
8. Tran DQ, Salinas FV, Benzon HT, Neal JM. Lower extremity regional anesthesia: essentials of our current understanding. Reg Anesth Pain Med. 2019;44(2):143–80.
9. Bendtsen TF, Lopez AM, Clark TB. Ultrasound-guided saphenous (subsartorius/adductor canal) nerve block. In: Hazdic's textbook of regional anesthesia and acute pain management. 2nd ed. New York: McGraw-Hill Education; 2017.

Further Reading

Migirov A, Vilella RC. Anatomy, abdomen and pelvis, adductor canal (subsartorial, hunter's canal). Treasure Island, FL: StatPearls; 2021.

Vora MU, Nicholas TA, Kassel CA, Grant SA. Adductor canal block for knee surgical procedures: review article. J Clin Anesth. 2016;35:295–303. https://doi.org/10.1016/j.jclinane.2016.08.021.

Sciatic Nerve Blockade

Drew Jensen and Ashley Shilling

Essential Concepts

- The sciatic nerve is the largest peripheral nerve in the body and provides the majority of sensation to the lower leg as well as providing innervation to the muscles of the lower leg and most of the hamstrings.
- Blockade of the sciatic nerve can be used to provide anesthesia for lower extremity procedures and analgesia for acute or chronic pain of the lower extremity.
- Many approaches to sciatic nerve blockade have been described, with the subgluteal and popliteal approaches being two common techniques to block the sciatic nerve.
- Whenever feasible, ultrasound guidance should be utilized when performing sciatic nerve blocks.

1 Overview

The sciatic nerve is the largest peripheral nerve in the body and originates from the sacral plexus, specifically the ventral rami of the L4–S3 nerve roots. Although called the sciatic nerve, this nerve is largely composed of two distinct nerves (the

D. Jensen
Columbia Anesthesia Group, Vancouver, WA, USA
e-mail: djensen@cagmed.com; dj6kr@virginia.edu

A. Shilling (✉)
Department of Anesthesiology, University of Virginia Health System, Charlottesville, VA, USA
e-mail: ABM5F@hscmail.mcc.virginia.edu; abm5f@virginia.edu

D. Souza et al. (eds.), *Bedside Pain Management Interventions*,
https://doi.org/10.1007/978-3-031-11188-4_65

tibial nerve and common peroneal nerve) which share a common connective tissue sheath from their point of origin in the sacral plexus until they diverge and separate at the level of the popliteal fossa [1]. The sciatic nerve provides most of the motor function and sensation to the lower leg. Given its long course in the posterior aspect of the thigh, many approaches to sciatic nerve blockade have been described [2]. Knowledge of anatomy and approaches to the sciatic nerve can make this nerve block useful for management of acute or chronic lower extremity pain.

2 Indications and Contraindications

Sciatic nerve blockade is useful when anesthesia or analgesia of the lower leg or posterior thigh is desired. Common indications include anesthesia and analgesia for foot and ankle surgery, lower leg surgery, lower extremity amputations, or as adjunct analgesia to knee surgery. Chronic lower extremity pain has also been treated with sciatic nerve blockade.

Absolute contraindications for performing a sciatic nerve block are similar for other peripheral nerve blocks, namely patient refusal and active infection at the nerve block site. Many relative contraindications exist and include coagulopathy, history of peripheral or central nervous system pathology, and aberrant or distorted anatomy. However, reports exist of successful sciatic nerve blockade in coagulopathic patients and in patients with nervous system disease [1]. Informed consent should be obtained, when possible, prior to performing a sciatic nerve block, with particular attention paid to discussion of the risks associated with peripheral nerve blockade, namely bleeding, infection, risk of peripheral nerve injury, and local anesthetic systemic toxicity.

3 Clinical Anatomy

The sciatic nerve exits the pelvis through the greater sciatic foramen and enters the gluteal region, inferior to the piriformis. In the gluteal region, it descends inferiorly towards the posterior compartment of the thigh, passing between the bony landmarks of the greater trochanter of the femur and the ischial tuberosity. Here, the sciatic nerve lies deep to the gluteus maximus muscle and superficial to the quadratus femoris and superior and inferior gemellus muscles (Fig. 1).

In the posterior thigh, the sciatic nerve continues inferiorly towards the popliteal fossa, traveling on the dorsal surface of the adductor magnus and ventral surface of the long head of the biceps femoris, which passes obliquely across the sciatic nerve in a medial to lateral fashion. Upon reaching the popliteal fossa, the sciatic nerve branches into the common peroneal nerve and tibial nerve. Although this bifurcation usually occurs above the popliteal fossa, anatomic variation does exist.

The sciatic nerve (via its terminal branches) provides sensation to the entirety of the foot, ankle, and leg below the knee, with the exception of the medial aspect of the lower leg and ankle which is supplied by the saphenous nerve, the terminal branch of

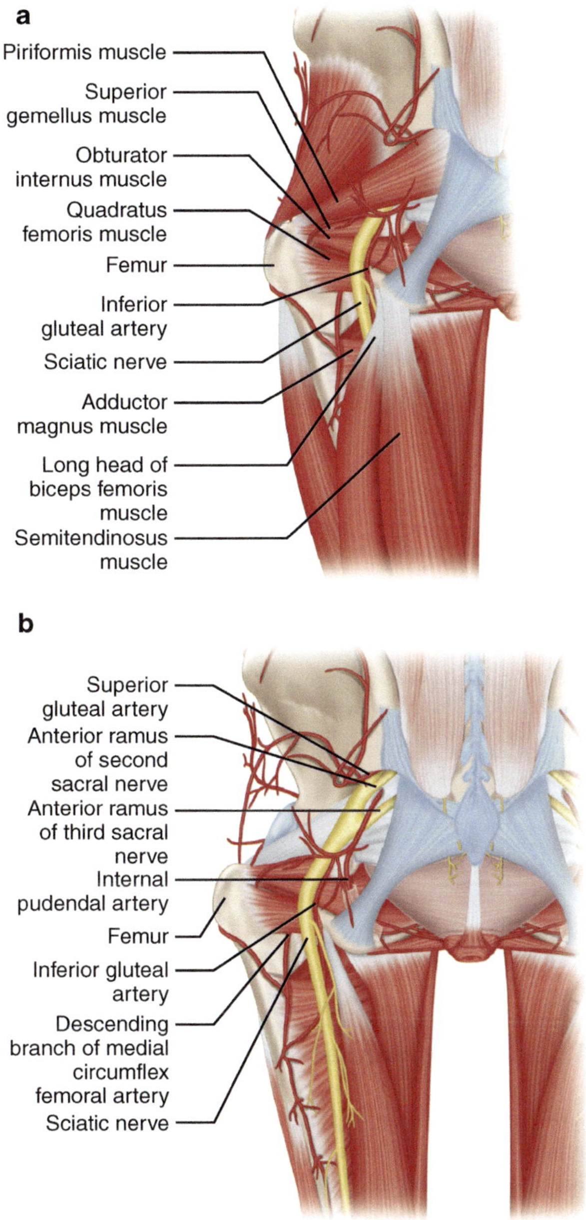

Fig. 1 Sciatic nerve anatomy. (**a**) Muscles in proximity to the sciatic nerve, as labeled. Gluteus maximus muscle overlying sciatic nerve is not shown. (**b**) Vascular structures around the sciatic nerve, as labeled

the femoral nerve. The terminal branches of the sciatic nerve also innervate the muscles of the foot and lower leg. The sciatic nerve itself innervates most of the hamstring muscles and gives off articular branches to both the knee and hip joint (Fig. 2). Of note, the skin of the posterior thigh is innervated by the posterior femoral cutaneous nerve and may not be anesthetized with proximal sciatic nerve blockade.

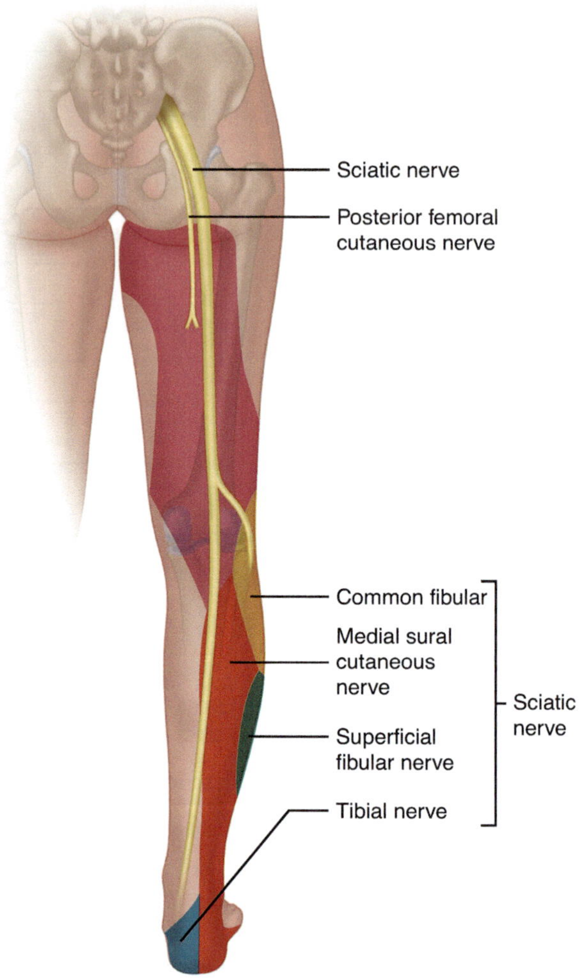

Fig. 2 Sensory innervation of the posterior lower extremity, as labeled

4 Equipment and Supplies

While performing any peripheral nerve block, standard monitors including ECG, pulse oximeter, and blood pressure cuff should be used to monitor the patient throughout the block. Mild sedation, with either a benzodiazepine or opioid, while not preferable, could potentially be employed for patient comfort. The choice of local anesthetic and additives will depend on the patient and indication for the procedure, but often 10–30 cc of 0.2–0.5% ropivacaine or bupivacaine is used. An 80–100 mm nerve block needle is usually sufficient to reach the sciatic nerve in most patients. A low-frequency curvilinear ultrasound probe is often used while performing proximal sciatic nerve blocks, while a high-frequency linear ultrasound probe is used for the popliteal approach to the sciatic nerve [3, 4]. Some practitioners utilize nerve stimulation in-lieu of, or in addition to, ultrasound guidance.

5 Subgluteal Sciatic Nerve Block, Ultrasound Technique

The subgluteal approach to sciatic nerve blockade is best accomplished with the patient in the lateral decubitus position, with the side to be blocked superior [3, 5]. The hip and knee are flexed (Fig. 3).

The greater trochanter and ischial tuberosity are palpated and can be marked with a marking pen, along with a line connecting these two palpated structures. A point 2–4 cm caudal to the midpoint of this line often serves as a good approximation for the location of the sciatic nerve and can guide initial ultrasound probe placement [3, 5–7]. The lateral and posterior proximal thigh and gluteal area is prepped in a standard sterile fashion. With a low-frequency curvilinear ultrasound

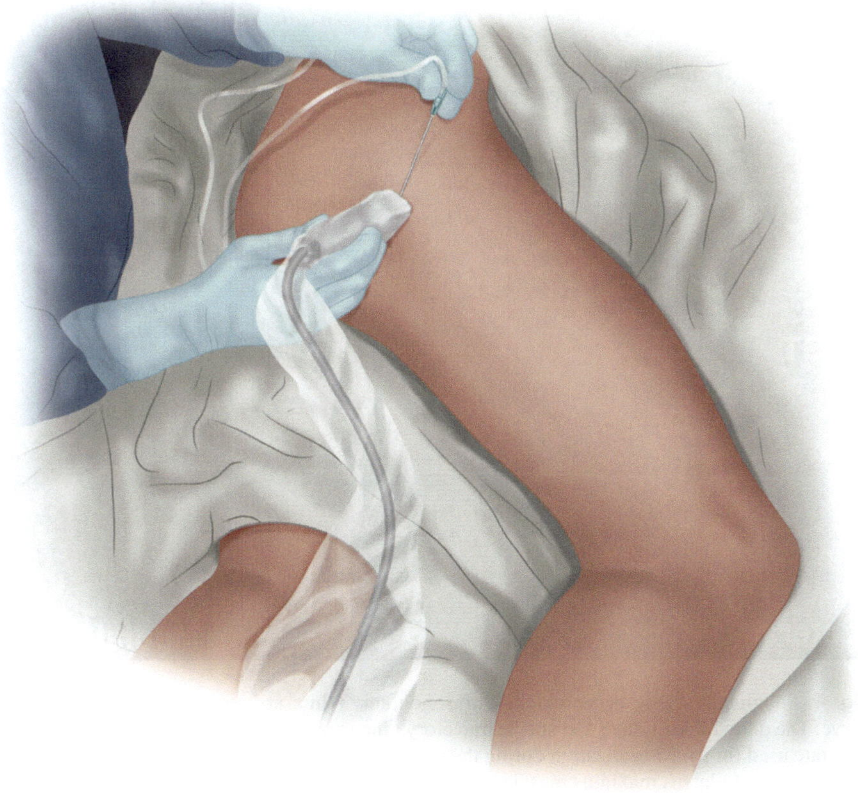

Fig. 3 Subgluteal sciatic nerve block. Ultrasound probe, needle, and patient positioning

probe in a transverse orientation on the posterior thigh, the sciatic nerve can be found deep to the gluteus maximus and superficial to the quadratus femoris (Fig. 4).

Identification of the ischial tuberosity and greater trochanter with the ultrasound probe can help with sciatic nerve identification. The nerve appears hyperechoic and often flat or triangle-shaped [3, 5]. Using an in-plane technique, the nerve block needle is passed from lateral to medial, with the goal of placing the tip of the nerve block needle adjacent to the sciatic nerve in the fascial plane between the gluteus maximus and the quadratus femoris. After aspiration to ensure the needle has not inadvertently been placed intravascularly, local anesthetic is injected. Depending on needle placement, the sciatic nerve may move superficial or deep to the tip of the needle, so additional needle repositioning may be necessary. Local anesthetic volumes of 10–20 cc are usually sufficient for adequate sciatic nerve blockade [3].

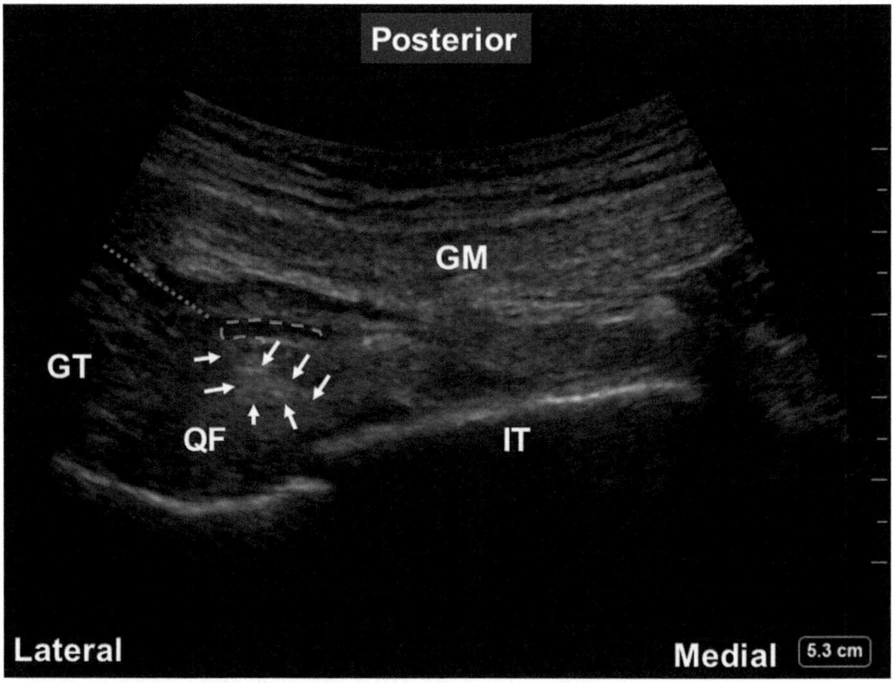

Fig. 4 Subgluteal sciatic nerve block. Ultrasonogram. White arrows point towards the sciatic nerve. The dotted line outlines the needle trajectory. The area within the blue dashed line indicates injectate used for hydrolocalization during the needle advancement towards the target. *GT* greater trochanter, *GM* gluteus maximus muscle, *IT* ischial tuberosity, *QF* quadratus femoris muscle

6 Subgluteal Sciatic Nerve Block, Landmark Technique

Although ultrasound guidance is commonly used during sciatic nerve blocks and has benefits, sciatic nerve blockade can be accomplished by a landmark technique as well [1, 6]. Nerve stimulation is used for nerve localization and may be added to ultrasound techniques if the nerve is unclear. As described above, the patient is placed in the lateral decubitus position with hips and knees flexed. The gluteal region is prepped in a sterile fashion. The point of needle insertion will be the point described above, namely 2–4 cm caudal to the midpoint of the line connecting the greater trochanter and ischial tuberosity [6]. Needle insertion is perpendicular to the skin. The current in the nerve stimulator is set to 1.0 mA. The needle is advanced through muscle towards the sciatic nerve. As the needle approaches the nerve, stimulation of the sciatic nerve via the nerve stimulator should elicit contraction of the hamstring muscles and motor response in the foot. The current through the nerve stimulator should be reduced until sciatic nerve stimulation is appreciated at 0.3–0.5 mA; stimulation at currents greater than this can lead to an increased risk of block failure while stimulation at currents less than this could indicate intraneural needle placement [6, 8]. After negative aspiration, local anesthetic can be incrementally injected. Sciatic nerve response should diminish after injection of local anesthetic.

7 Popliteal Sciatic Nerve Block, Ultrasound Technique

The popliteal approach to the sciatic nerve can be accomplished from a variety of patient positions, including supine, lateral, and prone [1, 2, 4, 5, 9]. The supine approach will be described. With the patient in the supine position, the lower leg is elevated on a leg rest. The lateral aspect of the of the lower thigh is prepped in a sterile fashion. A linear, high-frequency probe is placed in a transverse orientation at the popliteal crease (Fig. 5).

The sciatic nerve is identified just as it bifurcates into the tibial and common peroneal nerves, but with each nerve still enveloped in its common nerve sheath (Fig. 6).

This bifurcation often occurs several centimeters proximal to the popliteal crease between the semimembranosus and biceps femoris and posterolateral to the popliteal artery [1, 4, 5]. Under ultrasound guidance, the nerve block needle is introduced using an in-plane technique in a lateral to medial fashion towards the sciatic nerve. Ideal needle placement occurs with the tip of the needle within the common nerve sheath but between or outside the tibial and common peroneal nerves. Injection of local anesthetic (after aspiration) should demonstrate deposition of medication within the common nerve sheath and separation of the tibial and common peroneal nerves. Local anesthetic volumes of 15–30 cc are usually sufficient for adequate nerve coverage [1, 4].

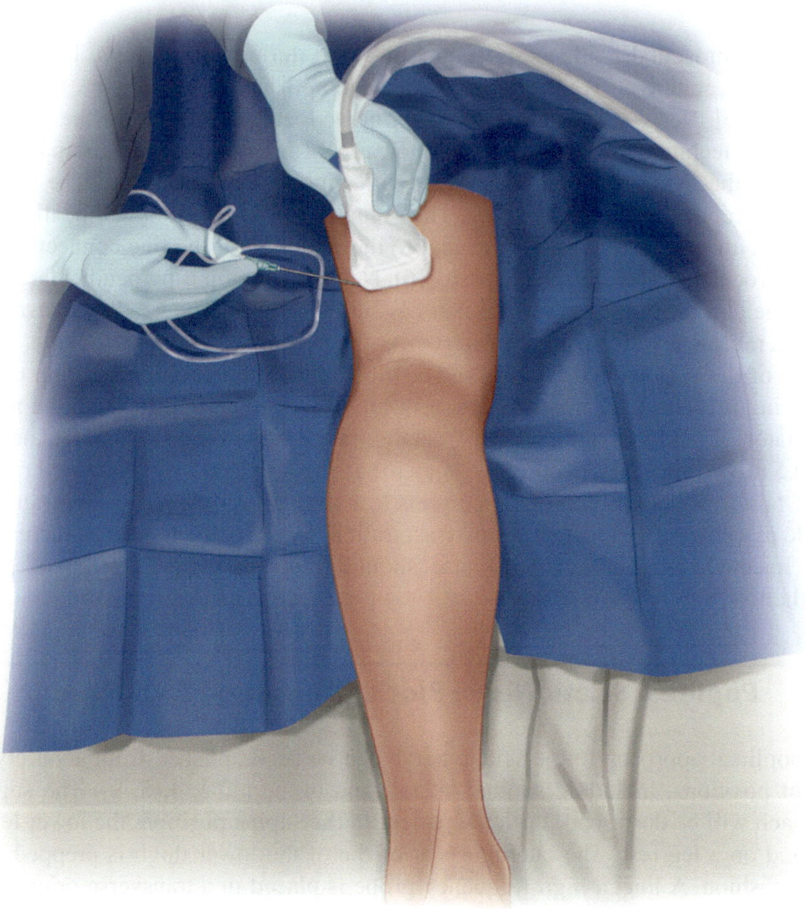

Fig. 5 Sciatic nerve block in the popliteal fossa. Ultrasound probe, needle, and patient positioning

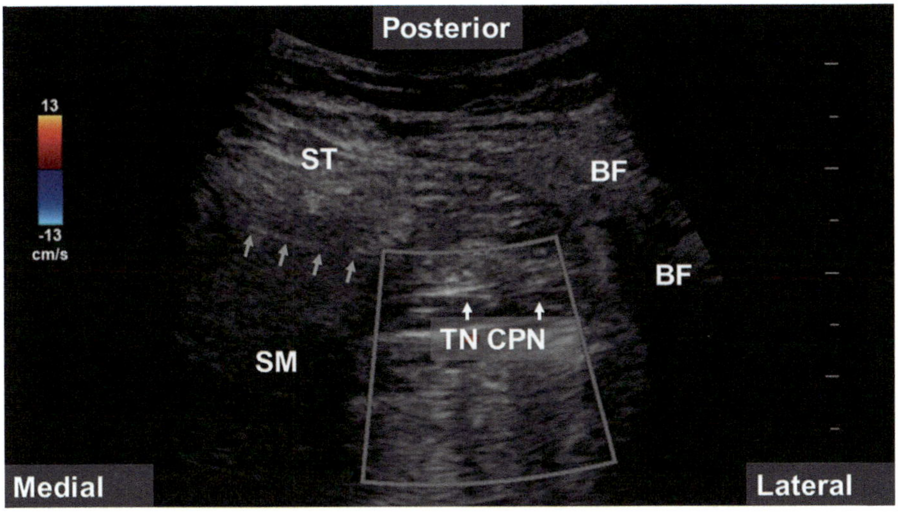

Fig. 6 Sciatic nerve block popliteal fossa. Ultrasonogram. Grey arrows point towards the needle. *TN* tibial nerve, *CPN* common peroneal nerve, *ST* semitendinosus muscle, *SM* semimembranosus muscle, *BM* biceps femoris muscle

8 Popliteal Sciatic Nerve Block, Landmark Technique

As mentioned previously, ultrasound is largely the standard of care when performing peripheral nerve blocks. However, the lateral approach to the sciatic nerve at the level of the popliteal fossa can be accomplished with a landmark-based technique with the assistance of nerve stimulation [9, 10]. The patient can be positioned similarly to the ultrasound-guided approach as described above. Palpation of the lateral thigh will demonstrate a plane between the vastus lateralis and biceps femoris muscles. The distal lateral thigh should be prepped in a sterile fashion. The initial point of needle insertion will be perpendicular to the skin in this muscular plane, approximately 8–10 cm proximal from the popliteal crease. As the needle is advanced, it should come into contact with the femur. At this point, the needle is withdrawn and redirected posteriorly behind the femur, at an angle approximately 30° from the perpendicular [10, 11]. Initial current on the nerve stimulator is set to 1.0 mA and the needle advanced along its new trajectory. Stimulation of the sciatic nerve will demonstrate plantar flexion or dorsiflexion at the ankle. The current on the nerve stimulator is decreased until sciatic nerve stimulation is apparent at 0.3–0.5 mA of current. After negative aspiration, local anesthetic is injected.

9 Potential Complications and Adverse Effects

As with any procedure, informed consent should be obtained and should include a discussion of complications associated with the procedure. As with other peripheral nerve blocks, complications of sciatic nerve block include bleeding, infection, or block failure. Local anesthetic systemic toxicity is a rare but potentially deadly complication arising from systemic absorption of local anesthetic. Although rare, toxic doses of local anesthetics should be known and intralipid should be readily available whenever local anesthetics are administered. Of additional concern is the risk of peripheral nerve injury associated with peripheral nerve blocks. Although rare, a peripheral nerve injury to the sciatic nerve can be a devastating complication of sciatic nerve blockade [1].

Clinical and Technical Pearls

- Whenever available, ultrasound guidance should be used to improve needle localization and provide direct visualization of local anesthetic spread around the sciatic nerve.
- Nerve stimulation can be used in combination with ultrasound guidance or by itself when ultrasound guidance is unavailable. Knowledge of nerve stimulation and interpretation of motor response to stimulation at various current intensities is necessary for performance of a sciatic nerve block with nerve stimulation localization.
- Aspiration should precede any injection of local anesthetic through a nerve block needle. The presence of blood on aspiration should prompt needle readjustment and injection of local anesthetic should not occur until a negative aspiration is visualized.
- If resistance on injection of local anesthetic is appreciated, the needle should be readjusted, as this can be indicative of intraneural needle placement which can increase the risk of nerve injury.

References

1. Tran DQ, Salinas FV, Benzon HT, Neal JM. Lower extremity regional anesthesia: essentials of our current understanding. Reg Anesth Pain Med. 2019;44:143–80.
2. Tran DQ, Clemente A, Finlayson RJ. A review of approaches and techniques for lower extremity nerve blocks. Can J Anesth. 2007;54:922–34.
3. Hadzic A. Chapter 33F, Ultrasound-guided sciatic nerve block. In: Hadzic's textbook of regional anesthesia and acute pain management. 2nd ed. New York: McGraw-Hill Education; 2017.
4. Hadzic A. Chapter 33G, Ultrasound-guided popliteal sciatic block. In: Hadzic's textbook of regional anesthesia and acute pain management. 2nd ed. New York: McGraw-Hill Education; 2017.
5. Grant SA, Auyong DB. Chapter 3, Lower limb ultrasound guided nerve block. In: Ultrasound guided regional anesthesia. 2nd ed. Oxford: Oxford University Press; 2016.
6. Hadzic A. Chapter 82D, Sciatic nerve block. In: Hadzic's textbook of regional anesthesia and acute pain management. 2nd ed. New York: McGraw-Hill Education; 2017.
7. Nwawka OK, Meyer R, Miller TT. Ultrasound-guided subgluteal sciatic perineural injection. J Ultrasound Med. 2017;36:2319–24.
8. Hadzic A, Vloka J, Hadzic N, Thys DM, Santos AC. Nerve stimulators used for peripheral nerve blocks vary in their electrical characteristics. J Am Soc Anesthesiol. 2003;98:969–74.

9. Vloka JD, Hadzic A, Koorn R, Thys D. Supine approach to the sciatic nerve in the popliteal fossa. Can J Anesth. 1996;43:964–7.
10. Hadzic A. Chapter 82E, Block of the sciatic nerve in the popliteal fossa. In: Hadzic's textbook of regional anesthesia and acute pain management. 2nd ed. New York: McGraw-Hill Education; 2017.
11. Grasu RM, Costelloe CM, Boddu K. Revisiting anatomic landmarks: lateral popliteal approach for sciatic nerve block based on magnetic resonance imaging. Reg Anesth Pain Med. 2010;35:227–30.

Further Reading

Hadzic A. Hadzic's textbook of regional anesthesia and acute pain management. 2nd ed. New York: McGraw-Hill Education; 2017.

Lateral Femoral Cutaneous Nerve Block

Matthew R. Thames and Brett J. Elmore

Essential Concepts

- The lateral femoral cutaneous nerve (LFCN) is a purely sensory nerve that innervates the lateral thigh.
- LFCN block can be useful to provide analgesia for hip or leg procedures, and to diagnose and treat meralgia paresthetica.
- LFCN block is a straightforward and low-risk procedure when performed with ultrasound guidance.

1 Overview

Lateral femoral cutaneous nerve (LFCN) block provides analgesia to the lateral thigh, and is most commonly performed in conjunction with femoral nerve blockade to facilitate surgical intervention upon the hip or lower extremity. A branch from the lumbar plexus, the nerve is purely sensory and blockade is considered a low risk procedure. Ultrasound guidance is recommended to identify either the nerve itself or the appropriate surrounding landmarks.

M. R. Thames · B. J. Elmore (✉)
Department of Anesthesiology, University of Virginia, Charlottesville, VA, USA
e-mail: Mrt5ry@virginia.edu; Be7k@virginia.edu

D. Souza et al. (eds.), *Bedside Pain Management Interventions*,
https://doi.org/10.1007/978-3-031-11188-4_66

2 Indications and Contraindications

The LFCN may be blocked to provide analgesia for hip procedures, soft tissue surgery of the thigh such as skin graft harvesting or muscle biopsy, or as a component of total lower extremity blockade along with the femoral, sciatic, and obturator nerves. Cryoneurolysis of the LFCN has also been described in recent literature as a means to provide more extended analgesia for the skin graft or burn patient [1].

The LFCN block may also be utilized in the diagnosis and treatment of meralgia paresthetica, a condition of numbness and/or pain most classically caused by compression of the nerve such as that from a low lying belt across the hips or, in recent times, arising from tight-fitting pants (earning the nickname "skinny jeans syndrome").

There are few contraindications to lateral femoral cutaneous nerve block, which is considered a superficial peripheral block, when applying American Society Regional Anesthesia guidelines regarding anticoagulants. Total dosing of local anesthetic should be considered in every patient, in particular those receiving multiple peripheral nerve blocks or having multiple sources of medication.

3 Clinical Anatomy

The lateral femoral cutaneous nerve arises from the lumbar plexus, which is composed of the ventral rami of spinal nerves L1–L4. More specifically, its origins lie in the posterior divisions of the L2 and L3 ventral rami. Along with the rest of the lumbar plexus and its branches, the LFCN descends caudally within the psoas major muscle. By the L4–L5 level, it is distinctly lateral to the femoral and obturator nerves that also travel inferiorly within the same fascial plane. After exiting the psoas major, the LFCN continues its caudad and lateral course across the iliacus muscle in the direction of the anterior superior iliac spine (ASIS), before entering the thigh deep to the inguinal ligament and dividing into 3–5 terminal cutaneous branches [2, 3].

The LFCN has no motor function and is solely a sensory nerve, innervating the lateral and anterior thigh. Its cutaneous distribution can be highly variable but may extend as far down as the knee (Fig. 1).

4 Equipment and Supplies

LFCN blocks are performed with standard monitoring of pulse oximetry, blood pressure, and electrocardiography as for any substantial injection of local anesthetic. The procedure may be performed sterilely or, more commonly, under clean conditions after prepping the area with antiseptic solution. The block is typically well tolerated with or without subcutaneous lidocaine prior to inserting the block needle. Small doses of midazolam or dexmedetomidine may be useful in the patient with significant anxiety, especially when performing in conjunction with other nerve blocks (Table 1).

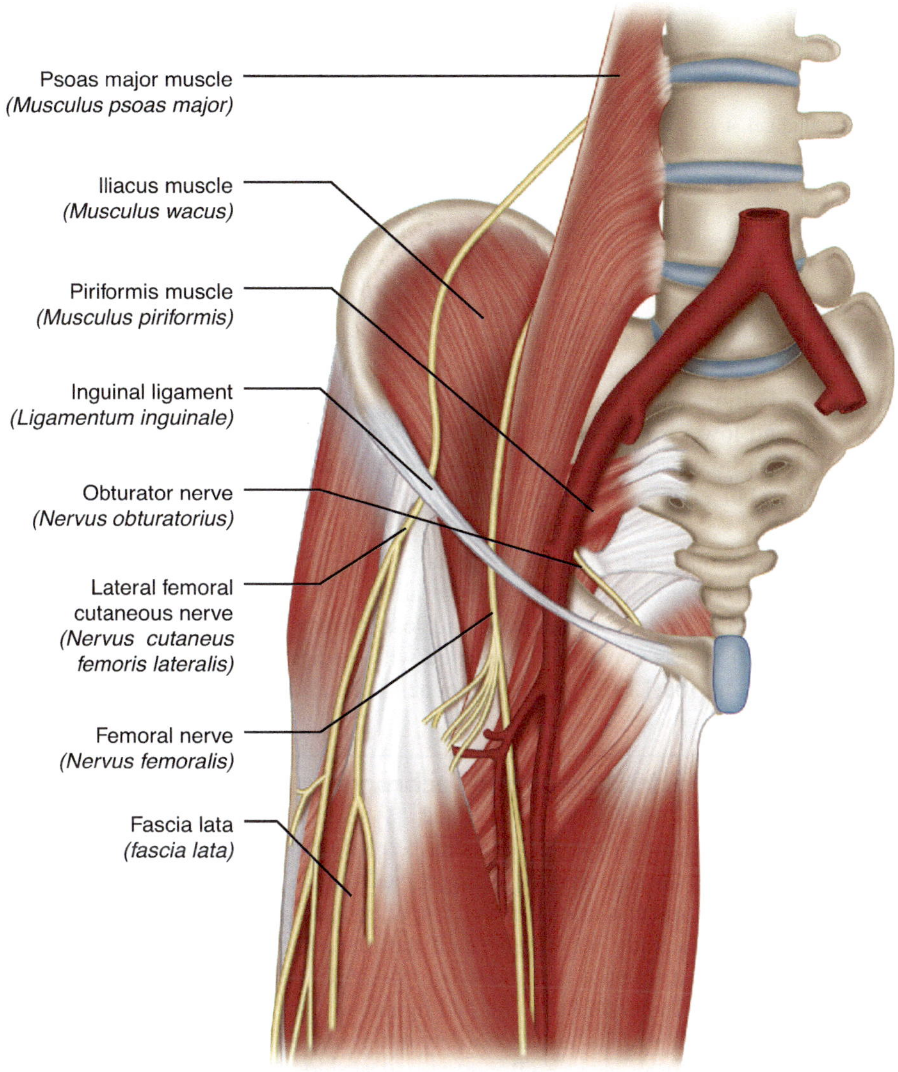

Fig. 1 Anatomy of the lateral femoral cutaneous nerve (LFCN)

5 LFCN Block, Landmark Technique

Due to anatomic variability, precise blockade of the LFCN based upon landmark techniques alone can be challenging. The nerve has classically been described as coursing deep to the inguinal ligament about 1–2 cm inferior and medial to the ASIS, and traveling further inferiorly within the thigh in the plane between the fascia lata and fascia iliaca, typically 0.5–1 cm below the skin [2]. In the absence of

Table 1 Equipment and supplies for LFCN block

Supplies	Institution-specific practice/preference
Ultrasound machine	Linear 15–6 MHz transducer
Antiseptic prep stick	2% Chlorhexidine gluconate/70% isopropyl alcohol
Gloves	Nitrile gloves used under clean conditions
Ultrasound gel, 4 × 4 gauze	Sterile gel applied after prepping skin. 4 × 4 gauze used to blot insertion site and clean gel after procedure
Syringe with local anesthetic	5–10 mL 0.5% Ropivacaine ± 1 mg preservative-free dexamethasone as adjunct to prolong the block
Block needle	22 g B bevel echogenic needle

ultrasound guidance, a fanning infiltration of local anesthetic in this region or loss of resistance technique to inject below the fascia lata can be utilized.

Peripheral nerve stimulation (PNS) can also be used to confirm proximity to the nerve by eliciting a paresthesia in the LFCN distribution, and boasts a higher success rate and lower complication rate than a landmark based fan infiltration technique [2]. PNS seems to match ultrasound guidance with regards to success rate and onset time, but at the expense of a threefold increase in the number of needle passes [2].

In regards to other non-selective approaches, the LFCN does appear to be somewhat reliably blocked along with the femoral nerve by a landmark based fascia iliaca block relying on tactile feedback and loss of resistance upon penetrating the fascia iliaca. It is less consistently reached with a traditional "three-in-one" block (targeting the femoral, LFCN and obturator nerves) performed using PNS (Fig. 2) [2].

6 LFCN Block, Ultrasound Technique

Ultrasound visualization of the LFCN may be challenging especially in postoperative patients with surgical related changes such as fluid extravasation from hip arthroscopy, but typically the relevant fascial planes and surrounding muscular landmarks can be readily identified. With the patient supine, the probe is placed approximately 2 cm inferior and medial to the ASIS and oriented transversely or with slight angling to parallel the inguinal ligament. The sartorius muscle is identified in cross section and its lateral border distinguished. If visualized, the LFCN appears in cross section as a small oval structure with a hyperechoic outline, and may lie atop the lateral tip of the sartorius or within the connective tissue between the sartorius and the tensor fascia lata muscle that is seen laterally [2, 4]. In the absence of visualization (or electively), the so called fat-filled flat tunnel (FFFT) between the muscles may be targeted and also provides a high rate of block success [5]. The needle is advanced in plane from lateral to medial to approach the nerve or, alternatively, to enter the FFTF/plane between the muscles, which may be confirmed by a tactile loss of resistance. Five to ten milliliters of local anesthetic in this plane is sufficient for reliable blockade; while as little as 0.3 mL has been proven effective if the nerve itself is visualized and targeted [3].

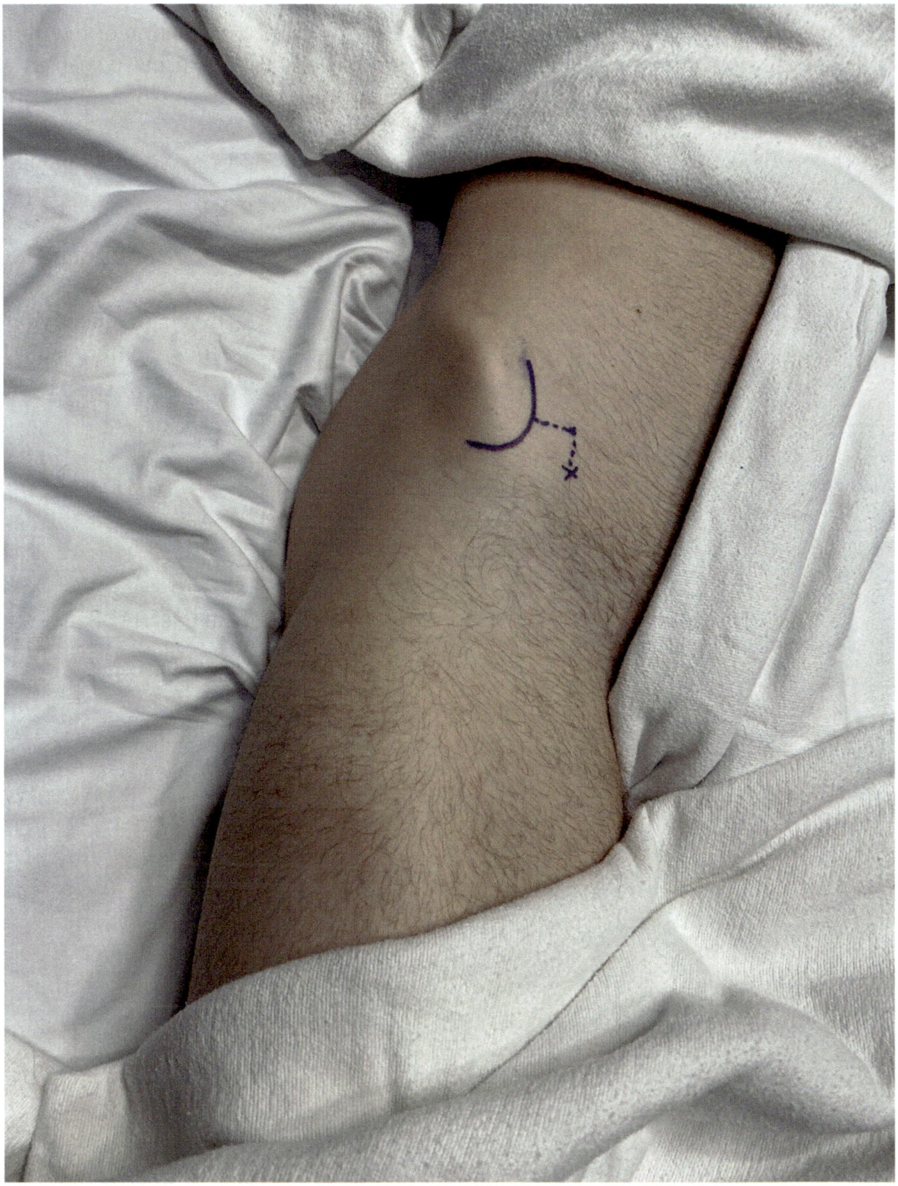

Fig. 2 While ultrasound guidance is preferred, a landmark-based approach is achieved by subcutaneous infiltration of the area 2 cm inferior and 2 cm medial to anterior superior iliac spine (ASIS)

Alternatively, ultrasound guided deposition of local anesthetic just deep to the inguinal ligament (similarly 1–2 cm medial to the ASIS) has also been described and in one study was found to have a higher success rate (Figs. 3, 4, 5 and 6) [2, 4].

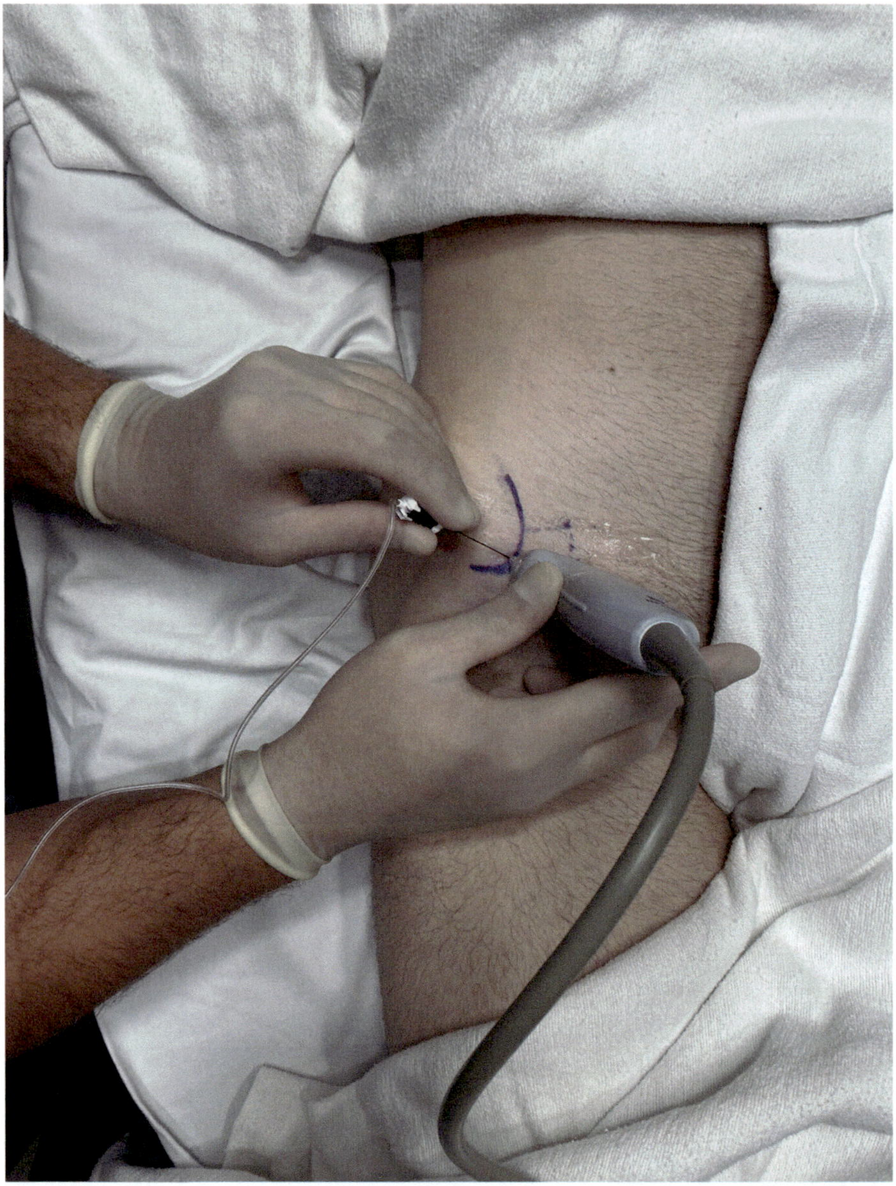

Fig. 3 The ultrasound probe is placed parallel to the inguinal ligament just inferior and medial to the ASIS, and the needle is advanced in the plane from a lateral to medial direction

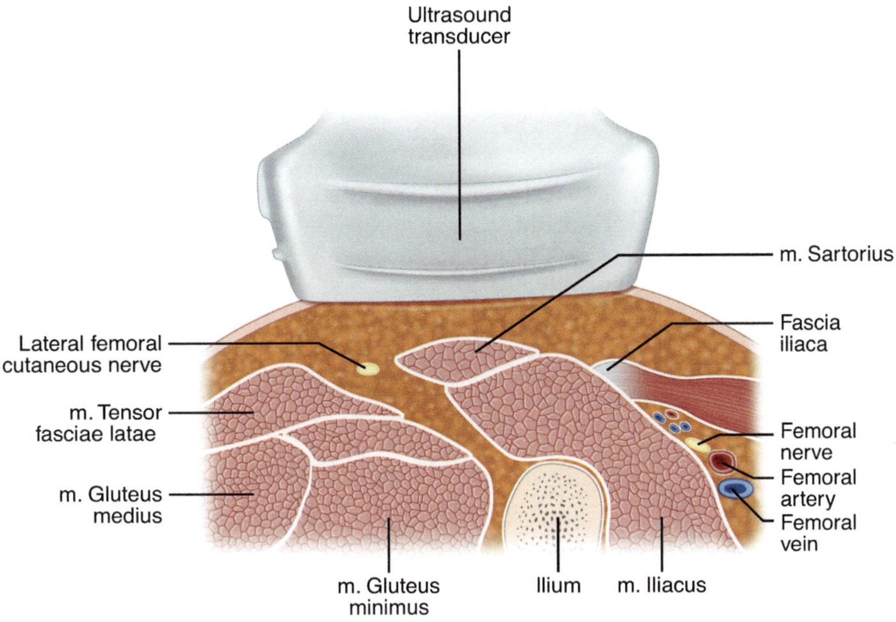

Fig. 4 Relevant cross-sectional anatomy, as labeled

7 Potential Complications and Adverse Effects

Blockade of the LFCN is a minimally invasive peripheral procedure with standard low level risk related to bleeding and infection. As with all blocks, care should be taken to avoid intravascular injection and to limit total doses of local anesthetic to reduce the risks of local anesthetic systemic toxicity.

With low volumes and sufficient lateral distance from the femoral nerve, isolated block of the LFCN presents minimal risk of motor blockade or residual weakness. As with any block, residual paresthesia in the LFCN distribution may occur following the block, although etiology may be difficult to determine given the high frequency of such paresthesias following hip surgery.

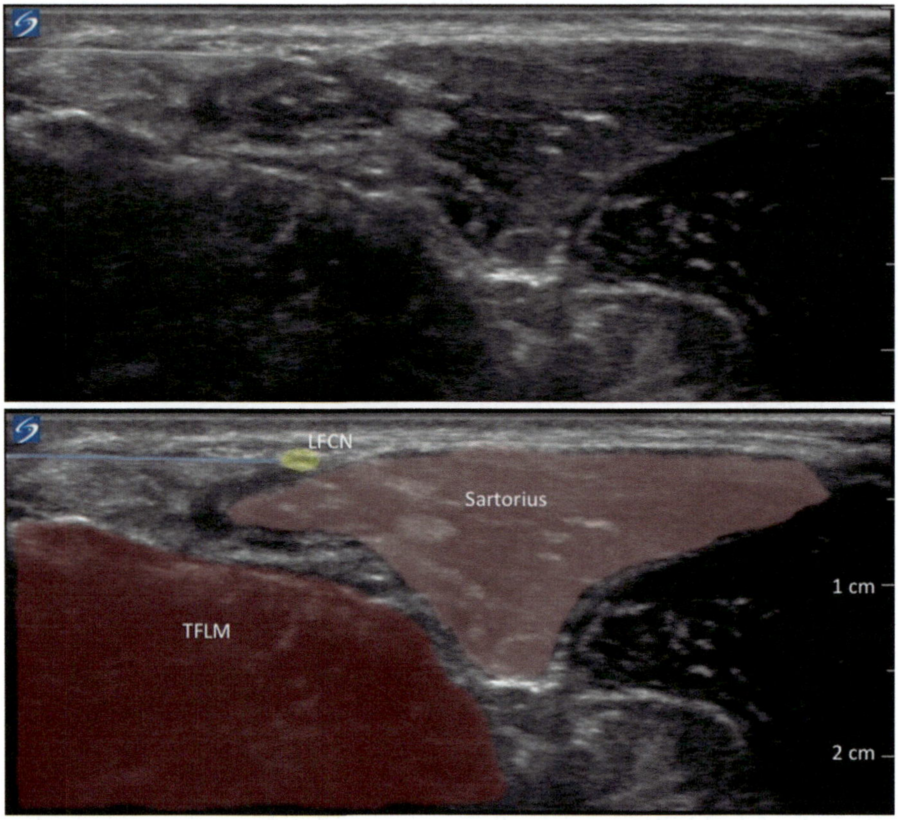

Figs. 5 and 6 Ultrasound image of needle approaching the LFCN shown on Fig. 5, The LFCN located atop the sartorius muscle. Landmarks delineated in Fig. 6 (*LFCN* lateral femoral cutaneous nerve, *TFLM* tensor fasciae latae muscle)

Clinical and Technical Pearls

- LFCN and femoral nerve blocks are often performed simultaneously for patients undergoing hip surgery; the nerves can be targeted individually or with a single injection via a fascia iliaca block.
- Although quite superficial, the LFCN has significant anatomic variability and therefore ultrasound guidance offers an advantage over a landmark-only approach for this block.
- LFCN block is a low risk procedure and complications are limited by the nature of the nerve being superficially located and solely sensory in function.

References

1. Finneran JJ IV, et al. Ultrasound-guided lateral femoral cutaneous nerve cryoneurolysis for analgesia in patients with burns. J Burn Care Res. 2019;41(1):224–7.
2. Tran DQ, et al. Lower extremity regional anesthesia: essentials of our current understanding. Reg Anesth Pain Med. 2019;44:143143–80.
3. Bodner G, et al. Ultrasound of the lateral femoral cutaneous nerve: normal findings in a cadaver and in volunteers. Reg Anesth Pain Med. 2009;34(3):265–8.
4. Hadzic A. Hadzic's textbook of regional anesthesia and acute pain management. 2nd ed. New York: McGraw-Hill Education; 2017.
5. Nielsen TD, et al. The lateral femoral cutaneous nerve: description of the sensory territory and a novel ultrasound-guided nerve block technique. Reg Anesth Pain Med. 2008;43(4):357–66.

Further Reading

Tran DQ, et al. Lower extremity regional anesthesia: essentials of our current understanding. Reg Anesth Pain Med. 2019;44:143143–80.

Saphenous Nerve Block

Prentiss A. Lawson Jr and William A. Potter

Essential Concepts

- Saphenous nerve block (SNB) may be useful for procedural and postoperative pain control in knee and medial foot and ankle surgery, as well as for the diagnosis and treatment of saphenous neuralgia.
- Single injection and continuous catheter techniques may be used for SNB.
- SNB is generally well tolerated, technically easy to perform, and without high incidence of complications.

P. A. Lawson Jr (✉)
Pain Medicine Division, Department of Anesthesiology and Perioperative Medicine, University of Alabama School of Medicine, University of Alabama at Birmingham, Birmingham, AL, USA
e-mail: palawson@uabmc.edu

W. A. Potter
Multispecialty Anesthesia Division, Department of Anesthesiology and Perioperative Medicine, University of Alabama School of Medicine, University of Alabama at Birmingham, Birmingham, AL, USA
e-mail: wapotter@uabmc.edu

D. Souza et al. (eds.), *Bedside Pain Management Interventions*,
https://doi.org/10.1007/978-3-031-11188-4_67

1 Overview

Saphenous nerve block (SNB) may be useful for procedural and postoperative pain control in knee and medial foot and ankle surgery, as well as for the diagnosis and treatment of saphenous neuralgia. Multiple sites for blockade and injection techniques have been described. It is now common practice to utilize ultrasound guidance when SNB is performed at proximal sites, while the landmark technique is still commonly used to block the saphenous nerve at the level of the ankle.

2 Indications for Saphenous Nerve Block

- Diagnostic: saphenous nerve block (SNB) may be used for diagnosing persistent knee or medial foot and ankle pain associated with saphenous neuralgia, or persistent neuropathic pain in the distribution of the saphenous nerve.
- Therapeutic: SNB may be used in the treatment of procedural or postoperative pain related to knee surgery, or procedural or postoperative pain related to medial foot and ankle surgery. The block may be performed at the level of upper to mid-thigh, distal thigh, or at the ankle. There may also be therapeutic utility in treating cases of saphenous neuralgia.

3 Contraindications to Saphenous Nerve Block

- Absolute contraindications: patient refusal, uncooperative patient, infection at the site of injection, allergy to medications necessary for the procedure.
- Relative contraindications: untreated bacteremia (risk may be higher with nerve catheters); bleeding diatheses or use of anticoagulants (nerve block may still be performed with informed consent and appropriate caution during and after the procedure); peripheral neuropathy, peripheral demyelinating disease, or pre-existing sensory deficits in the distribution of the saphenous nerve (Table 1).

Table 1 Indications, contraindications, and techniques for saphenous nerve block

Procedure	Indications	Techniques	Contraindications
Saphenous nerve block	Knee surgery (adductor canal/ femoral triangle) Medial lower leg or foot/ankle surgery Saphenous neuralgia	Landmark Ultrasound guided (± peripheral nerve stimulation with either technique)	Absolute: Patient refusal or inability to cooperate Allergy to medications Infection at site of injection Relative: Untreated bacteremia (esp. continuous catheters) Bleeding diatheses or anticoagulant use Pre-existing neurologic disorders or deficits in distribution of nerve block

4 Anatomy

The saphenous nerve (SN) is a sensory branch of the femoral nerve supplying sensation to the anterior and medial distal thigh and knee to the medial lower leg and foot (Fig. 1). It is found immediately lateral to the femoral artery, and in between the sartorius and vastus medialis muscles, at the apex of the femoral triangle in the upper leg [1]. The SN is then present throughout the adductor canal, which is the intramuscular compartment between the sartorius, adductor longus, adductor magnus, and vastus medialis muscles, from the femoral triangle to the adductor hiatus in the distal thigh. The SN has an anterior and then more medial position with respect to the femoral artery as it courses distally to the adductor hiatus [1–6]. The SN, along with muscular branches from the nerve to the vastus medialis, eventually forms a deep plexus leading to the anterior and medial genicular nerves innervating the deep anteromedial knee joint [1, 2, 6–8]. The SN courses through the vasoadductor membrane and superficially between the sartorius and gracilis muscles in the distal thigh [1, 7–10]. Continuing down the leg, infrapatellar and sartorial branches arise [3], with the infrapatellar branch providing sensation to the skin over the anterior knee and medial knee joint [1, 2, 7, 8]. The sartorial branch follows and supplies sensation to the medial leg below the knee, eventually giving off branches that innervate the capsule of the ankle joint [11, 12]. The SN is found anteromedial to the medial malleolus at the level of the ankle [3].

Fig. 1 Cutaneous sensory distribution of the saphenous nerve

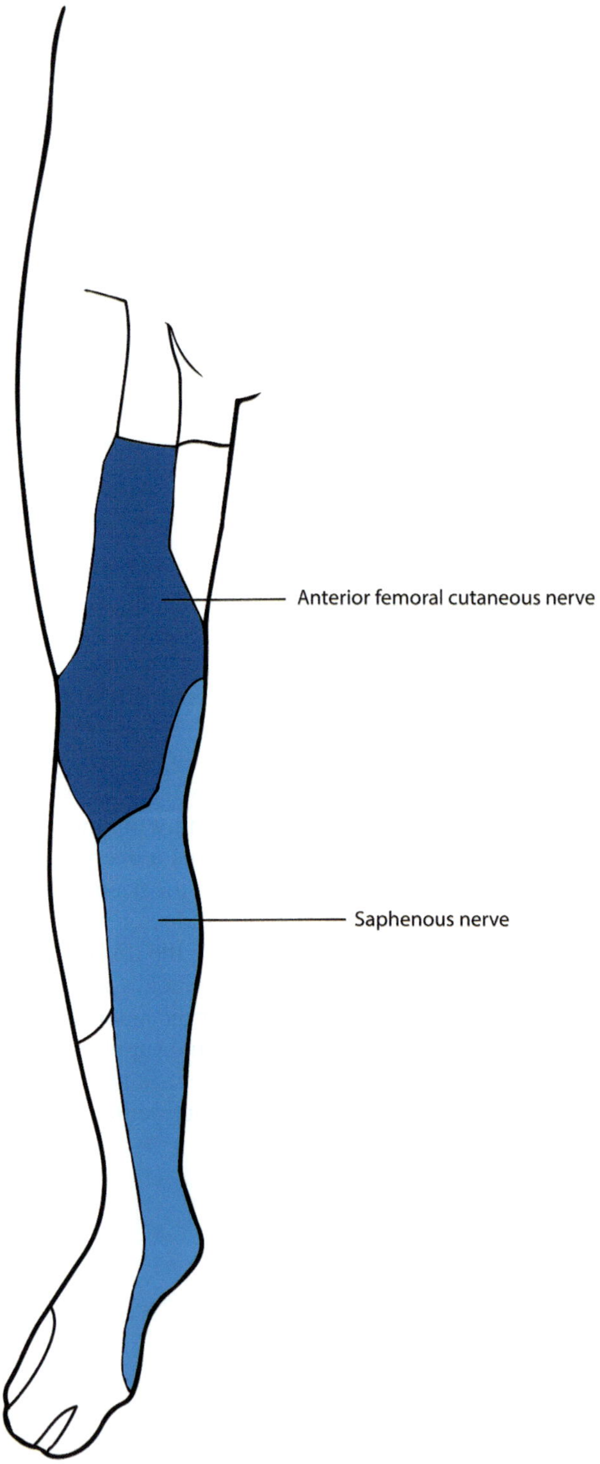

5 Equipment and Supplies

- Personal protective equipment (hat, mask, glasses) and gloves (sterile if catheter technique)
- Skin prep solution such as chlorhexidine gluconate 2% with isopropyl alcohol 70%
- Ultrasound machine with linear transducer (10–12 MHz) and sterile sleeve
- 5–8 cm 20 or 22 G blunt-tip needle with 10–20 cc syringe (single shot mid- or distal-thigh technique); 25 G skin needle for ankle technique
- Peripheral nerve block catheter tray (catheter technique)
- Appropriate long-acting local anesthetic (0.2–0.5% ropivacaine or 0.25% bupivacaine)
- Short acting local anesthetic (1% lidocaine) for anesthetizing skin with syringe and needle
- Peripheral nerve stimulator (if desired for mid- or distal-thigh technique)

6 Procedure Technique

The saphenous nerve (SN) may be blocked at several anatomic locations along the thigh and distal leg. In current clinical practice, blockade at the mid-thigh within the adductor canal is common for total knee arthroplasty and lower extremity surgeries involving the medial leg/foot. The block can also be performed at the distal thigh after the SN has left the adductor canal or at the ankle proximal to the medial malleolus.

Mid-Thigh/Adductor Canal

With the patient in the supine position and the leg slightly externally rotated at the hip, place a linear or curvilinear probe (based on patient habitus) in an orientation that is perpendicular to the long axis of the thigh at the mid-point between the anterior superior iliac spine and the base of the patella and midway between the anterior and posterior thigh.

Identify the relevant anatomy including the superficial femoral artery (SFA), sartorius muscle, vastus medialis muscle laterally, and the adductor longus muscle medially (Fig. 2). After cleaning and anesthetizing the skin with a short acting local anesthetic, a needle is inserted in-plane from the lateral side with an endpoint below the sartorius muscle and anterolateral to the superficial femoral artery. After negative aspiration, 10–20 cc of long acting local anesthetic is deposited adjacent to the SFA, with aspiration after every 3–5 cc of injectate, and confirmation of spread via ultrasound image. A catheter may be threaded under ultrasound guidance, if desired, with final placement antero-lateral to the SFA.

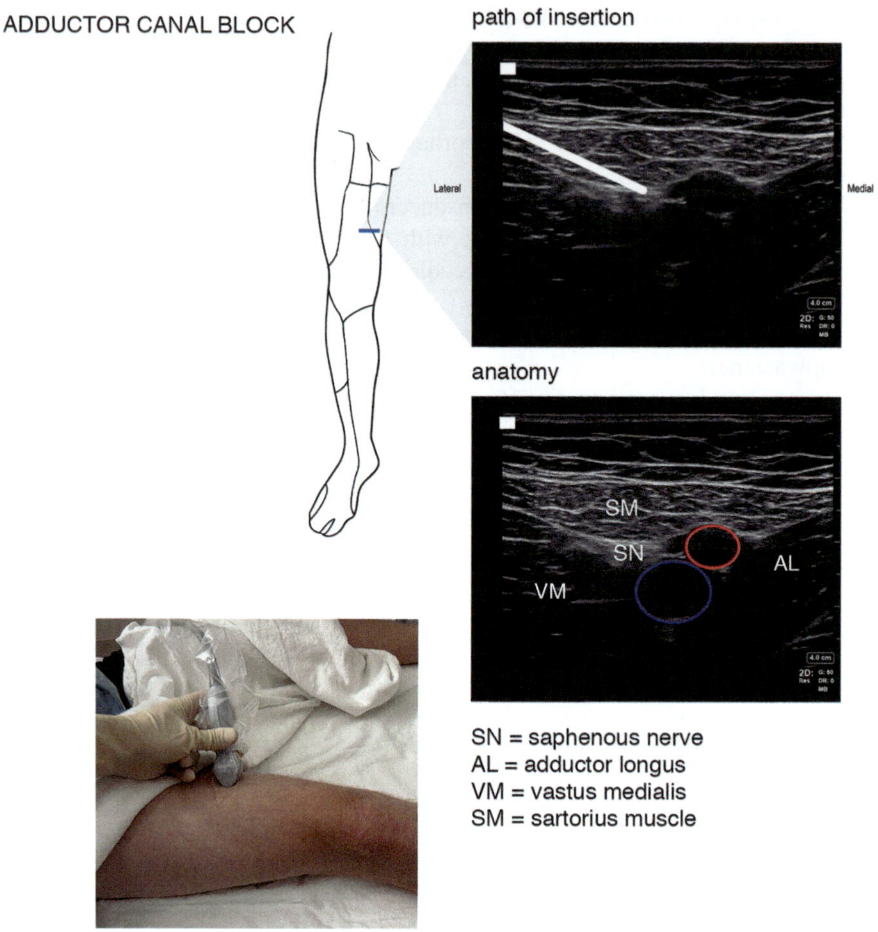

Fig. 2 Blockade of the saphenous nerve within the adductor canal

Distal Thigh/Trans-Sartorial

With the patient in the supine position and the leg slightly externally rotated at the hip, place a linear or curvilinear probe (based on patient habitus) in an orientation that is perpendicular to the long axis of the thigh, approximately 10 cm proximal to the popliteal crease and midway between the anterior and posterior thigh. Identify the relevant anatomy including the superficial femoral artery (SFA), sartorius muscle, vastus medialis muscle laterally and the adductor longus muscle medially (Fig. 3). Trace the SFA distally until it exits the adductor canal deep to the popliteal fossa. The saphenous nerve can generally be visualized between the sartorius and vastus medialis muscles at this location. The descending femoral artery may also be visualized in this plane using color mode Doppler.

After cleaning and anesthetizing the skin with a short acting local anesthetic, a needle is inserted in-plane from the lateral side, with an endpoint between the

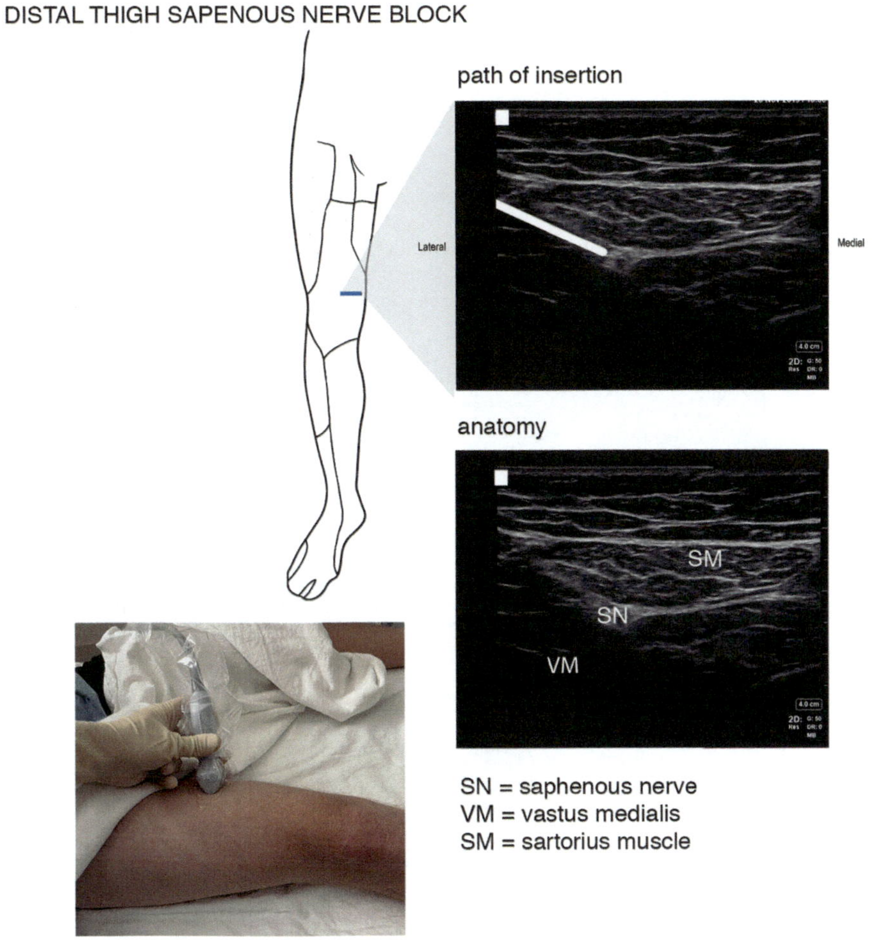

Fig. 3 Blockade of the saphenous nerve in the distal thigh

posterior-lateral border of the sartorius muscle and anteromedial border of the vastus medialis muscles. After negative aspiration, 10–20 cc of long-acting local anesthetic is deposited into this plane, with aspiration every 3–5 cc of injectate, and confirmation of spread via ultrasound image.

Ankle

At the level of medial malleolus, the saphenous nerve is superficial and can thus be blocked using a subcutaneous injection of local anesthetic. After cleaning the skin, a wheal is created by injecting local anesthetic subcutaneously 2–3 cm anterior and also posterior to the saphenous vein, at a level just cranial to the medial malleolus (Fig. 4).

SAPHENOUS NERVE BLOCK
LANDMARK TECHNIQUE AT ANKLE MEDIAL MALLEOLUS

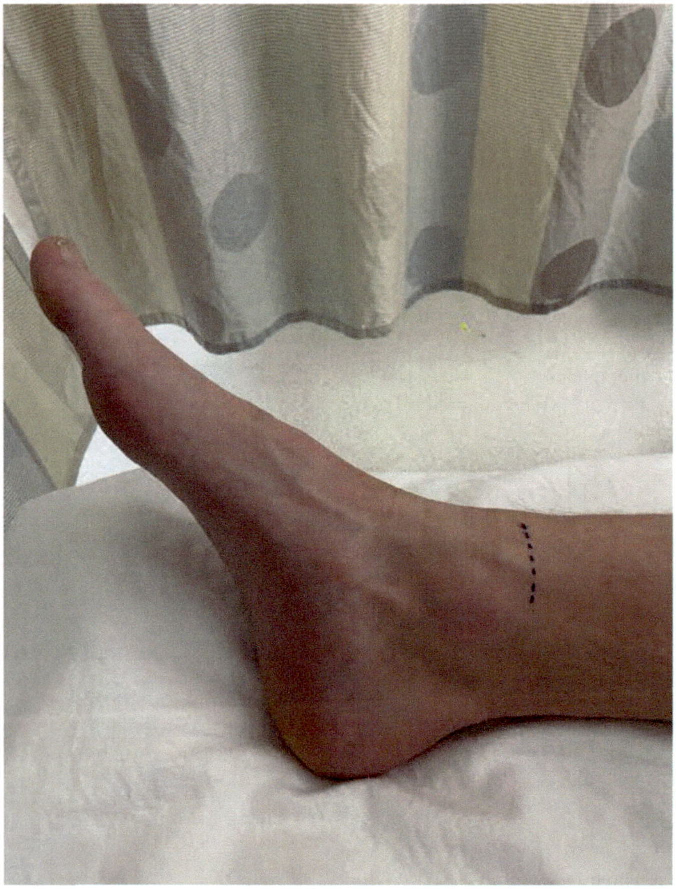

Fig. 4 Blockade of the saphenous nerve at the ankle. The dashed line just proximal to the medial malleolus represents the path for subcutaneous injection to block the saphenous nerve at the level of the ankle.

7 Potential Complications and Adverse Effects

Saphenous nerve block is a generally well tolerated procedure, though not completely without risk of complication.

- Infection may be rare with single injection or continuous catheter technique. The risk may be higher with catheter placement and directly related to catheter duration [13].
- SNB is a superficial/compressible block with low potential for bleeding complication [14].
- Persistent neurologic symptoms (pain, paresthesia, sensory or motor deficit) are infrequent with lower extremity nerve blocks [3, 15]. Deficits normally resolve and the incidence of long term (>6–12 months) neurologic symptoms in ultrasound guided regional anesthesia is rare (2–4 per 10,000 nerve blocks) [16].
- Allergic reaction to agents used for skin disinfection, local anesthetics, adjuvant medications used to prolong blockade, and medications used for sedation is possible.
- Local anesthetic systemic toxicity (LAST) after lower extremity nerve blocks has low incidence. Delayed presentation is possible, and precautions should be taken during and after the procedure. Any symptoms of LAST should be treated according to ASRA recommendations [17].
- Though in most cases strength is well preserved, significant quadriceps weakness can occur with adductor canal/femoral triangle block if there is retrograde spread of local anesthetic to the femoral nerve [18, 19].
- Though not common, myotoxicity has been reported with adductor canal/femoral triangle block [20]. Pain aggravated by stretch and relieved by shortening of the muscle, swelling, and weakness may be signs of myotoxicity. Recovery may take months [3].

Clinical and Technical Pearls

- The use of ultrasound guidance is recommended when blocking the saphenous nerve at proximal sites and facilitates continuous catheter technique.
- Sedation is not necessary but can be useful in anxious patients and for altering the seizure threshold when larger volumes of local anesthetic are used. Appropriate monitoring and maintaining a level of arousal where the patient can report any paresthesia or severe pain is recommended.
- Fall precautions should be taken when utilizing saphenous nerve block at proximal sites where muscular weakness can be a potential complication from inadvertent spread of local anesthetic.
- Steroid, such as preservative free dexamethasone 2–4 mg, may be added to single injection techniques to prolong blockade or potentially treat cases of saphenous neuralgia.

References

1. Burckett-St Laurant D, Peng P, Girón Arango L, et al. The nerves of the adductor canal and the innervation of the knee. Reg Anesth Pain Med. 2016;41:321–7.
2. Bendtsen TF, Moriggl B, Chan V, et al. The optimal analgesic block for total knee arthroplasty. Reg Anesth Pain Med. 2016;41:711–9.
3. Tran DQ, Salinas FV, Benzon HT, Neal JM. Lower extremity regional anesthesia: essentials of our current understanding. Reg Anesth Pain Med. 2019;44:143143–80.
4. Andersen HL, Andersen SL, Tranum-Jensen J. The spread of injectate during saphenous nerve block at the adductor canal: a cadaver study. Acta Anaesthesiol Scand. 2015;59:238–45.
5. Tubbs RS, Loukas M, Shoja MM, et al. Anatomy and potential clinical significance of the vasoadductor membrane. Surg Radiol Anat. 2007;29:569–73.
6. Runge C, Moriggl B, Børglum J, Bendtsen TF. The spread of ultrasound-guided injectate from the adductor canal to the genicular branch of the posterior obturator nerve and the popliteal fossa: a cadaveric study. Reg Anesth Pain Med. 2017;42:725–30.
7. Horner G, Dellon AL. Innervation of the human knee joint and implications for surgery. Clin Orthop Relat Res. 1994;301:221–6.
8. Kennedy JC, Alexander IJ, Hayes KC. Nerve supply of the human knee and its functional importance. Am J Sports Med. 1982;10:329–35.
9. Saranteas T, Anagnostis G, Paraskeuopoulos T, et al. Anatomy and clinical implications of the ultrasound-guided subsartorial saphenous nerve block. Reg Anesth Pain Med. 2011;36:399–402.
10. Horn J-L, Pitsch T, Salinas F, et al. Anatomic basis to the ultrasound-guided approach for saphenous nerve blockade. Reg Anesth Pain Med. 2009;34:486–9.
11. Mentzel M, Fleischmann W, Bauer G, et al. Ankle joint denervation. Part 1: anatomy—the sensory innervation of the ankle joint. Foot Ankle Surg. 1999;5:15–20.
12. Eglitis N, Horn J-L, Benninger B, et al. The importance of the saphenous nerve in ankle surgery. Anesth Analg. 2016;122:1704–6.
13. Capdevila X, Pirat P, Bringuier S, et al. Continuous peripheral nerve blocks in hospital wards after orthopedic surgery: a multicenter prospective analysis of the quality of postoperative analgesia and complications in 1416 patients. Anesthesiology. 2005;103:1035–45.
14. Horlocker TT, Vandermeuelen E, Kopp SL, et al. Regional anesthesia in the patient receiving antithrombotic or thrombolytic therapy: American society of regional anesthesia and pain medicine evidence-based guidelines (fourth edition). Reg Anesth Pain Med. 2018;43:263–309.
15. Farber SJ, Saheb-Al-Zamani M, Zieske L, et al. Peripheral nerve injury after local anesthetic injection. Anesth Analg. 2013;117:731–9.
16. Neal JM. Ultrasound-guided regional anesthesia and patient safety: update of an evidence-based analysis. Reg Anesth Pain Med. 2016;41:195–204.
17. Neal JM, Barrington MJ, Fettiplace MR, et al. The third American Society of Regional Anesthesia and Pain Medicine Practice advisory on local anesthetic systemic toxicity. Reg Anesth Pain Med. 2018;43:113–23.
18. Veal C, Auyong DB, Hanson NA, et al. Delayed quadriceps weakness after continuous adductor canal block for total knee arthroplasty: a case report. Acta Anaesthesiol Scand. 2014;58:362–4.
19. Chen J, Lesser JB, Hadzic A, et al. Adductor canal block can result in motor block of the quadriceps muscle. Reg Anesth Pain Med. 2014;39:170–1.
20. Neal JM, Salinas FV, Choi DS. Local anesthetic-induced myotoxicity after continuous adductor canal block. Reg Anesth Pain Med. 2016;41:723–7.

Further Reading

Arnold C, Alvarado AC, Brady MF. Saphenous nerve block. Treasure Island, FL: StatPearls; 2021. p. 2022.

Sebastian MP, Bykar H, Sell A. Saphenous nerve and IPACK block. Reg Anesth Pain Med. 2019;45(1):100750. https://doi.org/10.1136/rapm-2019-100750.

Femoral Nerve Block

Grant A. Neely and Brett J. Elmore

Essential Concepts

- Femoral Nerve Blocks are technically simple and relatively safe procedures to provide short term pain relief of the anterior hip, thigh, and knee in the perioperative setting.
- The femoral nerve originates from the posterior division of the ventral rami of L2–L4 and is the largest branch of the lumbar plexus. It provides cutaneous sensory innervation to the anterior thigh and medial lower leg as well as osseous sensory innervation to the majority of the femur and knee joint.
- Short- and intermediate-acting local anesthetics are primarily used to provide acute pain relief by blocking nociceptive afferent nerve fibers of the femoral nerve. Pain relief is achieved rapidly and may last up to 24 h.
- Femoral Nerve Block is performed with ultrasound guidance by locating the femoral nerve at the level of the inguinal crease and depositing local anesthetic adjacent to the nerve where it courses deep to the fascia iliaca.

1 Overview

A Femoral Nerve Block (FNB) is primarily utilized to provide cutaneous and osteotomal analgesia to the hip, thigh, and knee via nociceptive blockade with local anesthetic medications [1]. FNB is most commonly performed preoperatively for

G. A. Neely
Department of Anesthesiology, University of West Virginia, Morgantown, WV, USA
e-mail: BE7K@hscmail.mcc.virginia.edu

B. J. Elmore (✉)
Department of Anesthesiology, University of Virginia, Charlottesville, VA, USA

D. Souza et al. (eds.), *Bedside Pain Management Interventions*,
https://doi.org/10.1007/978-3-031-11188-4_68

Table 1 Femoral Nerve Block overview

Procedure	Technique	Indications	Contraindications	Notes
Femoral Nerve Block	Landmark Ultrasound-guided	Outpatient knee arthroscopy [6] Knee arthroplasty [7] Total knee replacement [8] Anterior cruciate ligament reconstruction [9] Analgesia in ED for femoral fractures [10] Major knee surgery [11] Leg amputation [12] Patellar realignment surgery [13]	Patient refusal Concurrent hemodynamic instability Active infection at the insertion site	Can be used in an anticoagulated patient Comprehensive analgesia to lower extremity requires additional nerve blocks to thee obturator, lateral femoral cutaneous and sciatic nerves [14]

orthopedic procedures involving the hip, femur, and knee [2, 3], but can be useful for rescue analgesia after surgery or for treating patients with acute injuries in the emergency department or admitted to the hospital with acute pain [4]. The femoral nerve can be easily located with ultrasound guidance and local anesthetic is deposited adjacent and lateral to the nerve with 10–20 mL of local anesthetic to provide short term analgesia, typically less than 24 h [5].

2 Indications and Contraindications

Indications and contraindications for Femoral Nerve Block are described in Table 1.

3 Clinical Anatomy

The femoral nerve originates from the posterior division of the ventral rami of the L2–L4 nerve roots and is the largest terminal branch of the lumbar plexus. It runs lateral to the psoas muscle in the pelvis and then passes underneath the inguinal ligament to enter the anterior compartment of the thigh where it quickly branches to provide innervation the femur, muscles, bones, joints, and skin in the anterior thigh (Fig. 1) [14].

Distal to the knee, via the sensory saphenous branch, it innervates the medial cutaneous leg and medial calcaneus. At the level of the inguinal crease in the femoral triangle, the nerve is positioned lateral to the femoral artery and vein [15] (Table 2).

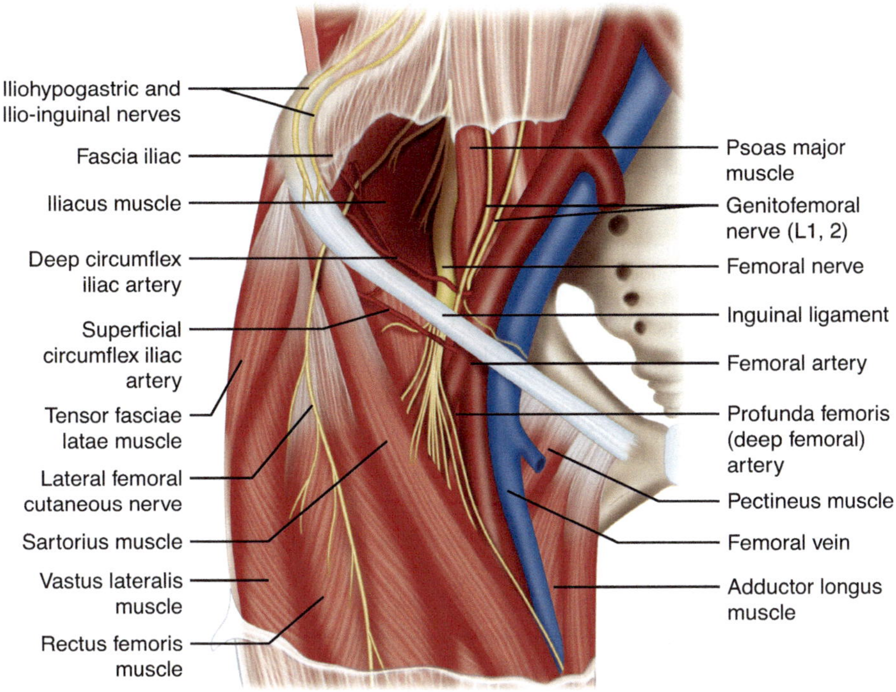

Fig. 1 Femoral nerve and anterior leg anatomy, as labeled

Table 2 Nerve distribution of the femoral nerve [14]

Spinal segments	Distribution
L2–L4	Anterior muscles of the thigh providing flexion and lateral rotation of the hip, extension of the knee, and flexion of the knee (quadriceps, sartorius, pectineus, iliopsoas muscles) Osteotome sensory branches to part of the femoral neck, femur, knee joint, proximal tibia, and distal medial tibia Articular sensory branches to hip and knee Cutaneous sensory branches to the skin over the anteromedial surface of the thigh and medial surface of leg and foot (via saphenous branch)

The femoral nerve lies under the fascia lata and fascia iliaca fascial planes, sits above and slightly medial to the iliacus muscle, and is typically 1–2 cm lateral to the femoral artery. The fascia iliac continues underneath the femoral artery and vein providing an anatomic separation between nerve and artery [15, 16].

4 Equipment and Supplies

Femoral Nerve Blocks are performed at the bedside with the patient in the supine position and the table flat with the patient's legs extended. The ultrasound machine should be positioned on the opposite side of the bed facing the operator. Standard

Table 3 Position, monitoring, equipment, and supplies for femoral nerve blockade

Position	Supine. Bed flat. Legs extended. Inguinal crease exposed
Monitors	Electrocardiogram (ECG), pulse oximeter (SpO_2), non-invasive blood pressure monitor (NIBP)
Equipment	Ultrasound machine with high-frequency linear probe (8–15 MHz) Supplemental oxygen if needed (nasal cannula, facemask) Emergency resuscitation equipment available
Syringe and needle	20–30 mL with 50–80 mm short-bevel nerve block needle
Skin preparation	Chlorhexidine with alcohol
Local anesthetic	Dependent on surgical indication and duration Short duration (2–6 h): mepivacaine 1.5% or lidocaine 1.5% Longer duration (12–18 h): bupivacaine or ropivacaine 0.25–0.5% [14]
Adjuvants	Minor prolongation of blockade. Each associated with unique side effects Dexamethasone (4 mg) Dexmedetomidine (1–2 μg/kg) Clonidine (25–50 μg) Epinephrine (2.5–5 μg/mL)

American Society of Anesthesiologists monitors are applied and equipment is readily available near the operator (Table 3).

5 Ultrasound Technique

1. Apply standard monitors noted above
2. Perform procedure timeout:
   (a) Identify patient: name, date of birth, medical record number
   (b) Confirm correct surgery, surgeon, and laterality of surgery
   (c) Confirm correct nerve block and laterality
   (d) Review allergies and anticoagulation/antiplatelet medication
3. Administer appropriate sedation medication if indicated
4. Disinfect femoral crease with chlorhexidine and alcohol
5. Place high-frequency linear ultrasound transducer at the femoral crease at the level of the inguinal ligament
6. Scan proximally (cephalad) and distally to locate the femoral artery and vein prior to the division of the femoral artery into the deep, superficial femoral artery
7. At the level of the femoral artery prior to branching, identify femoral nerve 1–2 cm lateral to the artery
8. The femoral nerve should be superficial to iliacus muscle and deep to fascia iliaca
9. Apply skin wheal of 1–2 mL local anesthetic (lidocaine 1–2%) on the lateral aspect of the ultrasound probe
10. 50–80 mm block needle inserted in-plane under ultrasound probe and advanced deep to fascia iliaca towards the lateral aspect of the femoral nerve (Figs. 2 and 3)

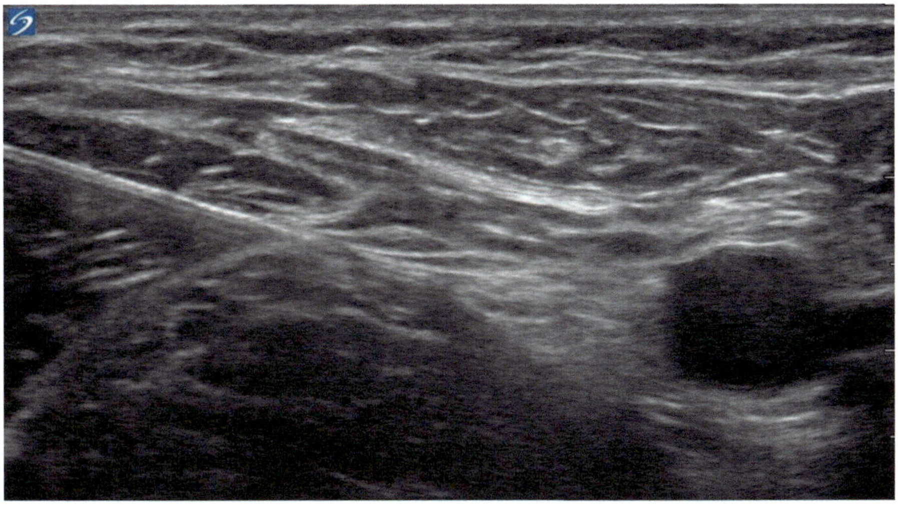

Fig. 2 Femoral Nerve Block ultrasonogram

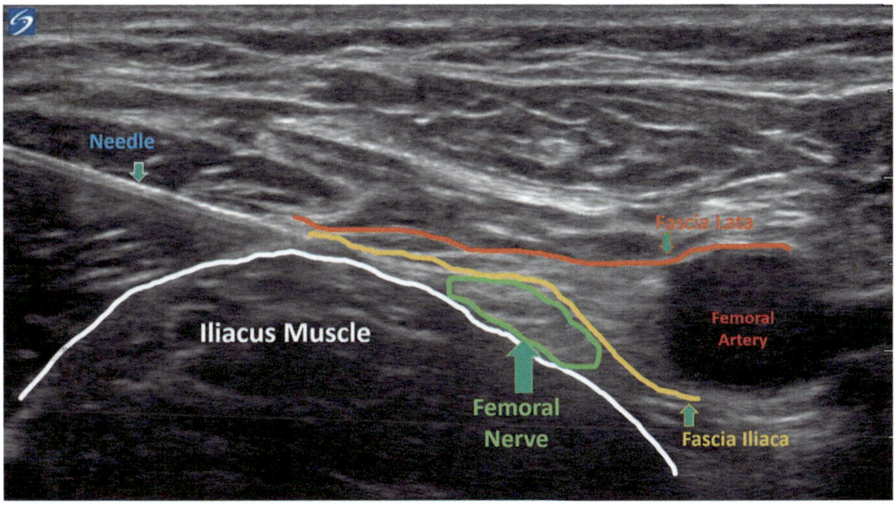

Fig. 3 Femoral Nerve Block sonography, as labeled

11. Inject 1–2 mL local anesthetic to confirm the proper location of the needle with spread underneath fascia iliaca that envelopes the femoral nerve
12. Administer 10–20 mL of local anesthetic 5 mL at a time after gentle aspiration prior to each injection
13. Local anesthetic should be seen surrounding the femoral nerve under fascia iliaca and tracking below the femoral artery (Fig. 4) [14–19]

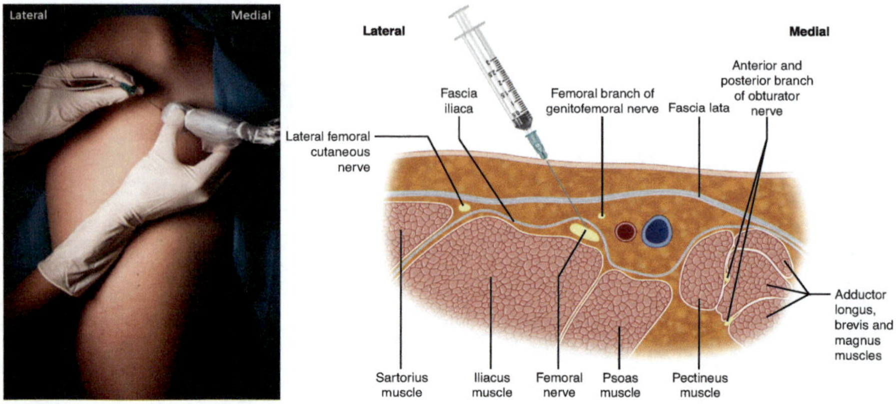

Fig. 4 Femoral Nerve Block. Patient positioning and ultrasound probe orientation on the left. Femoral Nerve Block, cross-section schematic on the right, as labeled

6 Potential Complications and Adverse Effects

FNBs are typically well-tolerated and performed without significant complications or adverse side effects. It is important to review the potential risks and benefits with patients to allow autonomous decision making while emphasizing patient safety. General complications and side effects shared by most peripheral nerve blocks apply to the Femoral Nerve Block including the risk of bleeding and hematoma, superficial infection, neuritis, temporary or permanent nerve injury with sensory and motor involvement, and local anesthetic systemic toxicity for intravascular injection or infiltration [20, 21] (Table 4).

Clinical and Technical Pearls

- Optimizing the position of the patient is of vital importance to block performance. For morbidly obese patients, consider using wide tape to retract pannus. Retract the pannus superiorly by attaching the tape to the contralateral bed rail.
- Identify where formal artery branches at the level of the inguinal ligament. Block performance and subsequent analgesia will be improved if the block is performed at the anatomic location proximal to the bifurcation of the femoral artery.
- Ensure the proper spread of local anesthetic below the fascia iliaca and adjacent to the femoral nerve by observing the medial spread of local anesthetic deep to the femoral artery. Circumferential and/or superficial spread of local anesthetic suggests incorrect placement between fascia lata and fascia iliaca.

Table 4 Complications and adverse effects unique to Femoral Nerve Block

• Hematoma formation secondary to femoral artery puncture in patients on anticoagulation/antiplatelet agents or with bleeding disorders	• Good compressibility of femoral vessels at inguinal crease • Apply firm pressure for greater than 5 min
• Increased incidence of infection secondary to the location in close proximity to groin	• More of a concern with femoral nerve catheters that are in place for longer than 48 h
• Risk of falling with numb limb due to quadriceps muscle group weakness	• Important to understand the patient's baseline mobility and assistance at home if outpatient surgery • May consider adductor canal block as alternative for knee surgeries

References

1. Ishiguro S, Yokochi A, Yoshioka K, et al. Anatomy and clinical implications of ultrasound-guided selective femoral nerve block. Anesth Analg. 2012;115:1467–70.
2. Li J, Dai F, Chang D, Harmon E, Ibe I, Sukumar N, et al. A practical analgesia approach to fragility hip fracture: a single-center, retrospective, cohort study on femoral nerve block. J Orthop Trauma. 2019;33(4):175–9.
3. Hadzić A, Houle TT, Capdevila X, Ilfeld BM. Femoral nerve block for analgesia in patients having knee arthroplasty. Anesthesiology. 2010;113:1014–5.
4. Ritcey B, Pageau P, Woo MY, Perry JJ. Regional nerve blocks for hip and femoral neck fractures in the emergency department: a systematic review. CJEM. 2016;18(1):37–47.
5. Salinas FV. Ultrasound and review of evidence for lower extremity peripheral nerve blocks. Reg Anesth Pain Med. 2010;35(2 Suppl):S16–25.
6. Montes FR, Zarate E, Grueso R, et al. Comparison of spinal anesthesia with combined sciatic-femoral nerve block for outpatient knee arthroscopy. J Clin Anesth. 2008;20:415–20.
7. Brodner G, Buerkle H, Van Aken H, et al. Postoperative analgesia after knee surgery: a comparison of three different concentrations of ropivacaine for continuous femoral nerve blockade. Anesth Analg. 2007;105:256–62.
8. Allen HW, Liu SS, Ware PD, Nairn CS, Owens BD. Peripheral nerve blocks improve analgesia after total knee replacement surgery. Anesth Analg. 1998;87:93–7.
9. Iskandar H, Benard A, Ruel-Raymond J, Cochard G, Manaud B. Femoral block provides superior analgesia compared with intra-articular ropivacaine after anterior cruciate ligament reconstruction. Reg Anesth Pain Med. 2003;28:29–32.
10. Mutty CE, Jensen EJ, Manka MA Jr, Anders MJ, Bone LB. Femoral nerve block for diaphyseal and distal femoral fractures in the emergency department: surgical technique. J Bone Jt Surg Am. 2008;90(Suppl):218–26.
11. Fowler SJ, Symons J, Sabato S, Myles PS. Epidural analgesia compared with peripheral nerve blockade after major knee surgery: a systematic review and meta-analysis of randomized controlled trials. Br J Anaesth. 2008;100:154–64.
12. Raith C, Kolblinger C, Walch H. Combined transgluteal ischial and femoral nerve block: retrospective data on 65 risk patients with leg amputation [in German]. Anaesthesist. 2008;57:555–61.
13. Luhmann SJ, Schootman M, Schoenecker PL, Gordon JE, Schrock C. Use of femoral nerve blocks in adolescents undergoing patellar realignment surgery. Am J Orthop. 2008;37:39–43.
14. Tran DQ, Salinas FV, Benzon HT, et al. Lower extremity regional anesthesia: essentials of our current understanding. Reg Anesth Pain Med. 2019;44:143–80.

15. Vloka JD, Hadzić A, Drobnik L, et al. Anatomical landmarks for femoral nerve block: a comparison of four needle insertion sites. Anesth Analg. 1999;89:1467–70.
16. Ty Muhly W, Orebaugh SL. Ultrasound evaluation of the anatomy of the vessels in relation to the femoral nerve at the femoral crease. Surg Radiol Anat. 2011;33:491–4.
17. Tran de QH, et al. Ultrasonography and stimulating perineural catheters for nerve blocks: a review of the evidence. Can J Anaesth. 2008;55(7):447–57.
18. Mariano ER, Loland VJ, Sandhu NS, et al. Ultrasound guidance versus electrical stimulation for femoral perineural catheter insertion. J Ultrasound Med. 2009;28:1453–60.
19. Tran DQ, Munoz L, Russo G, Finlayson RJ. Ultrasonography and stimulating perineural catheters for nerve blocks: a review of evidence. Can J Anaesth. 2008;55:447–57.
20. Sharma S, Iorio R, Specht LM, Davies-Lepie S, Healy WL. Complications of femoral nerve block for total knee arthroplasty. Clin Orthop Relat Res. 2010;468(1):135–40.
21. Widmer B, Lustig S, Scholes CJ, Molloy A, Leo SPM, Coolican MRJ, et al. Incidence and severity of complications due to femoral nerve blocks performed for knee surgery. Knee. 2013;20(3):181–5.

Further Reading

Hadzic A. Hadzic's textbook of regional anesthesia and acute pain management. 2nd ed. New York: McGraw-Hill; 2017.

Tran DQ, Salinas FV, Benzon HT, et al. Lower extremity regional anesthesia: essentials of our current understanding. Reg Anesth Pain Med. 2019;44:143–80.

Intra-Articular Knee Injections

Chinyere Archie, Anish Sethi, and Rany T. Abdallah

Essential Concepts

- Intra-articular knee (IA) injections are a useful therapeutic intervention for treatment of chronic knee pain, particularly that due to osteoarthritis
- Goals for initial IA injections are significant decrease in pain and improvement in functional performance
- IA injections may provide up to several months of pain relief
- IA injections are technically simple to perform, well-tolerated, and may be repeated serially. Practitioners should be familiar with the common approaches to IA knee injections
- IA knee injections may be performed at the bedside or under fluoroscopic guidance
- An array of injectable materials is approved for intraarticular knee administration

C. Archie · A. Sethi
Department of Anesthesiology, Temple University Hospital, Philadelphia, PA, USA
e-mail: chinyere.archie@tuhs.temple.edu; anish.sethi@tuhs.temple.edu

R. T. Abdallah (✉)
Division of Interventional Pain Medicine, Department of Anesthesiology, University of Vermont Medical Center, Burlington, VT, USA
e-mail: ranyabdallah@apicopain.com

D. Souza et al. (eds.), *Bedside Pain Management Interventions*,
https://doi.org/10.1007/978-3-031-11188-4_69

1 Intraarticular Knee Injections

Overview

Knee pain of varying etiologies is estimated to affect up to 25–30% of adults, with higher prevalence in the elderly population. The impaired mobility and overall functional status associated with frequent and chronic knee pain adversely affects quality of life [1–3]. Its prevalence, of varying etiologies, is expected to increase as the population ages. Knee osteoarthritis (OA) is a leading source of chronic pain [4], responsible for over 80% of the disease burden of osteoarthritis and it is the most common cause of knee pain in adults over 50 years of age [5, 6]. Other causes of knee pain include acute trauma causing bony and soft tissue disruption, surgery, and infections. Interventional treatments are useful in acute settings and are gaining popularity for treatment of knee osteoarthritis. Specifically, intraarticular knee injections appear to be a safe and effective alternative for those who have failed more conservative management of knee osteoarthritis, and in many cases, is used as a bridge to surgical intervention [7]. These injections may be a useful alternative for patients who are poor surgical candidates. IA knee injections of various materials are also gaining popularity as bedside procedures for temporary alleviation of knee pain due to other causes, including psoriatic arthritis, juvenile idiopathic arthritis, rheumatoid arthritis, and acute monoarticular gout.

Indications and Contraindications

Differential diagnoses of knee pain may be obtained by evaluating the chronicity, inciting factors, and location of the patient's painful symptoms (Table 1). This information, combined with a thorough history and physical can assist in assessing the etiology for acute and chronic knee pain. Osteoarthritis is the most common cause of knee pain, while other etiologies are seen less commonly.

Etiology of Knee Osteoarthritis

The etiology of knee osteoarthritis is considered multifactorial and is attributed to a combination of biochemical, genetic, and mechanical factors. Pathophysiology involves progressive degradation of the joint's articular cartilage, leading to matrix fibrillation, fissuring, ulceration, and eventual full-thickness loss of articular

Table 1 Common causes of knee pain based on anatomical location

Location	Differential diagnoses
Anterior	Patellofemoral pain syndrome (PFPS), patellar tendonitis, anterior cruciate ligament (ACL) rupture
Posterior	Baker/popliteal cyst, biceps femoris tendonitis
Lateral	Lateral cruciate ligament (LCL) rupture, lateral meniscus injury, iliotibial band syndrome
Medial	Medical cruciate ligament (MCL) rupture, medical meniscus injury, pes anserine bursitis, medial plica irritation

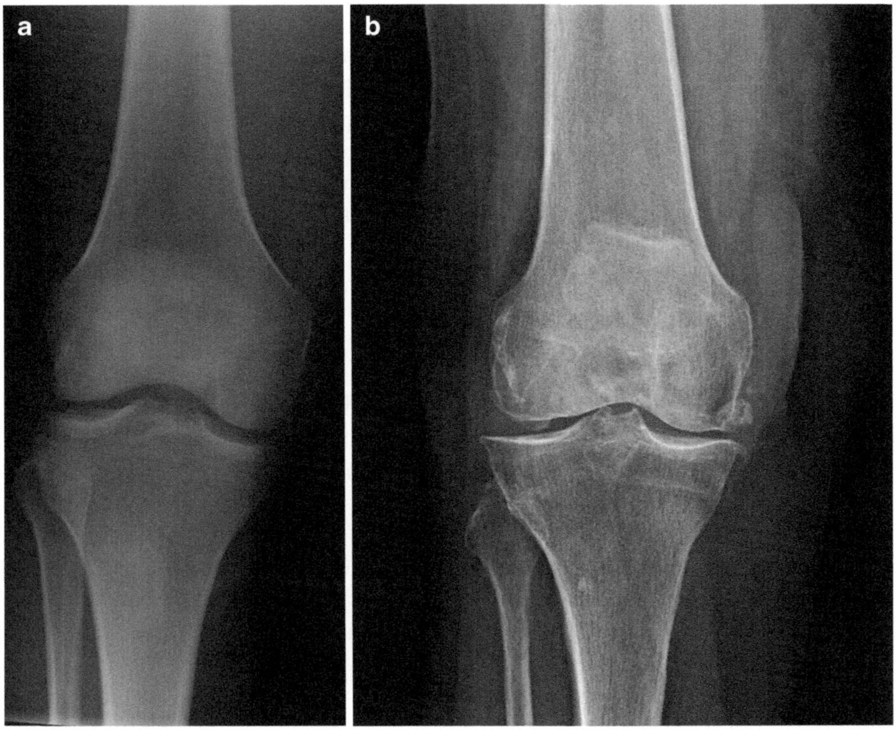

Fig. 1 (**a**) Normal AP knee radiograph in adult male illustrating preserved joint space. (**b**) Abnormal AP knee radiograph in adult female with tricompartmental osteoarthritis with joint space narrowing

surfaces. Osteophyte formation, subchondral bony thickening, and other hypertrophic changes accompany the disease, with eventual chronic synovial inflammation [8]. Diagnostic criteria include knee pain, crepitus, joint stiffness, bony tenderness, and the presence of pathological changes on radiographic imaging [9].

Plain film radiographs (Fig. 1a, b) can be utilized to assist in the diagnosis of knee pain. When compared to a normal knee X-ray (Fig. 1a), an abnormal knee X-ray indicative of osteoarthritis (Fig. 1b) will exhibit joint space narrowing, osteophyte formation, subchondral sclerosis, and cysts.

Intrarticular Knee Injection Candidates, Indications and Contraindications

The IA injection may be performed as a bedside technique in the outpatient clinic or inpatient setting. The substance injected is tailored to the patient's diagnosis and needs. Corticosteroids, blood-derived materials such as platelet-rich plasma, and viscosupplements such as hyaluronic acid or synovial fluid may be chosen.

Candidates for IA injections are those with knee pain, often times with some form of symptomatic arthritis, who have failed conservative management or who are poor candidates for surgery.

Absolute contraindications to IA injections include patient refusal, inability of a patient to cooperate, and allergy to the injectate material. Other contraindications include inherent coagulopathy or use of anticoagulant medications, active infection at the planned procedure site, bacteremia, and preexisting neurological deficits within the distribution of blockade. Extreme precaution must be used in patients with immunocompromised states such as the presence of malignancy, immune deficiency syndromes, and malnutrition. These patients have an increased relative risk of infection.

Clinical Anatomy

The knee joint is formed by the articulation of four bones: the femur, tibia, fibula and patella. The opposing surfaces of the first three bones are lined with articular cartilage to reduce friction. Functionally, the knee is comprised of two joints; the femoro-tibial and femoro-patellar joints. The entire knee joint is lined by a ligamentous capsule, which is covered in a synovial membrane that secretes synovial fluid. This viscous fluid, in addition to fat pads, bursae, and menisci help to alleviate shock and frictional forces. Any, or several, of these joint components may be eroded, fractured, chronically inflamed, or otherwise compromised in advanced arthritic disease [10].

The joint receives sensory and motor innervation from branches of three different nerves—the sciatic, obturator, and femoral nerves—all of which originate from the lumbar plexus. The obturator nerve contributes a genicular branch from its posterior division.

The sciatic nerve bifurcates into the common peroneal and tibial nerves at the popliteal fossa. The common peroneal nerve contributes three branches (superolateral genicular, inferolateral genicular, and recurrent genicular nerves) to the anterior aspect of the knee. The tibial nerve contributes the superomedial genicular, inferomedial genicular, and middle genicular nerves to supply the posterior aspect of the knee joint.

The femoral nerve contributes small branches from the nerves to the three vasti. One of its cutaneous sensory branches, the saphenous nerve, contributes suprapatellar and infrapatellar genicular branches to the anterior aspect of the knee [11].

There are several approaches to carrying out intraarticular knee joint injections. This chapter will focus on six commonly used approaches which can be performed by a pain practitioner. The approaches are named based on the point of needle entry relative to the patella. Often, severity of disease in one aspect of the joint may limit its range of motion and adequate exposure of needle trajectory pathways. This may preclude the use of one approach and necessitate utilization of an alternate approach.

Equipment and Supplies

The procedure should be carried out in compliance with strict sterile techniques and all necessary equipment, medication, and tools should be readily available (Table 2). Standard ASA monitors (non-invasive blood pressure, pulse oximetry,

Table 2 Equipment and supplies for intraarticular knee injections

- Syringes (3–10 mL)
- Small gauge needles (e.g., 18 G, 20 G, 22 G, 25 G, 1–1.5 in.)
- Local anesthetic for topical use (e.g., 1% lidocaine)
- Intraarticular injectate
  - Corticosteroid
    - Methylprednisolone acetate
    - Triamcinolone acetate
    - Triamcinolone hexacetonide
    - Dexamethasone
    - Betamethasone acetate
  - Hyaluronic acid
  - Platelet-rich plasma
- Sterile drapes, gloves
- Sterile cleaning solution
- Sterile gauze
- Sterile marker
- +/– Sedation/anxiolytic medications
- +/– Fluoroscopic source
- +/– Radiation protective clothing/outerwear
- +/– Radiopaque contrast material for injection

electrocardiography) should be available, although they need not be applied if no sedatives or systemic anxiolytics are used. Sedation may be used to facilitate patient compliance, but is typically not necessary as the procedure is well-tolerated and minimally invasive.

The procedure may also be performed under fluoroscopic guidance. In this case, the practitioner and patient should don appropriate outerwear for radiation protection, such as eyewear, leaded thyroid shield, and leaded gowns. However, fluoroscopic guided procedures are not typically performed at the bedside.

Intraarticular Knee Injection Techniques

The common approaches to intraarticular knee injections can be divided primarily into three categories—superior, lateral, and inferior. The choice of each approach is based upon a patient's disease pathology and pain etiology. Specific indications for each approach are further discussed later in this section. Additionally, specific anatomical landmarks and injection trajectories are reviewed in detail for each injection approach.

The general injection technique for the intraarticular knee injection remains the same, regardless of needle entry site. Prior to performing the injection, the clinician must prepare the skin with a sterile cleaning solution and allow it to dry completely. Following this, the clinician should don sterile gloves and stabilize the patella in the non-dominant hand, between the thumb and index finger. Using a 25 G needle, 1–2 mL of 1% lidocaine should be injected for topical anesthesia. Along the same trajectory, a 20 G needle attached to a syringe is inserted into the knee joint, applying constant negative pressure as the needle is advanced. The needle is advanced until a flashback of synovial fluid enters the syringe, providing confirmation that the needle is in the joint space. The needle may require redirection in order to optimize positioning within the joint space. Following this, the syringe is removed and another syringe containing the injectate medication is attached to the needle. The medication is then injected slowly in small aliquots with frequent aspiration to monitor for inadvertent intravascular spread. Throughout the injection process, the patient should be encouraged to provide feedback regarding pain or discomfort during the injection process. Once the injection is complete, the needle is withdrawn and properly disposed. Pressure may be held over the injection site to ensure proper hemostasis. Once hemostasis is adequately achieved, a sterile dressing should be placed over the injection site.

Superior Approach

The superior (lateral) approach (Fig. 2) may be utilized in patients with knee pain associated with a large effusion present within the suprapatellar bursa. With this approach, fluid may be aspirated with greater ease when compared to alternative approaches.

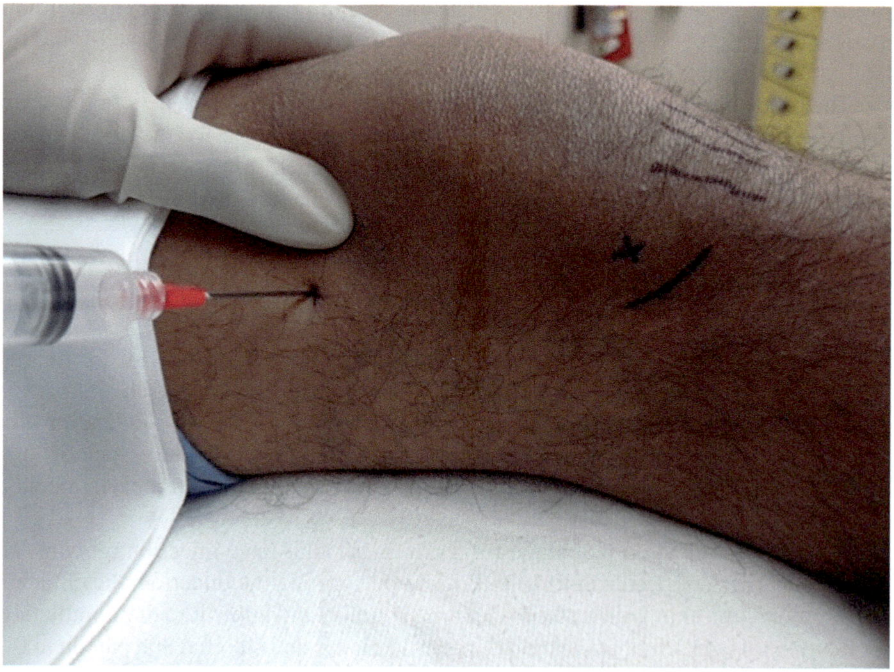

Fig. 2 Superior (lateral) approach for intraarticular knee injection: needle tip is placed at injection site on right knee. Straight lines represent the patellar tendon and curved line represents the lateral tibial plateau

This injection is performed with the patient lying supine and the knee slightly flexed and supported on a pillow or rolled towel. The entry site can be located by palpating the superolateral border of the patella. Mark the point that lies 1 cm lateral and 1 cm superior to this bony edge. This will be the point of needle entry. The needle is then advanced in a medial direction to a depth of approximately 1–2 in., or until joint fluid may be aspirated. Once this occurs, the injection of medication may be performed in a slow and continuous fashion.

Lateral Midpatellar Approach

The lateral midpatellar approach (Fig. 3) is utilized to effectively access the patellofemoral joint. This approach may be used for both joint aspiration and joint injection.

This injection is performed with the patient lying in the supine position, with the knee extended but relaxed. The lateral border of the patella is palpated, and the needle entry point is located 1–2 cm lateral to the midpoint of the lateral border of the patella. When performing the injection, the needle is directed medially at a 45° angle towards the midpoint of the medial compartment of the joint at a depth of

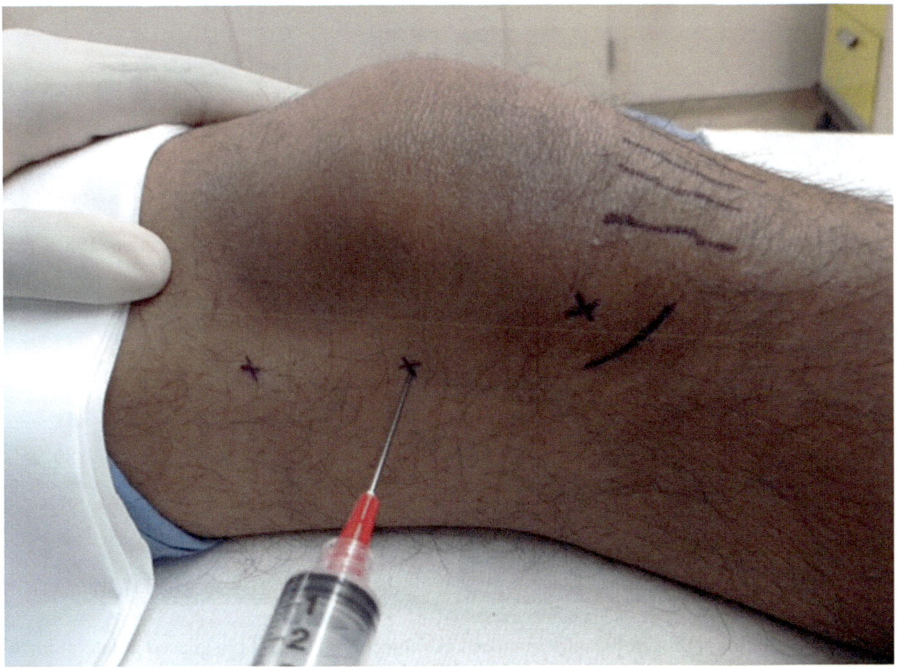

Fig. 3 Lateral (midpatellar) approach for intraarticular knee injection: needle tip is placed at injection site on right knee. Straight lines represent the patellar tendon and curved line represents the lateral tibial plateau

1–1.5 in. The patella may be translated medially or laterally in order to facilitate needle placement under the patella.

Access to the knee joint via this approach may be difficult in patients with severe patellofemoral osteoarthritis or obesity; additionally, due to discomfort during needle placement, patients may tense the thigh extensor muscles, causing further technical difficulty during the procedure.

Inferior Approach

The inferior (or infrapatellar) approaches (Fig. 4a, b) can be utilized for intraarticular knee injections. This approach may be used when the patient is unable to fully extend the affected knee due to pain or joint stiffness; however, this approach typically limits the ability to aspirate joint fluid.

This injection is performed with the patient seated, with the knees flexed to approximately 90°. The medial tibial plateau, lateral tibial plateau, and patellar ligament are palpated.

The lateral injection site (Fig. 4a) is located 1 cm above the lateral tibial plateau and 1 cm lateral to the patellar ligament. The needle is advanced slightly upwards in a posteromedial direction to a depth of approximately 1–1.5 in.

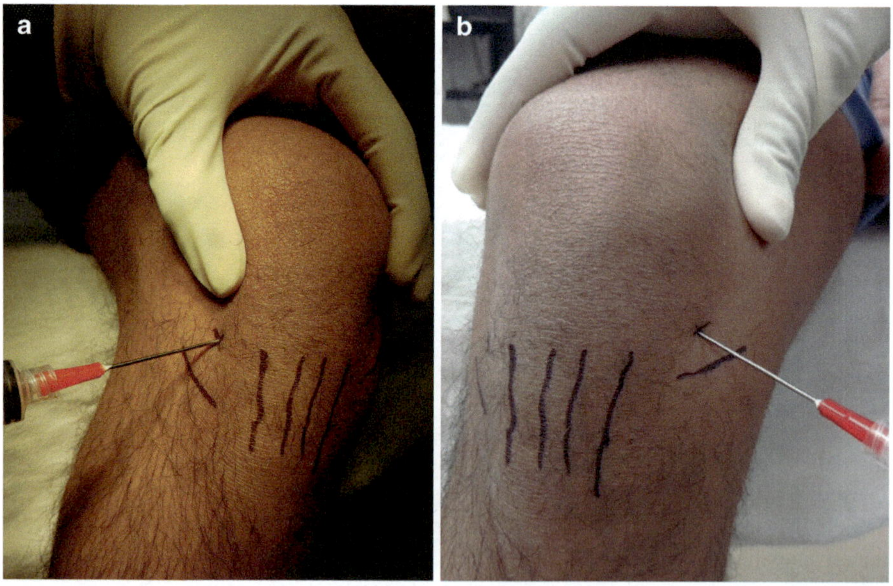

Fig. 4 (**a**) Inferior approach for intraarticular knee injection: needle tip is placed at lateral injection site on right knee. Straight lines represent the patellar tendon and curved line represents the lateral tibial plateau. (**b**) Inferior approach for intraarticular knee injection: needle tip is placed at medial injection site on right knee. Straight lines represent the patellar tendon and curved line represents the medial tibial plateau

The medial injection site (Fig. 4b) is located 1 cm above the medial tibial plateau and 1 cm medial to the patellar ligament. The needle is advanced slightly upward in a posterolateral direction to a depth of approximately 1–1.5 in.

Ultrasound-Guided Approach

Suprapatellar Bursa Technique

Ultrasound guidance may be utilized to perform the intraarticular knee joint injection. A common approach is via the suprapatellar bursa (Fig. 5a, b). The suprapatellar bursa lies directly cephalad to the patella and is located between the anterior surface of the distal femur and quadriceps tendon.

The patient should be placed in a supine position with the knee slightly flexed with the assistance of a pillow or rolled towel (Fig. 5a). A high-frequency linear transducer is utilized to perform the injection. An initial ultrasound survey scan can be obtained by placing the probe in a longitudinal position superior to the patella. The hyperechoic patella and femur are noted, with the suprapatellar bursa located deep to the quadriceps tendon.

Once the suprapatellar bursa is visualized, the ultrasound transducer is then rotated to a transverse position just above the patella in order to perform the injection (Fig. 5b). In this view, the suprapatellar bursa is noted deep to the quadriceps tendon, and is the target site for the injection. The femur is noted deep within the ultrasound field as a curved echogenic line casting a shadow. With advanced knee joint degeneration, there may be the presence of a moderate amount of fluid in the suprapatellar bursa, which can be aspirated with this approach if necessary.

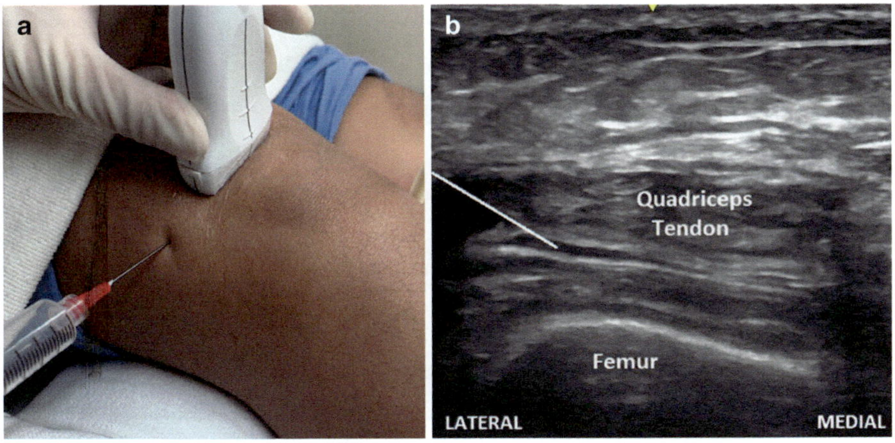

Fig. 5 (**a**) Positioning of transducer and needle for performance of suprapatellar approach to knee injection. (**b**) Ultrasound view of suprapatellar region with solid white line depicting the trajectory of the needle tip into suprapatellar bursa. Note a minimal amount of fluid present within the bursa

The skin overlying the lateral knee is prepped with sterile solution. After instilling topical anesthetic to create a skin wheal, a 3.5 in. needle is advanced just posterior to the superolateral border of the patella with an in-plane approach under live ultrasound-guidance to the suprapatellar bursa (Fig. 5b). Once the needle tip is visualized within the suprapatellar bursa, a combination of local anesthetic and steroid is slowly instilled. Following this, the needle is removed and a sterile dressing should be placed over the injection site.

Medial Intraarticular Technique

An alternative approach to the intraarticular knee injection under ultrasound guidance is the medial intraarticular technique (Fig. 6a, b). This approach can provide direct access deep within the joint space.

In order to perform this injection technique, the patient is placed in the supine position with the lower extremity slightly externally rotated (Fig. 6a). A high-frequency linear transducer is placed over the medial aspect of the knee joint in a longitudinal configuration. The bony contours of the distal femur and proximal tibia are noted in the ultrasound view as they form the knee joint (Fig. 6b). The medial meniscus is visualized as a triangular-shaped structure between the margins of the femur and tibia. This articulation provides access to the medial knee joint for the purposes of this injection.

The skin over the medial knee joint is prepped with sterile solution. After instilling topical anesthetic to create a skin wheal, a 3.5 in. needle is advanced over the mid-point of the ultrasound probe in an out-of-plane approach under live ultrasound-guidance to enter the knee joint via the medial borders of the distal femur and proximal tibia. Once the needle tip is within the joint space, a combination of local anesthetic and steroid is slowly instilled. Following this, the needle is removed and a sterile dressing should be placed over the injection site.

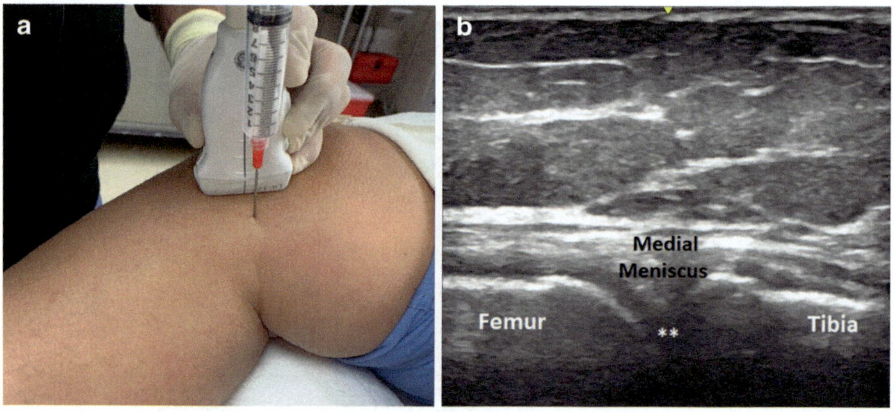

Fig. 6 (**a**) Positioning of transducer and needle for performance of medial intraarticular approach to knee injection. (**b**) Ultrasound view of the medial knee joint with the triangular-shaped medial meniscus at the confluence of the distal femur and proximal tibia, providing an entry-point to the knee joint. The asterisks depict the target point for the needle tip

Potential Complications and Adverse Effects

This procedure is generally well-tolerated, and most patients experience some degree of pain relief within minutes. However, several potential complications and adverse effects must be considered by the clinician. Mild discomfort or muscle spasm may occur surrounding the knee joint. These should resolve within a few hours. Unintended injury to surrounding structures is rare, but neurovascular and tendinous injury may occur. Temporary weakness or numbness of leg muscles may occur and should resolve within a few hours. During this period, patients should be advised to ambulate with assistance, to minimize falls or other injury. Inadvertent intravascular injection of local anesthetic may lead to local anesthetic systemic toxicity (LAST), manifesting with headaches, dizziness, perioral numbness, tinnitus or even seizures, loss of consciousness and cardiac arrest. The clinician should be familiar with the institutional policy for management of LAST, have a high index of suspicion should these symptoms occur, and act quickly to resuscitate the patient. Anaphylactic reactions can occur in response to any of the materials or medications used. In the event of such a reaction, emergent supportive therapy must be instituted depending upon the reaction. Other adverse effects include bleeding or hematoma formation and development of intraarticular or periarticular knee infections. Patients should be educated on the signs and symptoms of procedural complications, and should be advised to seek medical care immediately if any of these adverse events occur.

Clinical and Technical Pearls

- Intraarticular knee injections may be used in cases of suboptimal response to conservative management for knee pain.
- Intraarticular knee injections can be utilized as a bridge to knee replacement, or can be an effective ongoing treatment for patients who are poor surgical candidates.
- These injections can be performed at the bedside, typically without the need for systemic sedation.
- Coagulopathy, local infections, and immuocompromised states are relative contraindications to use of intraarticular injections.
- The needle approach to the intraarticular space may be tailored depending upon the patient's knee pathology.
- Various injectate materials may be utilized based upon the patient's disease pathology.
- Potential complications may include hematoma formation, infection, musculoskeletal injury, or nerve injury.

References

1. Mannoni A, Briganti MP, Di Bari M, et al. Epidemiological profile of symptomatic osteoarthritis in older adults: a population based study in Dicomano, Italy. Ann Rheum Dis. 2003;62:576–8.
2. Grotle M, Hagen KB, Natvig B, Dahl FA, Kvien TK. Prevalence and burden of osteoarthritis: results from a population survey in Norway. J Rheumatol. 2008;35:677–84.
3. Peat G, McCarney R, Croft P. Knee pain and osteoarthritis in older adults: a review of community burden and current use of primary health care. Ann Rheum Dis. 2001;60:91–7.
4. Murray CJ, et al. The state of US health, 1990–2010: Burden of diseases, injuries, and risk factors. JAMA. 2013;310:591–608.
5. Vos T, et al. Years lived with disability (YLDs) for 1160 sequelae of 289 diseases and injuries 1990–2010: a systematic analysis for the Global Burden of Disease Study 2010. Lancet. 2012;380:2163–96.
6. Zeni JA Jr, Axe MJ, Snyder-Mackler L. Clinical predictors of elective total joint replacement in persons with end-stage knee osteoarthritis. BMC Musculoskelet Disord. 2010;11:86.
7. National Collaborating Centre for Chronic Conditions (UK). Osteoarthritis: national clinical guideline for care and management in adults. London: Royal College of Physicians; 2008.
8. Martel-Pelletier J. Pathophysiology of osteoarthritis. Osteoarthr Cartil. 2004;12:S31–3.
9. Salehi Abari I. ACR revised criteria for early diagnosis of knee osteoarthritis. Autoimmune Dis Ther Approach. 2016;3(1):118.
10. Narouze S, Raju S. Chapter 59: Interventional techniques for pain management. In: Benzon H, et al., editors. Essentials of pain medicine. Amsterdam: Elsevier; 2011.
11. Jamison DE, Cohen SP. Radiofrequency techniques to treat chronic knee pain: a comprehensive review of anatomy, effectiveness, treatment parameters, and patient selection. J Pain Res. 2018;11:1879–88. https://doi.org/10.2147/JPR.S144633.

Further Reading

Bellamy N, Campbell J, Robinson V, Gee T, Bourne R, Wells G. Intraarticular corticosteroid for treatment of osteoarthritis of the knee. Cochrane Database Syst Rev. 2006;2:CD005328.

Hurdle MFB. Ultrasound-guided knee injections. In: Narouze S, editor. Atlas of ultrasound-guided procedures in interventional pain management. New York: Springer; 2011.

Narouze S, Raju SVY. Joint injections. In: Benzon HT, Raja SN, Liu SS, Fishman SM, Cohen SP, editors. Essentials of pain medicine. 3rd ed. London: Elsevier Health Sciences; 2011. p. 423–30.

Periarticular Knee Injections

Karl J. Hinrichs, James E. Wolf, and Rany T. Abdallah

Essential Concepts

- Periarticular knee injections are an effective diagnostic and therapeutic tool in treating a variety of painful knee conditions.
- The pes anserinus bursa represents a significant cause of non-articular knee pain, and after appropriate workup may be treated with injections of steroid and local anesthetic.
- Careful history, physical exam, and judicious use of diagnostic imaging can help isolate pain syndromes that may be complex and overlapping.
- Injections are typically low risk and are often aided by ultrasound.

1 Pes Anserinus Bursa Injection

Overview

The pes anserinus ("goosefoot"; "pes anserinus syndrome") is the anatomic location where the sartorius, gracilis, semimembranosus and semitendinosus tendons connect to the medial aspect of the tibia. Along with the tendons, there is an underlying pes anserinus bursa, which was first described as a source of chronic pain by

K. J. Hinrichs
Department of Anesthesiology, University of Vermont, Burlington, VT, USA
e-mail: karl.hinrichs@uvmhealth.org

J. E. Wolf · R. T. Abdallah (✉)
Division of Interventional Pain Medicine, Department of Anesthesiology, University of Vermont, Burlington, VT, USA
e-mail: james.wolf@uvmhealth.org; ranyabdallah@apicopain.com

D. Souza et al. (eds.), *Bedside Pain Management Interventions*,
https://doi.org/10.1007/978-3-031-11188-4_70

Moschcowitz in 1937 [1]. As a pain syndrome, while there is some evidence in patients on ultrasound (US) and magnetic resonance imaging (MRI) [2–10], it remains primarily clinically diagnosed [1, 3, 4, 7, 8, 11, 12]. While surgery may be an option for some patients, injections with steroids have provided a less invasive alternative, and relief after injections can aid in diagnosis [8, 11].

Indications and Contraindications

Table 1 summarizes the associated conditions and clinical findings of pes anserinus. Pes anserinus remains a predominantly clinical diagnosis [1, 3, 4, 7, 8, 11, 12] and a diagnosis of pes anserinus syndrome should be considered in a patient presenting with these clinical findings without evidence of other pathology. Before considering an injection, a patient may consider rest, ice, medical therapy and physical therapy [8, 11]. Patient refusal, active infection or bleeding risk or inability to tolerate steroids or local anesthetic would be contraindications to this procedure.

Clinical Anatomy

The pes anserinus (PA) is the anatomic location where the sartorius, gracilis, semimembranosus and semitendinosus tendons connect to the medial aspect of the tibia (Fig. 1a). The PA bursa is typically immediately proximal to the tendon insertion [13], and typically does not communicate with the knee joint [6, 7]. Anatomically, studies have evaluated the distance from the PA bursa to the medial joint line of the knee (2.5–3 cm below the joint line) [2, 4, 10], or by using the tibial tuberosity as a reference point (2 cm medial, 1.2 cm superior from the inferomedial point of the tibial tuberosity) [14]. While anatomic approach for injection of the PA bursa is possible, ultrasound guidance can improve injection safety and accuracy while evaluating for other potential sources of knee pain [4, 8]. The PA is richly innervated and surrounded by the inferior medial genicular artery, the lateral genicular artery, and the anterior tibial recurrent artery [15].

Table 1 A summary of associated conditions and clinical finds of pes anserinus

Clinical findings	Associations
Medial knee pain	Type-2 diabetes mellitus [3]
Pain worse when ascending or descending stairs [3, 4]	Knee osteoarthritis [4]
Pain worse at night [3]	Rheumatoid arthritis [1]
Pain getting out of a chair/car [1, 3]	Fibromyalgia [1]
Pain for at least 2 weeks [3, 4]	Long-distance runners [1, 7]
Pain when performing weight-bearing activity [3, 4]	Overweight patients [1, 7]
Relief with rest and heat [1, 7, 11]	Women [1, 7]
Pain not better explained by other symptoms	Incidence peaks age 50 (+/– 13 years) [12]
Improvement with injection of local anesthetic [8, 11]	

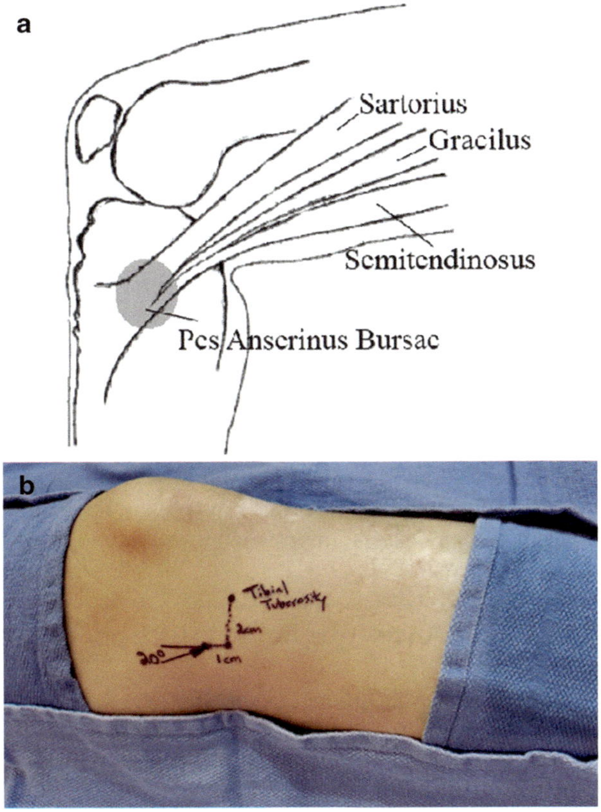

Fig. 1 (**a**) Example of pes anserinus bursae location (shaded circle) with tendon insertion as viewed from the medial aspect of the knee. (**b**) Left knee viewed from the medial aspect, with labeled tibial tuberosity and injection site (arrow)

Table 2 Equipment and supplies

Syringe	3 or 5 mL
Needle	25-gauge, 1.5″ (or 38-mm) needle [7]
Anesthetic	0.25 Bupivacaine 1–2% Lidocaine [1, 2, 13]
Corticosteroid	Triamcinolone 20–40 mg (t1/2 life: 18–36 h), betamethasone 6 mg (t1/2 life: 36–54 h) Methylprednisolone 20–40 mg (t1/2 life: 18–36 h) [1, 2, 12]
Ultrasound	Linear US probe [2–4]

Equipment and Supplies

Pes anserinus blocks are easily performed at bedside. A list of equipment and supplies is provided in Table 2. A syringe with a 25 gauge, 1.5 in. needle is utilized to inject 3 mL of the anesthetic solution. Anesthetic solution usually consists of the local anesthetic lidocaine or bupivacaine, with or without a corticosteroid. Local anesthetic only can be considered for diagnostic block [8, 11] and if there is a contraindication to steroid injection.

2 Pes Anserinus Bursa Injection, Landmark Technique

Before the patient is draped and prepped, consider a US survey to visualize for other soft tissue pathologies that may mimic pes anserinus [1, 4]. Patient is positioned supine with knee gently flexed and in slight external rotation [1, 8].

Using a surgical marker, delineate significant landmarks and injection site (Fig. 1b). Before ultrasound, injections were frequently performed at the point of maximal tenderness, where the needle would be advanced perpendicularly until bone was contacted, then withdrawn 2–3 mm and medications were injected [1, 12, 16]. Others have suggested an alternative method using the tibial tuberosity as a reference point (2 cm medial, 1.2 cm superior from the inferomedial point of the tibial tuberosity), angling the needle trajectory 20° from a front-facing view inferiorly and medially [14].

Always adhere to aseptic technique. Slight resistance to injection can be anticipated. Care should be taken to avoid injection into tendon [1]. Patients are unlikely to benefit from repeat injections if no benefit is noted. Injections can be repeated for those who demonstrate improvement (no more than three injections per year) [1].

3 Pes Anserinus Bursa Injection, Ultrasound Technique

Studies suggest US guidance can help decrease pain when compared to blind PA bursa injection [16]. The patient is positioned and prepared as previously described [1, 8]. The pes anserinus tendon insertion region (PA) is located 2.5–3 cm distal to the medial joint line with the transducer placed longitudinally (Fig. 2a) [2, 4]. The anatomy can be confirmed by keeping this in mind while tracing the tendons (sartorius, gracilis, semimembranosus and semitendinosus tendons) to their insertion point [1]. The tendons, which appear as echogenic, oval, fibrillar structures [1] can be traced from the posterior-medial thigh, where initially one may first identify the semitendinosus tendon. Scanning inferiorly and rotating the probe to keep the ligaments in a transverse view, the other tendons will come into view as they converge superficial to the medial collateral ligament (MCL) [1, 14, 16]. At this level the needle is slowly inserted in-plane (Fig. 2b) and is placed above the MCL, then aspirated. Injection must be slow, avoiding injection under pressure and watching spread above MCL on US (note: The inferior medial genicular artery is located deep to the MCL in this region [1, 14, 16]).

4 Potential Complications and Adverse Effects

Although generally well tolerated, occasional adverse reactions and complications can occur. Table 3 summarizes the potential complications and adverse effects of pes anserinus injection. Complications can be reduced by evaluating any potential patient-specific risk factors [1].

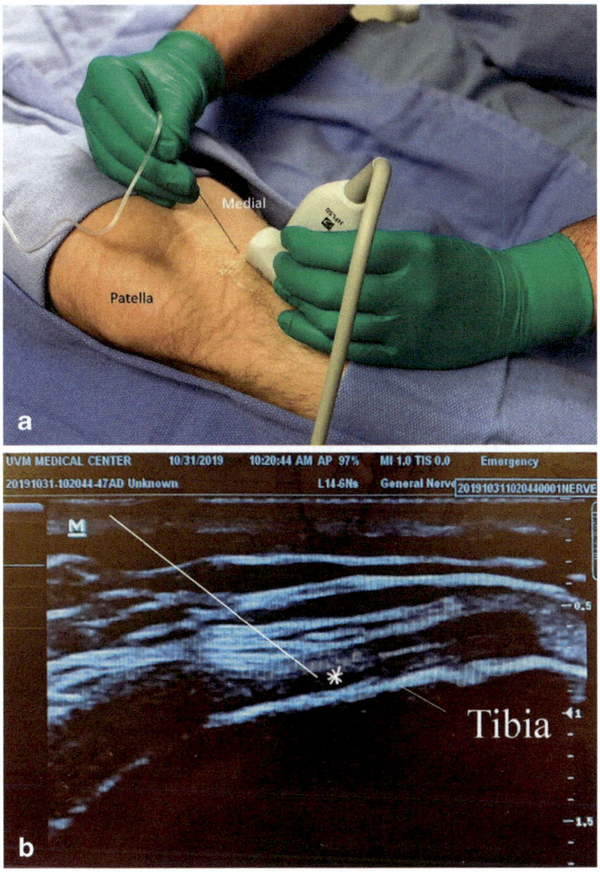

Fig. 2 (**a**) Example of US positioning and needle approach. (**b**) *Approximate location of pes anserinus bursae under ultrasound visualization with example needle path to pes anserinus bursae (solid white line). Notably, the pes anserinus bursae may not be detectable unless inflamed or swollen. US guidance can be used to help rule out other pathology and should be used in conjunction with anatomic landmarks, the point of maximal tenderness and there should be a lack of resistance to injection

Table 3 Summary of potential complications and adverse effects of pes anserinus injection

Bleeding
Infection [13]
Pain with injection and immediately following procedure (up to 30% of patients) [1]
Direct tendon injection, and in extreme cases tendon weakness/rupture [1]
Fat atrophy [1]
Skin depigmentation [1]
Anaphylaxis can occur with the use of lidocaine or bupivacaine anesthetic, and blocks should not be performed if there has been a prior allergic reaction to the anesthetic

Clinical and Technical Pearls

- Pes anserinus bursa injection is a bedside procedure that is aided by ultrasound and can provide prolonged relief while also providing diagnostic information.
- Pes anserinus remains a clinical diagnosis. Careful physical exam, ruling out other potential pathologies, and patient selection are important factors to consider before performing an injection.
- Avoid injecting under pressure.
- Counsel patients on the possibility of pain immediately following injection.

References

1. Helfenstein MJ, Kuromoto J. A síndrome anserina. Rev Bras Reumatol. 2010;50:313–27.
2. Yoon HS, Kim SE, Suh YR, Seo YI, Kim HA. Correlation between ultrasonographic findings and the response to corticosteroid injection in pes anserinus tendinobursitis syndrome in knee osteoarthritis patients. J Korean Med Sci. 2005;20:109–12.
3. Unlu Z, Ozmen B, Tarhan S, Boyvoda S, Goktan C. Ultrasonographic evaluation of pes anserinus tendino-bursitis in patients with type 2 diabetes mellitus. J Rheumatol. 2003;30:352–4.
4. Toktas H, Dundar U, Adar S, Solak O, Ulasli AM. Ultrasonographic assessment of pes anserinus tendon and pes anserinus tendinitis bursitis syndrome in patients with knee osteoarthritis. Mod Rheumatol. 2014;25:128–33.
5. Rennie W, Saifuddin A. Pes anserine bursitis: incidence in symptomatic knees and clinical presentation. Skelet Radiol. 2005;34:395–8.
6. Marra MD, Crema MD, Chung M, Roemer FW, Hunter DJ, Zaim S, et al. MRI features of cystic lesions around the knee. Knee. 2008;15:423–38.
7. Forbes JR, Helms CA, Janzen DL. Acute pes anserine bursitis: MR imaging. Radiology. 1995;194:525–7.
8. Finnoff JT, Nutz DJ, Henning PT, Hollman JH, Smith J. Accuracy of ultrasound-guided versus unguided pes anserinus bursa injections. PM&R. 2010;2:732–9.
9. Draghi F, Danesino GM, Coscia D, Precerutti M, Pagani C. Overload syndromes of the knee in adolescents: sonographic findings. J Ultrasound. 2008;11:151–7.
10. Alvarez-Nemegyei J, Canoso JJ. Evidence-based soft tissue rheumatology IV. JCR J Clin Rheumatol. 2004;10:205–6.
11. Sarifakioglu B, Afsar SI, Yalbuzdag SA, Ustaömer K, Bayramoğlu M. Comparison of the efficacy of physical therapy and corticosteroid injection in the treatment of pes anserine tendino-bursitis. J Phys Ther Sci. 2016;28:1993–7.
12. Larsson L, Baum J. The syndrome of anserina bursitis: an overlooked diagnosis. Arthritis Rheum. 1985;28:1062–5.
13. Hemler DE, Ward WK, Karstetter KW, Bryant PM. Saphenous nerve entrapment caused by pes anserine bursitis mimicking stress fracture of the tibia. Arch Phys Med Rehabil. 1991;72:336–7.
14. Lee JH, Kim KJ, Jeong YG, Lee NS, Han SY, Lee CG, et al. Pes anserinus and anserine bursa: anatomical study. Anat Cell Biol. 2014;47:127–31.
15. Zaffagnini S, Golanò P, Farinas O, Depasquale V, Strocchi R, Cortecchia S, et al. Vascularity and neuroreceptors of the pes anserinus: anatomic study. Clin Anat. 2003;16:19–24.
16. Lee JH, Lee JU, Yoo SW. Accuracy and efficacy of ultrasound-guided pes anserinus bursa injection. J Clin Ultrasound. 2019;47(2):77–82.

Further Reading

Waldman SD. Atlas of pain management injection techniques. 4th ed. Amsterdam: Elsevier; 2017.

Genicular Nerves Blocks

Priyanka Ghosh and Lynn Kohan

Essential Concepts

- Genicular nerve blocks are an effective tool to diagnose and treat osteoarthritic knee pain.
- The most common nerves targeted for nerve block are the superior medial, superior lateral, and inferior medial genicular nerves.
- The procedure can be performed with an ultrasound approach at the bedside.
- Treating OA causing knee pain is the main goal of a genicular nerve block.
- Genicular nerve blocks are relatively technically easy to perform and well tolerated, and patients experience relatively few side effects.
- Pain relief is rapid, and the duration of therapeutic benefit may last days to weeks, to months.

1 Genicular Nerve Blocks

Overview

Knee pain, including osteoarthritis of the knee, affects 250 million people worldwide, and 20–30% of those over the age of 65 have knee pain [1]. Treatment for knee pain includes conservative options such as physical therapy, anti-inflammatory

P. Ghosh
Department of Anesthesia, Weill Cornell Medicine, New York, NY, USA

L. Kohan (✉)
Department of Anesthesiology, University of Virginia Health System, Charlottesville, VA, USA
e-mail: Lrk9g@hscmail.mcc.virginia.edu

D. Souza et al. (eds.), *Bedside Pain Management Interventions*,
https://doi.org/10.1007/978-3-031-11188-4_71

drugs, and injections with steroids or hyaluronic acid. Total knee arthroplasty (TKA) remains the gold standard for advanced knee OA, however, even after surgery almost half of patients, approximately 44%, report persistent pain [1]. Unfortunately, knee pain has a lack of optimal treatment options, necessitating alternative methods to manage these patients. A relatively novel option is blockade of the genicular nerves, the sensory nerves which lie on the periosteum before entering the knee joint capsule and are easily located using bony landmarks and ultrasound guidance. More commonly, this procedure has been performed with the use of fluoroscopic guidance, however, the procedure may be done with ultrasound guidance thus enabling it to be performed at the bedside.

Indications and Contraindications

Patients who have refractory knee pain despite more conservative measures are good candidates for genicular nerve blocks. Other appropriate patients are patients with OA who want to avoid surgery, are not candidates for surgery, patients who have failed knee replacement and found to have no structural issues with their replacement, and patients who have had successful pain relief with genicular nerve blocks or radiofrequency ablation (RFA) in the past whose pain has returned (Table 1). Genicular nerve blocks are relatively safe and have relatively few contraindications, the majority falling into either active infection at the site of nerve block or unstable or unsuitable knee joint anatomy.

Clinical Anatomy

The innervation to the anterior knee capsule is complex (Fig. 1). Description of the trajectory of the genicular nerves supplying the anterior knee capsule has varied in the literature [2]. Three of the branches that supply the anterior knee capsule are the superior medial (SM), superior lateral (SL), and inferior medial (IM) genicular nerves.

The genicular nerves are traditionally thought to arise from branches of three major nerves: the sciatic, femoral, and obturator, which are all derived from the lumbar plexus [3, 4]; however, their anatomic origins can be somewhat variable [5].

Table 1 Patients suitable for genicular nerve block

Patients with refractory knee pain secondary to OA who have failed conservative treatment
Patients with all Kellgren–Lawrence grades can be considered
Patients with refractory OA knee pain who want to avoid surgery
Patients with refractory OA knee pain who are not good surgical candidates secondary to high body mass index (BMI)
Patients with refractory OA knee pain who are not good surgical candidates because of co-morbidities
Patients who have failed knee replacement and found to have no structural problems with their replacement
Patients who had previous successful genicular nerve block or RFA, whose pain has returned

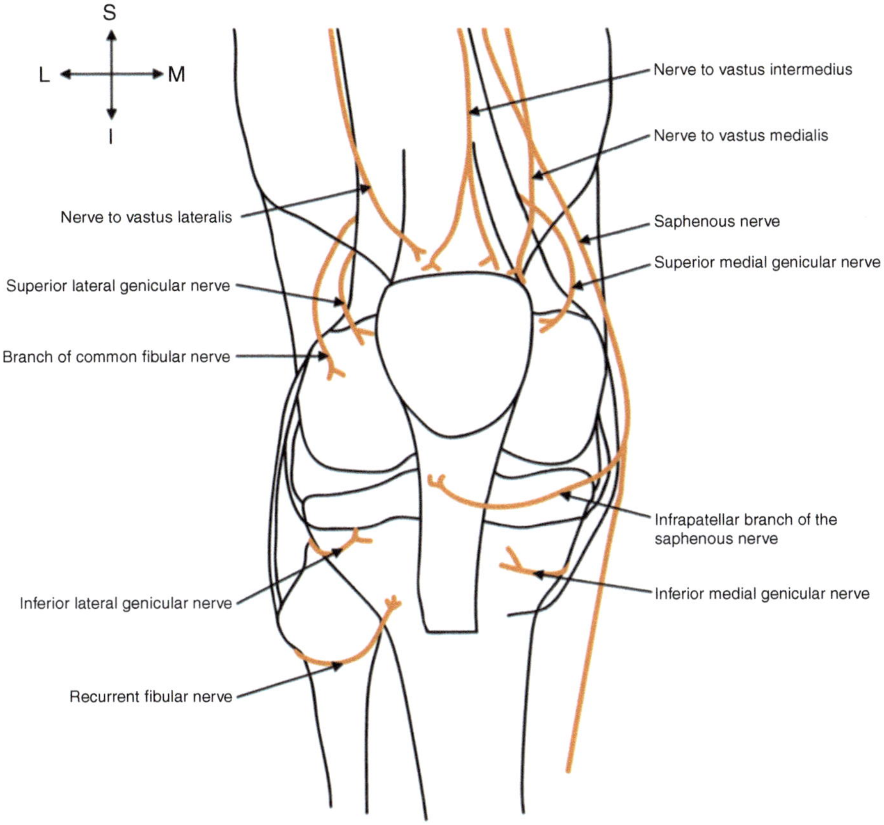

Fig. 1 Innervation of the anterior knee capsule. (Printed with permission from Vanneste B, Tomlinson J, Desmet M, Krol A. Feasibility of an ultrasound-guided approach to radiofrequency ablation of the superiorlateral, superiormedial, and inferiormedial genicular nerves: a cadaveric study. Regional Anesthesia Pain Medicine 2019; 0: 1–5)

Within the popliteal fossa, the sciatic nerve bifurcates into the tibial and common peroneal nerves. The tibial nerve remains posterior in the lower leg and gives rise to the SM and IM genicular nerves, which innervate the superior and inferior medial aspects of the knee joint respectively. The SM nerve may also arise from the femoral nerve [5]. The common peroneal nerve continues into the anterior compartment of the lower leg and gives rise to the SL genicular nerve, which innervates the anterior portion of the knee; it also gives off the inferior lateral genicular nerve (IL) which is not targeted due to its close proximity to the common peroneal nerve causing foot drop. The saphenous nerve, a cutaneous branch of the femoral nerve, gives off the suprapatellar and infrapatellar (IP) genicular nerves to the anterior portion of the knee. The obturator nerve has a more variable contribution than other nerves. Its posterior branch can provide an articular branch to the posterior knee. The main three targets for genicular nerve blocks are the SL, SM and IM genicular nerves.

Equipment and Supplies

Genicular nerve blocks are easily performed at the bedside, utilizing ultrasound-guidance or can be performed in the fluoroscopy suite. Depending on patient body habitus, you can utilize 22 or 25 G 2 or 3.5 in. needles. If 22 G needles are employed a small 25–27-gauge 1–1.5 in. needle is used to locally anesthetize the skin. The three procedure needles are inserted near the three sites of interest and injected with 0.5 mL of local anesthetic at each site, for a total of 1.5 mL of total injectate for three sites for a plane block. For a therapeutic block, utilize 2 mL of injectate per site (Table 2).

Ultrasound Technique

The patient is positioned supine with a pillow underneath the popliteal fossa to lessen discomfort. The area to be treated is prepped and draped in sterile manner. A 12 MHz linear transducer is utilized. The transducer should first be placed parallel to the long bone shaft and moved up or down to identify the epicondyle of the long bone (Fig. 2).

For the SL genicular nerve, the transducer can be placed in a coronal plane on the lateral side of the femoral shaft. The transducer should then be moved distally and centered on the junction of the between the lateral femoral condyle and the shaft [6]. For the SM genicular nerve, the transducer should be placed on the medial side of the femoral shaft and then moved distally to the junction of the medial femoral condyle and the shaft [6]. For the IM genicular nerve can be placed in a coronal plane on the medial side of the tibial shaft. The probe can then be moved proximally to the junction of the medial epicondyle and the shaft [6] (Fig. 2).

Next one can confirm the location of the genicular arteries with Doppler flow. Once the arteries are identified, the SM, SL, and IM genicular nerves can be identified adjacent to the arteries (Fig. 3).

Ultrasound-guided identification of the genicular nerve block target sites.

Insert the needle tip, in plane in the long-axis view next to each genicular artery, aspirate to assure no vascular puncture and inject 0.5 mL of injectate at each of the three sites. Remove the needles and place band-aid over injection site if warranted.

Table 2 Required supplies for genicular nerve blocks

Syringe	5 mL syringes [2]
Needle	25–27-Gauge (G) 1–1.5 in. needle [3] 25 G 2 in. or 3.5 in. **OR** 22 G 2 in. or 3.5 in. needles [3]
Ultrasound	Linear 12 MHz probe
Anesthetic	1–2% Lidocaine for numbing skin; 0.25–0.5% bupivacaine for injectate
Corticosteroid	Triamcinolone 5–40 mg (t1/2 life: 18–36 h), betamethasone 10 mg (t1/2 life: 36–54 h), dexamethasone 4 mg (t1/2 life: 36–54 h) Methylprednisolone 80–125 mg (t1/2 life: 18–36 h)
Adjuncts	Can consider adding clonidine

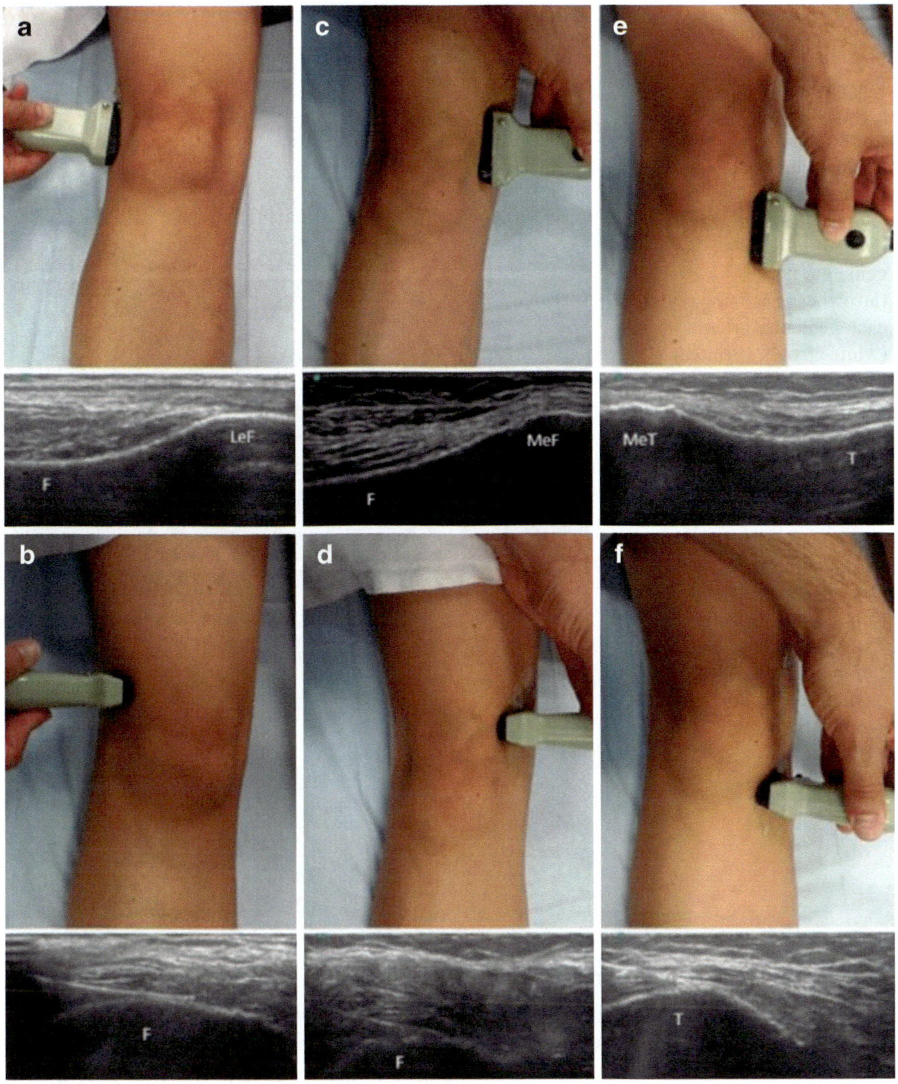

Fig. 2 (**a**–**c**) Probe positioning (in healthy volunteer) and ultrasound images (in cadaver) with the RF cannula in the final position. (**a**) Target point for the SLGN in the coronal plane. (**b**) Final position of the RF cannula for the SLGN in the transverse plane. (**c**) Target point for the SMGN in the coronal plane. (**d**) Final position of the RF cannula for the SMGN in the transverse plane. (**e**) Target point for the IMGN in the coronal plane. (**f**) Final position of the RF cannula for the IMGN in the transverse plane. Left is proximal, right is distal (**a**, **c**, **e**); left is anterior, right is posterior (**b**, **d**, **e**). *F* femur, *IMGN* inferomedial genicular nerve, *LeF* lateral epicondyle femur, *MeF* medial epicondyle femur, *MeT* medial epicondyle tibia, *RF* radiofrequency, *SLGN* superolateral genicular nerve, *SMGN* superomedial genicular nerve, *T* tibia. (Printed with permission from Vanneste B, Tomlinson J, Desmet M, Krol A. Feasibility of an ultrasound-guided approach to radiofrequency ablation of the superiorlateral, superiormedial, and inferiormedial genicular nerves: a cadaveric study. Regional Anesthesia Pain Medicine 2019; 0: 1–5)

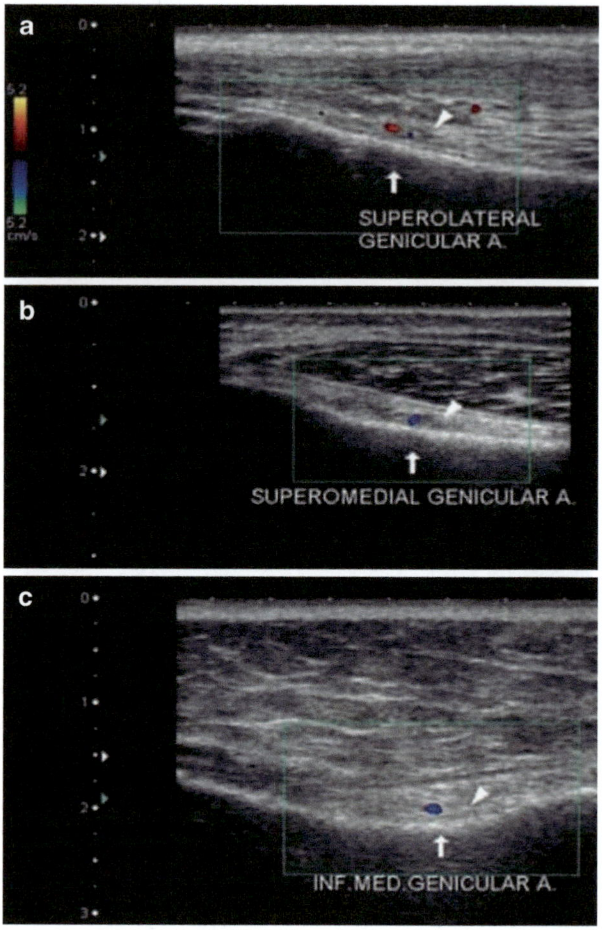

Fig. 3 Ultrasound-guided identification of GNB target sites. Representative longitudinal images of the knee at the level of the distal femoral condyle and medial tibial metaphysis are shown. The superior lateral (**a**), superior medial (**b**), and inferior medial (**c**) genicular nerves (arrowhead) accompany each genicular artery (white arrow). (Printed with permission from Choi W, PhD, Shin JW, MD, Lee IG, MD, Seo DK, MD, Lee SH, MD, Kim DH, Choi SS, Yoon SH. Ultrasound-Guided Genicular Nerve Block for Knee Osteoarthritis: A Double-Blind, Randomized Controlled Trial of Local Anesthetic Alone or in Combination with Corticosteroid Randomized Trial Pain Physician 2018; 21: 41–52)

Potential Complications and Adverse Effects

Although generally well tolerated by patients, occasional adverse reactions and complications can occur which the clinician should be aware of when performing the genicular nerve blockade (Table 3). Aside from the discomfort of pain or muscle spasms, adverse events are relatively rare. They include vascular injection of local anesthesia given proximity to genicular arteries, increased pain, decreased mobility and increased stiffness.

Table 3 Additional potential complications and adverse effects

Pressure should be applied to prevent hematoma production in patients with bleeding disorders or on anticoagulation
Due to the risk of vasoconstriction of the genicular artery resulting in necrosis, local anesthetic with epinephrine should not be used
Risks should be weighed against potential benefits when utilizing genicular nerve blocks during pregnancy
Anaphylaxis can occur with use of lidocaine or bupivacaine anesthetic, and blocks should not be performed if there has been a prior allergic reaction to the anesthetic
Patients receiving frequent injections or perhaps using corticosteroids, either orally or as a result of other interventional procedures, are at risk for developing Cushing syndrome or adrenal insufficiency. Clinicians must be diligent in questioning patients specifically about the potential recent use of steroids as this medication history is often not reported by the patient
Meticulous attention should be paid in patients with bony defects or prior TKR while performing this block

Clinical and Technical Pearls

- Genicular nerve blocks, performed via ultrasound, are guided by identification of the genicular arteries next to the superior medial, superior lateral, and inferior medial genicular nerves.
- Imperative to utilize Doppler flow on ultrasound and very carefully aspirate before each injection to avoid intravascular injection given the proximity to the arteries.

References

1. Crawford DC, Miller LE, Block JE. Conservative management of symptomatic knee osteoarthritis: a flawed strategy? Orthop Rev (Pavia). 2013;5:e2.
2. Franco CD, Buvanendran A, Petersohn JD, et al. Innervation of the anterior capsule of the human knee: implications for radiofrequency ablation. Reg Anesth Pain Med. 2015;40:363–8.
3. Hirasawa Y, Okajima S, Ohta M, Tokioka T. Nerve distribution to the human knee joint: anatomical and immunohistochemical study. Int Orthop. 2000;24(1):1–4.
4. Kennedy JC, Alexander IJ, Hayes KC. Nerve supply of the human knee and its functional importance. Am J Sports Med. 1982;10(6):329–35.
5. Tran J, Peng PWH, Lam K, et al. Anatomical study of the innervation of anterior knee joint capsule: implication for image-guided intervention. Reg Anesth Pain Med. 2018;43:407–1.
6. Vanneste B, Tomlinson J, Desmet M, Krol A. Feasibility of an ultrasound-guided approach to radiofrequency ablation of the superolateral, superomedial, and inferomedial genicular nerves: a cadaveric study. Reg Anesth Pain Med. 2019;2019:100381.

Further Reading

Fonkoue L, Behets CW, Steyaert A, et al. Accuracy of fluoroscopic-guided genicular nerve blockade: a need for revisiting anatomical landmarks. Reg Anesth Pain Med. 2019;44(10):950–8. https://doi.org/10.1136/rapm-2019-100451.

Ankle Block

Peter Merjavy

Essential Concepts

Ankle blocks can be performed easily at the bedside using either the landmark technique or with ultrasound guidance.

Ultrasound guidance may improve block success compared with the landmark technique.

The ankle blocks provides anesthesia/analgesia to the foot and toes.

The foot is supplied by five nerves. Two of them are deep and three are superficial.

- **TD**—The **T**wo **D**eep are the **T**ibial nerve and **D**eep Peroneal nerve.
- **SSS**—Three **S**uperficial are the **S**ural, **S**aphenous and **S**uperficial Peroneal nerves.
- All nerves are branches of sciatic nerve (sacral plexus) except the saphenous nerve, which is the terminal branch of femoral nerve (lumbar plexus) (Fig. 1).

P. Merjavy (✉)
Anaesthetic Department, Craigavon Area University Teaching Hospital, Southern Health and Social Care Trust, Portadown, Co.Armagh, Northern Ireland, UK

D. Souza et al. (eds.), *Bedside Pain Management Interventions*,
https://doi.org/10.1007/978-3-031-11188-4_72

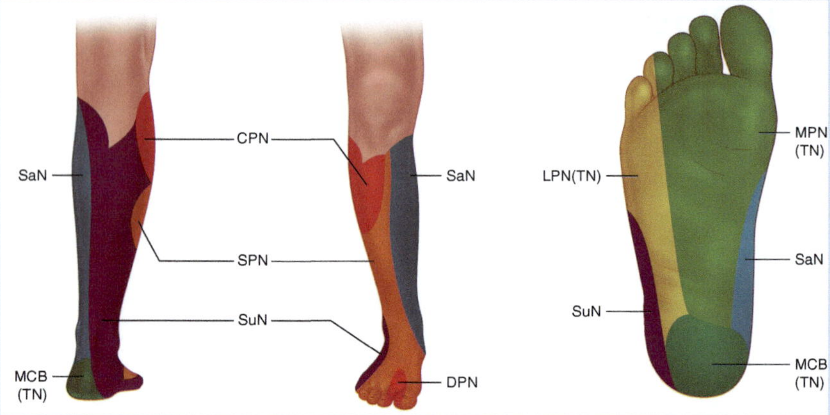

Fig. 1 Dermatomes of Saphenous Nerve (SaN), Sural Nerve (SuN), Medial Calcaneal Branch (MCB) of Tibial Nerve (TN), Medial Plantat Nerve (MPN) of TN, Common Peroneal Nerve (CPN), Superficial Peroneal Nerve (SPN), and the Deep Peroneal Nere (DPN)

1 Overview

Regional anesthesia to the foot can be challenging secondary to the complicated nerve supply of the foot and varied locations of the nerves around the ankle. Anesthesia and analgesia, however can be adequately achieved via the use of an ankle block either via a landmark or ultrasound guided technique. An advantage of the ankle block over other lower-limb blocks is that it is associated with minimal motor block, allowing early mobilization especially in the ambulatory surgery setting [1]. An ankle block can be safely offered to patients undergoing foot surgery as it can provide both intraoperative anaesthesia and postoperative analgesia. Ankle blocks can also be used for analgesia after various foot injuries. Traditionally the landmark technique has been considered as an infiltration block. Advantages of the ultrasound technique include the potential for more reliable surgical anaesthesia and reduction of local anaesthetic volume required [1].

2 Indications and Contraindications

Indications

An ankle block can be used to provide anesthesia/analgesia for most types of foot surgeries including forefoot reconstruction, bunionectomies, arthroplasty, osteotomy, and amputation [2–4]. Ankle blocks can also be used to provide analgesia for foot fractures, and pain from soft tissue injuries. Additionally, ankle blocks can be utilized for diagnostic or therapeutic purposes for spastic equinovarus or sympathetically mediated pain. Ankle blocks are ideal for outpatient surgery since motor block of the proximal leg and calf does not occur [2–4].

Contraindications

- Absolute contraindications: patient refusal, infection at the site of injection, allergy to local anaesthetics and/or adjuvants [4].
- Relative contraindications: bleeding disorders or active effect of anticoagulants (ankle block may still be performed with informed consent and appropriate caution during and after the procedure); peripheral neuropathy, peripheral demyelinating disease, or pre-existing sensory deficits in the distribution of the nerves involved. Ankle tourniquet is generally well tolerated by patients up to 90 min. Calf or thigh tourniquets are relatively contraindicated as the area of tourniquet is not covered by the nerve block and will require more proximal block, neuraxial block or general anaesthesia. Solutions containing adrenaline (epinephrine) should be avoided for the ankle block because of potential risk of compromising the distal vascular supply if the foot [4].

3 Equipment and Supplies

- Patent IV access
- Anxiolysis—pharmacological (Midazolam 0.5–1 mg, Fentanyl 50–75 μg) or non-pharmacological (music via headphones, virtual reality glasses … etc.) if needed.
- Personal protective equipment (hat, mask) and sterile gloves
- Skin prep solution such as Chlorhexidine gluconate 2% with isopropyl alcohol 70%
- Ultrasound machine with high frequency linear transducer (12–15 MHz) and sterile ultrasound probe cover (transparent dressing or sleeve) and sterile ultrasound gel
- Trolley with sterile tray or sterile drape
- 4 cm 27 G needle (25G needle can be used as well) with 2 × 10 or 1 × 20 mL (cc) syringe
- Long-acting local anesthetic (0.75–1% Ropivacaine, 0.5% Bupivacaine or 0.5–0.75% Levobupivacaine)
- Short acting local anesthetic (1% lidocaine) for anesthetizing skin is usually not necessary.
- Sterile dressings to cover the injection points

4 Ankle Block

Tibial Nerve

Anatomy

The tibial nerve TN (*nervus tibialis*) is the larger of the two terminal branches of the sciatic nerve. It continues further caudally within the popliteal fossa toward the popliteal skin crease and lies posterior and lateral to the popliteal vessels. Within the lower aspect of the popliteal fossa, it sends sensory and muscular branches to the major ankle flexors (the gastrocnemius and soleus muscles) as well as articular branches to the knee joint. The TN then courses distally with the popliteal vessels deep to the tendinous arch of the soleus and runs along the dorsal surface of the tibialis posterior muscle. At the distal third of the lower leg, the TN emerges from beneath the soleus and enters the foot through the tarsal tunnel behind the medial malleolus and lies posterior to the posterior tibial vessels [5, 6].

Proximal to the medial malleolus, the TN (often wrongly named in this location as posterior tibial nerve) gives off its medial calcaneal branch (be aware, that lateral calcaneal branch comes from the sural nerve), which supplies the medial part of the heel. At the level of the medial malleolus, the TN lies on and superficial to the belly and tendon of flexor hallucis longus (FHL) muscle, covered by superficial and deep fascia, and is typically found immediately dorsal to the posterior tibial artery [5, 7]. As the TN crosses over to the plantar aspect of the foot, it gives off the medial and lateral plantar nerves, which provide sensory and motor innervation to the foot and ankle. The medial plantar nerve supplies digital nerves to the medial 3 1/2 toes, whereas the lateral plantar nerve sends digital nerves to the lateral 1 1/2 toes [7].

Sonoanatomy

The nerve typically appears hyperechoic with honeycomb pattern. A useful mnemonic for the relevant structures seen from anterior to posterior is "Tom, Dick ANd Harry", which refers to the **T**ibialis posterior tendon, flexor **D**igitorum longus tendon, **A**rtery + **N**erve + (typically) two veins and flexor **H**allucis longus tendon (FHL) lying deep to these structures. The nerve's intimate relationship with the artery should be kept in mind to avoid misidentification as TN usually lies posterior to the posterior tibial vessels but occasionally lies anteriorly. The tibial nerve can be confused with the FHL tendon. In case of doubt, scan proximally and distally to identify the structures again. The tibial nerve can be seen lying on the sheath of FHL, which appears as a hyperechoic (white) line. The FHL tendon is seen within the muscle [4, 6] (Fig. 2).

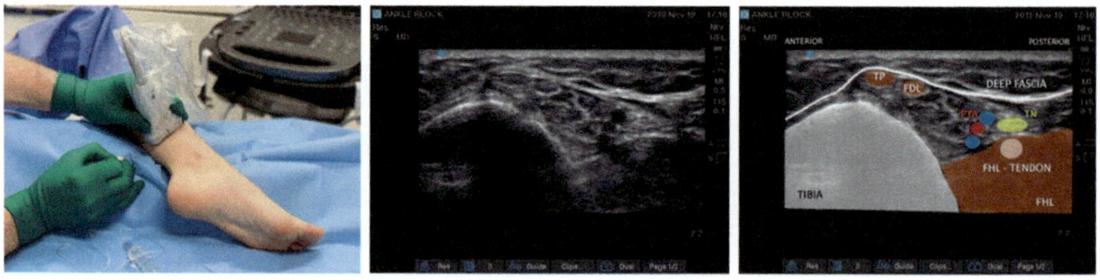

Fig. 2 Patient position and needle approach for U/S guided tibial nerve (TN) block. U/S image shows relationship of posterior tibial (PT), flexor digitorum longus (FDL), flexor hallucis longus (FHL) muscles as well as posterior tibial artery (PTA) with associates veins and deep fascia

Block Performance

- Scan just above the level of the medial malleolus, from tibia to Achilles tendon.
- Identify all the structures described above, by scanning up and down the leg.
- Approach the nerve from posterior to anterior (to avoid tibialis posterior and flexor digitorum longus tendons) at a level where the nerve is most easily visible; which may be up to 10 cm proximal to the ankle.
- Aim for a 6 o'clock position then a 12 o'clock position to get a circumferential spread of local anaesthetic (LA); 5–7 mL is a typical volume.
- Ensure that your probe rests proximally enough to ensure the needle approach will not pierce the Achilles tendon.
- Caution must be used when the tibial nerve lies anterior to the vessels as the tendon of FHL then lies posterior to vessels and may easily be mistaken for the nerve.

Deep Peroneal Nerve

Anatomy

The deep peroneal nerve DPN (*nervus peroneus profundus*) is a branch of common peroneal nerve CPN, which is the lateral terminal branch of the sciatic nerve. It travels obliquely along the lateral border of the popliteal fossa just medial to the tendon of the long head of the biceps femoris muscle. It exits the popliteal fossa by crossing over the lateral head of the gastrocnemius and can be found subcutaneously between the fibular head and the peroneus longus muscle.

As it runs around the neck of the fibula, the CPN divides into its two terminal branches: the superficial and deep peroneal nerve. The deep peroneal nerve passes posterior to the extensor digitorum longus and anterior to the interosseous membrane, where it is joined by the anterior tibial artery [5].

The deep peroneal nerve enters the dorsal aspect of the foot, deep to the extensor retinaculum between the tendons of extensor hallucis and digitorum longus and usually lateral to the dorsalis pedis artery (continuation of anterior tibial artery). Along its course, the deep peroneal nerve supplies the anterior muscle group of the lower leg and provides an articular branch to the ankle joint as well as a cutaneous branch to the first interdigital space [5, 6].

Sonoanatomy

In the leg the deep peroneal nerve descends on the anterior surface of the interosseus membrane (*membrana interossea*) before passing medially over the anterolateral surface of the distal tibia. Throughout its course the nerve is associated with the anterior tibial vessels. As it descends, it is commonly described as lying lateral to the vessels then anterior then reverts to lateral. However, the nerve may also lie medial to the vessels [7].

Proximal to the ankle joint the structures seen from medial to lateral are tibialis anterior, extensor hallucis longus, anterior tibial artery, deep peroneal nerve and extensor digitorum longus. The nerve usually appears hypoechoic with a hyperechoic rim, but it is small and often difficult to distinguish from the surrounding tissue [4, 6] (Figs. 3 and 4).

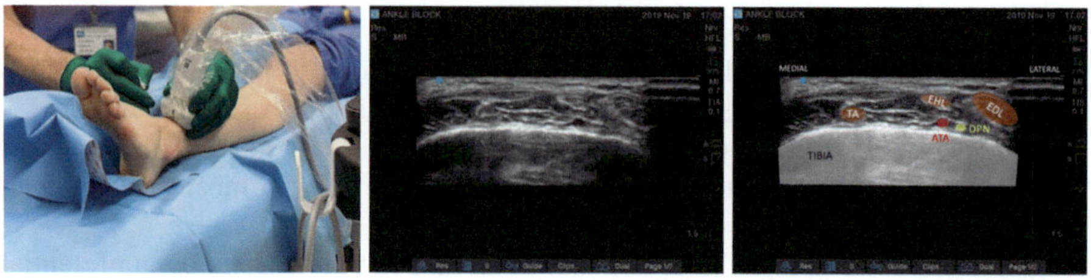

Fig. 3 Patient position and needle approach for U/S guided deep peroneal nerve (DPN) block. U/S image shows relationship of tibialis anterior (TA), extensor hallucis longus (EHL) and extensor digitorum longus (EDL) muscles with anterior tibial artery (ATA) at the distal part of tibia

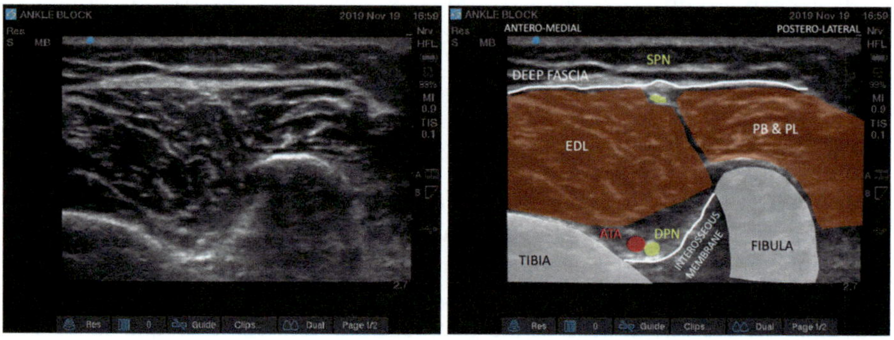

Fig. 4 U/S image shows both superficial peroneal nerve (SPN) and deep peroneal nerve (DPN) and their relationship with extensor digitorum longus (EDL), peroneus brevis (PB), peroneus longus (PL) muscles, anterior tibial artery (ATA), deep fascia and interosseous membrane in the middle of the calf. One needle insertion point can be used to block both nerves

Block Performance

- Use a high resolution and low depth setting of your ultrasound probe
- Place the probe in transverse axis over the ankle joint.
- Identify the pulsatile anterior tibial artery/dorsal pedis artery (it is often accompanied by two veins). Do not apply too much pressure as the vessel is easily compressed.
- Trace the artery proximally and use the bright hyperechoic reflection of the tibia to contrast the nerve and vessel. The deep peroneal nerve is usually seen as a small hypoechoic structure rolling over the top of the vessels from medial to lateral.
- Approach the nerve in-plane from lateral to medial, try to avoid tendons and periosteum as this is quite painful.
- After negative aspiration give 1–2 mL of local anaesthetic (LA).
- If you can't see the nerve, then carefully inject LA on either side of the anterior tibial artery
- You may choose to block the DPN more proximally. In this case place your probe in short axis over middle of shin. Visualise interosseous membrane and

anterior tibial artery. Place your needle tip just lateral to artery and inject 5–7 mL of LA.

- There is a possibility to use same injection point at skin for SPN and proximal approach to DPN.

Superficial Peroneal Nerve

Anatomy

After bifurcation from CPN, the superficial peroneal nerve SPN (*nervus peroneus superficialis*) travels down through the leg lying first between peroneus longus and brevis and then in the groove between peroneus brevis and extensor digitorum longus underneath the cover of deep fascia (*fascia cruris*) to supply the ankle eversion muscles. In the lower third of the anterolateral surface of the leg (10–20 cm above the ankle joint) it pierces the deep fascia and divides into two or three small branches that provide cutaneous sensory innervation to the dorsal aspect of the ankle and foot [4, 5, 7].

Sonoanatomy

In the distal two-thirds of the leg, this nerve emerges between peroneus longus and brevis proximally to lie between peroneus brevis and extensor digitorum longus distally. The nerve pierces the deep fascia to lie superficially in the lower part of the leg before dividing and passing onto the foot.

Proximal to the lateral malleolus, in the anterolateral aspect of the distal third of leg, the structures seen from anteromedial to posterolateral are extensor digitorum longus and peroneus brevis muscle and longus tendon (overlying the fibula). The nerve usually lies in the groove formed by the junction of the two muscles. It can be seen traversing the deep fascia to lie superficially before flattening and dividing as one scans proximally to distally [6].

Be aware that this is a small nerve and there are no helpful vascular landmarks therefore a good understanding of the sono-anatomy is essential for block success [7] (Fig. 5).

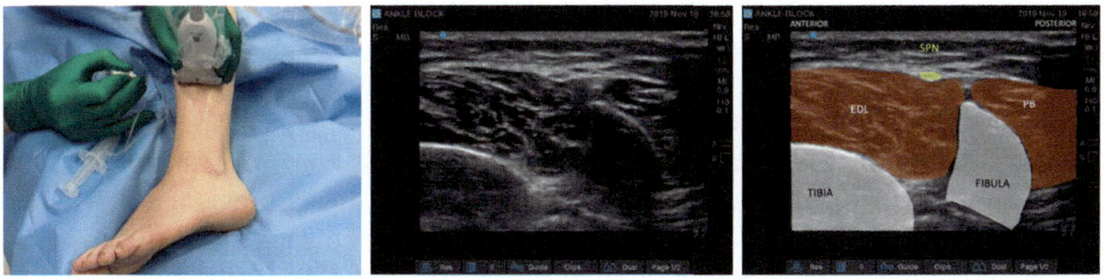

Fig. 5 Patient position and needle approach for U/S guided superficial peroneal (SPN) block. U/S image shows relationship with extensor digitorum longus (EDL) and peroneus brevis (PB) muscles at distal third of the lateral calf

Block Performance

- Aim to block the nerve before it gives off any proximal branches
- Place the probe in the anterolateral aspect of the distal third of the leg in transverse axis (approximately 5–10 cm proximal and anterior to the lateral malleolus).
- Scan up and down and from medial to lateral to identify the above structures.
- As the fibula dives deep two muscle bellies merge towards each other. The anterior muscle is extensor digitorum longus and posteriorly is peroneus brevis (at this level you can usually see the tendon of peroneus longus lying superficial to it as a thin dark band surrounded by a bright connective tissue).
- As you scan proximally keep the junction of these two muscles in the centre of your screen
- The superficial peroneal nerve can be seen passing posteriorly, superficial to the deep fascia over the belly of EDL, before penetrating fascia to lie in the groove formed between the two muscles.
- It lies within this groove for a variable distance before diving between peroneus brevis and longus.
- Scan the course of the nerve until you are confident of its relationship to the other structures

Sural Nerve

Anatomy

The sural nerve SuN (*nervus suralis*) is formed by the union of the medial sural cutaneous nerve MSCN from TN and lateral sural communicating branch LSCN of the CPN at the knee joint (*nervus cutaneus surae medialis et lateralis*). In the majority (81%) of cases, the MSCN descends between the two heads of the gastrocnemius muscles where it receives the peroneal communicating branch (LSCN) to form the common sural nerve. Occasionally, the common sural nerve is derived solely from the TN (18% of cases) or the CPN (1% of cases). SuN then continues distally and courses between the dorsal aspect of the Achilles tendon and the dorsal aspect of the lateral malleolus in close proximity and either anterior or posterior to the small saphenous vein (*vena saphena parva*). The sural nerve provides cutaneous innervation to the posterolateral aspects of the lower leg and ankle, lateral part of the heel as well as the dorsolateral aspect of the foot [5, 6].

Sonoanatomy

Proximal to the lateral malleolus, the sural nerve can be visualized as a small hyperechoic structure that is usually anterior to the compressible small saphenous vein, lying on a fascial plane (deep fascia) between the peroneus brevis anteriorly and Achilles tendon posteriorly. The sural nerve, can be traced back along the posterior aspect of the leg, running in the midline superficial to the Achilles tendon and two bellies of gastrocnemius muscles. A calf tourniquet can be used to increase the size of the vein and facilitate its imaging; the nerve is often found in the immediate vicinity of the vein [4, 6] (Fig. 6).

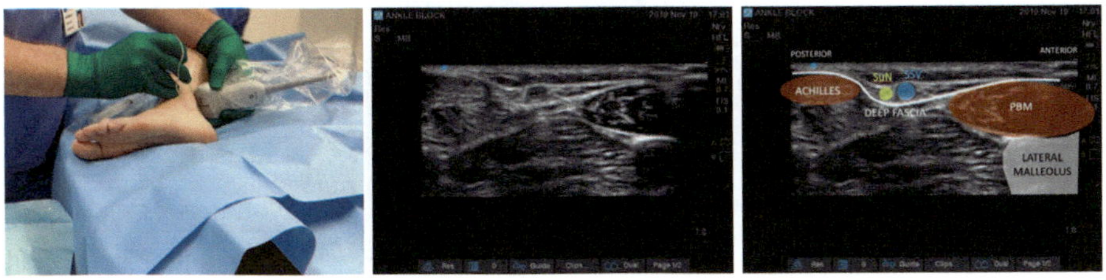

Fig. 6 Patient position and needle approach for U/S guided sural nerve (SuN) block. U/S image shows relationship with Achilles tendon, peroneus brevis (PB) muscle, small saphenous vein (SSV) and deep fascia

Block Performance

- Place the probe over the posterolateral aspect of the leg, just proximal to the lateral malleolus.
- Scan up and down and from anterior to posterior to identify the structures described above and the fascial plane between the peroneus brevis and Achilles tendon to locate the small saphenous vein.
- Tendon of peroneus longus is visible as a dark oval structure, superficial and lying over the belly of peroneus brevis
- Apply only gentle pressure as the vein is easily compressed. The nerve is usually visualized just anterior to the vein.
- Follow the nerve proximally as it passes posteriorly over the Achilles tendon and observe its relationship to the vein to make sure you will block the correct structure
- Using an in-plane approach, inject 1–4 mL of LA.
- Aim to direct your needle with an anterior in-plane approach taking care to avoid the tendon of peroneus longus.

Saphenous Nerve

Anatomy

The saphenous nerve (SaN) is the terminal cutaneous branch of the femoral nerve. It descends the leg medially in close relationship to the great saphenous vein (*vena saphena magna*) before passing anteriorly to the medial malleolus [6].

The SaN innervates the medial part of the lower leg below the knee and medial malleolus down to the first tarsometatarsal joint (usually 5–7 cm distal to medial malleolus). Occasionally (3%) it extends 1–1.5 cm distally, but not to the base of the great toe. It is therefore necessary for medial ankle surgery, but not for forefoot surgery [8].

Sonoanatomy

The saphenous nerve travels down the medial aspect of the leg usually posterior and in close proximity to the great saphenous vein. At the ankle it passes in front of the

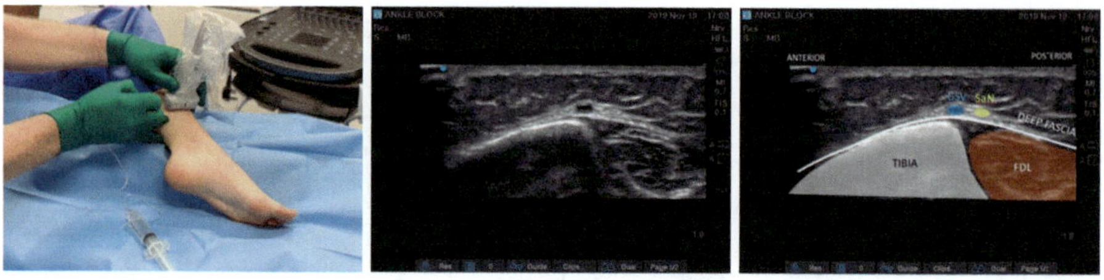

Fig. 7 Patient position and needle approach for U/S guided saphenous nerve (SaN) block. U/S image shows relationship with flexor digitorum longus (FDL) muscle, great saphenous vein (GSV), deep fascia and tibia approximately 5 cm above medial malleolus

medial malleolus. Identifying and visualizing this nerve with ultrasound is often difficult as it is very small and variable. If the surgical site requires the saphenous nerve to be blocked then performing a peri-venous injection around the great saphenous vein proximal to the ankle will suffice.

If the vein has been harvested for coronary grafting a more proximal saphenous block above the knee (true adductor canal block) may be easier to perform [6, 7] (Fig. 7).

Block Performance

- Gently place the probe over the anteromedial aspect of the ankle in the transverse axis, taking care not to compress the vein.
- Scan up and down and try to identify the nerve in close proximity to the vein and inject 1–2 mL of LA
- If not identified, perform a careful peri-venous injection of 3–5 mL of LA.
- The saphenous nerve block is not routinely performed for forefoot surgery, as it rarely supplies sensation this far distally.

Ergonomics

- The injection point for all nerves is more proximal than the landmark technique. This is because of the bony prominence of the malleoli, which compromise good probe to skin contact.
- Whatever the position of the patient, the operator should maintain in-line with the probe and ultrasound screen, so there is no need to turn the head during needle insertion
- If needling with right hand stand, stand on the left-hand side of the patient, all nerves on both legs are accessible from this position so it avoids moving the equipment around the room.
- The patient may be positioned supine with the leg supported off the bed or supine with leg to be blocked crossed over the other leg, lateral decubitus or prone.
- We prefer position the patient supine with leg to be blocked crossed over the knee in a figure '4' position.
- Always start with the tibial nerve, it is the largest nerve and therefore takes the longest for the block to develop (up to 20 min).

- Position your needle initially deep to the nerve in the 6 o'clock position, inject, if spread is not circumferential then reposition your needle to the 12 o'clock position.

Landmark Technique

The tibial nerve is located just behind the medial malleolus, usually posterior to posterior tibial artery. A sharp 25–27G needle is inserted posterior to medial malleolus and posterior tibial artery perpendicular to the skin. Needle is advanced deep to superficial fascia until the contact with the bone is observed. (After withdrawal of 1–2 mm and 5–10 mL (cc) op LA is injected after negative aspiration).

Practitioner should be cautious as tibial nerve can occasionally be found on the other side of the artery and there are frequently one or two veins attached to posterior tibial artery.

Deep peroneal nerve is located immediately lateral to the external hallucis longus muscle tendon (between tendons of extensor hallucis longus EHL and extensor digitorum longus EDL muscles). Anterior tibial artery (caudally known as dorsalis pedis artery) pulse can be usually found medially to the nerve. Index finger of non-dominant hand is used to palpate the groove between EHL and EHL tendons. Needle is inserted just lateral to pulse of the anterior tibial artery with slight cranial orientation until contact with the bone is observed. Needle is then withdrawn 1 mm and 2–3 mL (cc) of LA is injected. This is repeated with redirection of the needle slightly laterally and further 2–3 mL of LA is injected, both after negative aspiration.

Deep peroneal nerve runs on the medial side of the anterior tibial artery in the proximal part of the ankle and moves over to the lateral side approximately at the level of intermalleolar line. However in couple of occasions the nerve is found with significant distance lateral to the artery (1–1.5 cm).

Three superficial nerves—Saphenous, Sural and Superficial peroneal nerves—can be located by subcutaneous infiltration of local anaesthetic from medial edge of Achilles tendon, over the medial malleolus, front part of the intermalleolar space, lateral malleolus to the lateral aspect of the Achilles tendon. As this circumferential LA infiltration is technically a field block, larger volume—17–20 ml (cc)—of LA is often required.

Caution

Ankle block using landmark technique does not take into consideration anatomical variations of the nerves, does not address difficult landmarks (obesity, oedema), is associated with lower success rate, slower block onset times and larger LA volumes required [9–12]. Landmark technique is therefore not recommended to be used in clinical practice when ultrasound is readily available.

5 Potential Complications and Adverse Effects

The complication rate after ankle block is low. Complications include bleeding, infection, and transient paresthesias. Local anesthetic toxicity is rare given the low volume of local anesthetic used [3].

Clinical and Technical Pearls

- Use a 40 mm 27-G hypodermic needle with a extension tube for remote injection. This needle reduces discomfort during injection, however, we would recommend that anaesthesiologists perfect their ‘in-plane’ needle technique before using these very sharp needles.
- Spray the small area immediately before each injection with Ethyl Chloride spray to cool the skin, which reduces the pain on injection.
- A 20-mL Luer-lock syringe does not result in unduly high injection pressures and obviates the need to change syringe during the procedure (potentially allowing air into the system), but we have also used 10-mL syringes.
- We prefer the in-plane technique to ensure excellent visualization of the whole needle shaft and tip at all times during insertion (this is particularly important with 27-G hypodermic needles, which do not possess a short bevelled tip) [6].
- When using veins as landmarks, use as little pressure as possible on the transducer in order to permit the veins to fill.
- The deep peroneal nerve is sometimes difficult to identify on ultrasound. An injection of small amount of LA around the artery may help with visualization.
- If the smaller superficial nerves (sural, saphenous and superficial peroneal) are not seen, these nerves can be blocked using the anatomical landmark technique—injecting local anaesthetic into the subcutaneous tissue as a “skin wheal”; for the sural nerve, inject from the Achilles tendon to the lateral malleolus; for the superficial peroneal and the saphenous, inject anteriorly from one malleolus to the other, taking care to avoid injuring the great saphenous vein [4].
- When testing the block, remember to inform the patient that the lateral border of the foot (sural) or the medial/proximal foot (saphenous) will feel normal if you have not blocked these nerves.
- We offer ultrasound-guided ankle blocks to our patients undergoing day-case forefoot surgery. The advantages of the technique in our experience are rapid onset of reliable surgical anaesthesia, efficiency of placement (the nerves are found swiftly), and reduction of local anaesthetic volume required (we routinely use a total volume of 15 mL of local anaesthetic, but have reduced these volumes to 10 mL for bilateral surgery).
- Effective anxiolysis can be easily achieved before performing multiple LA injections using 0.5–1 mg of i.v. midazolam and 50–75 μg of i.v. fentanyl or other short-acting opioid.
- By avoiding general anaesthesia, our patients can step off the operating table, bypass the recovery unit and be ready for discharge immediately, which is ideal in the day-case unit [6].
- Block duration is related to type and concentration of LA used. We use 0.5–0.75% Levobupivacaine and the duration of block is 20–28 h. It is

important to inform the patient about the rebound pain when nerve block wears off. In one study most of patients (78%) felt pain on block regression was acceptable but (22%) patients experienced difficult pain management. Patients appreciated avoiding GA: 'no nausea', 'not woozy.' Some reported pre-operative apprehension, however all patients said they would have the same anaesthetic technique again [13].

- 8 mg of systemic (i.v.) dexamethasone is equivalent to perineural dexamethasone (4 mg) in prolonging the analgesic duration of an ankle block with ropivacaine 0.375%. We see the protective effect against nausea or vomiting using the systemic route and therefore favour the systemic route given the possibility for increased risk of neurotoxicity of perineural dexamethasone [14].

Take Home message

- Ultrasound-guided ankle block provides reliable anaesthesia and postoperative analgesia for awake forefoot surgery, allowing early mobilization in the day-care setting.
- Ankle block performed using ultrasound-guidance may improve block success, when compared with anatomic landmark-guided technique.
- A good knowledge of anatomy and sono-anatomy is essential.
- Block the tibial nerve first; as this nerve block takes the longest time to develop.
- Use of a 27-G needle reduces the discomfort of using a standard block needle in awake patients (however, great care is required with this sharp needle).

References

1. Fredrickson MJ. Ultrasound-guided ankle block. Anaesth Intensive Care. 2009;37(1):143–5.
2. Delbos A, Philippe M, Clément C, Olivier R, Coppens S. Ultrasound-guided ankle block. History revisited. Best Pract Res Clin Anaesthesiol. 2019;33(1):79–93. https://doi.org/10.1016/j.bpa.2019.05.002. Epub 2019 May 7. PMID: 31272656.
3. Albaqami MS, Alqarni AA. Efficacy of regional anesthesia using ankle block in ankle and foot surgeries: a systematic review. Eur Rev Med Pharmacol Sci. 2022;26(2):471–84.
4. Vandepitte C, Lopez AM, Boxstael SV, Jalil H. Ultrasound-guided ankle block. In: Hadzic's texbook of regional anesthesia and acute pain management. 2nd ed. McGraw-Hill Education; 2017. p. 636–41. ISBN 978-0-07-174122-4.
5. Tran DQ, Salinas FV, Benzon HT, Neal JM. Lower extremity regional anesthesia: essentials of our current understanding. Reg Anesth Pain Med. 2019;44:143143–80.
6. Purushothaman L, Allan A, Bedforth N. Ultrasound-guided ankle block. Contin Educ Anaesth Crit Care Pain. 2013;13(5):174–8.
7. Allan A, Scarfe M. Ankle block: landmark and ultrasound techniques. Anaesthesia Tutorial of the Week 178. www.totw.anaesthesiologists.org. Accessed 10 May 2010.

8. Lopez AM, Sala-Blanch X, Magaldi M, Poggio D, Asuncion J, Franco CD. Ultrasound-guided ankle block for forefoot surgery: the contribution of the saphenous nerve. Reg Anesth Pain Med. 2012;37:554–7.
9. Chin KJ, Wong NWY, Macfarlane AJR, Chan WWS. Ultrasound-guided versus anatomic landmark-guided ankle blocks: a 6-year retrospective review. Reg Anesth Pain Med. 2011;36:611–8.
10. Redborg KE, Antonakakis JG, Beach ML, Chinn CD, Sites BD. Ultrasound improves the success rate of a tibial nerve block at the ankle. Reg Anesth Pain Med. 2009;34:256–60.
11. Redborg KE, Sites BD, Chinn CD, et al. Ultrasound improves the success rate of a sural nerve block at the ankle. Reg Anesth Pain Med. 2009;34:24–8.
12. Shah A, et al. Landmark technique vs ultrasound-guided approach for posterior tibial nerve block in cadaver models. Indian J Orthop. 2020;54(1):38–42.
13. Sadler A, Raju P. Awake ankle surgery under ultrasound-guided ankle block: patient experience. Reg Anesth Pain Med. 2019;44(Suppl 1):A268–9.
14. Marty P, et al. Perineural versus systemic dexamethasone in front-foot surgery under ankle block: a randomized double-blind study. Reg Anesth Pain Med. 2018;43:732–7.

Further Reading

Bigeleisen PE, et al. Section III, Chapter 23—Ultrasound guided ankle blocks. In: Ultrasound guided regional anesthesia and pain medicine. Baltimore: LWW; 2010. p. 140–4.

Georgiou A, et al. Chapter 8—The lower limb. In: Applied anatomy for anaesthesia and intensive care. Cambridge: Cambridge University Press; 2014. p. 178–83.

Marhofer P. Chapter 14.8—Ankle blocks. In: Ultrasound guidance in regional anaesthesia. 2nd ed. Oxford: Oxford University Press; 2010. p. 163–9.

Wells M. Chapter 9—Ankle block. In: Local and regional anaesthesia in the emergency department made easy. Amsterdam: Elsevier; 2010. p. 165–75.

Intra-Articular Injections of the Foot and Ankle

Minton Truitt Cooper

Essential Concepts

- Intra-articular injections of the foot and ankle are effective tools for both treating and diagnosing a variety of joint pathologies of the foot and ankle
- Essentially any joint in the foot or ankle may be injected. The larger joints such as the ankle or subtalar joint are frequently injected with image guidance. Smaller joints are typically injected under ultrasound or fluoroscopic guidance
- Therapeutic benefit may last from weeks to months
- Injections may be used for diagnostic purposes when the source of pain is unclear
- Although complications are rare, they may include infection or systemic effects of corticosteroids.

1 Overview

Injections of the foot and ankle are common procedures that can be useful for providing pain relief as well as diagnostic information. Essentially any joint may be injected, and it is useful to divide the foot and ankle into segments including the ankle/hindfoot, midfoot and forefoot. Each of these segments are susceptible to injury and other pathology, such as focal chondral lesions, osteoarthritis, inflammatory arthritis, and synovitis. Osteoarthritis of the foot may occur in as much as 16.7% of the population [1], with ankle arthritis occurring in over 3% of the

M. T. Cooper (✉)
Department of Orthopaedic Surgery, University of Virginia, Charlottesville, VA, USA
e-mail: Mtc2d@hscmail.mcc.virginia.edu

D. Souza et al. (eds.), *Bedside Pain Management Interventions*,
https://doi.org/10.1007/978-3-031-11188-4_73

population, with the majority being post-traumatic [2]. Improvement in pain and function may persist for 4 months to a year [3, 4]. If successful, injections may be repeated, however it is recommended to limit the number of injections to the same joint to 3–4 per year, attempting to space them out with 3–4 months between repeat injections.

Typically, glucocorticoids are used when therapeutic improvement is sought. The benefit is derived from the decrease in arachidonic acid derived pro-inflammatory chemicals within the joint fluid and synovium [5].

2 Indications and Contraindications

Indications for intra-articular injections of the foot and ankle include osteoarthritis, inflammatory conditions (including rheumatoid arthritis, psoriatic arthritis, gout), synovitis, and focal osteochondral lesions. Diagnostic injections may be performed when the source of a patient's pain is unclear; this may be done with local anesthetic only, or in combination with corticosteroid. Contraindications: Contraindications to corticosteroid injections include infectious processes, acute injuries or fractures, neuropathic joints. Other considerations must include coagulopathies in which hemostasis cannot be maintained, uncontrolled diabetes mellitus where systemic effects may cause transient increase in blood glucose levels, or immunosuppressed patients.

3 Clinical Anatomy

The ankle joint is made up of the articulation between the tibia, fibula and talus (Fig. 1), and is primarily responsible for dorsiflexion and plantarflexion. The hind-foot joints include the subtalar joint, the talonavicular joint, and the calcaneocuboid joint, which are responsible for inversion/eversion or supination/pronation. The midfoot consists of the naviculocuneiform joints, the intercuneiform joints, and the tarsometatarsal joints. The forefoot includes the metatarsophalangeal joints, the interphalangeal joints, as well as the articulation between the first metatarsal and sesamoids.

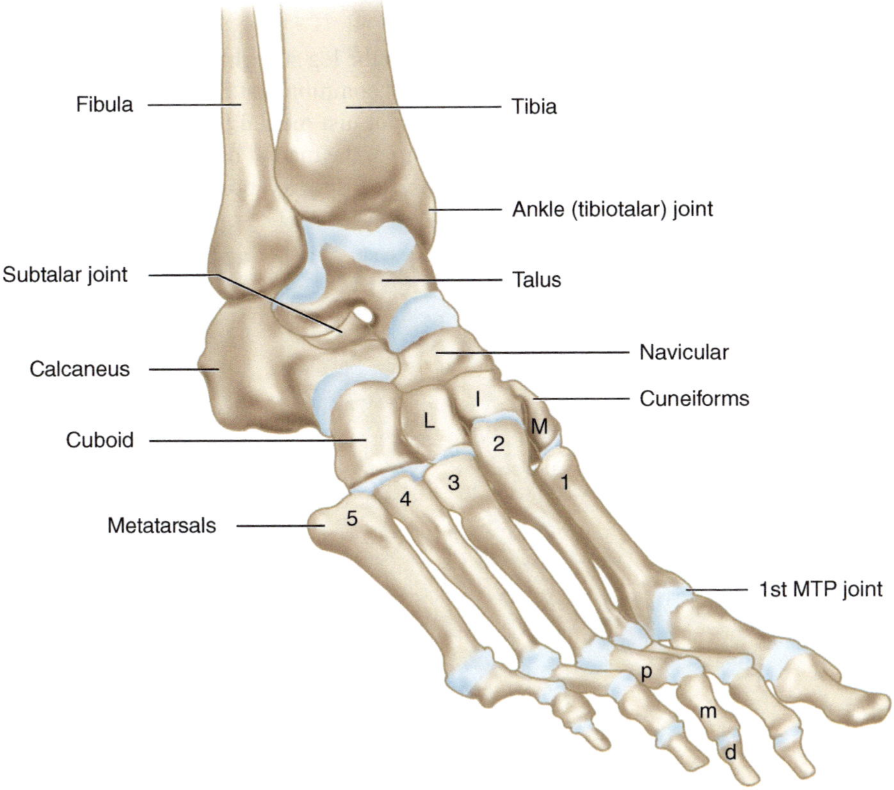

Fig. 1 Osseous anatomy of the foot and ankle. *L* lateral cuneiform, *I* intermediate or middle cuneiform, *M* medial cuneiform, *P* proximal phalanx, *M* middle phalanx, *D* distal phalanx

Table 1 Required supplies for intra-articular injection of the foot or ankle

Syringe	5 or 10 mL
Needle	25 g, 1.5 in.
Anesthetic	0.5% Bupivacaine or 1% lidocaine without epinephrine
Corticosteroid	Triamcinolone (2.5–5 mg) or methylprednisolone (10–40 mg)

4 Equipment and Supplies

Joints of the foot and ankle are performed with a 25 gauge 1.5 in. needle. Medications may include a mixture of local anesthetic without epinephrine (lidocaine or bupivacaine) and corticosteroid (usually in a 1:1 volume ratio), or local anesthetic alone in the case of a diagnostic injection. Commonly used corticosteroids include methylprednisolone (10–40 mg) or triamcinolone (2.5–5 mg) (Table 1). For the ankle or subtalar joint, typically 2 mL total are injected, whereas in the other smaller joints of the foot, typically the volume will be 1 mL or less. For the ankle or subtalar joint, imaging is not typically needed, however for the other joints, guidance with ultrasound or fluoroscopy may be used to ensure precise placement of the injection.

5 Ankle Joint Injection

The patient is placed in the supine position with the leg straight and the foot near the end of the bed. The ankle joint is accessed most commonly at the anteromedial joint line—this is identified by palpating the soft spot just medial to the tibialis anterior tendon, approximately 1 cm proximal to the tip of the medial malleolus (Fig. 2). The area is sterilely prepped and the needle is inserted directed postero-laterally.

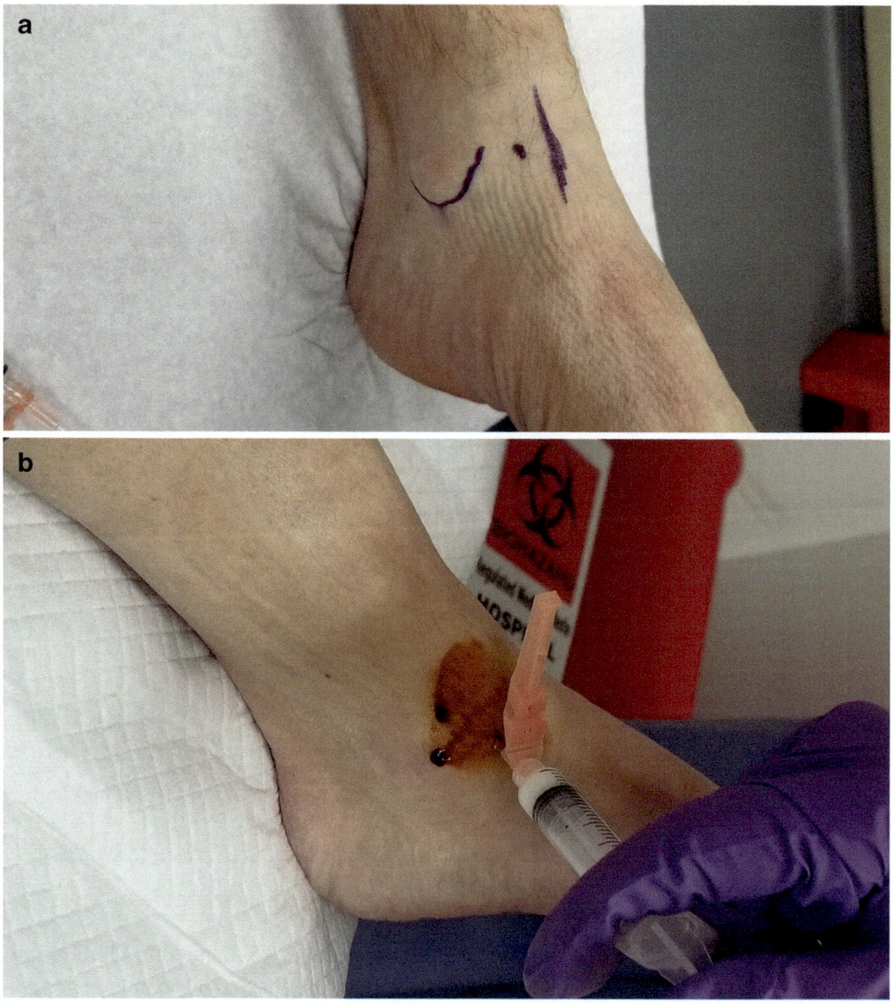

Fig. 2 Ankle (tibiotalar joint) injection. (**a**) The medial malleolus and tibialis anterior tendon have been marked. The location of the injection is just medial to the tibialis anterior and slightly proximal to the tip of the medial malleolus. (**b**) The needle is inserted directed posterolaterally at an approximately 45° angle

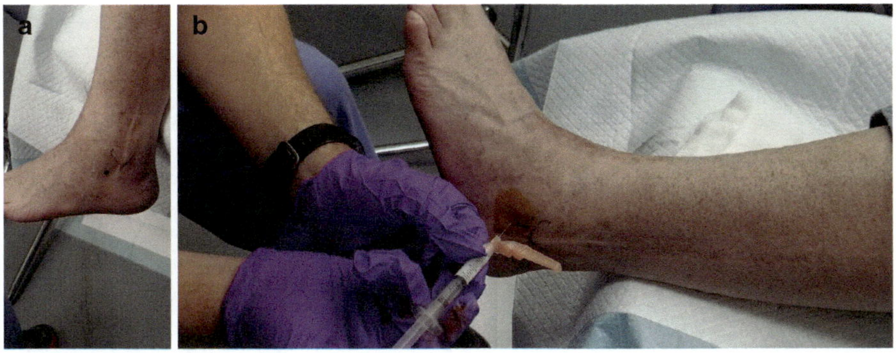

Fig. 3 Subtalar joint injection. (**a**) The distal end of the lateral malleolus has been outlined. The site of injection is just anterior and inferior to this point. (**b**) The needle is inserted and directed cephalad at approximately 30°

6 Subtalar Joint Injection

The patent is placed in the supine position with the leg slightly internally rotated. The site of the injection is palpated just inferior to and anterior to the tip of the lateral malleolus, at the ankle of Gissane (Fig. 3a). The needle is directed 30°–45° cephalad (Fig. 3b).

7 Other Foot Intra-articular Injections

The other joints of the foot, including talonavicular, calcaneocuboid, tarsometatarsal joints, as well as the first metatarsophalangeal joint are typically injected under fluoroscopic imaging (Fig. 4) or ultrasound guidance. The joint to be injected identified and most commonly entered from a dorsal approach, as these joints all lie just beneath the subcutaneous tissue. If special attention is directed at the articulation between the sesamoid and the metatarsal head, this may be accessed from a medial approach, however this joint communicates with the first metatarsophalangeal joint. Steroid injection into the lesser metatarsophalangeal joints should be performed with caution, as there is significant risk of damage to the soft tissue restraints of the joint and a high incidence of complication (dislocation or the development of a hammertoe) [6].

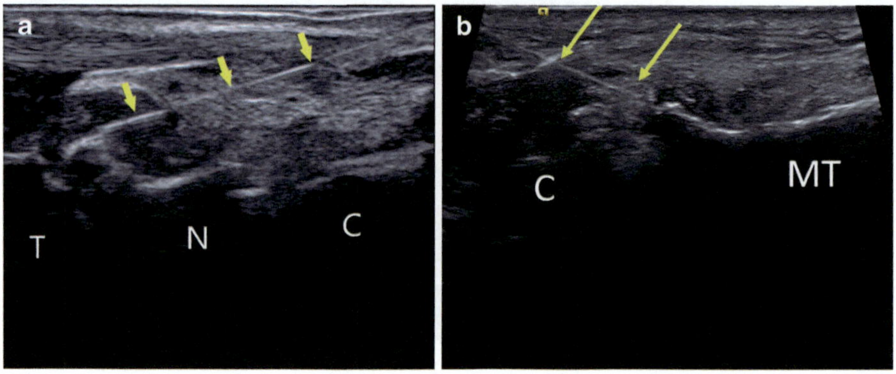

Fig. 4 Fluoroscopic imaging demonstrating talonavicular (**a**) and tarsometatarsal (**b**) joint injections. It is noted that the second and third tarsometatarsal joints communicate

8 Potential Complications and Adverse Effects

Although rare, patients may occasionally sustain adverse effects from intra-articular corticosteroid injections. The most common of these include post-injection flare, with an increase in pain and erythema beginning within several hours, which typically subsides in several days. Treatment may consist of rest and ice. Skin changes are most common with longer acting medications such as triamcinolone, and occur more often when the joint is missed and the injection is performed subcutaneously. Damage to the surrounding ligaments and tendons may occur as corticosteroids have been shown to weaken the tensile strength of ligaments for up to 1 year [7]. This is primarily a concern with injection of the lesser MTP joints which may lead to disruption of the plantar plate and dislocation. In patients with diabetes, elevated blood glucose may be observed for several days following and injection and should be counseled to monitor their glucose carefully. Among the most serious complications is septic arthritis, the risk of which may be minimized by using careful sterile technique.

Clinical and Technical Pearls

- Ankle and subtalar joints are typically easily performed at the bedside without ultrasound or fluoroscopic guidance. These may be more difficult in obese patients or those with significant ankyloses of the joints.
- Although not a contraindication, extra care should be taken for patients on anticoagulation and they should be monitored for at least 15 min following the injection.
- When using injections to obtain diagnostic information about the source of a patient's pain, it is recommended to only perform one joint injection at a setting.
- Care should be taken to avoid over-distension of joints, particularly the smaller joints of the foot and ankle such as the less metatarsophalangeal joints.

References

1. Roddy E, Thomas MJ, Marshall M, Rathod T, Myers H, Menz HB, et al. The population prevalence of symptomatic radiographic foot osteoarthritis in community-dwelling older adults: cross-sectional findings from the clinical assessment study of the foot. Ann Rheum Dis. 2015;74(1):156–63.
2. Saltzman CL, Salamon ML, Blanchard GM, Huff T, Hayes A, Buckwalter JA, et al. Epidemiology of ankle arthritis: report of a consecutive series of 639 patients from a tertiary orthopaedic center. Iowa Orthop J. 2005;25:44–6.
3. Protheroe D, Gadgil A. Guided intra-articular corticosteroid injections in the midfoot. Foot Ankle Int. 2018;39(8):1001–4.
4. Ward ST, Williams PL, Purkayastha S. Intra-articular corticosteroid injections in the foot and ankle: a prospective 1-year follow-up investigation. J Foot Ankle Surg. 2008;47(2):138–44.
5. Creamer P. Intra-articular corticosteroid treatment in osteoarthritis. Curr Opin Rheumatol. 1999;11:417–21.
6. Reis ND, Karkabi S, Zinman C. Metatarsophalangeal joint dislocation after local steroid injection. J Bone Jt Surg Br. 1989;71(5):864.
7. Brand C. Intra-articular and soft tissue injections. Aust Fam Physician. 1990;19(5):671–82.

Further Reading

de Cesar NC, da Fonseca LF, Simeone Nascimento F, O'Daley AE, Tan EW, Dein EJ, et al. Diagnostic and therapeutic injections of the foot and ankle—an overview. Foot Ankle Surg. 2018;24(2):99–106.

Pekarek B, Osher L, Buck S, Bowen M. Intra-articular corticosteroid injections: a critical literature review with up-to-date findings. Foot (Edinb). 2011;21(2):66–70.

Soft Tissue Injections of the Foot and Ankle

Minton Truitt Cooper

Essential Concepts

- Soft tissue injections of the foot and ankle (including tendon sheaths, plantar fascia, and peripheral nerves) are effective tools for both treating and diagnosing conditions affecting these structures.
- Ultrasound guidance may be useful for increasing the accuracy of placement of these injections, preventing intra-tendinous or intra-neural injections, and to provide additional diagnostic data.
- When injecting tendinous structures, care must be taken not to place injections directly into the tendon, but rather into the sheath surrounding the tendon, as corticosteroid injection directly into the tendon may lead to further damage or rupture.
- Injections for the tarsal tunnel (for posterior tibial nerve irritation) may be extremely helpful in diagnosing this condition, as well as providing significant symptomatic improvement.
- Although complications are rare, they may include infection, nerve damage, or systemic effects of corticosteroids.

M. T. Cooper (✉)
Department of Orthopaedic Surgery, University of Virginia, Charlottesville, VA, USA
e-mail: Mtc2d@hscmail.mcc.virginia.edu

D. Souza et al. (eds.), *Bedside Pain Management Interventions*,
https://doi.org/10.1007/978-3-031-11188-4_74

1 Overview

Injections of soft tissue structures of the foot and ankle are common procedures that can be useful for providing pain relief as well as diagnostic information. Common injections include the tarsal tunnel, plantar fascia origin, tendon sheaths, or Morton's neuroma. These injections may be performed with ultrasound guidance to improve accuracy and safety. A case series by Ostergaard et al. [1] reviewing 365 patients who underwent corticosteroid injections of the foot and ankle found that they were safe, with 86% reporting improvement in symptoms. However, they found that they were ineffective at providing relief greater than 3 months for certain conditions, such as plantar fasciitis.

When injections are to be performed for tenosynovitis or tendinitis, they should be performed in the tendon sheath, not directly into the tendon, due to the detrimental effect of corticosteroid on tendon strength, and possible resultant tendon rupture—it has been shown that corticosteroid injection into ligaments leads to loss of tensile strength for 1 year [2]. In the foot and ankle, common tendon sheath injections include the peroneal tendons and the posterior tibial tendon. Injections for Achilles tendinitis have not been shown to be beneficial [3] and may lead to rupture, therefore are not recommended. In general tendon sheath injections should be used sparingly.

Plantar fasciitis is another common foot condition for which injections are performed [4, 5]. Plantar fasciitis is a degenerative condition, with thickening of the plantar fascia, most typically at the origin of the medial cord off of the calcaneus (Fig. 1). Recent

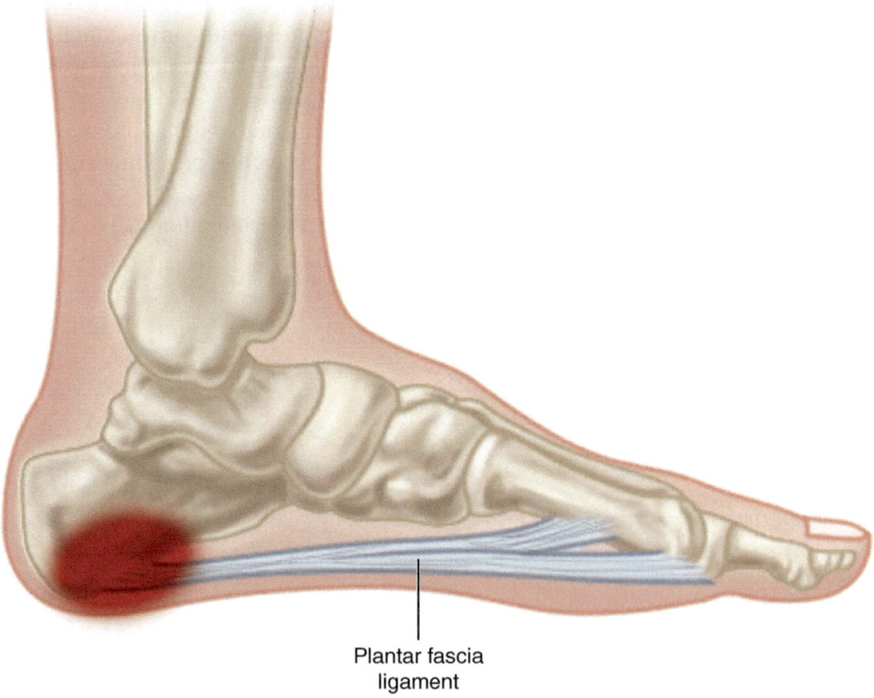

Fig. 1 Plantar fasciitis most commonly develops at the origin of the medial band of the plantar fascia off of the calcaneal tuberosity

meta-analyses [5, 6] found corticosteroid injections may be effective at providing short term relief, however no medium to long term benefits have been shown. Despite a concern for plantar fascia rupture, they did not find any adverse events aside from post-injection pain.

Tarsal tunnel syndrome occurs due to compression of the posterior tibial nerve beneath the flexor retinaculum or abductor hallucis muscle fascia at the posterior medial and ankle and medial hindfoot. This injection may be performed under ultrasound guidance to ensure appropriate placement of the injection and avoid intraneural injection. Baxter's nerve is the first branch of the lateral plantar nerve, which courses under the heel and is a common cause of heel pain. This nerve may also be injected under ultrasound guidance.

Lastly, Morton's neuroma is a common cause of forefoot pain. Patients may report a variety of symptoms including pain, paresthesia or numbness radiating to the affected toe, or a clicking that represents the nerve snapping between the metatarsal heads. The affected interspace may be injected with or without ultrasound guidance. These injections may be particularly helpful at differentiating pain originating from a neuroma versus other pathologies such as metatarsophalangeal joint synovitis.

2 Indications and Contraindications

Indications for soft tissue injection of the foot and ankle include tenosynovitis of the peroneal or posterior tibial tendons, plantar fasciitis, tarsal tunnel syndrome, Baxter's nerve compression, or Morton's neuroma. Injections are typically performed after other conservative management such as shoe orthoses, physical therapy, and oral non-steroidal anti-inflammatory medications have been attempted. These injections are also indicated to obtain confirmation of the exact etiology of the patient's pain. *Contraindications*: Contraindications to corticosteroid injections include infectious processes or acute injuries or fractures. Injection of degenerative tendon disorders or the Achilles tendon in general is relatively contraindicated. Other considerations must include coagulopathies in which hemostasis cannot be maintained, uncontrolled diabetes mellitus where systemic effects may cause transient increase in blood glucose levels, or immunosuppressed patients.

3 Clinical Anatomy

The posterior tibial nerve travels along the posterior medial aspect of the ankle beneath the flexor retinaculum along with the posterior tibial, flexor digitorum longus and flexor hallucis longus tendons (Fig. 2). It branches into the medial and lateral plantar nerves and then travels beneath the abductor hallucis muscle

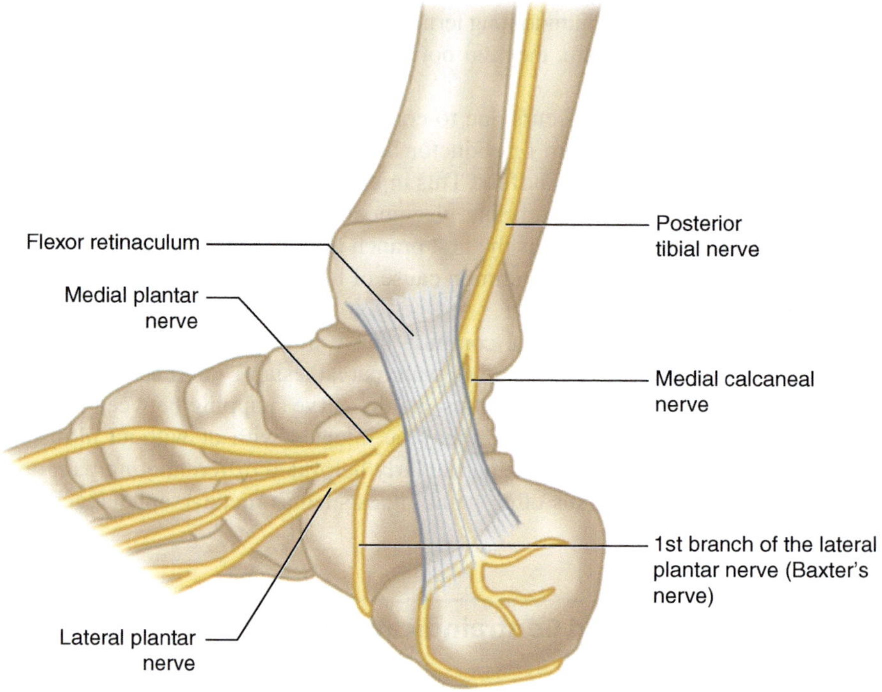

Fig. 2 Depiction of the posterior tibial nerve and its branches as it course along the posteromedial ankle beneath the flexor retinaculum to the plantar aspect of the foot

where it may also be compressed. The first branch of the lateral plantar nerve (Baxter's nerve) travels beneath the heel between the quadratus plantae and flexor digitorum brevis muscles, where it may be compressed leading to heel pain (Fig. 3).

The plantar fascia originates from the plantar aspect of the calcaneus, inserting on the toes to create support for the arch during the gait cycle. The origin of the medial aspect of the plantar fascia is the most common site for plantar fasciitis, and thus is where most injections are placed.

Morton's neuroma is not a true "neuroma," but rather a perineural fibrosis of a common interdigital nerve of the forefoot, most commonly affecting the nerve between the third and fourth metatarsal heads (Fig. 4).

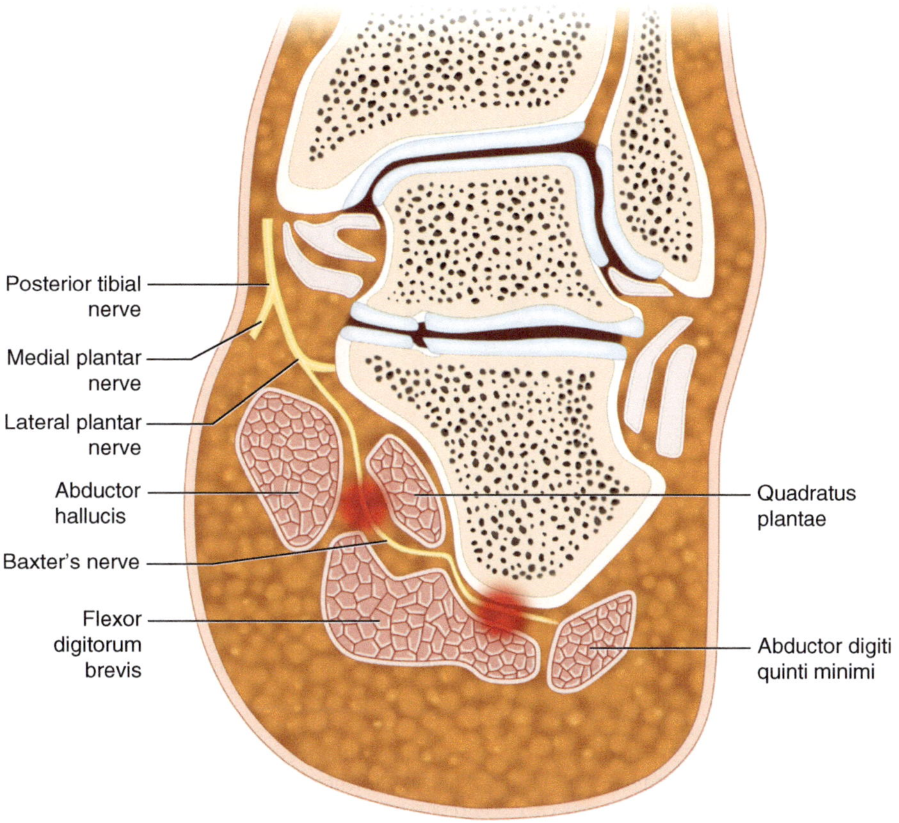

Fig. 3 The first branch of the lateral plantar nerve (Baxter's nerve) may be compressed between the fascia surrounding the quadratus plantae and flexor digitorum brevis muscles in the plantar heel

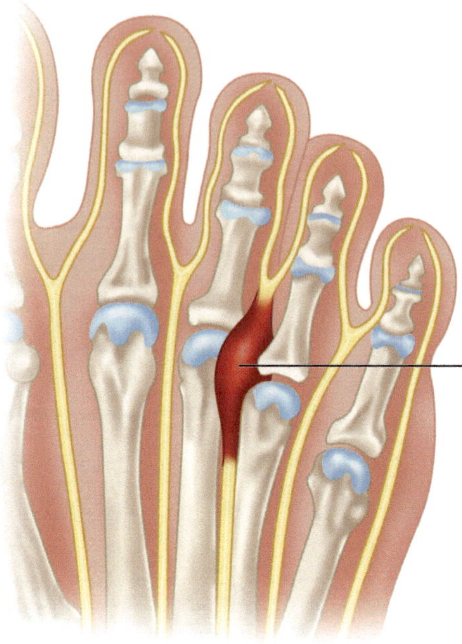

Fig. 4 Morton's neuroma arises from the common interdigital nerve as it passes between the lesser metatarsal heads, most commonly between the third and fourth metatarsals

Table 1 Required supplies for soft tissue injections about the foot and ankle

Syringe	5 or 10 mL
Needle	25 g, 1.5 in.
Anesthetic	0.5% Bupivacaine or 1% lidocaine without epinephrine (0.5 mL for neuroma, 1 mL for tarsal tunnel or plantar fascia)
Corticosteroid	Triamcinolone (2.5–5 mg) or methylprednisolone (10–40 mg). 0.5 mL for neuroma, 1 mL for tarsal tunnel or plantar fascia

4 Equipment and Supplies

Most injections of the foot and ankle are performed with a 25 gauge 1.5 in. needle (Table 1). Medications may include a mixture of local anesthetic without epinephrine (lidocaine or bupivacaine) and corticosteroid (usually in a 1:1 volume ratio), or local anesthetic alone in the case of a diagnostic injection. Commonly used corticosteroids include methylprednisolone (10–40 mg) or triamcinolone (2.5–5 mg). In general, soft tissue injections will be performed with 2 mL or less total volume. Although these injections may be performed without image guidance, ultrasound guidance may be used to enhance accuracy, as well as to prevent intra-neural injection of the posterior tibial nerve for tarsal tunnel injections.

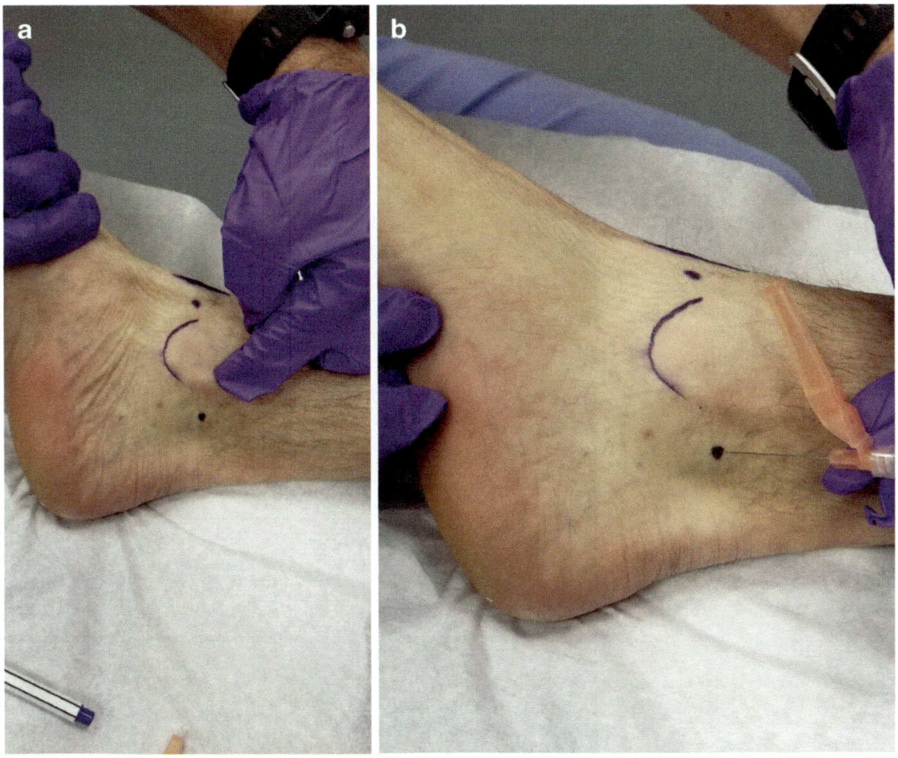

Fig. 5 Technique for tarsal tunnel injection. (**a**) The location is identified 1 cm posterior to the posterior tibial tendon, which may be visualized by having the patient invert the foot. (**b**) The needle is inserted, directed proximal to distal, through the flexor retinaculum

5 Tarsal Tunnel Injection

The patient is placed in the supine position with the intended lower extremity externally rotated. The medial malleolus is identified and the posterior tibial tendon may be identified by having the patient invert the foot (Fig. 5a). The injection is placed with a 25-gauge needle 1 cm posterior to the posterior tibial tendon, directed from proximal to distal (Fig. 5b). Aspiration should be performed to ensure that the needle is not in a vascular structure. Significant resistance likely indicates an intratendinous position and the needle should be slightly redirected prior to injection. Typically 2 cc of a mixture of corticosteroid and anesthetic will be administered.

6 Plantar Fascia Injection

The plantar fascia origin is readily injected without image guidance. The patient is placed in the supine position with the affected lower extremity allowed to externally rotate. Most typically it is the origin of the medial band of the plantar fascia that is affected. The plantar medial calcaneal tuberosity is palpated to verify the point of maximum tenderness (Fig. 6). A 25-gauge needle is inserted from the plantar medial surface directed proximally and slightly laterally. Resistance of the thick plantar fascia is felt and the injection is placed at both the deep and superficial surfaces, often redirecting the needle in different trajectories.

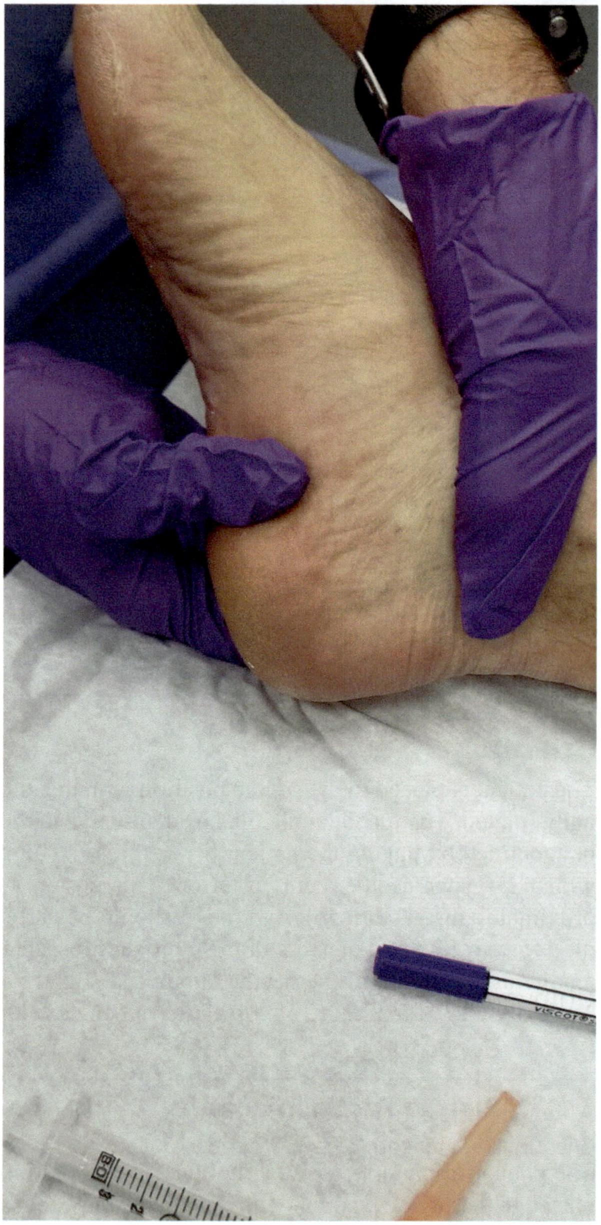

Fig. 6 The plantar medial heel is palpated to locate the site of maximal tenderness for plantar fascia injection, just distal to its attachment at the calcaneal tuberosity

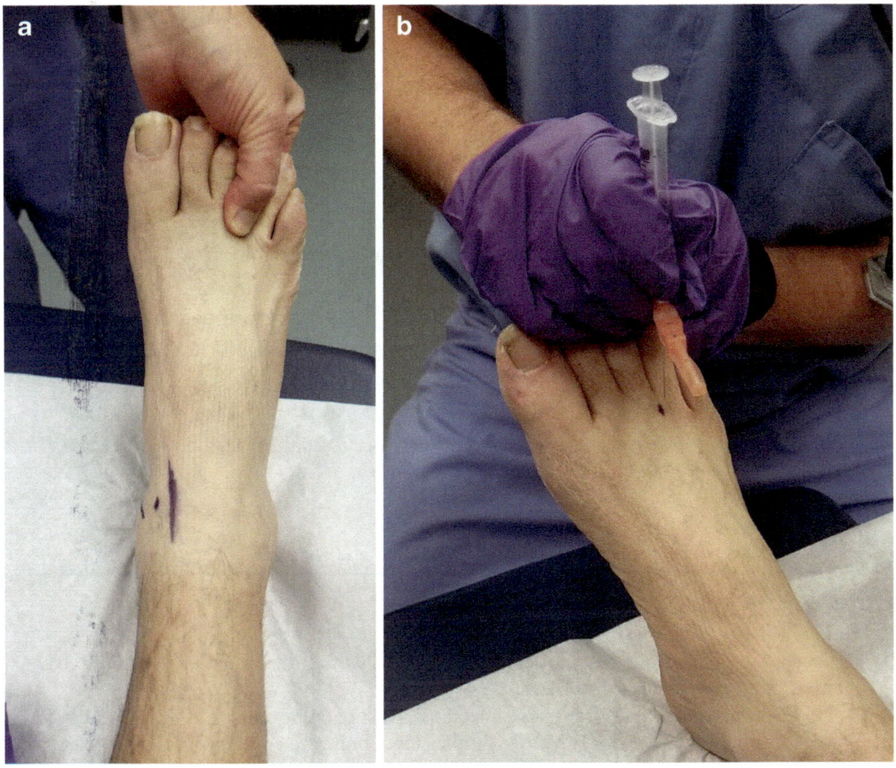

Fig. 7 Technique for injection of Morton's neuroma. (**a**) The targeted interspace is compressed with the thumb and index finger, (**b**) the needle is inserted from the dorsal foot between the metatarsal heads to the plantar aspect of the foot, deep to the intermetatarsal ligament

7 Injection for Morton's Neuroma

Injection without imaging has been shown to be as effective as those performed with ultrasound guidance [7]. The patient is positioned in a supine position and the targeted interdigital space is palpated by compressing the interspace with the thumb and index figure (Fig. 7). A 25-gauge needle is inserted from distal-dorsal to proximal-plantar. Resistance is felt from the intermetatarsal ligament and 1 mL of fluid is injected plantar to this structure.

8 Potential Complications and Adverse Effects

Although rare, patients may occasionally sustain adverse effects from corticosteroid injections of the soft tissues. When injecting the plantar fascia, plantar fascia rupture has been shown to occur at a rate of 1.5%, with heel pad atrophy occurring in 1.4% [8]. Skin depigmentation is also possible with corticosteroid injection.

Infections are extremely rare with soft tissue injections using sterile technique. Intra-tendinous injection should be avoided as they may weaken tendon strength and lead to rupture, particularly in already damaged tendons.

Clinical and Technical Pearls

- Injection to the foot may be painful, particularly injections of the origin of the plantar fascia. The patient should be in a comfortable position with the foot well supported to avoid movement.
- Caution should be used with patients on anti-coagulation, particularly in tarsal tunnel injections where there may be complex venous network around the tibial nerve.
- Care should be taken when injecting soft tissues of the foot and ankle to avoid intra-tendinous injections as these may weaken tendons and lead to rupture.

References

1. Ostergaard M, Halberg P. Intra-articular corticosteroids in arthritic disease: a guide to treatment. BioDrugs. 1998;9(2):95–103.
2. Brand C. Intra-articular and soft tissue injections. Aust Fam Physician. 1990;19(5):671–82.
3. Shrier I, Matheson GO, Kohl HW 3rd. Achilles tendonitis: are corticosteroid injections useful or harmful? Clin J Sport Med. 1996;6(4):245–50.
4. Jain SK, Suprashant K, Kumar S, Yadav A, Kearns SR. Comparison of plantar fasciitis injected with platelet-rich plasma vs corticosteroids. Foot Ankle Int. 2018;39(7):780–6.
5. Whittaker GA, Munteanu SE, Menz HB, Bonanno DR, Gerrard JM, Landorf KB. Corticosteroid injection for plantar heel pain: a systematic review and meta-analysis. BMC Musculoskelet Disord. 2019;20(1):378.
6. Chen CM, Lee M, Lin CH, Chang CH, Lin CH. Comparative efficacy of corticosteroid injection and non-invasive treatments for plantar fasciitis: a systematic review and meta-analysis. Sci Rep. 2018;8(1):4033.
7. Mahadevan D, Attwal M, Bhatt R, Bhatia M. Corticosteroid injection for Morton's neuroma with or without ultrasound guidance: a randomised controlled trial. Bone Jt J. 2016;98-B(4):498–503.
8. Johnson JE, Klein SE, Putnam RM. Corticosteroid injections in the treatment of foot and ankle disorders: an AOFAS survey. Foot Ankle Int. 2011;32(4):394–9.

Further Reading

de Cesar NC, da Fonseca LF, Simeone Nascimento F, O'Daley AE, Tan EW, Dein EJ, et al. Diagnostic and therapeutic injections of the foot and ankle—an overview. Foot Ankle Surg. 2018;24(2):99–106.

Johnson JE, Klein SE, Putnam RM. Corticosteroid injections in the treatment of foot and ankle disorders: an AOFAS survey. Foot Ankle Int. 2011;32(4):394–9.

Paavola M, Kannus P, Jarvinen TA, Jarvinen TL, Jozsa L, Jarvinen M. Treatment of tendon disorders. Is there a role for corticosteroid injection? Foot Ankle Clin. 2002;7(3):501–13.

Index

D. Souza et al. (eds.), *Bedside Pain Management Interventions*,
https://doi.org/10.1007/978-3-031-11188-4

B

C

GPSR Compliance

The European Union's (EU) General Product Safety Regulation (GPSR) is a set of rules that requires consumer products to be safe and our obligations to ensure this.

If you have any concerns about our products, you can contact us on ProductSafety@springernature.com

In case Publisher is established outside the EU, the EU authorized representative is:

Springer Nature Customer Service Center GmbH
Europaplatz 3
69115 Heidelberg, Germany

Batch number: 10726131

Printed by Printforce, the Netherlands